THE FAT-SOLUBLE VITAMINS

Proceedings of a symposium

in honor of

HARRY STEENBOCK

1969

Sponsored by the Wisconsin Alumni Research Foundation

The FAT-SOLUBLE VITAMINS

Edited by

H. F. DeLuca

and

J. W. Suttie

THE UNIVERSITY OF WISCONSIN PRESS

Madison, Milwaukee, and London

Published by
The University of Wisconsin Press
Box 1379, Madison, Wisconsin 53701
The University of Wisconsin Press, Ltd.
27–29 Whitfield Street, London, W.1

Printed in the United States of America by the
North Central Publishing Company
St. Paul, Minnesota

ISBN *0–299–05600–7*
LC *70–106038*

CONTENTS

CONTRIBUTORS

Gordon F. Anderson, Associate Professor, Department of Physiology and Pharmacology, Wayne State University, College of Medicine, Detroit, Michigan 48207

Louis V. Avioli, Associate Professor of Medicine, Division of Endocrinology and Medicine, Jewish Hospital of St. Louis, 216 South Kings Highway, St. Louis, Missouri 63110

Marion I. Barnhart, Professor, Department of Physiology and Pharmacology, Wayne State University, College of Medicine, Detroit, Michigan 48207

F. C. Bartter, Chief, Endocrinology Branch, National Heart Institute, National Institutes of Health, Bethesda, Maryland 20014

Werner Baumgartner, Veterans Administration Hospital, Long Beach, California 90804

John G. Bieri, Chief, Nutritional Biochemistry Section, National Institute of Arthritis and Metabolic Diseases, National Institutes of Health, Bethesda, Maryland 20014

John W. Blunt, Department of Chemistry, University of Canterbury, Christchurch 1, New Zealand

Moussa Cohanim, Department of Medicine, Queens University, Kingston, Ontario, Canada

A. Saari Csallany, Professor of Nutritional Biochemistry, Department of Animal Science, University of Illinois, Urbana, Illinois 61801

H. F. DeLuca, Harry Steenbock Research Professor of Biochemistry, Department of Biochemistry, University of Wisconsin, Madison, Wisconsin 53706

L. De Luca, Department of Nutrition and Food Science, Massachusetts Institute of Technology, Cambridge, Massachusetts 02139

H. H. Draper, Professor of Nutritional Biochemistry, Division of Nutritional Biochemistry, Department of Animal Science, University of Illinois, Urbana, Illinois 61801

Honor B. Fell, Director, Strangeways Research Laboratory, Cambridge, England

Diosdado A. Garcia, Department of Medicine, Queens University, Kingston, Ontario, Canada

DeWitt S. Goodman, Professor, Department of Medicine, Columbia University College of Physicians and Surgeons, New York, New York 10032

J. Green, Beecham Research Laboratories, Vitamins Research Station, Walton Oaks, Dorking Road, Tadworth, Surrey, England

Harold E. Harrison, Pediatrician-in-Chief, Department of Pediatrics, Johns Hopkins University, School of Medicine, Baltimore City Hospital, Baltimore, Maryland 21224

Helen C. Harrison, Assistant Professor, Department of Pediatrics, Johns Hopkins Medical School, Baltimore, Maryland 21205

Y. F. Herman, Chemical Division, U.S.A. Medical Research and Nutrition Laboratory, Fitzsimmons General Hospital, Denver, Colorado 80240

B. Connor Johnson, Professor and Chairman, Department of Biochemistry, University of Oklahoma Medical Center, 800 N.E. 13th, Oklahoma City, Oklahoma 73104

E. Kodicek, Director, Dunn Nutritional Laboratory, University of Cambridge and Medical Research Council, Cambridge, England

M. R. Lakshmanan, Faculty of Sciences, University of Medical Sciences, Bangkok, Thailand

Julius Lowenthal, Professor, Department of Pharmacology and Therapeutics, McGill University, Montreal, Quebec, Canada

E. G. McDaniel, Laboratory of Nutrition and Endocrinology, National Institute of Arthritis and Metabolic Diseases, National Institutes of Health, Bethesda, Maryland 20014

John T. Matschiner, Department of Biochemistry, College of Medicine, University of Nebraska, Omaha, Nebraska 68105

Mark J. Melancon, Jr., Department of Pharmacy, University of Wisconsin–Milwaukee, Milwaukee, Wisconsin 53201

H. Morii, Third Department of Internal Medicine, University of Tokyo, Hongo, Tokyo, Japan

Sharon M. Noonan, Department of Physiology and Pharmacology, Wayne State University, College of Medicine, Detroit, Michigan 48207

Anthony W. Norman, Department of Biochemistry, University of California, Riverside, California 92502

James Allen Olson, Visiting Professor and Acting Chairman, Faculty of Sciences, University of Medical Sciences, Bangkok, Thailand

Robert E. Olson, Professor and Chairman, Department of Biochemistry, St. Louis University School of Medicine, St. Louis, Missouri 63104

Charles Y. C. Pak, Endocrinology Branch, National Heart Institute, National Institutes of Health, Bethesda, Maryland 20014

N. Raica, Jr., Chemical Division, U.S.A. Medical Research and Nutrition Laboratory, Fitzsimmons General Hospital, Denver, Colorado 80240

Lawrence G. Raisz, Associate Professor, School of Medicine and Dentistry, University of Rochester, Rochester, New York 14620

Anita B. Roberts, Postdoctoral Fellow, Department of Pharmacology, Harvard University, Cambridge, Massachusetts 02115

William E. Rogers, Jr., Acting Chief, Dental Caries and Hard Tissues Program, Extramural Programs, National Institute of Dental Research, National Institutes of Health, Bethesda, Maryland 20014

H. E. Sauberlich, Chief, Chemical Division, U.S.A. Medical Research and Nutrition Laboratory, Fitzsimmons General Hospital, Denver, Colorado 80240

David Schachter, Associate Professor of Physiology, Department of Physiology, Columbia University College of Physicians and Surgeons, Presbyterian Hospital, New York, New York 10022

Howard A. Schneider, Director, Institute of Nutrition, University of North Carolina, Chapel Hill, North Carolina 27514

Klaus Schwarz, Chief, Laboratory for Experimental and Metabolic Diseases, Veterans Administration Hospital, Long Beach, California 90801

M. L. Scott, Professor of Animal Nutrition, Department of Poultry Science, Cornell University, Ithaca, New York 14850

M. A. Stedham, Chemical Division, U.S.A. Medical Research and Nutrition Laboratory, Fitzsimmons General Hospital, Denver, Colorado 80240

J. W. Suttie, Professor, Department of Biochemistry, University of Wisconsin, Madison, Wisconsin 53706

A. L. Tappel, Professor and Biochemist, Department of Food Science and Technology, University of California, Davis, California 95616

J. N. Thompson, Department of National Health and Welfare, Food and Drug Directorate, Tunney's Pasture, Ottawa, Ontario, Canada

Clarence L. Trummel, School of Medicine and Dentistry, University of Rochester, Rochester, New York 14620

R. H. Wasserman, Professor, Department of Physical Biology, New York State Veterinary College, Cornell University, Ithaca, New York 14850

George Wolf, Associate Professor of Physiological Chemistry, Department of Nutrition and Food Science, Massachusetts Institute of Technology, Cambridge, Massachusetts 02139

Edmund R. Yendt, Professor and Head, Department of Medicine, Queens University, Kingston, Ontario, Canada

PREFACE
HARRY STEENBOCK IN SCIENTIFIC PERSPECTIVE

Howard A. Schneider

Harry Steenbock, to whom the symposium was dedicated, was permitted a long life, some 81 years. As a biochemist his interests over a long professional career ranged far, but in all their scope nothing more epitomizes Harry Steenbock's most important interest, and his most important contributions, than the subject of the fat-soluble vitamins. It is appropriate that this volume marks this vital connection, and the trenchant studies presented here give rich promise of a renaissance in interest and achievement after a period of some fallow years. The record thus being written by present and future workers will, in a sense, be its own commentary, but it seems fitting that we also mark what it was about Harry Steenbock and his work that compels us to so memorialize him.

A man who thus commands our respect and admiration must have been, as the scholar of another day would have said, a "man of many parts." It may be philosophically foolhardy to fragment a man, for only the *whole* man was truly a man, but for my special purpose I beg permission to briefly delineate that part of Harry Steenbock which was Harry Steenbock, the scientist. All can share our humanity with Harry Steenbock, but, at first glance, only scientists can share and understand Harry Steenbock the scientist. This I regard as regrettable, and to hide behind Lord Snow and say, "Alas, it's the Two Culture trap again," is to evade an historical imperative. And so I propose to discuss, first, what a scientist is, and second, why Harry Steenbock was a great one. This would be a difficult task, and one which I would never begin, if Harry Steenbock's intellect were that of an ordinary man. The task is really easier when it comes to an extraordinary man. It is much like our delight when, on some occasion made bold enough, we read one of the classics. Bedazzled and, yes, intimi-

Taken from a speech given prior to the Harry Steenbock Symposium on the Fat-Soluble Vitamins.

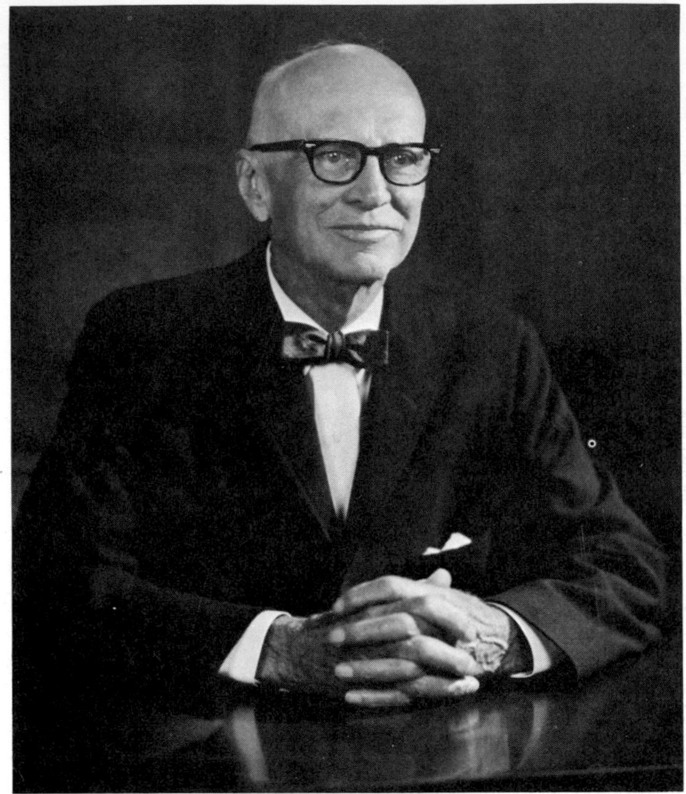

Photograph by Edgar L. Obma

Harry Steenbock, 1886–1967

dated by the towering reputation, we are also overcome by diffidence. What can this great man have to say to us in our insignificance? But, having made the plunge, what do we find in the classic: A discussion and an analysis of some important issue so cogent, so clear, so supple, so incisive, that no one can ever discuss the subject again without taking the view thus presented into account. And, of course, that is precisely why it is a classic – a work of the highest excellence, enduring, and rising forever above provincialism and the niggling, demeaning dialect of the brief allotted time of its composition. Harry Steenbock's science, in a word, was classic.

What, however, is science? The Age of Science, as we know it, is approximately three hundred years old and my question might seem to come a little late in the day. It turns out, really, that there are several levels of answer to that seemingly simple question. For Harry Steenbock,

I believe, *his* answer was, that science was an unending, never-to-be-finished task of searching for an understanding of the natural world. It was because, in his view, the search for understanding never ended, but only deepened, that, I believe, he never wrote a book. Publish, yes. Write scientific papers, yes. But never a book. Book writing, I suggest, smacked of finality to him. And he knew better.

Science, then, for Harry Steenbock was a search for understanding. But what is understanding? Perhaps we can get to the heart of that query if we turn to a philosopher for help. I would prefer the American philosopher William James, who characteristically directs our approach to the aims of science by emphasizing the idea of purpose. "What is the purpose of scientific understanding?" would be a Jamesian question. And in answering that, William James provides a touchstone for our estimate of Harry Steenbock. According to James, the purpose of scientific understanding is twofold—to conceive simply and to foresee, to predict. And this achievement, the pinnacle of scientific understanding, was exactly what recommends Harry Steenbock, the scientist, to us today. My thesis can now be stated quite pointedly: Harry Steenbock was a great scientist because he developed ideas of great and powerful simplicity, because these ideas fulfilled the Jamesian ideal of fully predicting the operation of a part of the natural world, and because he thereby gave us a tool to remake and master the environment which molds us all.

I wish now to depart from generalities and specifically attempt to recapture the intellectual excitement of one of the climactic peaks in Harry Steenbock's career which, it seems to me, demonstrated his capacity for extracting from a puzzling array of facts with powerful simplicity that critical insight which reduced chaos and enigma to order, and thereby, at the same stroke, achieved predictability over the subject matter. As another American philosopher, F. S. C. Northrop, has observed, "For what characterizes a genius like Galilei, Lavoisier or Einstein is the economy of thought and effort by means of which he achieves his result. Each one of these men found the key factor in the situation and went directly to the heart of the problem which had been baffling his predecessors." It was precisely this economy of thought, seizing on what was relevant and important and discarding the rest, that steered Harry Steenbock on his course.

No one reading this needs reminding of Harry Steenbock's greatest discovery, the generation in foods of antirachitic properties by ultraviolet light. How simple! Push the tray of food under the ultraviolet lamp for a few minutes, and then have the food heal the softened bones of rickets. All the rest is detail. Others had observed that ultraviolet light somehow benefited the rachitic subjects who were directly exposed to it. It was gossiped about in the scientific journals, and it was conjectured to operate in some mysterious and arcane ways, the very air under the lamp was changed, electrical fields possibly were involved, electrical charges grew or were discharged, the very dance of the electrons may have changed — and it was all puzzling. When Harry Steenbock finished with it, it was not mysterious and the puzzle was solved. How did he do it?

In 1924 the situation in the biological properties of ultraviolet light was something like this: There was a general agreement that ultraviolet light from a carbon-arc or a mercury vapor lamp, as from the sun, was capable of healing rickets in an experimental animal, promoting growth and maintaining normal levels of calcium and phosphorus in the blood. But cod-liver oil did that too. This now can be restated very simply: "Light equals oil." That there is a special "light" here, ultraviolet radiation, and a special oil, the liver oil of a fish, doesn't save the situation. The relationship still flies in the face of common sense. One might as well accept such nonsensical statements as "apples equal music." But let us return to "light equals oil." If we cast about a bit and read the scientific journals of the day, as, of course, did Harry Steenbock, one can read that the usefulness of cod-liver oil depends, not on the oil, but on its content of what was called "the fat-soluble vitamine." But if we accept this we are still not much better off: "Light equals fat-soluble vitamine." However, there were at that time some indications that "fat-soluble vitamine" was not one entity, but two. Harry Steenbock was not accepting that as yet, however. He wanted more evidence. And now he began to provide that evidence himself, slowly, cautiously, but inevitably. A critical insight came quite simply: irradiating the rats improved their growth only temporarily, and though the rickets healed, the familiar and the telltale signs of ophthalmia, an inflammation of the eyes, made their appearance whether the rats were irradicated or not. It was a neat trick: irradiating the rats prevented the rickets, but eventually growth ceased and ophthalmia made its inexorable appearance. Materials such as butter or cod-liver oil provided for both the healing of the rickets and the cure of the ophthalmia. A new clarity in viewing these matters now came to Harry Steenbock. There were indeed two fat-soluble vitamins, and light was somehow related to only one of these, the one that prevented and cured rickets.

And for a while Harry Steenbock used the irradiation of his rats as a kind of dissecting instrument: by its means he would supply solely the antirachitic vitamin and thus allow the other fat-soluble vitamin that dealt with the eye disease — scientists were beginning to call it vitamine A — to become limiting. This raised the intriguing possibility that now, with the antirachitic factor supplied by these independent means, the rats would be solely responsive in their growth to the still-missing vitamin A. A means of measuring vitamin A, of assaying, was now at hand,

and that was important, for quantifying now could truly begin. For the moment, and though not articulated, there was now a change in the paradox: Now, "light equals the antirachitic vitamine" was the new statement. Curiously, for a short while little attention was paid to this, and I believe Harry Steenbock tended to put it aside. He was, at this time, more deeply interested in vitamin A, and his ambition was now to make some precise measurements of vitamin A activity, using the ultraviolet irradiation of the animals to provide the antirachitic activity in ample amounts so that variation in antirachitic effects would not plague his experiments with *their* uncertainties. One thing at a time! There can be little doubt that Harry Steenbock was a full disciple of Justus von Liebig, the great founder of agricultural chemistry and the propounder of the Law of the Minimum: When multiple factors are limiting, biological response will occur only when the factor in greatest demand is supplied first.

But just as he started on the new program, the unexpected happened. Harry Steenbock set out to remeasure the vitamin A content of butter by his improved technique. In order to be sure that his irradiation levels were doing what they were supposed to do, Harry Steenbock wisely included some controls, some rats on each test diet that were not irradiated. Time after time, dozens of times, these nonirradiated rats had, of course, grown poorly compared with their irradiated brothers; but to be absolutely sure, these so-called negative controls were included once again. Now disaster struck. All the rats grew equally well, irradiated or not! The difference between irradiation and no irradiation had vanished.

It would be inaccurate to say that, when carefully planned experiments collapse, gloom and despair do not descend on the hapless experimenter. But it is also true that, if mere technical blundering can be eliminated, then an opportunity exists for discovery. As I heard Dr. Oswald T. Avery of the Rockefeller Institute, the discoverer of DNA in the genes, once say to his younger assistants, "When you fall down, pick something up." Harry Steenbock did just that.

First, he went over all of his records of the dozens of preceding experiments and looked for some difference between those consistent experiences and the current and unexpected disaster. At length he thought he had found a possible explanation. The laboratory had been growing busier. Rat cages were being used to capacity, and in the last experiment, in contrast to all the preceding experiments, he had housed the irradiated animals and the nonirradiated animals together, feeding them the same diet of a given percentage of butterfat (these varying percentages were supposedly the meaningful and limiting source of vitamin A that was being supplied). Each day the marked irradiated animals were removed for their sunlamp bath, and then returned to their nonirradiated group members. It had not been planned for, but now it would have to be explained how irradiated rats had communicated their state of being irradiated to their nonirradiated cage mates. The vitamin A assay had to be put aside.

While Harry Steenbock pondered this, a publication arrived from England indicating that strange things indeed were going on in the area of irradiation. Hume and Smith reported that it was possible to give a rat the benefit of irradiation by *not* irradiating him—just by irradiating the empty glass jar and *then* putting the rat in. Astonishing! But even more astonishing was their report that if, before you put the rat into the irradiated jar you blew the air out of the jar, then the irradiation effect was lost. Indeed, they concluded, "it is the air and not some property impressed on the glass jars which is active."

Harry Steenbock was doubtful. If irradiated air was the means of conveying the effects of radiation, it was hard to see how irradiating rats away from a cage and then bringing the rat back to the cage brought irradiated air back with it. That didn't make much sense. There were a lot of questions he had for Hume and Smith. When they blew air into their irradiated jars, did they blow out the remnants of food and bedding, too? And come to think of it, when his own rats were carried back and forth from the cage to the irradiation area and back to the cage again, did some food go back and forth with them, on their whiskers and their hairy coats? It was a slender chance, but Harry Steenbock and his assistant Archie Black tried irradiating the food and feeding *that*. And, of course, it worked. By a single stroke, the whole tangled, confused, incomprehensible, mad mess was straightened out. Order was restored, and the paradox "Light equals fat-soluble vitamine" became a straightforward statement that was no longer a paradox. "The biological effect of ultraviolet light equals a photochemically activated material that has the biological properties of the fat-soluble antirachitic vitamin." How simple!

It was Harry Steenbock's most important triumph as an investigator. On this feat alone, Harry Steenbock could rightfully be called a great scientist. It was a time for greatness and Harry Steenbock measured up to his time. Times, of course, change. This volume records how Harry Steenbock's successors in the field are now meeting their challenges.

VITAMIN D

1

METABOLISM AND FUNCTION OF VITAMIN D

H. F. DeLuca

Introduction

The disease rickets was first described hundreds of years ago but was first produced experimentally by Sir Edward Mellanby in 1919. It was readily recognized as a nutritional disease, since it could be cured or prevented by the administration of cod-liver oil. Mellanby incorrectly ascribed this activity to the newly discovered vitamin A. McCollum and co-workers (1922), however, established that the antirachitic activity was due to another fat-soluble vitamin, vitamin D. Steenbock's discovery that antirachitic activity was induced by irradiation of foods, particularly of the sterol fraction, ultimately led to the identification of the structure of vitamin D and to the eradication of rickets as a major medical problem (Steenbock, 1924; Steenbock and Black, 1924, 1925).

Vitamin D_3 (Fig. 1.1), the natural or animal form of vitamin D, was not identified until 1936 (Windaus et al., 1936; Schenck, 1937), while vitamin D_2, that derived from ergosterol, was identified in 1931 (Askew et al., 1931; Windaus et al., 1932). From those times until very recently it had been assumed that the vitamin D molecule functioned as an unchanged molecule, a concept which has now been disproved, as will be shown in this chapter and others.

Overall physiologic action of vitamin D

Rickets can best be defined biochemically as a disease in which the calcification process cannot keep pace with the synthesis of the organic matrix of bone (DeLuca, 1967). The end effect of vitamin D, to bring about the calcification of bone, has led many investigators to suggest without support-

These studies were supported by a grant from the United States Public Health Service, AMO–5800–08, a grant from the Harry Steenbock Research Fund of the Wisconsin Alumni Research Foundation, and a contract from the United States Atomic Energy Commission AT–(11–1)–1668.

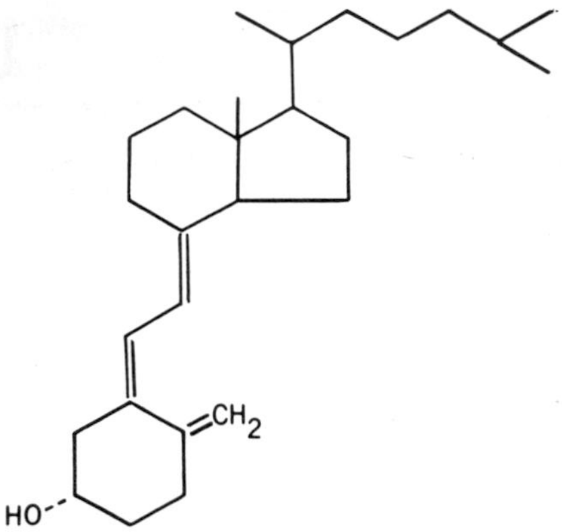

Fig. 1.1. Structure of vitamin D_3 (cholecalciferol).

ing evidence that vitamin D must participate in the calcification process. Experiments aimed at this point have failed to provide unequivocal evidence; instead, the weight of evidence is in opposition to this concept (DeLuca, 1967). It is now evident that blood and extracellular fluid are normally supersaturated with regard to bone mineral (Neuman and Neuman, 1958), whereas in rickets, blood is undersaturated with regard to bone mineral (Neuman, 1958). This fact, together with the early experiments of Shipley and co-workers (1925, 1926), indicate that in rickets the supply of calcium and phosphorus to the bone is defective and that the essence of vitamin D action is to elevate the plasma calcium and phosphate to supersaturation levels. On the basis of certain clinical cases, it seems that vitamin D may induce calcification of bone without changing the $[Ca^{++}] \times [HPO_4^{=}]$ product of the blood. It is possible, therefore, that the vitamin is active in the calcification mechanism, but this supposition lacks adequate experimental support.

The physiologic action of vitamin D in elevating plasma calcium and phosphorus is brought about by two basic effects, namely, increased intestinal absorption of calcium and increased bone mineral mobilization. Increased intestinal calcium absorption in response to vitamin D was first suggested in 1923 (Orr et al., 1923) and was finally established by Nicolaysen and co-workers (Nicolaysen, 1937*a*, 1937*b*, 1937*c*, 1937*d*, 1951). As will be discussed in considerable detail later in the book, it is evident that vitamin D induces a calcium transport system which is an active cation oriented system. Phosphate is transported secondarily (Martin and DeLuca, 1969*a*, 1969*b*; Martin, 1969; Wasserman, 1963).

Another more recently established action of the vitamin is the mobilization of bone mineral from the nonexchangeable fraction (Carlsson, 1952; Bauer et al., 1955). Although poorly understood biochemically, this process requires the presence of vitamin D and is greatly augmented by the parathyroid hormone. This process is most likely thermodynamically active, but no evidence is available on this point. In any case, this system also elevates plasma calcium and phosphorus. The actions of physiologic doses of vitamin D in the kidney are much less clear. Vitamin D may increase tubular reabsorption of calcium (Gran, 1960), but if that is true the action appears quantitatively of minor importance. The reported action of the vitamin on renal tubular reabsorption of phosphate (Harrison and Harrison, 1941) appears to be a secondary phenomenon (DeLuca, 1967). Thus, by increasing the intestinal absorption of calcium and phosphate as well as the mobilization of bone mineral, the vitamin elevates plasma calcium and phosphate to a point so that normal mineralization of bone can occur.

Metabolism of vitamin D

Very characteristic of vitamin D action is the extensive length of time between the administration of vitamin D and the appearance of its first physiological effect (Fig. 1.2) (DeLuca, 1967). Clearly, with an intravenous

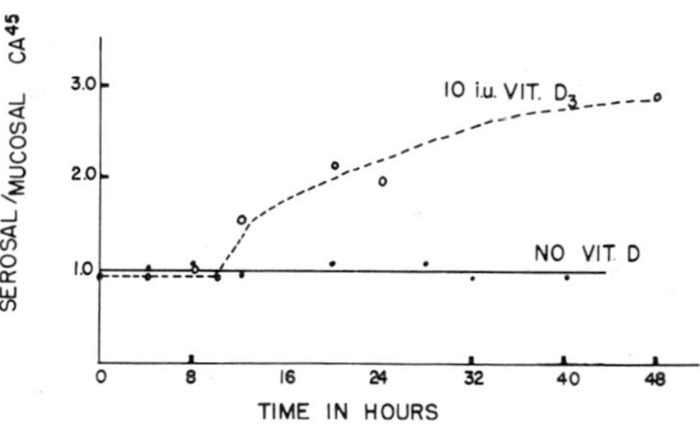

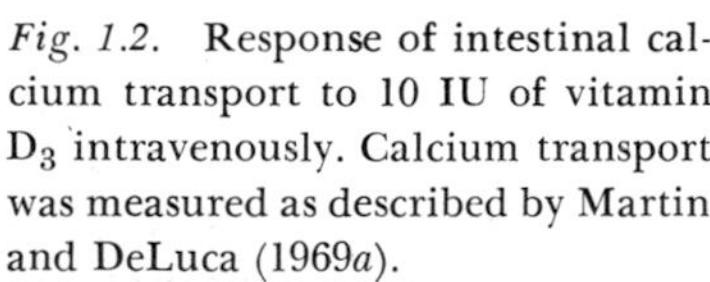
Fig. 1.2. Response of intestinal calcium transport to 10 IU of vitamin D_3 intravenously. Calcium transport was measured as described by Martin and DeLuca (1969*a*).

dose of 10 IU (0.25 μg), a lag of 10–12 hr occurs before the intestinal calcium-transport response appears (DeLuca, 1967; Blunt et al., 1968*c*). Our investigations were first pointed to the fate of the vitamin D during this time. For these studies it was necessary to synthesize vitamin D's of extremely high specific activity, namely, 1,2-^{3}H vitamin D_3 (Neville and DeLuca, 1966), 22,23-^{3}H vitamin D_4 (DeLuca et al., 1968), and random-^{14}C vitamin D_2 (Imrie et al., 1967). It was possible to show that the radioactive vitamin D was rapidly transported to the targets of vitamin D action, namely, intestine and bone. Parenthetically it should be noted that the vitamin and its major metabolite are transported in the blood bound to an α-globulin (Rikkers and DeLuca, 1967).

Vitamin D–deficient rats were given 10 IU of ^{3}H vitamin D_3 intravenously and were killed 24 hr later; the tissue extracts were chromatographed on silicic acid columns. It was evident that the vitamin is converted to a major polar metabolite (Fig. 1.3) (Lund and DeLuca, 1966). This major

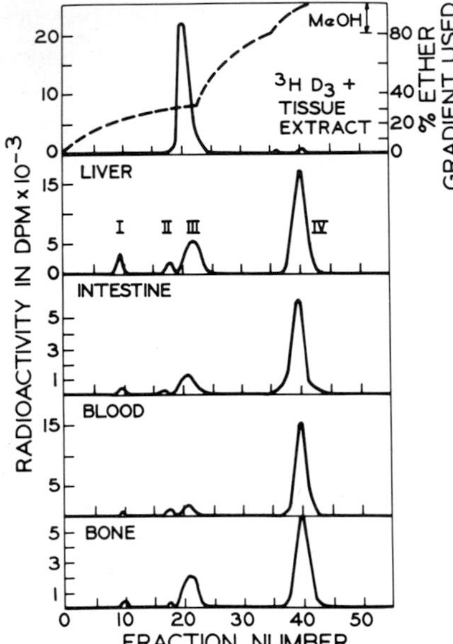

Fig. 1.3. Silicic acid column profiles of chloroform extracts of tissues taken from rats given 10 IU of 1,2-^{3}H vitamin D_3 intravenously 24 hr previously. Methods were as described by Lund and DeLuca (1966).

metabolite fraction was resolved into seven metabolites when the solvent gradient was modified (Fig. 1.4) (Ponchon and DeLuca, 1969*a*), but only the peak labeled IV retained biological activity. That metabolite has been identified as 25-hydroxycholecalciferol (25–HCC) and was later chemically synthesized (Fig. 1.5) (Blunt et al., 1968*a,* 1968*b*); Blunt and DeLuca, 1969) (see also Chapter 5). When tested in isolated bone systems (as discussed by Dr. Raisz in Chapter 7) (Trummel et al., 1968), the 25–HCC is markedly effective in inducing bone mobilization even at 0.9 IU/ml of medium, while as much as 380 IU of vitamin D_3 is without effect. An intestinal perfusion system has also been developed which transports calcium for a period of 4–6 hr (Fig. 1.6) (Olson and DeLuca, 1969). Intestines

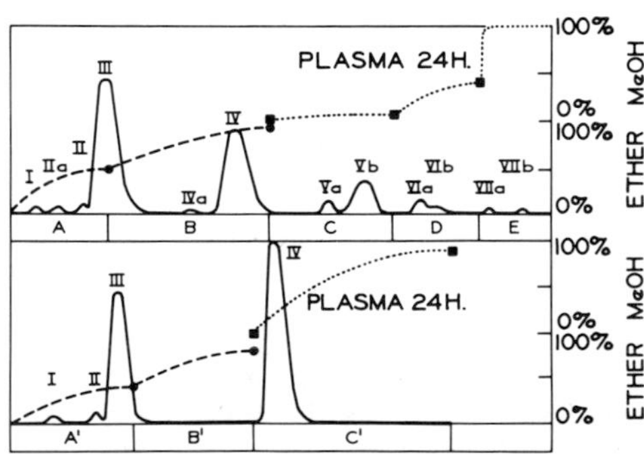

Fig. 1.4. Resolution of peak IV metabolite fraction (bottom) into seven components by a modified gradient elution procedure (top). The solid line represents the radioactivity plot and the dashed and dotted lines represent the solvent gradients used.

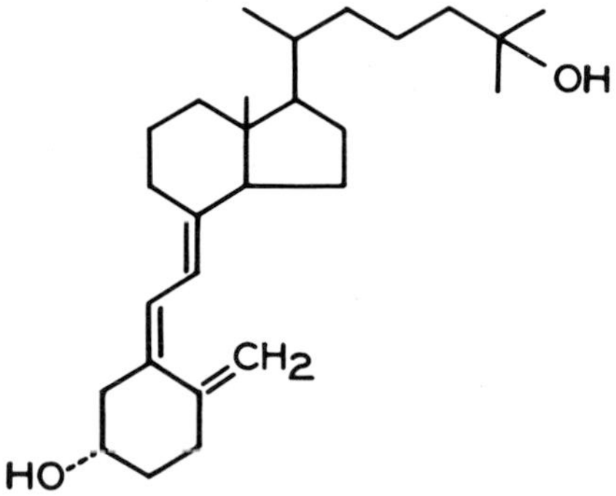

Fig. 1.5. Structure of 25-hydroxycholecalciferol (25–HCC).

from vitamin D–deficient rats that had been given 2000 IU of vitamin D 12 hr earlier show approximately a twofold increase in the rate of calcium transport. Infusion of 2.5 μg of 25–HCC into the arterial system of a vitamin D–deficient intestine brings about a rise in calcium transport within 1 hr to a level in excess of that of intestine from rats given vita-

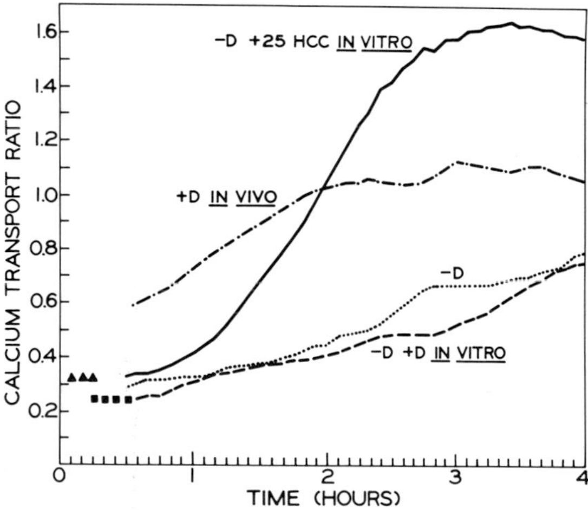

Fig. 1.6. Stimulation of calcium transport by 25–HCC in perfused intestine from vitamin D–deficient rats. The calcium transport ratios are shown for the intestine from the control rats (dotted line), from deficient rats that had received 2000 IU of vitamin D_3 12 hr earlier (dots and dashes), from deficient intestines into which 2.5 μg of 25–HCC was infused into the arterial system at 5 min (solid line), and from deficient intestines into which 250 μg of vitamin D_3 was infused at 15 min (dashed lines). (Olson and DeLuca, 1969. Reproduced from *Science 165*:405; © 1969 by the American Association for the Advancement of Science.)

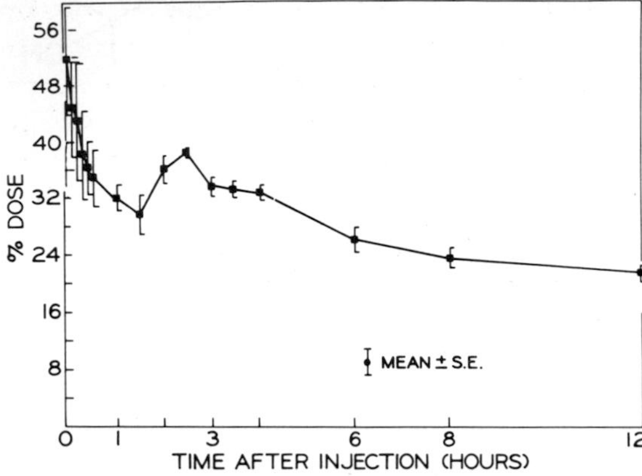

Fig. 1.7. Disappearance of ^3H in the plasma after an intravenous dose of 10 IU of 1,2-^3H vitamin D_3. (Ponchon and DeLuca, 1969*b*. Reproduced by permission of the *Journal of Clinical Investigation.*)

min D 12 hr earlier. Infusion of 10,000 IU (and sometimes 50,000 IU) of vitamin D_3 was without effect throughout the experiment. Thus, in both isolated bone and isolated intestine, 25–HCC is effective, whereas vitamin D is not, providing strong evidence that, at least at the tissue level, 25–HCC is the active form of the vitamin.

The time course of disappearance of radioactivity from the blood after ^3H vitamin D_3 is administered results in a triphasic curve (Fig. 1.7). the rapid, initial fall in radioactivity is due to both the mixing of the ^3H vita-

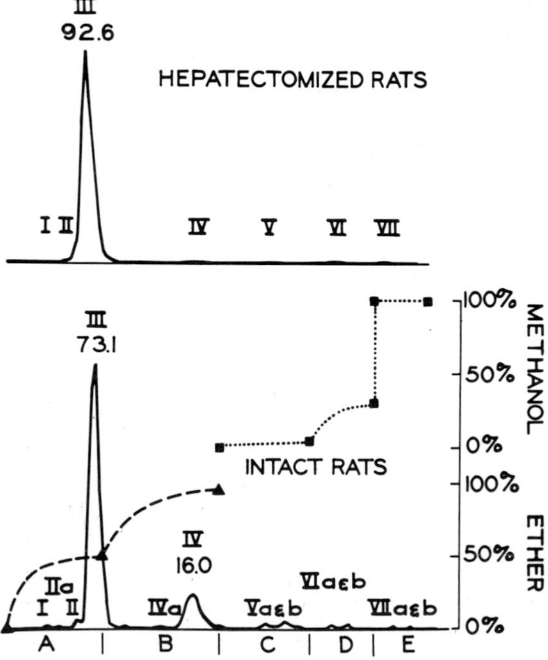

Fig. 1.8. Failure of hepatectomized rats to make 25–HCC. Control and hepatectomized rats received 10 IU of ^3H vitamin D_3 4 hr before they were killed. The plasma extracts were chromatographed on silicic acid columns as previously described. (Ponchon et al., 1969. Reproduced by permission of the *Journal of Clinical Investigation.*)

min D_3 in the plasma and extracellular fluid compartment and the uptake by the tissues. At this stage the liver takes up 60%–80% of the administered dose. At the time of the rebound of radioactivity of the plasma (1–2 hr after injection), the liver loses much of its radioactivity, which makes its appearance in the plasma (Ponchon and DeLuca, 1969*b*). The radioactivity that appears in the plasma is in the form of 25–HCC, suggesting that the liver is the major site of 25–HCC synthesis. Total hepatectomy (Fig. 1.8) prevents the appearance of 25–HCC in the plasma and other tissues; this is strong evidence that the liver is the major, if not the sole, site of

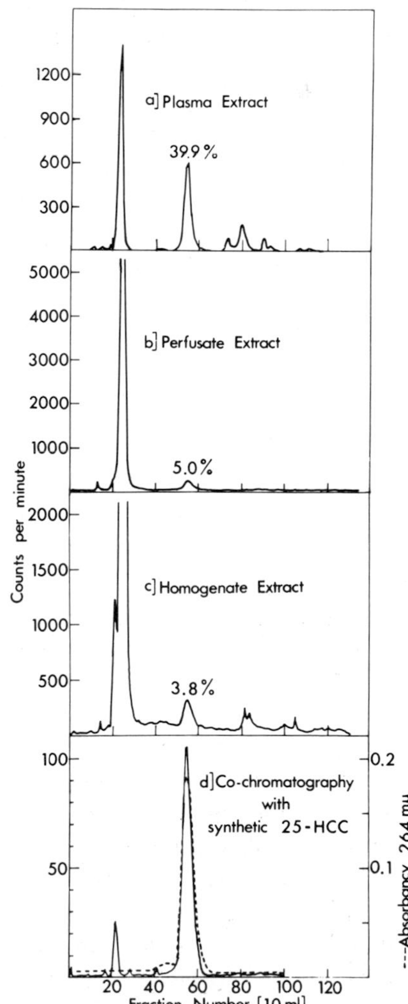

Fig. 1.9. Conversion of vitamin D_3 to 25–HCC by perfused liver and liver homogenates from vitamin D–deficient rats. The *d* plot is a cochromatography of 25–HCC produced by the homogenate reaction with synthetic 25–HCC. Conditions were as described by Horsting and DeLuca (1969).

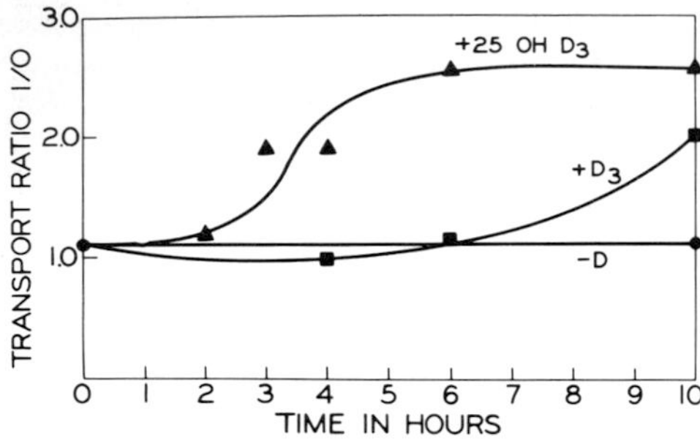

Fig. 1.10. Response of intestinal calcium transport to 0.25 μg of either 25–HCC or vitamin D_3 given intravenously to vitamin D–deficient rats. Experiments were described by Blunt and co-workers (1968*c*).

25–HCC synthesis (Ponchon et al., 1969). Perfused liver and liver homogenates are capable of converting vitamin D to 25–HCC (Fig. 1.9) (Horsting and DeLuca, 1969). The process requires oxygen and TPNH. It is strongly product inhibited providing an important control mechanism for the action of vitamin D. It may also result in the classification of vitamin D as a hormone, since the "secretion" of the active or hormonal form (25–HCC) may be controlled by a feedback inhibition by the product, 25–HCC.

The need to convert vitamin D_3 into an active form is responsible for a portion of the time lag in vitamin D action (Fig. 1.10). Nevertheless, some lag exists even when 25–HCC is administered intravenously (Blunt et al., 1968*c*).

RNA synthesis and protein synthesis in response to vitamin D

Insight into the lag in vitamin D action was first obtained in 1965 when Zull and co-workers demonstrated that the two physiologic actions of vitamin D – namely, the stimulation of intestinal calcium transport and bone mobilization – could be blocked by the prior administration of actinomycin D, an inhibitor of DNA transcription (Fig. 1.11) (Zull et al., 1965, 1966*a*; see also Norman, 1965). However, if the actinomycin D is given 4 hr after vitamin D, the action of the vitamin cannot be prevented. Other inhibitors of protein and RNA synthesis could also partially block the vitamin D actions. Thus it can be concluded that the action of vitamin D must involve both transcription of DNA and protein synthesis.

Confirmation of this was obtained when it could be demonstrated that the pulse labeling of intestinal nuclear RNA with ^3H orotic acid could be stimulated by administering vitamin D (Zull et al., 1966*b*; Stohs et al., 1967). Figure 1.12 shows that 3 hr after an intraperitoneal dose of 2000 IU of vitamin D_3 there is a maximum labeling of nuclear RNA of the intestine. This labeling decreases to nonsignificance at 8 hr. This RNA labeling could be blocked by prior administration of actinomycin D. When

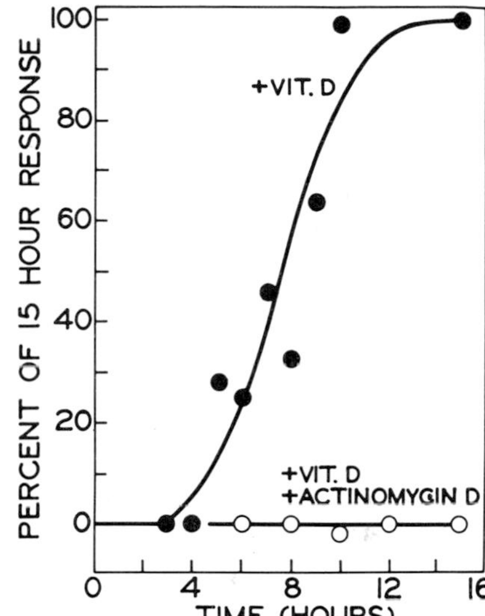

Fig. 1.11. Effect of actinomycin D on vitamin D–induced calcium transport in rat small intestine. (Zull et al., 1965. Reproduced from *Science 149*:182; © 1965 by the American Association for the Advancement of Science.)

10 IU of 25–HCC is given, the pulse labeling of RNA occurs in less than 30 min (Table 1.1) (Cousins and DeLuca, unpublished data).

When template activity of chromatin isolated from either vitamin D–deficient rats or from rats given 2000 IU of vitamin D_3 intraperitoneally is measured with an excess of highly purified RNA polymerase from *E. coli* nucleoside triphosphates including ^{14}C ATP, a marked increase due to vitamin D administration is found (Fig. 1.13) (Hallick and DeLuca, 1969). The increase is maximal when the chromatin is obtained from the rats 3

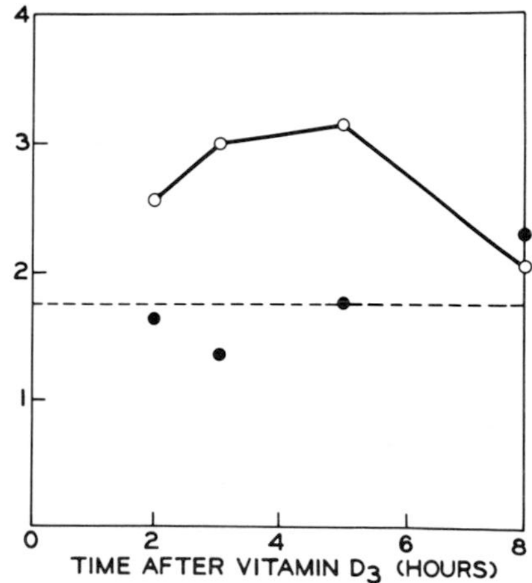

Fig. 1.12. Vitamin D–stimulated pulse labeling of nuclear RNA of rat intestine by ^3H orotic acid. (Stohs et al., 1967.) The solid line and open circles represent the incorporation of ^3H orotic acid into nuclear RNA at various times after 2000 IU of vitamin D_3 was given intraperitoneally to vitamin D–deficient rats. The solid circles and dashed lines represent incorporation into nuclear RNA of vitamin D–deficient rats.

TABLE 1.1. *Effect of 25–HCC on the pulse labeling of intestinal nuclear RNA by ³H orotic acid*

Time after 25–HCC	dpm/OD 260 mμ Control rats	dpm/OD 260 mμ 25–HCC rats	Increase due to 25–HCC
15 min[a]	6	16	2.7
30 min[a]	102	158	1.5
60 min[b]	36	32	1.0
60 min[a]	28	50	1.8

Source: Cousins and DeLuca, unpublished results.

Note: Vitamin D–deficient rats were given either 0.25 μg of 25–HCC or the vehicle alone intrajugularly. ³H orotic acid (50 μC_i) was given in the other jugular vein either at the same time or later. The rats were killed 15 min, 30 min, or 60 min after the 25–HCC injection, and their nuclear RNA was isolated by method described by Stohs and DeLuca, 1967.

[a] The orotic acid was given at the same time as the 25–HCC.

[b] The orotic acid was given 30 min after the 25–HCC.

hr after vitamin D is administered, in exact agreement with the in vivo RNA labeling experiments. Preliminary results suggest that, in minutes after 25–HCC is administered, template activity is increased. Thus it appears that 25–HCC in some way unmasks a specific DNA that codes for a calcium-transport substance.

Subcellular location of vitamin D and its metabolites

Of importance to this mechanism is the subcellular location of the active form of vitamin D. Table 1.2 shows that most of the ³H from ³H vitamin

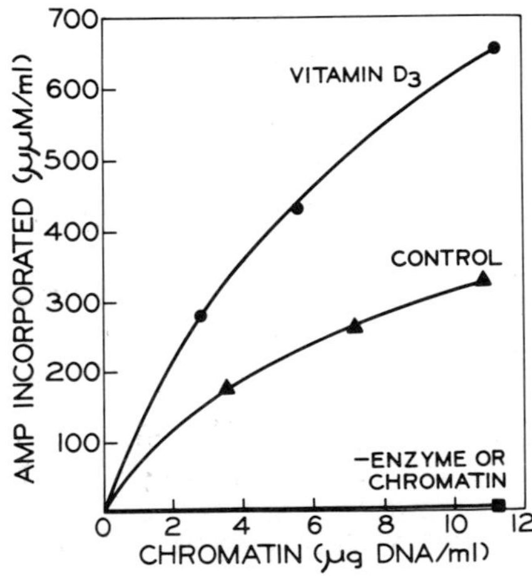

Fig. 1.13. Vitamin D–induced template activity of chromatin isolated from small intestine. Chromatin was isolated from rats given either 2000 IU of vitamin D or vehicle intraperitoneally 3 hr before being killed. (Hallick and DeLuca, 1969. Reproduced by permission of the National Academy of Sciences.)

TABLE 1.2. *Location of radioactivity in rat intestinal mucosa after 1,2-³H vitamin D_3*

Fraction	Percentage of total radioactivity of mucosa
Nuclei isolated from 1% citric acid solution	12.1 ± 3.8
Crude nuclei	57.6 ± 3.4
Mitochondria	6.7 ± 0.4
Microsomes	10.3 ± 1.2
Ribosomes	0.6 ± 0.2
Cytoplasm	22.8 ± 6.2

Notes: Rats were given, intravenously, 0.25 μg of 1,2-^{3}H vitamin D_3, and the radioactivity in the intestinal mucosa was determined 8 hr later. The method for cell fractionation was as described by Stohs and DeLuca (1967).

Values are given as mean ± SE.

D_3 in the intestine is found in two fractions—the crude nuclei and the cytoplasmic fraction (Stohs and DeLuca, 1967). When nuclei are isolated from intestinal mucosa in citric acid medium, little radioactivity remains in this fraction (Table 1.3). However, when the nuclei are isolated by means of 2.3 M sucrose, the radioactivity remains in the nuclear fraction (Table 1.3). If the nuclei are treated with citric acid or Triton X–100, the outer nuclear membrane is stripped off (Blobel and Potter, 1966; Gurr

TABLE 1.3. *Effect of preparation on ³H in nuclei from animals given 1,2-³H vitamin D_3*

Preparation and nuclei	Percentage of total ³H in tissue
Citric acid (1%)	
Rat mucosa	12.2 ± 3.8
Chick mucosa	14.8 ± 6.9
Sucrose (2.3 M)	
Rat liver	2.5 ± 0.6
Chick mucosa	52.1 ± 8.4
Rat mucosa	46.6 ± 11.3
Sucrose (2.3 M) + citric acid (1%)	
Chick mucosa	15.1 ± 6.7
Sucrose (2.3 M) + Triton X–100	
Chick mucosa	22.0 ± 7.4
EDTA + NaCl	
Rat mucosal DNA protein	9.6 ± 0.7

Notes: The data are from Stohs and DeLuca (1967). 10 IU of 1,2-^{3}H vitamin D_3 or of 22,23-^{3}H vitamin D_4 were injected intravenously. Rats were killed 8 hr later and chicks, 12 hr later.

Values are given as mean ± SE.

TABLE 1.4. *Intestinal nuclear radioactivity during isolation of chromatin*

Stage of procedure	Total dpm in preparation	Percentage of homogenate radioactivity
Crude nuclei	1600	65
EDTA supernatant fluid [a]	1159	50
EDTA (crude chromatin)	514	22
Crude chromatin after Tris wash	50	2
Sediment chromatin from 1.7 M sucrose (pure chromatin)	0	0

Note: The chromatin was prepared by the method of Marushige and Bonner (1966). Vitamin D–deficient rats received 0.25 μg of 1,2-^{3}H vitamin D_3 8 hr before being killed.

[a] Centrifugation of this fraction at 125,000 $\times$ g for 2 hr yielded a membrane (ppt) fraction which contained 1030 dpm and 45% of the homogenate radioactivity.

et al., 1963) and most of ^{3}H is lost; thus Stohs and DeLuca (1967) concluded that a major site of ^{3}H location from ^{3}H vitamin D is the nuclear membrane. Haussler and co-workers (1968) have concluded that the chromatin contains the ^{3}H from ^{3}H vitamin D. Our repeated attempts to confirm their data have failed. Instead, our results from experiments with either 26,27 ^{3}H 25–HCC or 1,2 ^{3}H vitamin D_3 show that the ^{3}H is found with the membrane fraction (Table 1.4) during the isolation of chromatin and that no radioactivity is associated with pure chromatin (Chen and DeLuca, unpublished data).

The question of whether 25–HCC is active as such or whether it is converted before it acts in the intestine has also been examined (Chen, Tanaka, Cousins, and DeLuca, unpublished results). The RNA-labeling experiments and the template-activity experiments indicate that the transformation would have to be rapid for it to be meaningful with respect to an active form. Experiments with ^{3}H 25–HCC (Fig. 1.14) showed three metabolites that are more polar than 25–HCC. One of these (peak V) appears after 2 hr and thus is unlikely to be an active form; peaks VI and VIa may appear early enough but they appear in the same proportion to 25–HCC regardless of dose. Only continued investigation can resolve this important point.

Calcium transport in intestine

The nature of the calcium-transport substance induced by vitamin D represents an important but as yet unknown area. It is important to realize first that, in addition to fructose and Mg^{++}, Na^+ is required for calcium

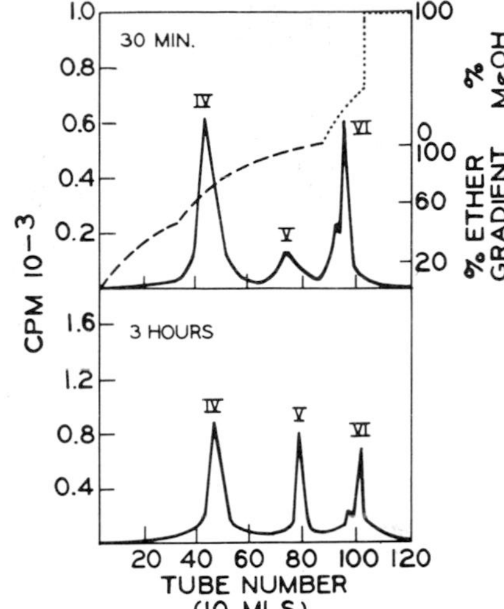

Fig. 1.14. Silicic acid column profiles of extracts of rat small intestine 30 min and 3 hr after an intravenous dose of 10 IU of 26,27-^{3}H 25–HCC.

transport by the small intestine (Martin and DeLuca, 1969*a*). When Na+ is absent, the intestine takes up calcium from the mucosal surface but is unable to extrude the calcium into the serosal medium. Results on uptake clearly revealed that Na+ does not influence the rate of calcium uptake across brush borders. In Na+-free medium, vitamin D nevertheless increases mucosal uptake of Ca++, even though it does not appreciably increase calcium transport into the serosal medium. A study of initial rates of calcium uptake across the brush-border surface show that vitamin D increases the earliest measurable uptake (Fig. 1.15) (Martin and DeLuca, 1969*b*). This mechanism is saturable; it has a K_m of about 2 mM; it does not require $HPO_4^{=}$; and it is decreased by a lack of O_2. These data suggest that vitamin D induces a substance which, by an energy-dependent process, effects the early transfer of Ca++ across the brush borders.

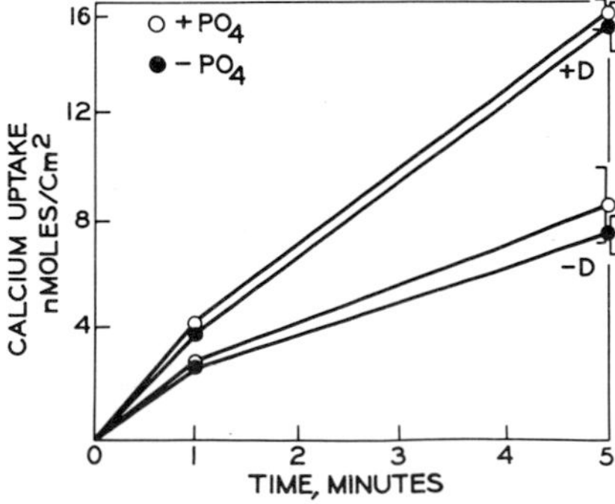

Fig. 1.15. Vitamin D–stimulated rate of calcium uptake by the mucosa of rat small intestine in the presence and absence of phosphate. (Martin and DeLuca, 1969*b*. Reproduced by permission of Academic Press.)

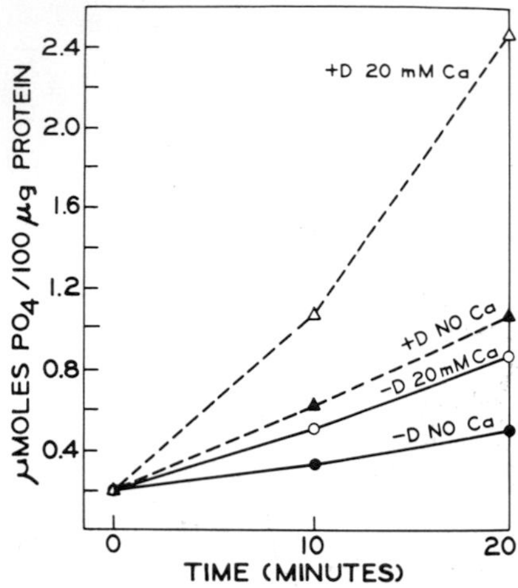

Fig. 1.16. Vitamin D–induced, calcium-dependent adenosine triphosphatase in isolated brush borders of small intestine of rats. (Martin et al., 1969. Reproduced by permission of Academic Press.)

Isolation of brush borders reveals a vitamin D–induced, Ca^{++}-dependent adenosine triphosphatase (Fig. 1.16). This system has a K_m of 2mM for free calcium, in agreement with the K_m for calcium uptake across brush borders. This adenosine triphosphatase appears at the same time as calcium absorption is increased in response to vitamin D. This adenosine triphosphatase is found in both rats and chicks and is under intensive study as the possible vitamin D–induced transport system. Its relationship to the calcium-binding protein of Wasserman and co-workers (Wasserman and Taylor, 1966; Taylor and Wasserman, 1967; Wasserman et al., 1968) is of great interest and is also under examination. It is sufficient to say that in our experiments the appearance of CaBP in response to vitamin D lags behind the appearance of calcium absorption (Fig. 1.17), a lag that cannot be accounted for by a lack of sensitivity of detection methods (Harmeyer and DeLuca, 1969).

The last figure (Fig. 1.18) demonstrates our current working hypothesis of how vitamin D functions: Vitamin D_3 is transported to the liver, where it is converted to 25–HCC. The 25–HCC is transported as a complex with α_2-globulin to the bone and intestine where it "unmasks" a specific DNA,

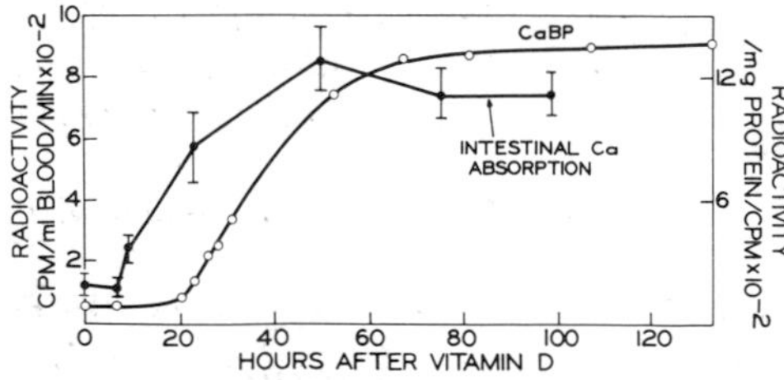

Fig. 1.17. Time course of appearance of calcium-binding protein and increased calcium absorption after a 500 IU oral dose of vitamin D_3 to rachitic chicks on a low-calcium diet. (Harmeyer and DeLuca, 1969. Reproduced by permission of Academic Press).

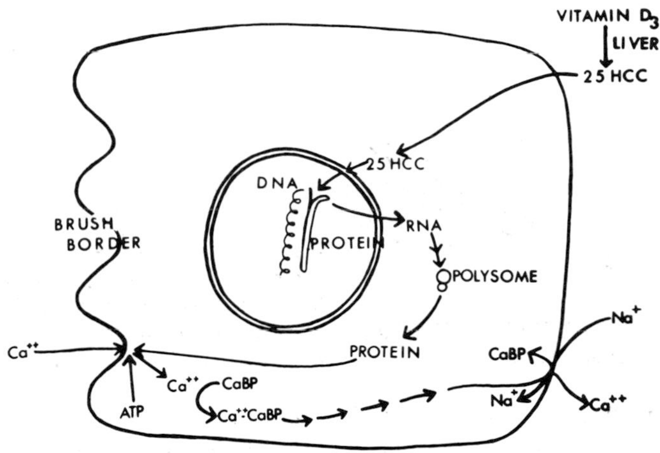

Fig. 1.18. Current hypothesis of vitamin D action on the intestine.

which is transcribed into a mRNA. Translation yields a protein or proteins, which makes its appearance at the brush border as an ATP requiring transport system. Calcium then traverses the cell facilitated in some way by CaBP and is extruded at the basement membrane aided by a Na+ gradient and exchange. Obviously, many facts remain to be learned, but it is clear that much progress has been made in our understanding of the function of vitamin D in recent years.

References

Askew, F. A., R. B. Bourdillon, H. M. Bruce, R. G. C. Jenkins, and T. A. Webster. 1931. The distillation of vitamin D. *Proc. Roy. Soc.* [*Biol.*] *107*:76.

Bauer, G. C. H., A. Carlsson, and B. Linquist. 1955. Evaluation of accretion, resorption, and exchange reactions in the skeleton. *Kungl. Fysiogr. Sallskäpets Lund Forh. 25*:3.

Blobel, G., and V. R. Potter. 1966. Nuclei from rat liver: Isolation method that combines purity with high yield. *Science 154*:1662.

Blunt, J. W., and H. F. DeLuca. 1969. The synthesis of 25–hydroxycholecalciferol — a biologically active metabolite of vitamin D. *Biochemistry 8*:671.

Blunt, J. W., H. F. DeLuca, and H. K. Schnoes. 1968. [Blunt et al., 1968*a*.] 25–Hydroxycholecalciferol: A biologically active metabolite of vitamin D_3. *Biochemistry* 7:3317.

Blunt, J. W., H. F. DeLuca, and H. K. Schnoes. 1968. [Blunt et al., 1968*b*.] 25–Hydroxycholecalciferol: A biologically active metabolite of cholecalciferol. *Chem. Commun. 14*:801.

Blunt, J. W., Y. Tanaka, and H. F. DeLuca. 1968. [Blunt et al., 1968*c*] Biological activity of 25–hydroxycholecalciferol a metabolite of vitamin D_3. *Proc. Nat. Acad. Sci. U.S.A. 61*:1503.

Carlsson, A. 1952. Tracer experiments on the effect of vitamin D on skeletal metabolism of calcium and phosphorus. *Acta Physiol. Scand. 26*:212.

DeLuca, H. F. 1967. Mechanism of action and metabolic fate of vitamin D. *Vitamins Hormones 25*:315.

DeLuca, H. F., M. Weller, J. W. Blunt, and P. F. Neville. 1968. Synthesis, biological activity and metabolism of 22,23 ^3H vitamin D_4. *Arch. Biochem. Biophys. 124*:122.

Gran, F. C. 1960. The retention of parenterally injected calcium in rachitic dogs. *Acta Physiol. Scand. 50*:132.

Gurr, M. I., J. B. Finean, and J. N. Hawthorne. 1963. Phospholipids of liver cell fractions. I. Phospholipid composition of the liver cell nucleus. *Biochim. Biophys. Acta 70*:406.

Hallick, R. B., and H. F. DeLuca. 1969. Vitamin D stimulated template activity of chromatin from rat intestine. *Proc. Nat. Acad. Sci. U.S.A. 63*:528.

Harmeyer, J., and H. F. DeLuca. 1969. Calcium binding protein and calcium absorption after vitamin D administration. *Arch. Biochem. Biophys. 133*:274.

Harrison, H. E. and H. C. Harrison. 1941. The renal excretion of inorganic phosphate in relation to the action of vitamin D and parathyroid hormone. *J. Clin. Invest. 20*:47.

Haussler, M. R., J. F. Myrtle, and A. W. Norman. 1968. The association of a metabolite of vitamin D_3 with intestinal mucosa chromatin *in vivo. J. Biol. Chem. 243*:4055.

Horsting, M., and H. F. DeLuca. 1969. Conversion of vitamin D_3 to 25–hydroxycholecalciferol by liver *in vitro. Fed. Proc. 28*:351.

Imrie, M. H., P. F. Neville, A. W. Snellgrove, and H. F. DeLuca. 1967. The metabolism of vitamin D_2 and vitamin D_3 in the rachitic chick. *Arch. Biochem. Biophys. 120*:525.

Lund, J., and H. F. DeLuca. 1966. Biologically active metabolite of vitamin D_3 from bone, liver, and blood serum. *J. Lipid Res.* 7:739.

Martin, D. L. 1968. The role of vitamin D in calcium transport by small intestine. Ph.D. thesis. University of Wisconsin.

Martin, D. L., and H. F. DeLuca. 1969*a*. The influence of sodium on calcium transport by the rat small intestine. *Amer. J. Physiol. 216*:1351.

Martin, D. L., and H. F. DeLuca. 1969*b*. Calcium transport and the role of vitamin D. *Arch. Biochem. Biophys. 134*:139.

Martin, D. L., M. J. Melancon, and H. F. DeLuca. 1969. *Biochem. Biophys. Res. Commun. 35*:819.

Marushige, K., and J. Bonner. 1966. Template properties of liver chromatin. *J. Mol. Biol. 15*:160.

McCollum, E. V., N. Simonds, J. E. Becker, and P. G. Shipley. 1922. Studies on experimental rickets. XXI. An experimental demonstration of the existence of a vitamin which promotes calcium deposition. *J. Biol. Chem. 53*:293.

Mellanby, E. 1919*a*. The part played by accessory food factors in the etology of rickets. *J. Physiol. 52*:LILI.

Mellanby, E. 1919*b*. An experimental investigation on rickets. *Lancet 196*:407.

Neuman, W. F. 1958. On the role of vitamin D in calcification. *Arch. Pathol. 66*:204.

Neuman, W. F., and M. W. Neuman. 1958. *The Chemical Dynamics of Bone Mineral.* University of Chicago Press, Chicago, Ill.

Neville, P., and H. F. DeLuca. 1966. The synthesis of [1,2 ^{3}H] vitamin D_3 and the tissue localization of a 0.25 μg (10 IU) dose per rat. *Biochemistry 5*:2201.

Nicolaysen, R. 1937*a*. Studies upon the mode of action of vitamin D. II. The influence of vitamin D on the fecal output of endogenous calcium and phosphorus in the rat. *Biochem. J. 31*:107.

Nicolaysen, R. 1937*b*. Studies upon the mode of action of vitamin D. III. The influence of vitamin D on the absorption of calcium and phosphorus in the rat. *Biochem. J. 31*:122.

Nicolaysen, R. 1937*c*. Studies upon the mode of action of vitamin D. IV. The absorption of calcium chloride, xylose and sodium sulfate from isolated loops of the small intestine and of calcium chloride from the abdominal cavity in the rat. *Biochem. J. 31*:323.

Nicolaysen, R. 1937*d*. Studies upon the mode of action of vitamin D. V. The absorption of phosphates from isolated loops of the small intestine in the rat. *Biochem. J. 31*:1086.

Nicolaysen, R. 1951. Influence of vitamin D on the absorption of calcium from the intestine of rats. Experiments with isolated loops. *Acta Physiol. Scand.* 22:260.

Norman, A. W. 1965. Actinomycin D and the response to vitamin D. *Science 149*:185.

Olson, E. B., and H. F. DeLuca. 1969. 25–Hydroxycholecalciferol. Direct effect on Ca transport. *Science 165*:405.

Orr, W. J., L. E. Holt, Jr., L. Wilkens, and F. H. Boone. 1923. The calcium and phosphorus metabolism in rickets with special reference to ultraviolet ray therapy. *Amer. J. Dis. Child. 26*:362.

Ponchon, G., and H. F. DeLuca. 1969*a*. Metabolites of vitamin D_3. *J. Nutr. 99*:157.

Ponchon, G., and H. F. DeLuca. 1969*b*. The role of the liver in the metabolism of vitamin D. *J. Clin. Invest. 48*:1273.

Ponchon, G., A. L. Kennan, and H. F. DeLuca. 1969. The activation of vitamin D by the liver. *J. Clin. Invest. 48*:2032.

Rikkers, H., and H. F. DeLuca. 1967. On *in vivo* study of the carrier proteins of ^{3}H-vitamin D_3 and D_4 in rat serum. *Amer. J. Physiol. 213*:380.

Schenck, F. 1937. Über das kristallisierte vitamin D_3. *Naturwissenschaften 25*:159.

Shipley, P. G., B. Kramer, and J. Howland. 1925. Calcification of rachitic bones *in vitro. Amer. J. Dis. Child. 30*:37.

Shipley, P. G., B. Kramer, and J. Howland. 1926. Studies upon calcification *in vitro. Biochem. J. 20*:379.

Steenbock, H. 1924. The induction of growth promoting and calcifying properties in a ration by exposure to light. *Science 60*:224.

Steenbock, H., and A. Black. 1924. Fat-soluble vitamins. XVII. The induction of growth-promoting and calcifying properties in a ration by exposure to ultra-violet light. *J. Biol. Chem. 61*:405.

Steenbock, H., and A. Black. 1925. Fat-soluble vitamins. XXIII. The induction of growth-promoting and calcifying properties in fats and their unsaponifiable constituents by exposure to light. *J. Biol. Chem. 64*:263.

Stohs, S. J., and H. F. DeLuca. 1967. Subcellular location of vitamin D and its metabolites in intestinal mucosa after a 10 IU dose. *Biochemistry 6*:3338.

Stohs, S. J., J. E. Zull, and H. F. DeLuca. 1967. Vitamin D stimulation of ^{3}H orotic acid incorporation into RNA of rat intestinal mucosa. *Biochemistry 6*:1304.

Taylor, A. N., and R. H. Wasserman. 1967. Vitamin D_3-induced calcium binding protein: Partial purification, electrophoretic visualization and tissue distribution. *Arch. Biochem. Biophys. 119*:536.

Trummel, C., L. G. Raisz, J. W. Blunt, and H. F. DeLuca. 1968. 25–Hydroxycholecalciferol, stimulation of bone resorption in culture. *Science 163*:1450.

Wasserman, R. H. 1963. Vitamin D and the absorption of calcium and strontium in vivo, pp. 211–28. *In* R. H. Wasserman (ed.), *The Transfer of Calcium and Strontium Across Biological Membranes.* Academic Press, New York.

Wasserman, R. H., R. A. Corradino, and A. N. Taylor. 1968. Vitamin D–dependent calcium-binding protein. *J. Biol. Chem. 243*:3978.

Wasserman, R. H., and A. N. Taylor. 1966. Vitamin D_3 induced calcium binding protein in chick intestinal mucosa. *Science 152*:791.

Windaus, A., O. Linsert, A. Lüttringhaus, and G. Weidlich. 1932. Crystalline-Vitamin D_2. *Justus Liebigs Ann. Chem. 492*:226.

Windaus, A., F. Schenck, and F. VonWerder. 1936. Über das antirachitisch wirksame bestrahlungsprodukt aus 7-dehydro-cholesterin. *Hoppe-Seyler's Z. Physiol. Chem. 241*:100.

Zull, J. E., E. Czarnowska-Misztal, and H. F. DeLuca. 1965. Actinomycin D inhibition of vitamin D action. *Science 149*:182.

Zull, J. E., E. Czarnowska-Misztal, and H. F. DeLuca. 1966. [Zull et al., 1966*a*.] On the relationship between vitamin D action and actinomycin-sensitive processes. *Proc. Nat. Acad. Sci., U.S.A. 55*:177.

Zull, J. E., S. J. Stohs, and H. F. DeLuca. 1966. [Zull et al., 1966*b*.] The relationship between vitamin D action and actinomycin sensitive processes. *Fed. Proc. 25*:545.

2

THE VITAMIN D–DEPENDENT CALCIUM-BINDING PROTEIN

R. H. Wasserman

Introduction

"*The history of rickets is that it has been enriched by a wealth of new hypotheses but few new facts.* This statement made [by Albu and Neuberg] in 1908 is no longer true since in the past four years facts of the greatest value have been discovered" (Park, 1923).

This quotation originates from a review written during the era when vitamin D was called X and when the connection between radiant energy and X was not precisely known. The year after Park's review appeared, Steenbock (1924) and Hess and Weinstock (1924) clarified the interrelationship between vitamin D and ultraviolet light. Subsequently there was a considerable surge in effort that resulted in an impressive body of information, particularly about the chemical and physical properties of the vitamin D molecule, its antirachitic and antiosteomalacic effect, its relationship to calcium and phosphorus metabolism, the distribution of the vitamin and provitamin throughout the plant and animal kingdoms, the nutritional requirements of various species for the vitamin, and the comparative efficacy in various species of the different forms of vitamin D and its derivatives.

There seems to have been a hiatus in innovative approaches for several years during and following World War II, and the opening quotation to

The author wishes to gratefully acknowledge the contributions to these studies by my colleagues, Dr. A. N. Taylor and Dr. R. A. Corradino, and to former graduate students who participated in several aspects of this research, including Dr. F. A. Kallfelz, Dr. R. L. Morrissey, and Dr. R. J. Ingersoll. The comments on the manuscript by Dr. Corradino and Dr. Taylor are greatly appreciated, as well as the continued interest by Dr. C. L. Comar.

These studies were supported by National Institutes of Health grants AM–04652 and AM–6271–NTN and United States Atomic Energy Commission Contract AT(30–1)–2147.

this chapter perhaps could have been justifiably restated five or six years years ago. Stimulation for the recent upswing in research interest in vitamin D, particularly at the molecular level, came from several quarters, not least of which was the in vitro demonstration of a calcium pump in intestinal tissue and the dependency of the calcium pump on vitamin D (Schachter and Rosen, 1959; Harrison and Harrison, 1960) and the isolation and identification of the more polar metabolite of vitamin D_3, 25-hydroxycholecalciferol (Blunt et al., 1968). Parallel development in related fields, such as molecular genetics and membrane biochemistry, provided concepts that allowed for the formulation of hypotheses of vitamin D action. As an example of this, it now appears that vitamin D acts by means of a DNA-directed mechanism, a concept that would have been difficult to develop prior to the discovery of the genetic effect of certain antibiotics such as actinomycin D and puromycin or prior to the delineation of the sequence of events in the synthesis of proteins. This and related matters have been adequately discussed in the preceding chapter by H. F. DeLuca.

Certain aspects of the intestinal absorption of calcium, vitamin D metabolism, and CaBP were the subject matter of recent reviews by our group (Wasserman, 1968; Wasserman, et al., 1969; Wasserman and Taylor, 1969; Wasserman and Kallfelz, 1970; Taylor and Wasserman, 1969). For this reason, the present chapter will emphasize newer information on the vitamin D–dependent, calcium-binding protein discovered in our laboratory a few years ago. The following topics will be covered: the tissue and species distribution, evidence associating CaBP with calcium absorption, localization of intestinal CaBP, some properties of CaBP, the possible role of CaBP in calcium absorption, and a comment on the control of CaBP synthesis.

Tissue and species distribution

When vitamin D_3 is administered to a rachitic chick, a calcium-binding protein (CaBP) is formed in intestinal mucosa (Wasserman and Taylor, 1966) and the kidney (Taylor and Wasserman, 1967). The same protein occurs in the uterine shell gland of the laying hen and is also dependent on vitamin D (Corradino et al., 1968), whereas the protein has not been detected in muscle, liver, blood, or pancreas (Taylor and Wasserman, 1967, 1970). Similar vitamin D–dependent, calcium-binding proteins have been found in the intestinal mucosa of the dog (Taylor et al., 1968), monkey (Wasserman and Taylor, 1970), calf (Wasserman, Wentworth, and Taylor, unpublished data, 1967), and rat (Kallfelz et al., 1967; Schachter et al., 1967; Moriuchi et al., 1969).

Evidence implicating CaBP in calcium absorption

A considerable body of evidence has accumulated which tends to suggest that CaBP has an important role in calcium absorption (Wasserman and Taylor, 1968; Taylor and Wasserman, 1969). Perhaps of most relevance is the relatively unique property of CaBP to bind calcium with a high affinity. This directly connects CaBP to the calcium translocation process and, further, suggests that the formation of the complex is in some way related to its function.

TIME RELATIONSHIPS

An important parameter is the time of appearance of CaBP as compared with the time required for vitamin D_3 to exert a physiological effect in a rachitic animal. Earlier data indicated that, in extracts of intestinal mucosa after vitamin D was administered to a rachitic animal, the enhancement of the calcium-binding activity occurred at about the same time that the absorption of calcium increased (Wasserman and Taylor, 1966). This matter was recently investigated in more detail with physiological (100 IU) and pharmacological (5000 IU) levels of vitamin D_3 (Ebel et al., 1969). It was demonstrated that CaBP was detectable in the supernatant fluid of intestinal mucosa homogenates at the same time that the first significant increase in ^{47}Ca absorption due to vitamin D was observed. This was true despite the fact that the larger amount of vitamin D (i.e., 5000 IU) reduced the lag time by about 10 hr.

Harmeyer and DeLuca (1969) purported to show that the enhanced absorption of calcium and the formation of CaBP could be distinguished on the basis of a time differential and a quantitative differential during the early phases of restoration of the calcium transport system in rachitic rats by vitamin D. Unfortunately, these investigators used only the ion-exchange procedure for CaBP detection (after Wasserman and Taylor, 1966) — which is the least sensitive of the three procedures currently used in our laboratory and which measures calcium-binding activity, and not CaBP specifically. The two other methods, gel electrophoresis and immunoassay, provide both of these essential features, specificity and sensitivity. As mentioned above, when the more sensitive and selective procedures are employed, CaBP has always been detected in intestinal mucosa at the same time that vitamin D_3 enhances calcium transport in rachitic chicks. Furthermore, in radioisotopic labeling experiments, MacGregor and co-workers (1970) clearly demonstrated that there was an increased incorporation of ^{3}H leucine into CaBP of vitamin D_3–deficient chicks (after being given supplemental vitamin D_3) before the absorption of calcium was increased. This latter experiment provides independent verification that the synthesis of CaBP is altered by vitamin D before the physiological response becomes manifest.

The lack of the apparent quantitative correlation between the rate of change of calcium absorption and the rate of calcium-binding activity noted by Harmeyer and DeLuca (1969) could be accounted for by: (a) the fact that the ion-exchange procedure measures calcium-binding activity and not CaBP per se; or (b) the observation that CaBP is localized in at least two distinct sites of the intestinal mucosa, the brush border region and the goblet cells; if only one of these sites is directly involved in calcium translocation, the measurement of total calcium-binding activity would not, for this reason, be expected to correlate with absorption.

An additional argument given by Harmeyer and DeLuca (1969) was that CaBP could be detected by only the more sensitive procedures at the time period that calcium absorption was affected, implying that too little is available to cause the effect. But how does one judge how much CaBP is required? Such an assessment requires knowledge of the mode of action of CaBP, which is certainly lacking at the present time. The conclusion by Harmeyer and DeLuca that their "data provide evidence that calcium absorption and CaBP formation as functions of vitamin D action are not directly related," therefore, is not yet solidly based and more convincing evidence must come from other quarters.

ADAPTATION

It has long been known that animals of various species can respond to low intakes of calcium by increasing the efficiency with which calcium is extracted from the diet. A question approached by us previously was whether the amount of CaBP in intestinal mucosa would also increase with the increased capacity to absorb calcium. This was found to be so in chicks (Wasserman and Taylor, 1968) and in rats (Schachter et al., 1967).

This matter was recently investigated in considerable detail in chicks (Morrissey, 1970; Morrissey and Wasserman, 1970). Part of the objective of the study was an attempt to gain an insight of control mechanisms as well as to quantitate the relationship between CaBP in intestinal mucosa and calcium absorption. In this situation, vitamin D_3 was not limiting. In one such experiment, groups of chicks were fed diets that differed in calcium and phosphorus contents. These diets contained either 0.08%, 1.2%, or 2.3% Ca and either 0.25%, 0.65%, or 1.2% P in a 3×3 factorial design. After the chicks had adapted to their respective diets, various measurements were made. The data clearly showed that the duodenal transfer of ^{47}Ca across a ligated duodenal segment *in situ* was directly related to the CaBP content of the duodenal mucosa, with a correlation coefficient of 0.99. Unlike the apparent discrepancies noted by Harmeyer and DeLuca

(1969), these data indicate that, at steady state, a highly significant correlation exists between these two parameters.

An important feature of these experiments was the determination of the effect of a phosphorus-deficient diet on calcium absorption, as was done by Carlsson in 1953 with rats. In brief, the following observations were made. Chicks receiving 1.2% Ca, 0.25% P (adequate Ca, deficient P) absorbed ^{47}Ca at a rate 2–3 times that of chicks receiving 1.2% Ca, 0.65% P (adequate Ca, adequate P), confirming the finding of Carlsson that phosphorus deficiency can affect the calcium absorptive system. Also, the group of phosphorus-deficient chicks had a comparably greater concentration of intestinal CaBP than the phosphorus-adequate group. Since the phosphorus-deficient group maintained a high serum calcium level and consumed a diet with the same concentration of calcium as the adequate group, it would seem unlikely that either of these two variables were involved in altering intestinal CaBP production or ^{47}Ca absorption. However, the degree of bone mineralization (bone ash) of the phosphorus-deficient group was significantly less than that of the adequate group (as expected), suggesting some inverse relationship with ^{47}Ca transfer. In fact, the correlation coefficient between ^{47}Ca absorption and bone ash over all groups was −0.94; between CaBP and bone ash, −0.95. Although a correlation coefficient indicates nothing about cause and effect relationships, other data from the experiment suggest that the degree of bone mineralization might be the responsible signaling parameter, but other factors, such as the calcium-regulating hormones, cannot yet be unequivocally eliminated.

A calcium-dependent adenosine triphosphatase associated with intestinal brush borders was recently studied by Melancon and DeLuca (1970). Their data suggested to them that the enzyme activity increased at about the same time that vitamin D_3 enhanced calcium absorption in rachitic chicks; but this aspect was not verified in this laboratory, where a considerable lag between these changes was noted (Taylor and Wasserman, 1970). In addition, CaATPase activity of brush border preparations of chicks adapted to a low-calcium diet was not significantly different from that of chicks fed a normal diet, whereas in the same experiment the concentration of intestinal calcium-binding protein was greater in the adapted chicks, as would be calcium absorption. Thus, an important feature of the vitamin D–dependent process, the capacity to adapt, does not seem to involve a change in CaATPase activity. Although CaATPase might have a significant role in the absorption process, the fact that the enzyme is already present in the rachitic chick (Melancon and DeLuca, 1970) suggests that it may be only indirectly related to the molecular events induced by vitamin D and to those associated with adaptation.

STRONTIUM RICKETS

The syndrome termed "strontium rickets" is produced in animals when they are fed a diet containing stable strontium as a substitute for most of the calcium. The earlier studies by Sobel (1935) suggested that there was a direct inhibition of the calcification mechanism, and Bartley and Reber (1961) observed that the retention of an oral dose of radiostrontium was decreased in pigs fed a stable strontium diet. This matter was investigated in some detail, and a brief report (Corradino and Wasserman, 1970) documented two findings in chicks: (a) the stable strontium diet reduced the absorption of ^{85}Sr (used as a tracer of calcium absorption) to a level seen in vitamin D–deficiency rickets; and (b) the CaBP content of intestinal mucosa was reduced to low or nonexistent levels by the strontium diet. Additional studies, done with ^{47}Ca tracer, verified these results and clearly demonstrated that, when CaBP concentrations decreased, calcium absorption decreased simultaneously and to about the same extent (Corradino et al., 1971). Again, a 1:1 correlation between CaBP and calcium absorption was observed under circumstances in which vitamin D_3 was not limiting. In addition, these observations might be of significance both in determining factors controlling the calcium translocation system and in explaining, in part, the molecular basis underlying the strontium rickets syndrome.

UREMIA

The first possible involvement of CaBP in a disease state arose from studies on uremic rats by Avioli and co-workers (1969). This experimentally induced situation results in the defective absorption of calcium, being comparable with one of the alterations occurring in patients with chronic renal insufficiency. Avioli and co-workers (1969) observed that, in the uremic rat, the capacity of the isolated everted gut sac to transport ^{45}Ca was reduced by about 50%; the calcium-binding activity of the intestinal mucosa was also decreased by about 50%. An interesting feature of this study was that ^{45}Ca transport could be restored by the administration of 25-hydroxycholecalciferol, but not by vitamin D_3 per se. The same pattern was noted with the enhancement of intestinal calcium-binding activity. It was suggested that alterations in vitamin D_3 metabolism in the uremic rat decreased, sequentially, the synthesis and concentration of intestinal CaBP, which then contributed to the defective absorption of calcium.

CONCLUSIONS

All of the above studies (and others not specifically cited in this chapter) strongly suggest that CaBP is a significant factor, if not the most significant factor, in the vitamin D–mediated absorption of calcium and, by inference, in the reabsorption of calcium by the kidney and the transfer of calcium across the uterus of the laying hen. As mentioned elsewhere (Wasserman et al., 1968), the two types of studies that would conclusively prove such a role have not been accomplished successfully to date, these being the restoration of the absorptive process by the addition of CaBP to rachitic intestinal tissue or the inhibition of the vitamin D process by the specific antibody formed against the protein.

Intestinal localization of CaBP

Using an immunofluorescent technique with cryostat-cut histological sections, it was shown that CaBP is localized in at least two identifiable sites of the intestinal mucosa, these being the goblet cells and the microvillar border of the absorptive cells (Taylor and Wasserman, 1970). The presence of CaBP in goblet cells was not anticipated from fractionation studies, and this locality is, for the present, assumed to represent a site of formation or concentration of nonfunctional CaBP. The CaBP situated in the microvillar region is more likely to be involved with calcium translocation, since physiological information strongly indicates that the transfer of calcium from lumen to mucosal tissue is one site that is significantly stimulated by the presence of vitamin D (Wasserman, 1963; Schachter et al., 1966; Wasserman and Taylor, 1969). It has not yet been possible to determine the exact site of localization of CaBP in the microvillar region. Because of the lack of resolution of present techniques, it has also not been possible to categorically state whether the protein is localized only in goblet cells and the microvillar border or whether it is also localized elsewhere in the mucosal tissue. Detailed information must await results from studies with the electron microscope.

The soluble leucine-binding protein of *E. coli* K–12 has been localized in a region apparently analogous to the microvillus, this being the cell envelope of the bacterial cell (Nakane et al., 1968). A surface localization of other binding proteins from bacteria has also been deduced because of their release by osmotic shock and their reactivity with diazotized aminonaphthylene-disulfonate, a nonpenetrating protein reagent (Pardee and Watanabe, 1968). This represents one similarity among several between CaBP and the soluble binding proteins from various bacteria (Pardee, 1966; Anraku, 1968; Piperno and Oxender, 1966). These proteins, as reviewed recently by Pardee (1968), have similar molecular sizes, similar binding affinities for their respective substrates, and each binds one molecule of substrate per molecule of protein.

Some properties of CaBP

The chick CaBP has been isolated in high purity, and some of its properties have been determined (Wasserman et al., 1968). The molecular size of the protein is of the order of 24,000–28,000; its formation constant with calcium is about 2.6×10^5 M^{-1}; and the binding capacity is one calcium atom per protein molecule. Its formation in response to vitamin D is inhibited by actinomycin D (Corradino and Wasserman, 1968).

Recent attention was given to assessing factors and conditions that might modify the binding affinity of CaBP and to determining the possible interaction of CaBP with certain amphiphilic compounds, particularly cetrimide and lysolecithin. Some of these investigations were done in collaboration with Dr. R. J. Ingersoll and will be reported in detail elsewhere.

*p*H OPTIMA OF THE BINDING REACTION

The influence of the ambient *p*H, with or without buffers, on the calcium-binding activity by purified CaBP was assessed by equilibrium dialysis. Purified CaBP (0.25 ml, containing about 0.013 mM protein in 0.15 M KCl and 5×10^{-6} M $CaCl_2$) was placed in small dialyzing sacs, and the latter suspended in flasks containing 150 ml of 0.15 M KCl and 5×10^{-6} M $CaCl_2$. Various buffers (10^{-3} M), when added, were chosen to cover the *p*H range of these experiments and included, in order of increasing *p*H, sodium acetate, 2-(*N*-morpholino) ethane sulfonic acid, piperazine-*N,N'*-bis(2-ethane sulfonic acid) monosodium monohydrate (PIPES), *N*-2-hydroxyethyl piperazine-*N'* ethane sulfonic acid, glycylglycine, and glycine. Tracer ^{45}Ca was added to the external solution and, after equilibration (5–6 hr), the inside and outside solutions were sampled and counted for ^{45}Ca by liquid scintillation. The *p*H was adjusted by additions of HCl or NaOH, and the *p*H measured initially and at the time of sampling.

The results of one of several replicates are depicted in Figure 2.1. Two maxima were usually observed, one at about *pH* 6.8 and the other in the range of *p*H 9.4–9.6; the intermediate minimum occurred at about *p*H 8.0. The assignment of specific amino acid residues to the binding site

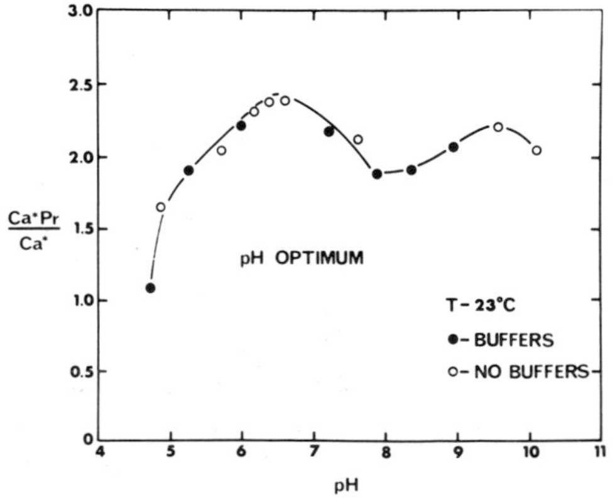

Fig. 2.1. Effect of *p*H on the binding of ^{45}Ca by CaBP, as determined by equilibrium dialysis. The data are expressed as the ratio of bound ^{45}Ca to unbound ^{45}Ca and represent the mean of triplicate determinations. (See text for experimental details; from Ingersoll and Wasserman, in preparation.)

and the physicochemical explanation of the two maxima are not feasible at the present time from these limited data. However, the binding site is certainly affected by the degree to which the molecule has been protonated, and since the ratio of bound ^{45}Ca to unbound ^{45}Ca is similar at *p*H values 6.8 and 9.5, it is tentatively suggested either that the chemical nature of a single binding site has changed as a function of *p*H or that a site buried at *p*H 6.8 becomes uncovered at *p*H 9.5 and that the *p*H 6.8 site becomes inaccessible at *p*H 9.5. Whatever the mechanism, the binding affinity of CaBP decreases by about 20% between *p*H values 6.8 and 8.0. This change could possibly be of significance as a mechanism for releasing CaBP-bound calcium at the absorptive surface, assuming that such a *p*H gradient exists across the microvillar membrane.

SULFHYDRYL GROUPS

The sequential oxidation-reduction of a key sulfhydryl moiety on the protein might provide a means to alter the binding capacity of the protein at an appropriate cytological site. Exposure of CaBP to *N*-ethylmaleimide, *p*-chloromercuribenzoate, or iodoacetate, however, did not affect calcium binding, indicating that sulfhydryl groups are not required for the formation of the calcium complex.

IONIC STRENGTH

The effect of ionic strength on the ^{45}Ca-binding capacity of CaBP was determined in the following way. Purified CaBP (0.013 mM) in buffer mixture was placed in one chamber of several equilibrium dialysis cells which was separated from the other chamber by Visking cellophane membrane. The second chamber contained the same volume (0.4 ml) of buffer mixture alone. The initial buffer mixture was 0.02 M KCl, 10^{-3} M PIPES, 5×10^{-6} M $CaCl_2$, *p*H 6.8. At zero time, 5 μCi tracer ^{45}Ca was added to one chamber and the cells were shaken at room temperature until equilibrium was attained. After sampling, sufficient KCl or NaCl was added to the appropriate cells to yield a total alkali metal concentration of 0.053 M. This sequence was repeated, yielding maximum total alkali metal concentrations of 0.10 M and 0.15 M.

Increasing the concentration of NaCl or KCl in the buffer solution from 0.02 M to 0.15 M decreased the binding of calcium to the protein by about 40% (Fig. 2.2). Thus there is the possibility that the responsiveness of the protein to ionic strength might have physiological significance. What makes such a proposal difficult to justify are the facts that Na^+ and K^+ are equally effective (i.e., there is no apparent alkali metal selectivity) and that the total concentration Na^+ and K^+ in cells in general is about equal to that of the extracellular environment (Maxwell and Kleeman, 1962). However, since CaBP is apparently located in the microvillar re-

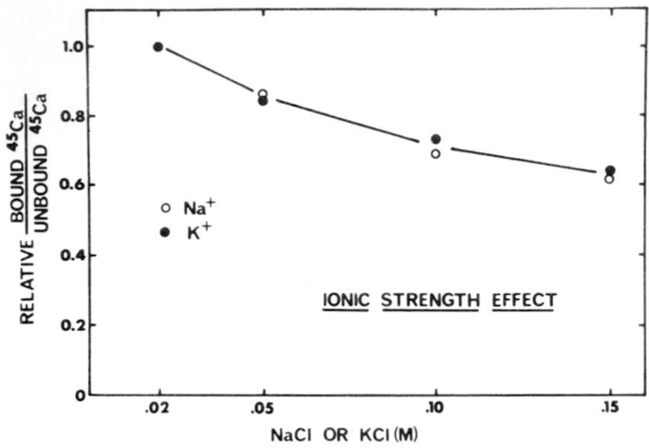

Fig. 2.2. Effect of ionic strength on the binding of ^{45}Ca by CaBP, as determined by equilibrium dialysis. The data are expressed as the ratio of bound ^{45}Ca to unbound ^{45}Ca relative to that of control cells. (See text for experimental details; from Ingersoll and Wasserman, in preparation.)

gion, it is conceivable that the status of total alkali metals in this area might differ, at least transiently, from that of the mucosal tissue.

PHOSPHOLIPID INTERACTION OF CaBP

Cetrimide, a cationic surface-active agent composed of a quaternary ammonium group and a 16-carbon alkyl side chain, was shown to depress the calcium-binding activity of the purified protein (Ingersoll and Wasserman, unpublished data, 1968). Certain other surface-active agents were ineffective in this regard; those tested thus far include taurocholic acid, glycocholic acid, and Tween 80. The observation that such other quaternary ammonium compounds as choline and acetylcholine did not affect the calcium-binding reaction suggested that both the hydrophobic group and the quaternary moiety are required. Since these requirements are similarly met by phosphatidylcholine, a component of many biological membranes, we obtained the soluble derivative of this type of phospholipid, lysolecithin, and examined its effect on CaBP by equilibrium dialysis (Wasserman, 1970).

It was shown that lysolecithin significantly depressed calcium binding by the protein (Fig. 2.3), presumably by forming a complex that has a lower affinity for the cation. A question of interest was whether the lysolecithin-induced inhibition of calcium binding was due to an irreversible denaturation of the protein. That this was not the case was demonstrated by the effect of adding taurocholate to lysolecithin-loaded equilibrium cells (Fig. 2.3). Taurocholate apparently was able to remove the lipid from CaBP; as a consequence of this, the binding capacity of the protein was restored. Furthermore, the ability of lysolecithin and CaBP to form a tight association was shown by the fact that the electrophoretic mobility of the CaBP-lysolecithin mixture in acrylamide gel was less than that of CaBP alone.

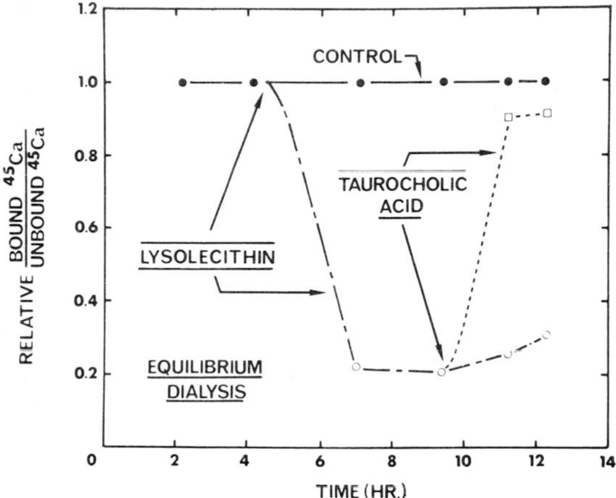

Fig. 2.3. Effect of lysolecithin on calcium binding by CaBP, and the reversal of this effect by taurocholate, as shown by equilibrium dialysis. Equilibrium dialysis cells, with Visking dialyzing membrane-separating 1-ml chambers, were loaded on one side with 0.4 ml buffer mixture (0.15 M KCl, 10^{-3} M PIPES, 5×10^{-6} M $CaCl_2$, *p*H 6.8) containing 5 μCi ^{45}Ca, and the other side with the same buffer mixture containing about 0.014 mM CaBP. At about 4 hr, lysolecithin was added to both sides of 4 of the 6 cells; at about 9.5 hr, taurocholate was added to 2 of the 4 lysolecithin-containing cells. The buffer mixture in which lysolecithin and taurocholate was dissolved was identical to that given above, except that the $CaCl_2$ was omitted. Buffer mixture alone without $CaCl_2$ was added to those cells not receiving lysolecithin or taurocholate in order to maintain the same volume in all cells. The final concentrations of lysolecithin and taurocholate were 1.52 mg/ml and 1.40 mg/ml, respectively. At the times indicated in the above figure, aliquots were taken from each side of all cells and counted by liquid scintillation detection. The results are expressed as the ratio of protein-bound ^{45}Ca to unbound ^{45}Ca relative to that of untreated controls. (Wasserman, 1970.)

Speculations on the role of CaBP in calcium translocation

The data and observations presented above clearly suggest that CaBP is, in some manner, involved in the total process of calcium absorption. Prior to the localization studies, one was tempted to consider CaBP as being cytoplasmic in origin and perhaps serving as a carrier of calcium through the intracellular milieu. This may be the case, but presently a role involving the microvillar localization of CaBP must be seriously considered. In this regard, Pardee (1968) offered two possible mechanisms with respect to the binding proteins in bacteria and animals. The first, termed the permease hypothesis, considered that these "recognition proteins are enzymes which catalyze the transfer of substrate in the external environment to a low-molecular weight membrane carrier." The second hypothesis was that the binding protein directly facilitates the movement of the substrate across the membrane, either by opening selective channels or by acting as a bona fide carrier. Pardee (1968) calculated that these macromolecules are long enough (70–120 Å) to stretch across the membrane, but he tended to discount such a mechanism because of the insolubility of the sulfate-binding protein in lipid solvents, including butanol and vegetable oil (Pardee, 1966). Despite this objection, a membrane-oriented role for CaBP was considered, at least hypothetically, because of its site of localization. In order for a molecule to act as a membrane carrier, three properties are required: (a) capacity to bind substrate, (b) ability to penetrate into and possibly through the lipid core of the membrane, and (c) capability of releasing the substrate at the appropriate site, by virtue of special conditions associated with the membrane-fluid interface, a conformational change of the protein, the presence of a receptor molecule, or the like. It has been adequately demonstrated that CaBP meets the first of these requirements.

The relevance of the lysolecithin studies to the function of CaBP (and perhaps other soluble binding proteins) is difficult to assess. However, it now becomes feasible to *at least* consider the possibility that CaBP can interact with components of the membrane and that this interaction is somehow related to the functional activity of the protein. One such possibility is depicted in Figure 2.4A in which CaBP, located in the surface coat close to the membrane, binds Ca^{++} and then transiently associates with the membrane. Through the protein-membrane interplay, the binding capacity of the protein is reduced and calcium is released in high concentration within or close to the membrane. The cation then diffuses through the membrane or, alternatively, interacts with a second substance within the membrane that further facilitates the transfer of the cation. A related proposal is one in which the protein actually penetrates into and through the lipid core of the membrane (Fig. 2.4B). When the binding groups of the protein are exposed to the aqueous environment external to the membrane, calcium becomes bound. Through thermal agitation of the protein or transitions of the membrane of the type proposed by Kavanau (1965), CaBP might enter the hydrophobic region of the membrane where the bound calcium is released and is thus available to

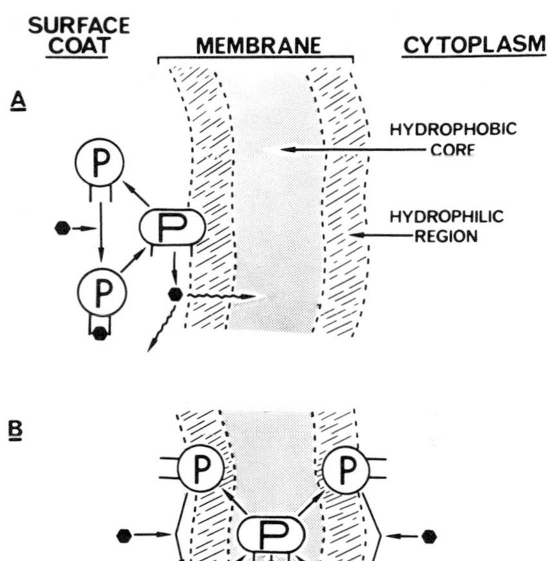

Fig. 2.4. Hypothetical models for a possible function of CaBP, based upon information concerning the localization of CaBP and recent observations on CaBP-lipid interactions.

A: The protein (CaBP) binds calcium ion external to the plasma membrane and, by a transient interplay with the more surface components of the membrane, releases the bound cation.

B: The protein actually penetrates into the hydrophobic core of the membrane and releases previously bound calcium.

diffuse into the cytoplasm or into the lumen. The rate and net direction of transfer would depend upon the concentration gradient of calcium across the membrane and the concentration of CaBP in a particular region of the surface coat–membrane complex. One could also incorporate the dependency of the binding reaction on *p*H and ionic strength into the same model as other means by which calcium might be released from CaBP.

Related to the second proposal is the concept that CaBP might act in a manner similar to such cyclic polyene antibiotics as valinomycin, opening specific calcium channels or, as thought by some, acting as bona fide membrane carriers (Bangham, 1968).

It must be emphasized that the fact that this particular protein reacts with a phospholipid is not, of itself, unique. Such protein-lipid interactions have been well-documented and have been investigated for many years. What inherently imparts specificity to CaBP is its special calcium-binding property and its particular localization. It should also be recognized that the hypotheses just proposed are highly speculative at present, and alternate roles for CaBP in the calcium translocation process have certainly not been excluded. For example, we had also suggested that CaBP may have a relatively passive role, functioning only as a collector of calcium at the microvillar border and providing substrate for the next step in the transport process (Wasserman et al., 1969). The present data available are insufficient to positively exclude one proposal over another.

Control of CaBP synthesis

The final topic of this chapter concerns the control of CaBP synthesis. The overwhelming evidence to date suggests that the critical event in vitamin D action occurs at the transcriptional level and results in the formation of a protein or proteins involved in calcium translocation. Since actinomycin D inhibits CaBP synthesis (Corradino and Wasserman, 1968), it may be inferred that CaBP is at least one of the proteins formed, either by *de novo* synthesis or indirectly by the action of a newly formed enzyme that modifies pre-existing cellular proteins. Without vitamin D, CaBP is not detectable in intestinal mucosa. The high concentration of CaBP in the goblet cell compels one to seriously consider that this specialized epithelial cell, involved in the formation of mucus, plays a significant role in the synthetic process.

Once vitamin D is available to the animal, what other factors control the amount of CaBP formed? In other words, how does one explain the ability of the animal to adapt to limited intakes of calcium or to such physiological needs for calcium as during growth or the formation of the egg shell? Is the controlling factor a known or unknown hormone, the calcium concentration in body fluids or in specific body cells, the degree of mineralization of the skeleton, the ionic environment of the nuclei of the responsive epithelial cells, or the amount of vitamin D_3 metabolite (such as 25-hydroxycholecalciferol) in the receptor cell? Teleologically, one may argue that the controlling point must be remote from the site of absorption, since the intestine represents only the means of making calcium available for the several critical reactions in which the divalent cation participates. Also, if the control is at the intestinal cell level, it is most likely mediated through the calcium activity of body fluids or that of the ingesta. However, the evidence obtained from studies on the adaptation mechanism indicated that phosphorus-deficient chicks can maintain a high absorption capacity for ^{47}Ca despite having a normal or above normal serum calcium level and when ingesting a diet with a normal or above normal level of calcium. In this series, the rate of ^{47}Ca absorption was best correlated (inversely) with the degree of bone mineralization, suggesting a cause-effect relationship between these two parameters. Although a search for a bone hormone comparable to Nicolaysen's (1943) endogenous factor has proven fruitless thus far, the skeletal origin of such a controlling substance cannot yet be disregarded. Serious consideration must also be given to the calcium-regulating hormones, but calcitonin has not been unequivocally demonstrated to affect calcium absorption (Krawitt and Wilson, 1967), and other information indicates that the parathyroidectomized animal can still adapt to low intakes of calcium (Kimberg et al., 1961). Certainly, the understanding of the mechanism of control of calcium absorption and net CaBP formation represents one of the more formidable and significant problems in this field today.

References

Anraku, Y. 1968. Transport of sugars and amino acids in bacteria. *J. Biol. Chem. 243*:3116.

Avioli, L. V., S. Scott, S. W. Lee and H. F. DeLuca. 1969. Intestinal calcium absorption: nature of defect in chronic renal disease. *Science 166*:1154.

Bangham, A. D. 1968. Membrane models with phospholipids. *In* J. A. V. Butler and D. Noble (eds.), *Progress in Biophysics and Molecular Biology*, Vol. 18, p. 31. Pergamon, Oxford.

Bartley, J. C., and E. F. Reber. 1961. Metabolism of radiostrontium in young pigs and in lactating rats fed stable strontium. *J. Dairy Sci. 44*:1754.

Blunt, J. W., H. F. DeLuca, and H. K. Schnoes. 1968. 25-hydroxycholecalciferol: A biologically active metabolite of vitamin D_3. *Biochemistry* 7:3317.

Corradino, R. A., J. G. Ebel, P. H. Craig, A. N. Taylor, and R. H. Wasserman. 1971. Calcium absorption and the vitamin D_3–dependent calcium binding protein. I. Inhibition by dietary strontium. *Calc. Tissue Res.* (in press).

Corradino, R. A., and R. H. Wasserman. 1968. Actinomycin D inhibition of vitamin D_3–induced calcium-binding protein (CaBP) formation in chick duodenal mucosa. *Arch. Biochem. Biophys. 126*:957.

Corradino, R. A., and R. H. Wasserman. 1970. Strontium inhibition of vitamin D–induced calcium-binding protein (CaBP) and calcium absorption in chick intestine. *Proc. Soc. Exp. Biol. Med. 133*:960.

Corradino, R. A., R. H. Wasserman, M. H. Pubols, and S. I. Chang. 1968. Vitamin D_3 induction of a calcium-binding protein in the uterus of the laying hen. *Arch. Biochem. Biophys. 125*:378.

Ebel, J. G., A. N. Taylor, and R. H. Wasserman. 1969. Vitamin D–induced calcium-binding protein of intestinal mucosa: Relation to vitamin D dose level and lag period. *Amer. J. Clin. Nutr. 22*:431.

Harmeyer, J., and H. F. DeLuca. 1969. Calcium-binding protein and calcium absorption after vitamin D administration. *Arch. Biochem. Biophys. 133*:247.

Harrison, H. E., and H. C. Harrison. 1960. Transfer of Ca^{45} across intestinal wall in vitro in relation to action of vitamin D and cortisol. *Amer. J. Physiol. 199*:265.

Hess, A. F., and M. Weinstock. 1924. Antirachitic properties imparted to inert fluids and to green vegetables by ultra-violet irradiation. *J. Biol. Chem.* *62*:301.

Kallfelz, F. A., A. N. Taylor, and R. H. Wasserman. 1967. Vitamin D–induced calcium-binding factor in rat intestinal mucosa. *Proc. Soc. Exp. Biol. Med.* *125*:54.

Kavanau, J. Lee. 1965. *Structure and Function in Biological Membranes*, 2 vols. Holden-Day, San Francisco.

Kimberg, D. V., D. Schachter, and H. Schenker. 1961. Active transport of calcium by intestine: Effects of dietary calcium. *Amer. J. Physiol.* *200*:1256.

Krawitt, E. L., and H. D. Wilson. 1967. Effect of thyrocalcitonin on duodenal calcium transport. *Proc. Soc. Exp. Biol. Med.* *125*:1084.

MacGregor, R. R., J. W. Hamilton, and D. V. Cohn. 1970. The induction of calcium binding protein biosynthesis in intestine by vitamin D_3. *Fed. Proc.* *29*:368.

Maxwell, M. H., and C. R. Kleeman. 1962. Dynamics of body water and electrolytes, p. 1. *In* M. H. Maxwell and C. R. Kleeman (eds.), *Clinical Disorders of Fluid and Electrolyte Metabolism.* McGraw-Hill, New York.

Melancon, M. J., Jr., and H. F. DeLuca. 1970. Vitamin D stimulation of calcium-dependent adenosine triphosphatase in chick intestinal brush borders. *Biochemistry* *9*:1658.

Moriuchi, S., K. Ooizumi, and N. Hosoya. 1969. Effect of vitamin D_3 on the calcium binding factor in rat intestinal mucosa. *J. Vitaminology (Japan)* *15*:178.

Morrissey, R. L. 1970. Ph.D. thesis. Cornell University.

Morrissey, R. L., and R. H. Wasserman. 1970. Adaptation, calcium binding protein and the intestinal absorption of calcium. *Fed. Proc.* *29*:847.

Nakane, P. K., G. E. Nichoalds, and D. L. Oxender. 1968. Cellular localization of leucine-binding protein from *Escherichia coli. Science* *161*:182.

Nicolaysen, R. 1943. The absorption of calcium as a function of the body saturation with calcium. *Acta Physiol. Scand.* *5*:200.

Pardee, A. B. 1966. Purification and properties of a sulfate-binding protein from *Salmonella typhimurium. J. Biol. Chem.* *241*:5886.

Pardee, A. B. 1968. Membrane transport proteins. *Science* *162*:632.

Pardee, A. B., and K. Watanabe. 1968. Location of sulfate-binding protein in *Salmonella typhimurium. J. Bacteriol.* *96*:1049.

Park, E. A. 1923. The etiology of rickets. *Physiol. Rev.* *3*:106.

Piperno, J. R., and D. L. Oxender. 1966. Amino acid-binding protein released from *Escherichia coli* by osmotic shock. *J. Biol. Chem.* *241*:5732.

Schachter, D., S. Kowarski, J. D. Finkelstein, and R.-I. W. Ma. 1966. Tissue concentration differences during active transport of calcium by intestine. *Amer. J. Physiol.* *211*:1131.

Schachter, D., S. Kowarski, and P. Reid. 1967. Molecular basis for vitamin D action in the small intestine. *J. Clin. Invest.* *46*:1113.

Schachter, D., and S. M. Rosen. 1959. Active transport of Ca^{45} by the small intestine and its dependence on vitamin D. *Amer. J. Physiol.* *196*:357.

Sobel, A. E., J. Cohen, and B. Kramer. 1935. The nature of the injury to the calcifying mechanism in rickets due to strontium. *Biochem. J. 29*:2640.

Steenbock, H. 1924. The induction of growth promoting and calcifying properties in a ration by exposure to light. *Science 60*:224.

Taylor, A. N., and R. H. Wasserman. 1967. Vitamin D_3–induced calcium-binding protein: partial purification, electrophoretic visualization and tissue distribution. *Arch. Biochem. Biophys. 119*:536.

Taylor, A. N., and R. H. Wasserman. 1969. Correlations between the vitamin D–induced calcium-binding protein and the intestinal absorption of calcium. *Fed. Proc.*, symposium issue. *28*:1834.

Taylor, A. N., and R. H. Wasserman. 1970. Immunofluorescent localization of vitamin D–dependent calcium-binding protein. *J. Histochem. Cytochem. 18*:107.

Taylor, A. N., R. H. Wasserman, and J. Jowsey. 1968. A vitamin D–dependent calcium-binding protein in canine intestinal mucosa. *Fed. Proc. 27*:675.

Wasserman, R. H. 1963. Vitamin D and the absorption of calcium and strontium in vivo, p. 211. *In* R. H. Wasserman (ed.), *The Transfer of Calcium and Strontium Across Biological Membranes.* Academic Press, New York.

Wasserman, R. H. 1968. Calcium transport by the intestine: A model and comment on vitamin D action. *Calc. Tissue Res. 2*:301.

Wasserman, R. H. 1970. Interaction of lysolecithin with vitamin D–induced calcium-binding protein: Possible relevance to calcium transport. *Biochem. Biophys. Acta 203*:176.

Wasserman, R. H., R. A. Corradino, and A. N. Taylor. 1968. Vitamin D–dependent calcium-binding protein: Purification and some properties. *J. Biol. Chem. 243*:3978.

Wasserman, R. H., R. A. Corradino, and A. N. Taylor. 1969. Binding proteins from animals with possible transport function. *J. Gen. Physiol. 54*:114s.

Wasserman, R. H., and F. A. Kallfelz. 1970. Transport of calcium across biological membranes, Chapter 6. *In* H. Schraer (ed.), *Biological Calcification: Cellular and Molecular Aspects.* Appleton-Century-Crofts, New York.

Wasserman, R. H., and A. N. Taylor. 1966. Vitamin D_3–induced calcium binding protein in chick intestinal mucosa. *Science 152*:791.

Wasserman, R. H., and A. N. Taylor. 1968. Vitamin D–dependent calcium-binding protein: Response to some physiological and nutritional variables. *J. Biol. Chem. 243*:3987.

Wasserman, R. H., and A. N. Taylor. 1969. Some aspects of the intestinal absorption of calcium, with special reference to vitamin D, Chapter 5. *In* C. L. Comar and F. Bronner (eds.), *Mineral Metabolism, An Advanced Treatise.* Academic Press, New York.

Wasserman, R. H., and A. N. Taylor. 1970. Evidence for a vitamin D_3–induced calcium-binding protein in new world primates. *Proc. Soc. Exp. Biol. Med.* (in press).

3

ROLE OF VITAMIN D, PARATHYROID HORMONE, AND CORTISOL IN INTESTINAL TRANSPORT OF CALCIUM AND PHOSPHATE

Harold E. Harrison and Helen C. Harrison

Extent of vitamin D action on intestinal calcium transport

In vivo studies utilizing standard balance techniques or intestinal uptake of radioactive calcium have established that vitamin D is essential for efficient absorption of calcium and of phosphate from the intestine. These studies have also established that parathyroid hormone and adrenocorticoids influence calcium absorption, an excess of the former increasing this function, and an excess of the latter decreasing the function. In vitro experiments have corroborated these observations and in addition have provided information of significance with regard to the nature of the transport systems and cellular mechanisms influenced by vitamin D, parathyroid hormone, and the corticoids.

The effect of vitamin D on calcium transport by intestine in vitro can readily be demonstrated; one of the questions which can be answered is the target tissue on which vitamin D acts, namely, whether the target tissue is a specific segment of the intestine or the entire length of the intestine. In the rat, as in other animals, there are important differences between the duodenum and the rest of the intestine with respect to in vitro calcium transport, but the action of vitamin D is not localized to the duodenum. However, unless the in vitro system used is suitable for the detection of calcium transport in distal intestine, the effect of vitamin D can be missed. We have employed two types of in vitro systems for calcium transport: (a) the active transport, from mucosal to serosal compartments, which effects higher concentrations of calcium in the serosal phase than in the mucosal phase, and (b) the passive movement of calcium from

This work was supported by National Institutes of Health Grant AM–00668.

mucosal to serosal compartments in the direction of the concentration difference. Both systems employ everted loops of intestine (Harrison and Harrison, 1960, 1965). Active transport of calcium requires metabolic energy and is also influenced by the sodium concentration of the medium that bathes the mucosal surface of the intestine. In the distal small intestine the transport is almost completely inhibited by sodium concentrations of 140–150 mEq/liter. Duodenal transport of calcium is less completely blocked by sodium and so can be demonstrated even in buffer media that contain sodium in concentrations equal to those of extracellular fluid. For the demonstration of vitamin D effect on active calcium transport, a buffer in which the sodium concentration is 50 mEq/liter is suitable for the entire length of the small intestine and the colon. Figure 3.1 shows the in-

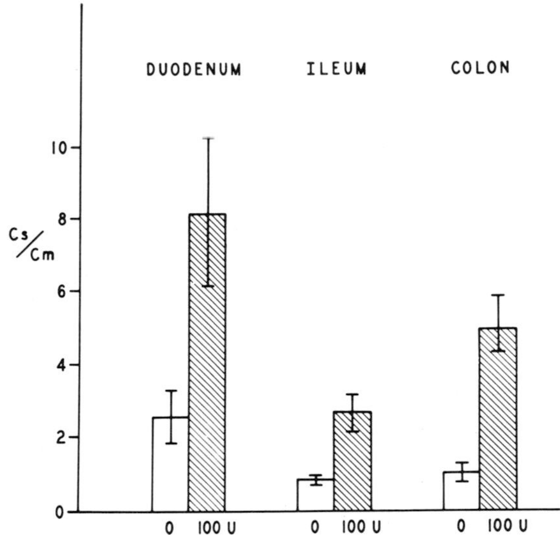

Fig. 3.1. Effect of vitamin D treatment on the efficiency (Cs-to-Cm ratio) of active transport of calcium in vitro in various segments of the small intestine and the colon.

Everted loops of each segment were incubated for 60 min at 37 C in a modified low-sodium K–H buffer containing 0.25 mM calcium labeled with ^{45}Ca aerated with 95% O_2, 5% CO_2. The concentrations of calcium and of ^{45}Ca were initially identical in serosal and mucosal fluids.

The preparations were made from vitamin D–deficient rats (unshaded areas) and from vitamin D–treated rats (shaded areas). The vitamin D–treated rats were deficient animals given 100 IU of calciferol 48–72 hr before calcium transport was measured.

The vertical lines indicate the 95% confidence limits for the data.

fluence of vitamin D treatment on the active transport of calcium in proximal and distal small intestine and colon. The efficiency of transport is measured by the ratio of Cs to Cm, i.e., the extent to which the concentration of calcium in the serosal fluid is increased beyond the concentration in the mucosal fluid. It is of somc importancc that the effect of vitamin D on the entire length of the intestine be recognized: if vitamin D action is explained by a specific vitamin D–induced intestinal factor, that factor must be found not only in the duodenum but also in the distal gut, including the colon. The soluble calcium-binding protein isolated by Wasserman and Taylor (1966) had been originally detected only in the duodenum, but more recently it has been detected in the distal intestine and colon of chick intestine (Taylor and Wasserman 1969). Similar studies in the rat are necessary to establish this protein as the specific vitamin D–induced factor that accelerates calcium transport.

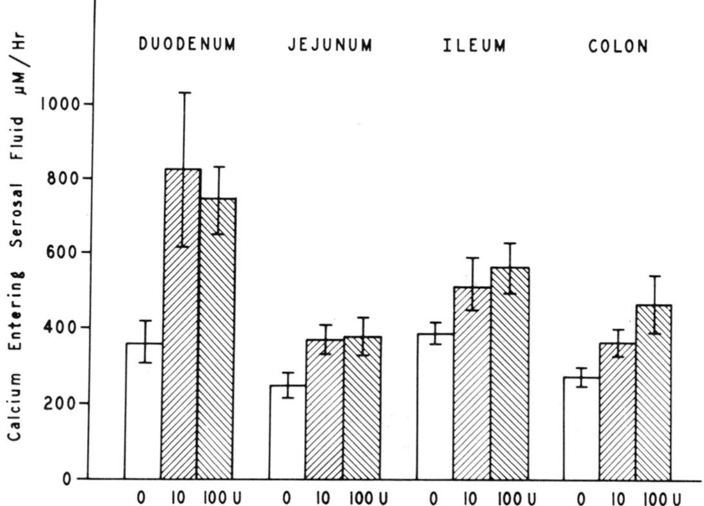

Fig. 3.2. Effect of vitamin D treatment on the passive transport of calcium across intestinal wall in vitro in various segments of the small intestine and the colon.

Everted loops of each segment were incubated for 60 min at 37 C in a K–H buffer with 0.5 mM *N*-ethyl maleimide to inhibit active transport of sodium and calcium. The initial concentration of calcium, labeled with ^{45}Ca, in the mucosal fluid was 0.5 mM, whereas the serosal fluid was initially calcium free.

The preparations were made from vitamin D–deficient rats (unshaded areas) and from vitamin D–treated rats (shaded areas). The vitamin D–treated rats were deficient animals given either 10 IU or 100 IU of calciferol 72 hr before transport studies were made.

The vertical lines indicate the 95% confidence limits for the data.

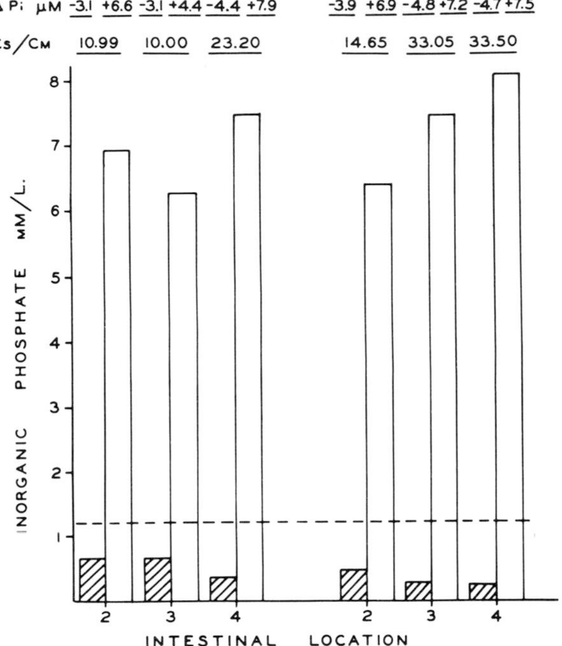

Fig. 3.3. Active transport of inorganic phosphate in vitro by everted loops of small intestine.

The concentrations of inorganic phosphate at the end of the incubation period are shown for the mucosal solution (unshaded areas) and for the serosal solution (shaded areas). The horizontal dashed line indicates the initial concentration of inorganic phosphate in both the serosal and the mucosal fluids.

The Cs-to-Cm ratios of inorganic phosphate are shown over each pair of columns.

The intestinal locations for the segments of the small intestine from which the loops were prepared proceed distally from the jejunum (location 2) to the beginning of the ileum (location 4).

(From Harrison and Harrison, 1961, Fig. 2.)

Passive movement of calcium, in the direction of the electrochemical gradient, can be demonstrated in vitro when metabolic energy generation is greatly inhibited by cyanide, *N*-ethyl-maleimide, anaerobiosis, or low temperature. Such inhibition of the production of metabolic energy blocks both the active transport of sodium and of calcium and the bulk movement of solution from the mucosal to the serosal phase. We have employed several systems for the measurement of passive, mucosa-to-serosa transfer of calcium, and all are suitable for the demonstration of an effect of vitamin D along the entire length of the intestine, including the colon (Fig. 3.2). The effect of vitamin D on this system is found after a physiologic dose (i.e., 10 IU) of vitamin D is administered to depleted rats, so this system is an indicator of the physiologic action of vitamin D. The postulated vitamin D–induced factor must therefore operate to enhance diffusion of calcium when the driving force is the concentration difference of calcium between two solution phases.

Phosphate transport in small intestine

In vivo studies of the effect of vitamin D on phosphate absorption suggested only that the effect on phosphate was in some way secondary to the increased efficiency of calcium absorption due to vitamin D (Nicolaysen et al., 1953). The in vitro intestinal preparation can transport inorganic phosphate against a concentration gradient from the mucosal to the serosal compartment (Harrison and Harrison, 1961) (Fig. 3.3). This system re-

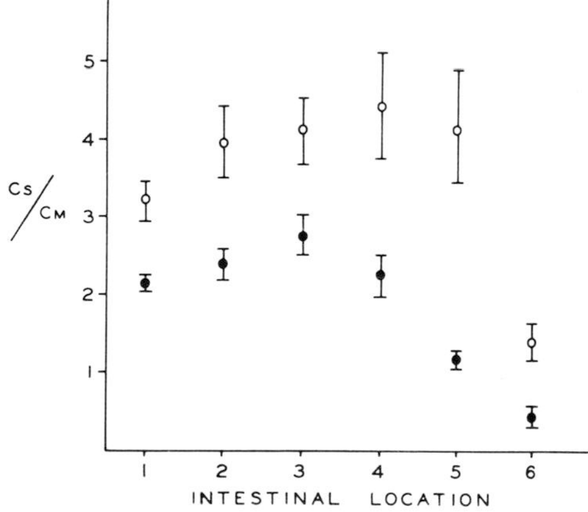

Fig. 3.4. Effect of vitamin D transport on the efficiency (Cs-to-Cm ratio) of the transport of inorganic phosphate in vitro by everted loops of small intestine.

The intestinal preparations were made from vitamin D–deficient rats (●) and from vitamin D–treated rats (○).

Values are given as mean ±SE.

The intestinal locations for the portion of the small intestine from which the everted loops were made proceed distally from the duodenum (location 1) to the terminal ileum (location 6).

(From Harrison and Harrison, 1961, Fig. 3.)

quires sodium and is inactivated by the removal of sodium from the buffer. The concentration of potassium in the medium is also important, and higher Cs-to-Cm ratios result by increasing the potassium concentration in the buffer from 4 mEq/liter to 16 mEq/liter. Phosphate transport by intestine in vitro is increased by treating the donor animal with vitamin D (Fig. 3.4). We have related this effect of vitamin D on phosphate to its effect on calcium (Fig. 3.5). Removal of calcium from the buffer reduced the Cs-to-Cm ratios for inorganic phosphate in intestine from both vitamin D–treated and vitamin D–deficient rats and greatly decreased the

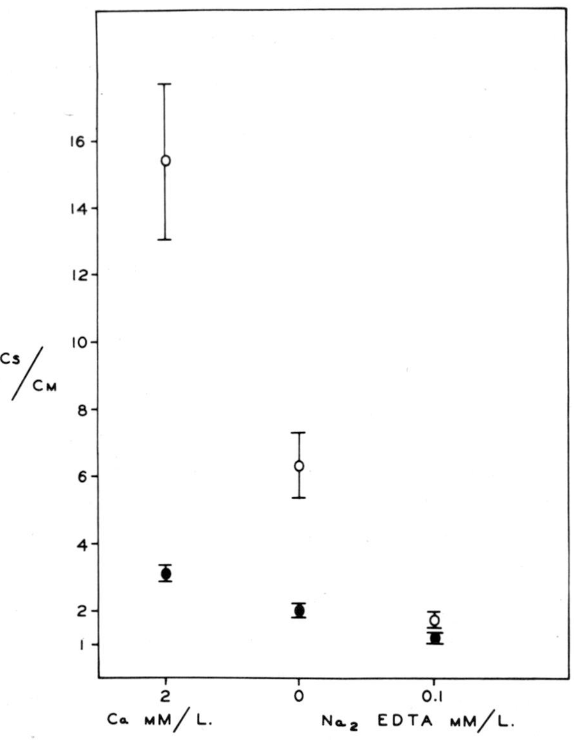

Fig. 3.5. Influence of calcium concentration of medium on active transport of inorganic phosphate by everted intestinal loops of vitamin D–treated rats (○) and of vitamin D–deficient rats (●).

Values are given as mean ± SE.

For the 3 series of experiments diagramed, the buffer had a high concentration of potassium, 16 mEq/liter, and a calcium concentration of 2 mM, 0 mM, or 0 mM with 0.1 mM Na_2EDTA.

(From Harrison and Harrison, 1961, Fig. 6.)

difference between the two groups. Further addition of a calcium-chelating agent, Na_2EDTA, completely inhibited phosphate transport and abolished the difference between intestine of depleted and treated rats. This concentration of Na_2EDTA did not inhibit glucose transport. Kowarski and Schachter (1969), using ^{32}P-labeled inorganic phosphate, also demonstrated a net mucosal-to-serosal flux of inorganic phosphate in everted intestinal sacs, but they were unable to show an effect of the calcium concentration on phosphate transport in their system. We have consistently found the effect due to calcium concentration at both high and low concentrations of potassium. For this reason we have postulated that the system for active transport of inorganic phosphate in the intestinal mucosa is dependent on the calcium concentration in a cell compartment. The action of vitamin D in enhancing inorganic phosphate transport could then be the result of an increased uptake of calcium by the mucosal cell. On the other hand, active transport of calcium by intestine in vitro can occur without inorganic phosphate in the bathing medium (Walling, 1968).

Effect of parathyroid hormone on calcium and phosphate transport

The action of parathyroid hormone on calcium transport across the intestinal mucosa has not been as unequivocally established as the action of vitamin D. Rasmussen (1959) reported that everted gut sacs from parathyroidectomized rats had less capacity for active transport of calcium than sacs from intact animals. In other laboratories, similar experiments have not given consistent results. We have restudied this problem in thyroparathyroidectomized or parathyroidectomized rats that were allowed to convalesce from the surgical procedure and to resume weight gain in order to eliminate nonspecific effects of surgical trauma (Lifshitz et al., 1969). Intestinal preparations from thyroparathyroidectomized rats and from parathyroidectomized rats were compared with preparations from rats that had been operated on and still had intact parathyroid function. The absence or presence of parathyroid function was measured by the concentrations of calcium, of magnesium, and of phosphate in the serum. Everted duodenal loops were used to determine active transport of calcium, and everted jejunal loops were used for the measurement of the transport of inorganic phosphate. The results are shown in Figures 3.6 and 3.7. It is evident that the Cs-to-Cm ratios for calcium and phosphate are less in the intestinal loops from hypoparathyroid rats. The effects of prior administration of parathyroid extract on in vitro measurement of intestinal calcium and phosphate transport in both hypoparathyroid and

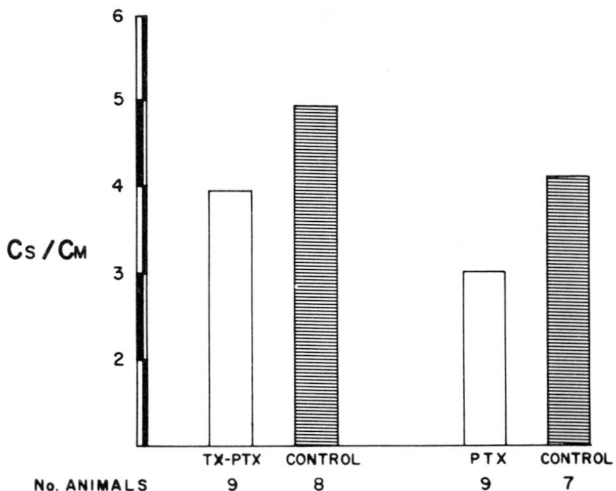

Fig. 3.6. Effect of thyroparathyroidectomy (TX–PTX) or parathyroidectomy (PTX) on the efficiency (Cs-to-Cm ratio) of calcium transport in vitro by everted rat duodenal loops.

The control animals were operated upon but had normal parathyroid function as measured by concentrations of calcium, of magnesium, and of phosphate in serum.

For both groups of experiments, the differences between the hypoparathyroid rats and the controls are statistically significant, $P < 0.05$.

(From Lifshitz et al., 1969, Fig. 1.)

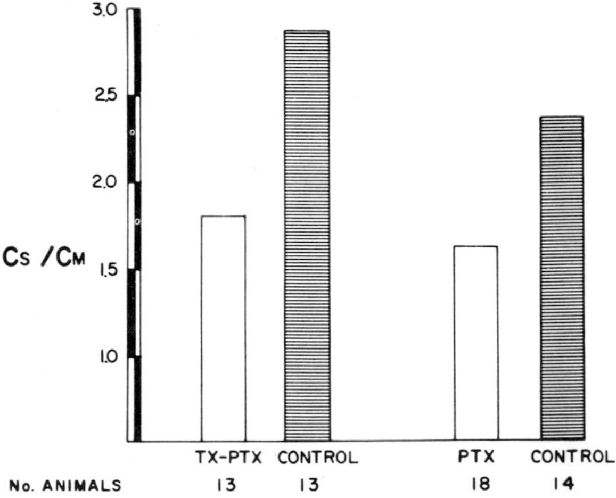

Fig. 3.7. Effect of thyroparathyroidectomy or parathyroidectomy on the efficiency (Cs-to-Cm ratio) of transport of inorganic phosphate in vitro by everted rat jejunal loops.

Control animals were as described in legend to Figure 3.6.

The differences are statistically significant, $P < 0.05$.

(From Lifshitz et al., 1969, Fig. 2.)

euparathyroid rats are given in Figures 3.8 and 3.9. The reduced calcium and phosphate transport of the intestine of the hypoparathyroid rat was restored to normal control values when parathyroid extract was administered, but it was not possible to further increase the transport by intestine from control rats by exogenous parathyroid hormone. The latter finding differs from the results of Borle and co-workers (1963), who were able to increase the uptake of ^{32}P by duodenum from intact rats by administering parathyroid extract. The data do indicate that the intestinal mucosa is a target tissue for parathyroid hormone and are compatible with, al-

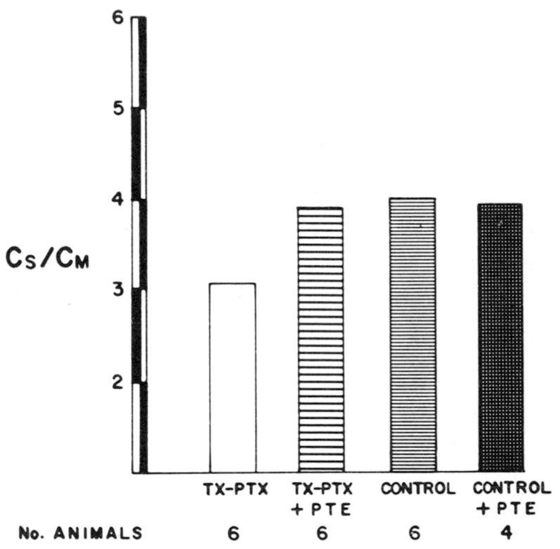

Fig. 3.8. Effect of administration of 100 U.S.P. units of parathyroid extract on the efficiency (Cs-to-Cm ratio) of calcium transport by everted duodenal loops of thyroparathyroidectomized rats (TX–PTX) or control, euparathyroid rats.

The differences between untreated and treated TX–PTX animals are statistically significant, $P < 0.05$.

(From Lifshitz et al., 1969, Fig. 3.)

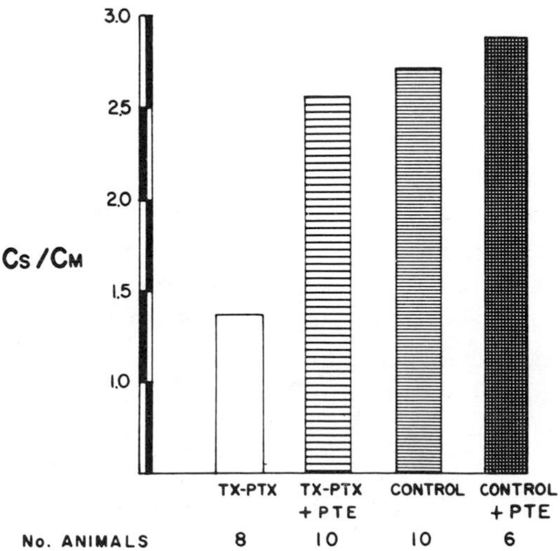

Fig. 3.9. Effect of administration of 100 U.S.P. units of parathyroid extract on the efficiency (Cs-to-Cm ratio) of transport of inorganic phosphate by everted jejunal loops of thyroparathyroidectomized (TX–PTX) rats or control, euparathyroid rats.

The differences between untreated and treated TX–PTX animals are statistically significant, $P < 0.05$.

(From Lifshitz et al., 1969, Fig. 4.)

though not proof of, the thesis that phosphate transport by intestinal mucosa is linked to calcium uptake by the cell.

There is an important difference between the actions of parathyroid hormone on the intestinal mucosa and on the renal tubule cell. In the intestinal preparations, parathyroid hormone increases mucosal-to-serosal transport of both calcium and phosphate. The in vivo studies of renal tubule function give evidence that parathyroid hormone increases renal tubule reabsorption of calcium but diminishes reabsorption of phosphate. A possible explanation for this seeming separation of calcium and phosphate transports has been suggested, namely, that the uptake of phosphate at the peritubular pole of the renal tubule cell is primarily increased when parathyroid hormone causes a net decrease in transfer of phosphate from lumen to peritubular space (Harrison et al., 1968). This is speculative, however, and at the moment no direct experimental approach to the solution of this problem has been developed.

We have shown that the vitamin D–depleted rat is apparently refractory to the action of parathyroid hormone (Harrison et al., 1958; Harrison and Harrison, 1965) and have suggested that vitamin D or an effect of vitamin D is needed to obtain a total response to parathyroid hormone. In an effort to apply this concept to the study of in vitro transport of calcium by the intestine, we have examined the effect of adenosine 3′,5′ cyclic monophosphate (CAMP) on the passive diffusion of calcium across the intestinal wall. Chase and Aurbach (1968) have shown that parathyroid hormone activates adenyl cyclase in homogenates of rat kidney cortex and increases CAMP output in urine. It is possible, therefore, that parathyroid hormone acts through a mediating factor, CAMP. The effect of this compound on the diffusion of calcium across the intestinal wall of everted duodenal loops from vitamin D–depleted and vitamin D–treated rats was measured by a modification of our everted-loop method. Short everted loops, 7 cm in length, were tied to lengths of fine polyethylene tubing, one of which was an influx tube and the other an efflux tube. The everted loop was filled with solution pumped through the influx tube and was emptied through the efflux tube. The everted loop was shaken while suspended in a reservoir of K–H buffer which contained ^{45}Ca in a total calcium concentration of 2.5 mM. The incubation temperature was 22 C, and the gas phase bubbled through the solution was 95% N, 5% CO_2. At 10-min intervals, 1 ml of calcium-free K–H buffer was pumped into the loop, and the previous aliquot was emptied into a collecting tube. The ^{45}Ca in the effluent was determined, and the transfer of calcium from mucosal to serosal fluid was calculated from the concentration of ^{45}Ca in the serosal fluid and the specific activity of the ^{45}Ca in the bathing solution. Figure 3.10 shows the result of experiments that compare the diffusion of calcium

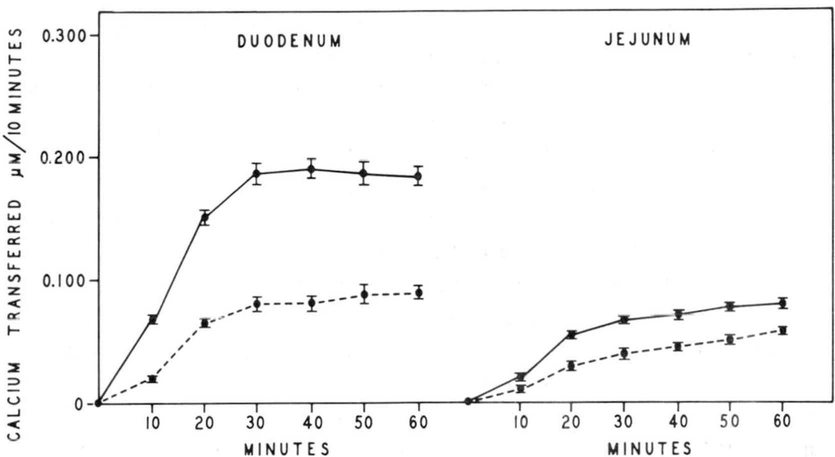

Fig. 3.10. Effect of vitamin D treatment on the in vitro transfer of calcium from mucosal to serosal compartments of intestinal loops under anaerobic conditions.

Intestinal preparations were made from vitamin D–treated rats (solid lines) and from vitamin D–deficient rats (dashed lines). The transfer of calcium is expressed in terms of ^{45}Ca accumulation in the serosal fluid per 10-min period.

Values are given as mean ± SE.

across duodenal and jejunal loops and the effect of the vitamin D status of the donor animal. The diffusibility of calcium across the duodenal wall is much greater than that across the jejunal wall. By the third 10-min period, the quantity of ^{45}Ca measured in the serosal fluid reached a relatively constant value; this indicates that a steady state had been attained, so the calcium entering the serosal fluid could be assumed to be equal to the calcium entering the mucosa from the outside solution. We can thus express the results in terms of calcium moving across the mucosal epithelium per 10-min period, since earlier studies have shown that the major permeability barrier to calcium in the intestinal wall is the mucosal epithelial layer (Harrison and Harrison, 1965). As emphasized above, this is a measure of passive diffusion of calcium when production of metabolic energy is inhibited by low temperature and anaerobiosis. The effect of vitamin D treatment in increasing diffusibility is apparent in both duodenal and jejunal segments. In another series of experiments, the everted loop was treated in vitro for 45 min with dibutyryl CAMP; this compound was added only to the serosal solution in a concentration of 10mM; 5 mM theophylline was added to inhibit phosphodiesterase. The preincubation period and the ^{45}Ca collection periods were all done at 22 C. The results of such pretreatment of duodenal loops with CAMP are shown in Figure 3.11. There is an increased rate of diffusion of calcium in the loops from

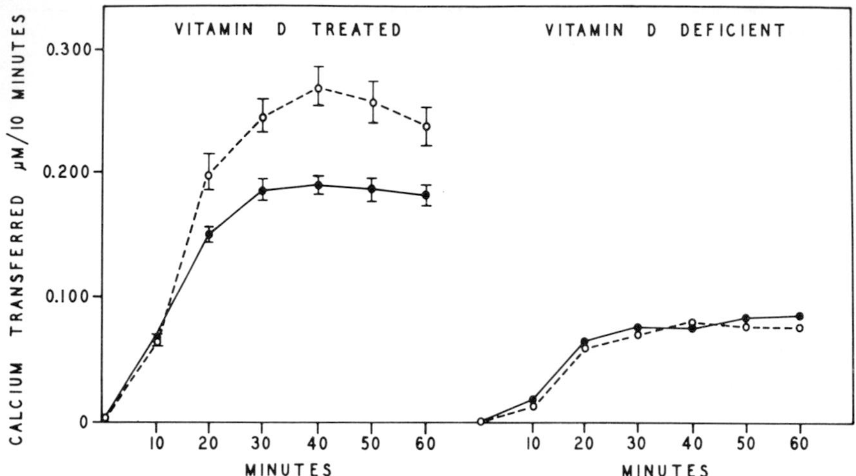

Fig. 3.11. Effect of in vitro exposure to dibutyryl CAMP on in vitro transfer of calcium from mucosal to serosal compartments of duodenal loops from vitamin D–treated and vitamin D–deficient rats.

The transfer of calcium (in terms of ^{45}Ca accumulation in the serosal fluid per 10-min period) is shown for duodenal loops treated with dibutyryl CAMP (dashed lines) and for control preparations (solid lines).

Values are given as mean ± SE.

vitamin D–treated rats, but not in those from vitamin D–deficient rats. There is evidence, therefore, that CAMP increases movement of calcium across the membrane formed by the intestinal wall, but only in the presence of a vitamin D–induced factor. If CAMP is the mediator of parathyroid hormone action – as suggested by Chase and Aurbach (1968), Dousa and Rychlik (1968) and Rasmussen and co-workers (1968), among others – this could be a model of the parathyroid hormone–vitamin D interaction in the enhancement of calcium transport. The results are in agreement with the in vivo experiments which indicate that the action of parathyroid hormone to raise serum calcium does not occur in vitamin D–depleted rats.

Effect of cortisol on intestinal calcium transport

Cortisol in suppressive doses, i.e., in amounts which suppress inflammatory reaction and inhibit growth, diminishes the in vivo intestinal absorption of calcium and of phosphate and increases the excretion of these ions in the urine by reduction of tubular reabsorption. The effect on the intestinal tract is opposite that of vitamin D. In vitro measurements with everted intestinal loops do indicate that treatment of the donor rats with cortisol for 3 days prior to the experiment does in fact reduce the vita-

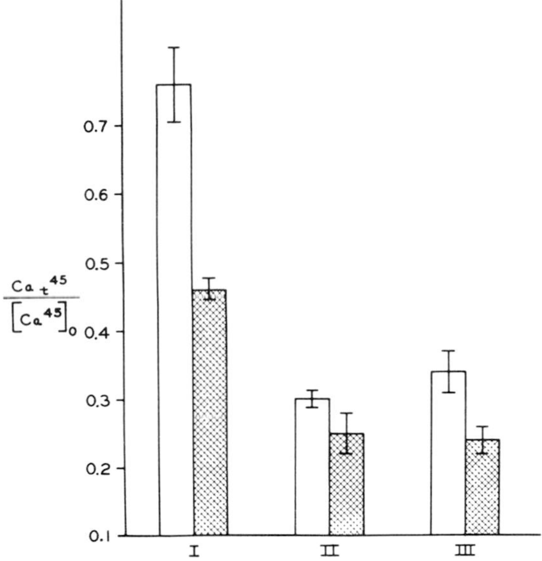

Fig. 3.12. Effect of cortisol treatment on the passive transport of calcium by everted intestine in vitro.

Rats previously given 1000 IU of vitamin D within a week of the experiment were either used as controls (unshaded areas) or were fed daily about 2 mg of cortisol per 100 g of body weight for 3 days before they were killed (shaded areas). The passive transport of calcium was measured by an exchange diffusion method. The height of the columns indicates the rate of mucosal-to-serosal diffusion of calcium.

Values are given as mean ± SE.

Intestinal locations were the duodenum (I), the jejunum (II), and the ileum (III).

min D augmentation of calcium transport (Harrison and Harrison, 1960), whether measured by passive transport (Fig. 3.12) or active transport (Fig. 3.13). We have not measured the effect of cortisol treatment on the in vitro transport of inorganic phosphate by intestinal preparations, but cortisol in the intact rat does reduce concentrations of inorganic phosphate in the serum, both in vitamin D–depleted and vitamin D–treated rats (Harrison et al., 1957).

Whether cortisol treatment has an effect on the concentration of a calcium binding protein in intestinal mucosal cell has not been studied. It is of possible significance that cortisol reduces the apparent permeability of cell membranes to citrate and increases the concentration gradient between intracellular and extracellular citrate (Harrison and Harrison,

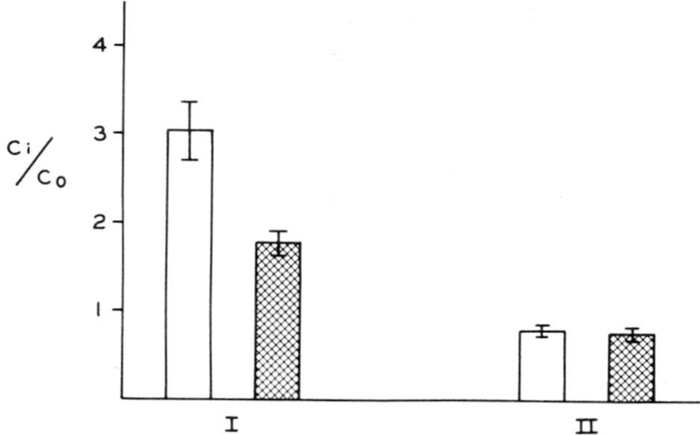

Fig. 3.13. Effect of cortisol treatment on the active transport of calcium in everted duodenum in vitro.

Control rats (unshaded areas) and cortisol-fed rats (shaded areas) were prepared as described in the legend to Figure 3.12. The height of the columns represents the ratio of the calcium concentration in the serosal fluid to that in the mucosal fluid, at the end of incubation time (initial ratio = 1).

Intestinal locations were the duodenum (I) and the jejunum (II).

The concentration of sodium in the buffer was 145 mEq/liter, which completely inhibits active transport of calcium by the jejunum but not by the duodenum.

1959). Whether this is related to the diffusibility of calcium across the plasma membrane is unknown.

We have proposed that the action of vitamin D on intestinal transport of calcium and of phosphate can be explained in terms of a single effect. It has been postulated by several investigators that a protein is induced in the intestinal mucosa as the result of the action of vitamin D or its metabolite. We suggest that such a vitamin D–induced factor increases the diffusion of calcium across the intestinal mucosal cells and enhances the active mucosal-to-serosal transport of calcium. The vitamin D–induced factor may act as a calcium carrier to mediate both passive diffusion and active transport, or it might primarily facilitate diffusion of calcium into and out of the mucosal epithelial cell with a net increase in the quantity of calcium available to an oriented energy-dependent calcium-transport system that pumps calcium into a space continuous with the extracellular space of the submucosa. The vitamin D–induced increase in calcium concentration in a cell compartment augments the transport of inorganic phosphate by a calcium-stimulated phosphate-transport system. The diffusibility of calcium across the intestinal mucosa is increased by CAMP, but only if the vitamin D–induced factor is also present. The effect of parathyroid hormone on both calcium and phosphate transport across the intestinal wall could be mediated by CAMP production in intestinal mucosa. Parathyroid hormone has been shown to activate adenyl cyclase in the proximal renal tubule, but similar studies have not yet been done for intestinal mucosal cells.

References

Borle, A. B., H. T. Keutmann, and W. F. Neuman. 1963. Role of parathyroid hormone in phosphate transport across rat duodenum. *Amer. J. Physiol. 204*:705.

Chase, L. R., and G. D. Aurbach. 1968. Renal adenyl cyclase: Anatomically separate sites for parathyroid hormone and vasopressin. *Science 159*:545.

Dousa, T., and I. Rychlik. 1968. The effect of parathyroid hormone on adenyl cyclase in rat kidney. *Biochim Biophys. Acta 158*:484.

Harrison, H. C., and H. E. Harrison. 1959. Cortisol and citrate metabolism. *Amer. J. Physiol. 196*:943.

Harrison, H. C., H. E. Harrison, and E. A. Park, 1957. Vitamin D and citrate metabolism: Inhibition of vitamin D effect by cortisol. *Proc. Soc. Exp. Biol. Med. 96*:768.

Harrison, H. C., H. E. Harrison, and E. A. Park. 1958. Vitamin D and citrate metabolism: Effect of vitamin D in rats fed diets adequate in both calcium and phosphorus. *Amer. J. Physiol. 192*:432.

Harrison, H. E., and H. C. Harrison. 1960. Transfer of Ca^{45} across intestinal wall in vitro in relation to action of vitamin D and cortisol. *Amer. J. Physiol. 199*:265.

Harrison, H. E., and H. C. Harrison. 1961. Intestinal transport of phosphate: Action of vitamin D, calcium and potassium. *Amer. J. Physiol. 201*:1007.

Harrison, H. E., and H. C. Harrison. 1964. The interaction of vitamin D and parathyroid hormone on calcium phosphorus and magnesium homeostasis. *Metabolism 13*:952.

Harrison, H. E., and H. C. Harrison. 1965. Vitamin D and permeability of intestinal mucosa to calcium. *Amer. J. Physiol. 208*:370.

Harrison, H. E., H. C. Harrison, and F. Lifshitz. 1968. The responses of vitamin D depleted and of thyroparathyroidectomized rats to ergocalciferol and dihydrotachysterol, p. 455. *In* R. V. Talmage and L. B. Belanger (eds.), *Parathyroid Hormone and Thyrocalcitonin (Calcitonin)*. Excerpta Medica Foundation, New York.

Kowarski, S., and D. Schachter. 1969. Effects of vitamin D on phosphate transport and incorporation into mucosal constituents of rat intestinal mucosa. *Amer. J. Physiol. 244*:211.

Lifshitz, F., H. C. Harrison, and H. E. Harrison. 1969. Influence of parathyroid function upon the in vitro transport of calcium and phosphate by the rat intestine. *Endocrinology 84*:912.

Nicolaysen, R., N. Eeg-Larsen, and O. J. Malm. 1953. Physiology of calcium metabolism. *Physiol. Rev. 33*:424.

Rasmussen, H. 1959. The influence of parathyroid function upon the transport of calcium in isolated sacs of rat small intestine. *Endocrinology 65*:517.

Rasmussen, H., N. Nagata, J. Feinblatt, and D. Fast. 1968. Parathyroid hormone, membranes and enzymes, p. 299. *In* R. V. Talmage and L. F. Belanger (eds.), *Parathyroid Hormone and Thyrocalcitonin (Calcitonin).* Excerpta Medica Foundation, New York.

Taylor, A. N., and R. H. Wasserman. 1969. Cellular localization of vitamin D–induced calcium-binding protein (CaBP) with fluorescent antibody. *Fed. Proc. 28*:759. (Abstr.)

Walling, M. W. 1968. Active transport of calcium across the small intestine in vitro. *J. Dent. Res. 47*:905.

Wasserman, R. H., and A. N. Taylor. 1966. Vitamin D_3–induced calcium-binding protein in chick intestinal mucosa. *Science 152*:791.

4

CALCIUM TRANSPORT, VITAMIN D, AND THE MOLECULAR BASIS OF ACTIVE TRANSPORT

David Schachter

Transport mechanisms

My interest in vitamin D grew out of a search for biological systems that might provide useful models for analyzing the molecular basis of active transport across membranes. Having had medical training, I was aware of the clinically important relationship of vitamin D to calcium absorption and normal bone growth. Inasmuch as vitamin D is related to sterols and sterols are important biochemical constituents of membranes, it seemed intriguing to study the mechanism of action of the vitamin at a cellular level. At the outset we suspected that the vitamin might serve as a prosthetic group for a membrane carrier or perhaps as a carrier itself.

At this point I should clarify explicitly the working premises we have adopted in considering the fundamental basis of membrane transport. A molecular picture of biological transport across membranes would entail a description in three dimensions of the membrane components involved, as well as a description of their mode of operation. This goal may be attained in the future when other fundamental processes such as the mechanism of enzyme action are understood in three-dimensional terms, but at present it seems wiser to ask simpler questions that are capable of solution in more conventional biochemical terms. We are considering two such questions: What is the biochemical nature of the membrane com-

Research presented here was supported by United States Public Health Service grants AM–01483 and AM–04407.

The work referred to in this report is the product of many co-workers, including Dr. Samuel Rosen, Dr. Eugene B. Dowdle, Dr. Daniel V. Kimberg, Dr. James D. Finkelstein, Dr. Gilbert S. Gordan, Dr. Geoffrey Berlyne and Dr. James Manis. In the past seven years it has been my good fortune to have Szloma Kowarski as co-worker and colleague.

ponents that are involved in many transport mechanisms, the so-called carriers? What are the energy-coupling reactions that permit such carriers to bring about transport against a concentration gradient?

The very notion of a membrane component, or carrier, requires elaboration. Physiologists often classify transport mechanisms into three general categories: *Passive diffusion* involves net transfer along electrochemical potential gradients, with no obligatory or specific interaction with specialized membrane components, and the net transfer follows Fick's law of diffusion. In *facilitated diffusion*, net transport also proceeds solely along electrochemical potential gradients, but it involves specific interaction with specialized membrane components termed carriers. Because of the interaction, such transfer mechanisms show specificity, rate-limiting kinetics, competitive inhibition, counter-flow phenomena, and inhibition by various protein reagents, e.g., reagents that inactivate sulfhydryl groups. Although the precise reactions involved in the carrier-substrate interaction are unknown, it is generally believed that the carrier is mobile, binding its substrate at one face of the cell membrane and releasing it at the opposite face. A carrier thus freed recirculates to transfer another molecule or ion of the substrate. *Active transport* is defined thermodynamically as net transfer against electrochemical potential gradients. From the mechanistic viewpoint, it appears reasonable to view active transport as fundamentally a carrier-mediated transfer, similar to facilitated diffusion, upon which energy-coupled reactions are imposed to permit the utilization of phosphate-bond energy for the movement.

The three types of transport just cited can be illustrated with reference to the mechanism for galactoside transport and accumulation in *E. coli* (Schachter, 1969). In strains which have a functioning *y* gene in the lactose operon, active accumulation of galactosides and of thiogalactosides can be observed. This active transport is clearly dependent on at least two factors: (1) the product of the *y* gene, now known to be a protein that is presumably the transport carrier (Fox and Kennedy, 1965), and (2) energy-coupled reactions that appear to function by dissociating the carrier-galactoside complex (Schachter and Mindlin, 1969). The carriers continue to function in the presence of inhibitors of energy metabolism (Koch, 1964; Winkler and Wilson, 1966). These inhibitors therefore convert the mechanism from an active transport to a facilitated diffusion, capable only of equilibrating the extracellular and intracellular galactoside concentrations. If the bacterial cells are grown in the absence of an inducer, so the *y* gene is inactive, the carrier function is lost and only passive diffusion, a very slow process in these cells, effects net transfer. Strains mutant for the *y* gene similarly fail to show either facilitated diffusion or active transport of galactosides.

Much of the crucial experimental evidence concerning the *E. coli* mechanism just described has appeared in the past five years, but we adopted the underlying premises, i.e., that active transport involves functioning carrier molecules plus energy-coupled reactions, in 1957, at the outset of our studies on the intestinal transport of calcium. The initial goals were to answer three questions: Is the calcium transport an active pump or one of the other transport mechanisms? If carrier molecules were involved, could we identify and isolate these, and how would they relate to vitamin D? If calcium absorption involves an active pump, what are the energy-coupled reactions? The twelve years since our first studies have been exciting ones in this area. The field is still in ferment, but at least partial answers to the three questions posed are now available; what follows is a summary of the current evidence and a model of what may be the molecular basis of a cation, active transport mechanism.

Calcium transport involves an active cation pump

At the outset of our studies it seemed desirable to develop in vitro techniques to define the nature of the intestinal calcium transport mechanism. When Samuel Rosen, then a medical student, came to the laboratory on an elective period, we set about adapting the everted gut-sac method of Wilson and Wiseman (1954). Using rabbits at first and rats subsequently, we were able to demonstrate net transport of ^{45}Ca and of total calcium against concentration gradients from the mucosal to the serosal surfaces of duodenal segments in vitro (Schachter and Rosen, 1959; Schachter et al., 1960). Estimations of the electrical potential differences across the intestinal segments in vitro indicated that the serosal surface is electrically positive with respect to the mucosal surface (Schachter and Britten, 1961), and hence calcium transport occurs against electrical potential gradients as well. Many of the typical features of active transport were noted for the calcium mechanism: a dependence on oxygen and a metabolizable hexose in the ambient medium; inhibition by metabolic blocking agents; competitive inhibition; relative specificity for calcium as compared to magnesium, barium, strontium, and potassium; rate-limited kinetics; and marked depression at low temperatures (Schachter, 1963). Subsequently these observations were confirmed in vitro by other investigators (Rasmussen, 1959; Harrison and Harrison, 1960), and evidence was also obtained to demonstrate the active transport across rat intestine in vivo (Wasserman et al., 1961).

The evidence cited thus far supports the existence of an active transfer of calcium, but inasmuch as the cation readily forms complexes, it was necessary to determine whether the mechanism is a cation pump or whether it merely involves complexing to some anionic species. Initially we adapted a murexide technique to estimate the concentration of ionized Ca^{++} (Schachter et al., 1960). This demonstrated that most of the cation transferred to the serosal surfaces of gut sacs in vitro was ionized, suggesting the operation of a cation pump. The conclusion was further supported by studies on the unidirectional fluxes of Ca^{++} across intestinal segments; in these studies, an apparatus enabled the electrical potential across the segment to be controlled according to the method of Ussing (Schachter, 1963). In the absence of an electrical potential, i.e., when the segment was "short-circuited," the mucosa-to-serosa flux exceeded the reverse flux approximately 10-fold. Increased positive electrical charge on the serosal surface caused the calcium flux toward that surface to decrease and the flux away from that surface to increase. When the serosal surface was approximately + 75 mv with respect to the mucosal surface, the two fluxes were equal. The behavior of the fluxes supported the conclusion that the calcium mechanism transferred a positively charged particle, presumably the calcium ion.

Recently, we have verified the foregoing conclusion more directly and definitively with a calcium-sensing divalent electrode (Orion) (Schachter et al., 1969). During the course of a typical experiment in which net transfer of calcium occurs across everted rat duodenal gut sacs in vitro, the potential of the calcium ion in the serosal medium, estimated directly with the specific electrode, increases in comparison with that in the mucosal medium. The result is the development of activity gradients for calcium ion serosal/mucosal in the range of 2.5–3.5. The evidence thus establishes definitely that the net transfer of a calcium ion occurs against its chemical potential, i.e., that the mechanism is a cation pump.

That calcium can be absorbed by means of a cation pump does not mean, of course, that every calcium ion must be pumped across the mucosa by the specific mechanism. Passive diffusion of calcium ions or diffusion of calcium complexes could, and probably does, play a role, particularly in certain species like the rat. In the rat, vitamin D deficiency, which severely impairs the calcium pump (see below), is compatible with considerable residual ability to absorb calcium, providing the ratio of calcium to phosphorus in the diet is optimal. Nonetheless, it appears that the calcium pump is of considerable physiological importance from the standpoint of regulation of the absorptive mechanism. In earlier studies (Schachter et al., 1960; Dowdle et al., 1960), evidence was obtained that an increased requirement for calcium for the organism as a whole results in activation of the specific intestinal mechanism. Thus, transport of calcium in vitro in intestinal segments is greater in young, growing rats than in old animals; it is enhanced in rats in the final week of pregnancy as compared with nonpregnant female controls; and it is greatly increased when the animals are placed on a low-calcium diet. More recently, studies with the calcium-specific electrode have shown the adaptive increases in each instance to involve greater activity of the calcium cation pump (Schachter et al., 1969). It is reasonable to suggest that the pump is, in fact, a major mechanism responsible for regulating calcium absorption to meet bodily requirements.

Vitamin D is crucial to the calcium cation pump. Intestinal segments from depleted rats were capable of some net transport of total calcium from mucosa to serosa in vitro, but gradients of activity of the calcium ion serosa/mucosa did not exceed 1.0 (Schachter et al., 1969).

Relationship of vitamin D to the calcium pump

As noted above, our original hope was that vitamin D might be the prosthetic group of a membrane carrier for calcium transport. Having developed some in vitro techniques for studying calcium transport, we were gratified to find that prior depletion of vitamin D in rabbits or rats markedly decreased the transfer and that repletion restored it (Schachter and Rosen, 1959). It was apparent from the early experiments that the restoration was a complicated process: Physiological doses, i.e., 0.1–1 IU for each rat, required approximately 48 hr for a maximal effect (Schachter et al., 1961). Large doses, i.e., 1000 IU or more, reduced the time required to approximately 6–8 hr. However, a lag period of 1½ hours ensued before increases in calcium transport were detectable, even after the large doses. The lag period intrigued us. Clearly an understanding of the events in this period was crucial to the elucidation of the role of vitamin D. We therefore designed experiments to determine whether the lag time was needed for accumulation of vitamin D in the intestinal mucosa. Using a bioassay, we demonstrated that, after a dose of 2000 IU, there was considerably more vitamin D activity in the duodenal mucosa after 4 hr than after 48 hr. The capacity to transport calcium, however, had increased only 50% after 4 hr, in contrast to an increment of almost 200% after 48 hr (Schachter et al., 1961). Subsequently we were able to confirm this result with ^{3}H vitamin D_3, prepared by a tritium-exchange technique and crystallized as the dinitrobenzoyl ester (Schachter et al., 1964). Two hours after ^{3}H vitamin D_3 was administered intravenously, a maximal level of the labeled vitamin was found in the duodenal mucosa, although restoration of the calcium transport mechanism occurred almost entirely after this time point, i.e., between 2 and 6 hr.

The lag period suggested to us that protein synthesis might be required in the response to the vitamin. Consequently we examined the effects of actinomycin D, an inhibitor of DNA-dependent synthesis of mRNA, and the effects of puromycin, an inhibitor of a later stage of protein synthesis, on the response to vitamin D. As reported in 1965 (Schachter and Kowarski, 1965), and independently by other groups (Zull et al., 1965; Norman, 1965), both inhibitors were effective in preventing the full response to the vitamins; we then changed our working hypothesis and suggested that vitamin D was essential for the formation or maintenance of one or more proteins essential to the calcium transfer mechanism. Such a protein might function as a transport carrier or in some other manner.

At least one candidate for such a protein has been identified and characterized by Wasserman and his colleagues in chick mucosal homogenates (Wasserman and Taylor, 1966). After their discovery of a soluble, calcium-binding protein, we began similar studies with rat mucosal homogenates. Initially we assayed such homogenates for calcium-binding activity, using trypsin-treated samples as controls. A striking correlation was found between this calcium-binding activity and the capacity of intestinal segments to transport calcium (Schachter et al., 1967). Indeed, in the rat we have found only a positive correlation between calcium-binding activity and transport when the transport is altered by a variety of parameters, including time after repletion with vitamin D, level of dietary calcium, age of the animal, pregnancy, and segment of the intestine involved. For some time we were concerned that the calcium-binding activity seemed to appear only in the duodenum. However, our prior studies on the response to low levels of dietary calcium had demonstrated that the distal ileum, after the duodenum, shows the greatest increase in calcium transport (Kimberg et al., 1961). We were thus able to assay ileal mucosa for calcium-binding activity after calcium deprivation. Here again the calcium binding correlated quite well with the transport.

The calcium-binding protein in rat mucosal homogenates has now been purified in our laboratory to approximately 75% purity. It has a molecular weight of approximately 13,000 as estimated by Sephadex-gel filtration. Preliminary studies indicate a dissociation constant for calcium of approximately 1.5×10^{-6} M. We have identified the protein band by acrylamide-gel electrophoresis and have demonstrated increased incorporation of ^{14}C-labeled amino acids into the band after vitamin D administration. As visualized by staining the acrylamide gels, there is considerably more of the protein in rat duodenal than in jejunal homogenates and more in mucosal preparations from vitamin D–repleted rats than from vitamin D–depleted rats.

Is the calcium-binding protein a transport carrier? We have adopted the tentative working hypothesis that it is, although the evidence based on correlations is clearly inconclusive. Indeed, we have come across one possible negative correlation between calcium transport and calcium-binding activity. In the golden hamster, net transport of calcium in vitro against concentration gradients is greater with ileal than with duodenal segments (Schachter et al., 1960). Recently we have demonstrated that the transport mechanism in hamster ileum is vitamin D dependent and functions as a calcium cation pump, similar to that in rat duodenum (Schachter et al., 1969). Despite the greater calcium transport in the hamster ileum, however, calcium-binding activity is consistently much greater with duodenal than with ileal homogenates. Further investigation is now in progress to clarify the apparent lack of correlation.

If the calcium-binding protein is the carrier, how can we visualize the energy coupling needed for active transport? Before presenting our current working model, it will be necessary to describe the evidence for the two-stage entry-exit model of calcium transfer.

THE ENTRY-EXIT MODEL

In 1961 we proposed that net transfer of calcium across the intestinal mucosa involved at least two steps: uptake at the mucosal surface (i.e., entry) and exit toward or to the serosal surface. Net entry was estimated by the decrease in calcium concentration in the mucosal bathing medium in vitro, and net exit by the increment in serosal fluid calcium. Prior experiments had demonstrated that the exit step was more readily rate limited with increasing calcium concentrations in the bathing media (Schachter et al., 1960). Moreover, the exit step was dependent on a metabolizable hexose in the medium, where entry was not similarly dependent (Schachter et al., 1961). We thus concluded that the exit step might involve energy coupling.

Subsequent studies have provided further evidence for the entry-exit model. Inasmuch as NaCl in the mucosal medium was found essential for active transport of hexoses and of amino acids (Crane, 1960; Csáky, 1961), we investigated the effects on calcium transport across rat duodenal gut sacs when the NaCl in the bathing media was replaced with isosmotic mannitol (Schachter et al., 1967, 1969). With replacement of 25% of the NaCl, both net entry and net exit of calcium were increased. Further replacement, however, markedly and progressively decreased the exit step with no change in entry. Thus the exit step appears to be dependent on ambient NaCl, a conclusion which suggests that exit is energy coupled. (It is noteworthy that the observations on NaCl replacement included measurements with the calcium-sensing electrode. Changes in total transport were throughout associated with, and could be explained by, parallel changes in calcium-ion transport.)

A relatively gross but simple procedure provided still further evidence for the model. Everted intestinal sacs were incubated with ^{47}Ca, and the mucosa was subsequently scraped from the underlying intestinal coats. The final ^{47}Ca concentrations in the mucosal and serosal media and in the tissue of the mucosal and underlying coats were estimated. In this way a profile of concentrations across the gut wall was obtained (Schachter et al., 1966). With respiring duodenal sacs, i.e., in the presence of the active-transport mechanism, two concentration differences were observed: (1) ^{47}Ca concentration in the mucosal tissue exceeded that in the mucosal medium, and (2) the serosal medium and underlying intestinal coats had greater ^{47}Ca concentrations than the mucosal tissue. The concentration profile after 2 hr of incubation represented a stationary state in which the serosal medium concentration could be considered as approximating a minimum value for the concentration in the interstitial fluid of the mucosal tissue compartment. Since the ^{47}Ca concentration in the serosal fluid, and hence in the interstitial fluid of the mucosal compartment, clearly exceeded that in the mucosal tissue compartment as a whole, it also exceeded the concentration within the mucosal cells. Hence transfer in the exit direction, i.e., from the mucosal cell to the interstitial fluid of the mucosal compartment, is apparently against a concentration gradient. Confirmation of this was obtained by demonstrating that the gradient from the mucosal tissue to the underlying coats and the serosal fluid was dependent on oxidative phosphorylation, a metabolizable hexose in the medium, and ambient NaCl (Schachter et al., 1966, 1969). Moreover, this gradient was observed with duodenal but not with jejunal segments (Schachter et al., 1966).

In summary, considerable experimental evidence indicates that net transport of calcium across intestinal mucosa by means of the specialized pump mechanisms involves two steps. Entry, or uptake at the mucosal surface, is rate limited (Schachter et al., 1961), but there is as yet no compelling evidence that energy coupling is involved at this stage. Exit, or release at the abmucosal face of the cell, occurs against apparent concentration gradients, is rate limited, and requires energy coupling and ambient NaCl. We have concluded, therefore, that the second step is the active transport in the thermodynamic sense, whereas entry may represent a carrier-facilitated diffusion or binding to a cell constituent (see below).

A WORKING MODEL OF THE CALCIUM PUMP

The critical reader will already have noted what I shall now state explicitly. The discussion unfolded to this point proceeds along a gradient of firm experimental evidence. The initial section deals with the evidence that establishes the existence of a calcium cation pump in intestinal mucosa. Confirmatory studies from many laboratories and from in vivo as well as in vitro studies leave little doubt about the existence and probable functional importance of the mechanism. In a subsequent section, the probable role of vitamin D in maintaining or stimulating the synthesis of one or more proteins essential to the calcium pump was considered. The calcium-binding protein is one, perhaps the major, candidate for this role. Clearly the evidence here is as yet less firm, and we can look forward to further discoveries in this area. In the third section above we refined the "black box" pump mechanism into two steps and suggested that energy coupling involves NaCl and occurs at the second, or exit, stage. These conclusions are perhaps the least well grounded in hard experimental evidence, and considerable work remains to be done.

In the final portion of this discussion I would like to tie together the various pieces of evidence into a working model of the calcium cation pump. Clearly this is sheer speculation, but it represents a considerable advance over the state of the field some dozen years ago. In the model we propose that vitamin D is essential for the synthesis or maintenance of the calcium-binding protein, which is a cytoplasmic protein (Schachter et al., 1967; Schachter, 1969). Hence the entry stage of the transcellular transport may represent binding to this cytoplasmic carrier, a process which is rate limited by the availability of unbound and accessible calcium-binding protein. The calcium-protein complex may then traverse the cell and enter the abmucosal membrane. When exposed to the ambient NaCl of the interstitial fluid, Ca^{++} may be displaced from the protein by Na^{+}. Thus the exit step might be coupled to energy metabolism indirectly, i.e., by maintenance of the normal gradient for Na^{+} extracellular/intracellular. In favor of this last conclusion is the demonstrable requirement for NaCl for the exit step. Moreover, using partially purified preparations of rat mucosal calcium-binding protein, we have demonstrated very effective displacement of Ca^{++} by Na^{+} at concentrations of Na^{+} comparable to those in extracellular fluid (Schachter et al., 1967).

From the standpoint of the problem of biological transport, the calcium-transfer mechanism and the role of vitamin D remain very useful areas for investigation, with considerable significance for several disciplines, including biochemistry, physiology, clinical medicine, and nutrition.

References

Crane, R. K. 1960. Intestinal absorption of sugars. *Physiol. Rev. 40*:789.

Csáky, T. Z. 1961. Significance of sodium ions in active intestinal transport of non-electrolytes. *Amer. J. Physiol. 201*:999.

Dowdle, E. B., D. Schachter, and H. Schenker. 1960. Requirement for vitamin D for the active transport of calcium by intestine. *Amer. J. Physiol. 198*:269.

Fox, C. F., and E. P. Kennedy. 1965. Specific labeling and partial purification of the M protein, a component of the β-galactoside transport system of *Escherichia coli. Proc. Nat. Acad. Sci. U.S.A. 54*:891.

Harrison, H. E., and H. C. Harrison. 1960. Transfer of Ca^{45} across intestinal wall *in vitro* in relation to action of vitamin D and cortisone. *Amer. J. Physiol. 199*:265.

Kimberg, D. V., D. Schachter, and H. Schenker. 1961. Active transport of calcium by intestine: Effects of dietary calcium. *Amer. J. Physiol. 200*:1256.

Koch, A. L. 1964. The role of permease in transport. *Biochim. Biophys. Acta 79*:177.

Norman, A. W. 1965. Actinomycin D and the response to vitamin D. *Science 149*:184.

Rasmussen, H. 1959. The influence of parathyroid extract upon the transport of calcium in isolated sacs of rat small intestine. *Endocrinology 65*:517.

Schachter, D. 1963. Vitamin D and the active transport of calcium by the small intestine, p. 197. *In* R. H. Wasserman (ed.), *The Transfer of Calcium and Strontium Across Biological Membranes.* Academic Press, New York.

Schachter, D. 1969. Toward a molecular description of active transport, p. 157. *In* R. M. Dowben (ed.), *Biological Membranes.* Little, Brown, Boston.

Schachter, D., and J. S. Britten. 1961. Active transport of nonelectrolytes and the potential gradients across intestinal segments in vitro. *Fed. Proc.* (Part. I) *20*:137.

Schachter, D., E. B. Dowdle, and H. Schenker. 1960. Active transport of calcium by the small intestine of the rat. *Amer. J. Physiol. 198*:263.

Schachter, D., J. D. Finkelstein, and S. Kowarski. 1964. Metabolism of vitamin D. I. Preparation of radioactive vitamin D and its intestinal absorption in the rat. *J. Clin. Invest. 43*:787.

Schachter, D., D. V. Kimberg, and S. Schenker. 1961. Active transport of calcium by intestine: Action and bioassay of vitamin D. *Amer. J. Physiol. 200*:1263.

Schachter, D., and S. Kowarski. 1965. Radioactive vitamin D: preparation, metabolism and mechanism of action. *Bull. N.Y. Acad. Med. 41*:241.

Schachter, D., S. Kowarski, J. D. Finkelstein, and R.-I. W. Ma. 1966. Tissue concentration differences during active transport of calcium by intestine. *Amer. J. Physiol. 211*:1131.

Schachter, D., S. Kowarski, and P. Reid. 1967. Molecular basis for vitamin D action in the small intestine. *J. Clin. Invest. 46*:1113.

Schachter, D., S. Kowarski, and P. Reid. 1969. Active transport of calcium by intestine: Studies with a calcium activity electrode, p. 108. *In* A. W. Cuthbert (ed.), *A Symposium on Calcium and Cellular Function.* Macmillan, London.

Schachter, D., and A. Mindlin. 1969. Dual influx model of thiogalactoside accumulation in *Escherichia coli. J. Biol. Chem. 244*:1808.

Schachter, D., and S. M. Rosen. 1959. Active transport of Ca^{45} by the small intestine and its dependence on vitamin D. *Amer. J. Physiol. 196*:357.

Wasserman, R. H., F. A. Kallfelz, and C. L. Comar. 1961. Active transport of calcium by rat duodenum *in vivo*. *Science 133*:883.

Wasserman, R. H., and A. N. Taylor. 1966. Vitamin D_3–induced calcium-binding protein in chick intestinal mucosa. *Science 152*:791.

Wilson, T. H., and G. Wiseman. 1964. The use of sacs of everted small intestine for the study of the transference of substances from the mucosal to the serosal surface. *J. Physiol. 123*:116.

Winkler, H. H., and T. H. Wilson. 1966. The role of energy coupling in the transport of β-galactosides by *Escherichia coli*. *J. Biol. Chem. 241*:2200.

Zull, J. E., E. Czarnowska-Misztal, and H. F. DeLuca. 1965. Actinomycin D inhibition of vitamin D action. *Science 149*:182.

5

BIOLOGICALLY ACTIVE METABOLITES OF VITAMIN D

J. W. Blunt and H. F. DeLuca

Introduction

For some time now, the existence of metabolites of vitamin D has been recognized (Kodicek, 1956), although the early reports claimed a complete lack of biological activity for any of the metabolites, all of which were unidentified. More recently, biologically active metabolites were detected by means of methanol-chloroform extraction of tissue from rats that had previously been given doses of tritium-labeled vitamin D_3 (Norman et al., 1964; Lund and DeLuca, 1966). Some radioactivity was found in the aqueous portion of the extracts, but no biological activity could be established for these metabolites. The chloroform extracts were chromatographed on silicic acid columns, and the radioactivity profiles from some tissues are shown in Figure 5.1. Peak I has been identified as long-chain fatty acids and esters of vitamin D (Lund et al., 1967; Fraser and Kodicek, 1965, 1966; Bell and Bryan, 1965). These esters were shown to have variable effectiveness, but always less than that of vitamin D, in curing rickets. (The function of the vitamin D esters will be discussed in more detail by Kodicek in Chapter 6). Peak II represents an as yet unidentified metabolite that has diminished biological activity. It is not previtamin D (Lund, 1966), and there is no evidence to suggest that it plays an important role in the function of vitamin D. Peak III is unchanged vitamin D_3. Peak IV material, as obtained in early experiments, was at least as effective as the parent vitamin in curing rickets in rats (Lund and DeLuca, 1966). Furthermore, when the isolated peak IV material was readministered to vitamin D–deficient rats, it, like vitamin D, stimulated calcium transport by the intestine and caused a rise in serum calcium

These studies were supported by grants from the National Institutes of Health, AMO–5800–08, and the Harry Steenbock fund of the Wisconsin Alumni Research Foundation.

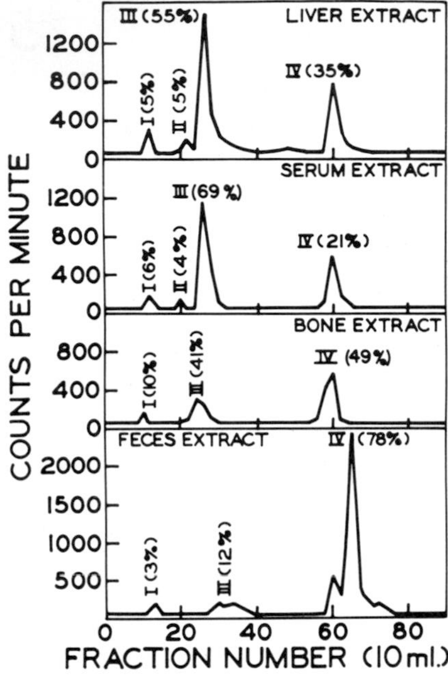

Fig. 5.1. Silicic acid column chromatography of lipid extracts from various tissues from rats given 500 IU of ^{3}H vitamin D_3 24 hr before the tissues were excised. (Lund and DeLuca, 1966. Reproduced by permission of the *Journal of Lipid Research.*)

(Morii et al., 1967). However, it acted much more rapidly than vitamin D in inducing calcium transport by the intestine. As the dosage of vitamin D to vitamin D–deficient rats was decreased to physiologic levels, the proportion of radioactivity found in the peak IV fraction increased (Fig. 5.2). Finally, virtually all of the radioactivity found in the nuclei of chick intestinal mucosa, the believed site of action of vitamin D (DeLuca, 1967), was present as peak IV (Stohs and DeLuca, 1967). These data are highly suggestive of the fact that some component of the peak IV fraction is the metabolically active form of the vitamin (DeLuca, 1967).

Isolation of 25–hydroxycholecalciferol

Clearly, it appeared essential to isolate and identify the active component of the peak IV fraction. In approaching this problem, it was necessary to find a source which would provide milligram quantities of the metabolite as free as possible from other, contaminating polar lipids. The peak IV material as originally obtained was effectively a methanol strip of the silicic acid columns used, and was thus heavily contaminated with lipids. It was also necessary to develop modified chromatographic procedures and a method of increasing at the source the amount of metabolite per gram of lipids. These problems were solved by obtaining the metabolite from

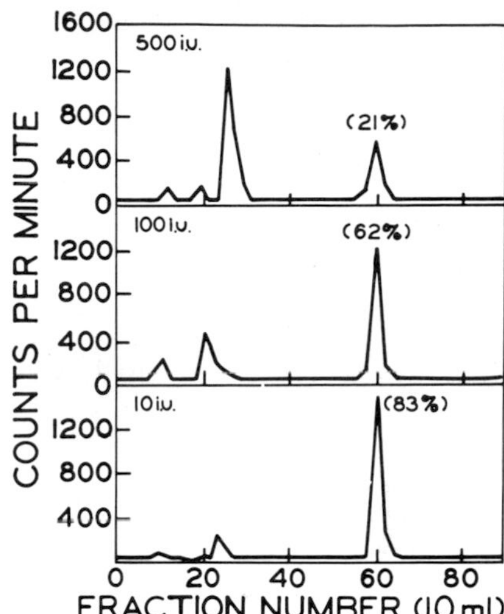

Fig. 5.2. Silicic acid column chromatography of rat serum lipids 24 hr after various oral doses of ^{3}H vitamin D_3. (Lund and DeLuca, 1966. Reproduced by permission of the *Journal of Lipid Research.*)

the plasma of pigs that had been maintained on high daily doses of vitamin D_3 (Blunt et al., 1968*a*, 1968*b*). Preliminary experiments indicated that such cumulative dosing of vitamin D_3 for several weeks could increase the circulating level of the peak IV metabolite some 100-fold above normal. Accordingly, four pigs were maintained on normal rations and given daily supplements of 250,000 IU of vitamin D_3 for 26 days. A total of 6.8 liters of plasma was then obtained. The next problem was to locate the biologically active metabolites without having to bioassay each fraction during subsequent chromatography of the plasma extract. We therefore prepared an extract containing radioactive metabolites by giving 2 mg of tritiated vitamin D_3 of suitable specific activity to a 50-lb pig and collecting the serum after 24 hr. The chloroform-soluble extract from this serum was combined with the similar extract from the four pigs. In order to reduce the volume of solvents used in the extraction of the large amounts of plasma, we first precipitated the plasma proteins by adding ammonium sulfate to reach 70% saturation. Earlier experiments with the radioactive serum had shown that this level of saturation was sufficient to precipitate nearly all of the radioactivity. The chloroform-soluble extract from the precipitated proteins was then obtained and the combined extracts were applied to a silicic acid column for chromatography (Fig. 5.3). By an extended gradient of diethyl ether in light petroleum, it was possible to separate the original peak IV into three components. Peaks IVa and V were both biologically inactive, while the new peak IV was fully active in curing rickets in rats. The material in this peak was then applied to a partition column consisting of methanol (80%) and water, as a stationary

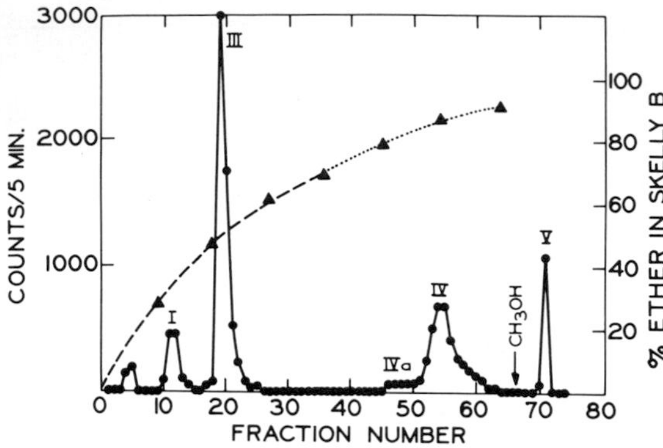

Fig. 5.3. Silicic acid column chromatography of combined extracts from pig plasma lipid. (Blunt et al., 1968*b*. Reproduced by permission of the American Chemical Society.)

phase on Celite, and a mobile phase of Skelly B (petroleum fraction, bp 65–67 C). The mobile phase was equilibrated 1:1 with the stationary phase. Figure 5.4 shows the radioactivity profile, on which is superimposed the weight of the metabolite as determined from its absorbance at 265 mμ. The material in this peak (1.3 mg) was shown to be pure by thin-layer and gas-liquid chromatography and was identified as 25–hydroxycholecalciferol as follows.

Identification of 25–hydroxycholecalciferol

Figure 5.5 shows the result of gas-liquid chromatography of the metabolite. Added to the sample was some vitamin D_3, which displays the two characteristic peaks (retention times of 10 min and 11 min) due to pyro- and isopyrocholecalciferol; these compounds arise from pyrolysis of the vitamin D_3 in the inlet heater (see Fig. 5.6, V and III). The material from the two peaks (retention times of 17 min and 19 min) due to the metabolite was collected and was shown to have ultraviolet absorption spectra identical with the spectra for pyro- and isopyrocholecalciferol. These data,

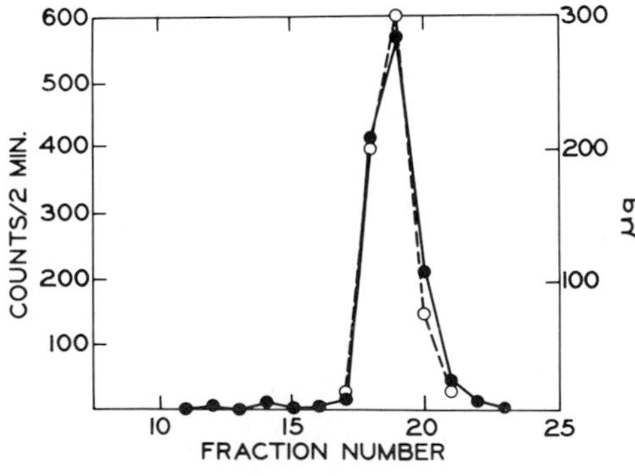

Fig. 5.4. Partition chromatography of peak IV (Fig. 5.3) material. The solid line indicates radioactivity, and the dotted line indicates fraction weights. (Blunt et al., 1968*b*. Reproduced by permission of the American Chemical Society.)

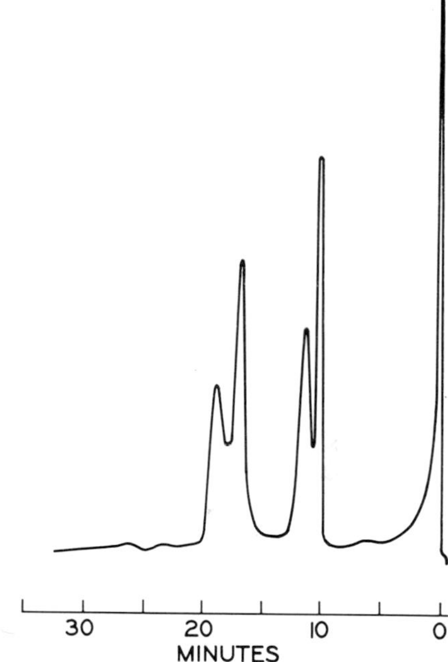

Fig. 5.5. Gas-liquid chromatography of 25-hydroxycholecalciferol and vitamin D_3. (Blunt et al., 1968*b*. Reproduced by permission of the American Chemical Society.)

together with the ultraviolet absorption maximum at 265 mμ for the metabolite and for vitamin D_3, suggested the presence of the unaltered calciferol triene system in the metabolite. A comparison of the mass spectra of the metabolite and of the parent vitamin was very informative (Fig. 5.7). The molecular ion at m/e 400.3340 indicated a molecular formula of $C_{27}H_{44}O_2$, i.e., a hydroxycholecalciferol. The location of the extra hydroxyl group in the sidechain was inferred from the presence in both spectra of a peak, m/e 271.2059, of composition $C_{19}H_{27}O$, i.e., the fragment remaining after loss of the sidechain by cleavage of the $C_{17\text{-}20}$ bond. Furthermore, a peak at m/e 59 (C_3H_7O) in the spectrum of the metabolite, but not in that of cholecalciferol, could have arisen by cleavage of the $C_{24\text{-}25}$ bond, with the hydroxyl group attached to C_{25}. Location

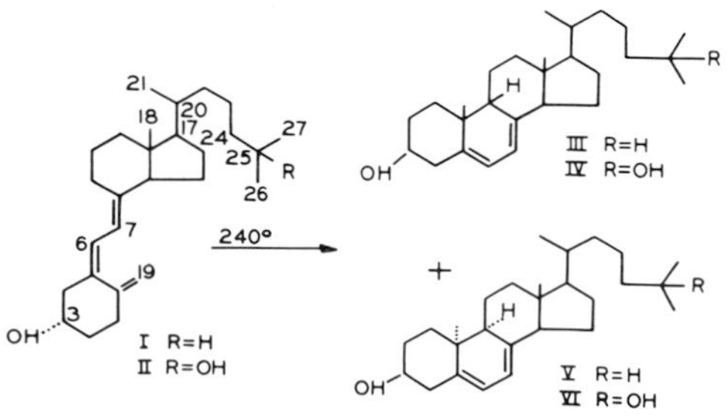

Fig. 5.6. Structures for I: cholecalciferol (vitamin D_3); II: 25-hydroxycholecalciferol; V: pyrocholecalciferol; III: isopyrocholecalciferol; and their respective 25-hydroxy derivatives (VI and IV). (Blunt et al., 1968*b*. Reproduced by permission of the American Chemical Society.)

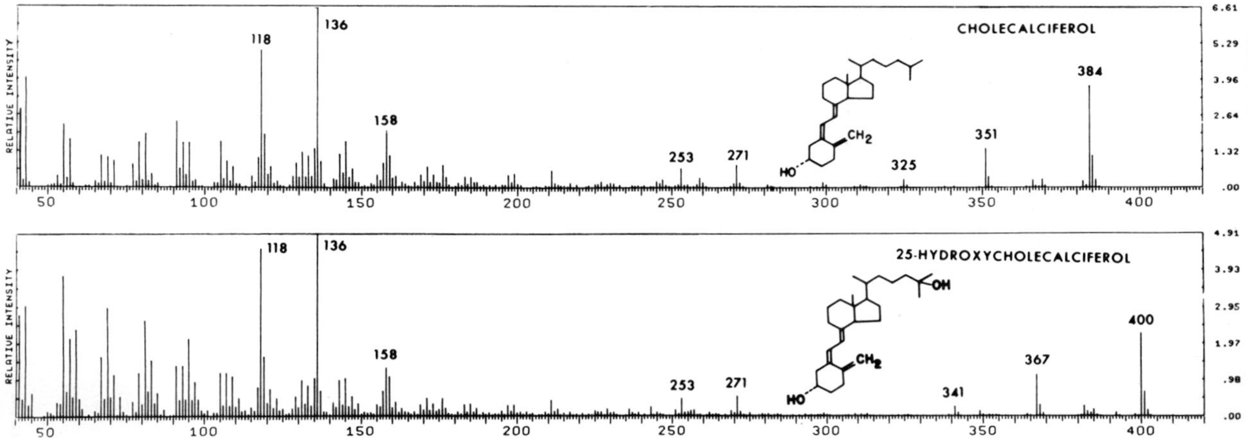

Fig. 5.7. Mass spectra of cholecalciferol and its 25-hydroxy derivative. (Blunt et al., 1968*b*. Reproduced by permission of the American Chemical Society.)

of the hydroxyl at C_{25} was verified by the 100 MHz nuclear magnetic resonance spectrum of the metabolite (Fig. 5.8). This exhibited a strong singlet peak at δ 1.20 ppm, due to the $C_{26,27}$-methyl protons, and an absence of a doublet peak at δ 0.87 ppm (J = 6.5 Hz) as found for the $C_{26,27}$-methyl protons of cholecalciferol, whose spectrum is shown in Figure 5.9. Thus the metabolite was identified as 25–hydroxycholecalciferol (25–OH–D_3) (Fig. 5.6, II).

Biological activity of 25–hydroxycholecalciferol

The biological activity of the pure isolated material was demonstrated in several systems (Blunt et al., 1968*c*). By the line-test assay in rats, 25–OH–D_3 was found to have an activity of 55–60 IU/μg, compared with the standard activity of 40 IU/μg of vitamin D_3. Intravenous administration of 2.5 μg of 25–OH–D_3 to vitamin D–deficient rats that had been maintained on a low-calcium diet elicited a more rapid elevation of serum calcium as a result of bone resorption than did a similar dose of vitamin D_3 (Fig. 5.10). Similarly, intrajugular administration of 0.25 μg of 25–OH–D_3 caused a more rapid onset of calcium transport as measured in isolated, everted rat gut sacs than a similar dose of vitamin D_3 (Fig. 5.11). In Chapter 7, Raisz and Trummel describe experiments in which bone resorption occurs in vitro in response to 25–OH–D_3, but not in response

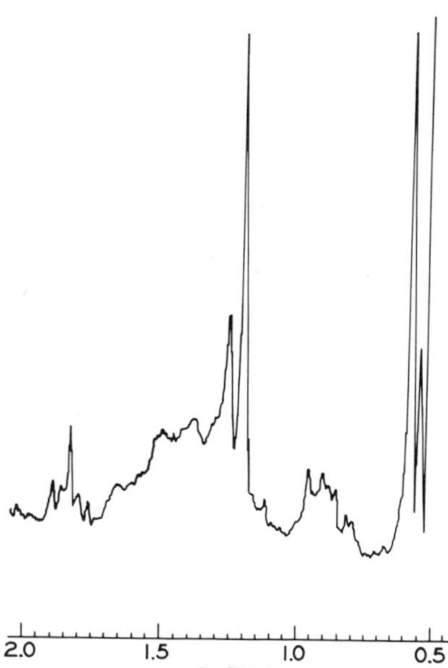

Fig. 5.8. Nuclear magnetic resonance spectrum (100 MHz) of 25-hydroxycholecalciferol. (Blunt et al., 1968*b*. Reproduced by permission of the American Chemical Society.)

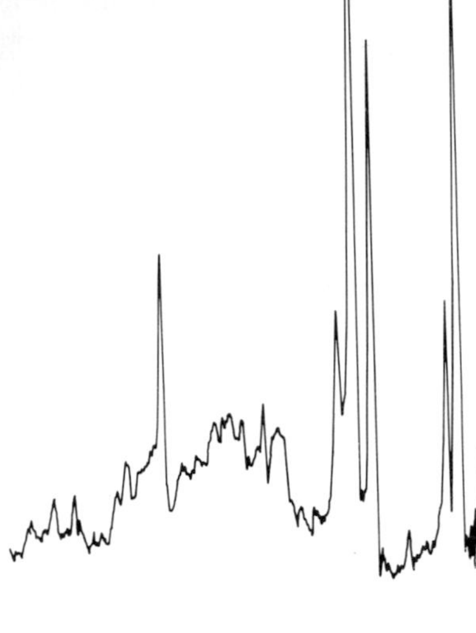

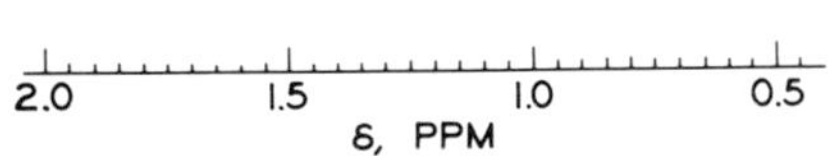

Fig. 5.9. Nuclear magnetic resonance spectrum (100 MHz) of cholecalciferol. (Blunt et al., 1968*b*. Reproduced by permission of the American Chemical Society.)

to vitamin D_3 (see also Trummel et al., 1969). Finally, increased calcium absorption by previously vitamin D–deficient chicks in response to 25–OH–D_3 has been demonstrated by the bone-ash assay (Fig. 5.12).

Isolation and identification of 25–hydroxyergocalciferol

It has been shown that vitamin D_2 also undergoes conversion to a peak IV metabolite that possesses biological activity (Drescher et al., 1969). By an extension of the methods we used for the isolation of 25–OH–D_3, we isolated this metabolite from pigs and showed it to be 25–hydroxyergocalciferol (25–OH–D_2) (Suda et al., 1969*a*, 1969*b*). (Fig. 5.13). In order

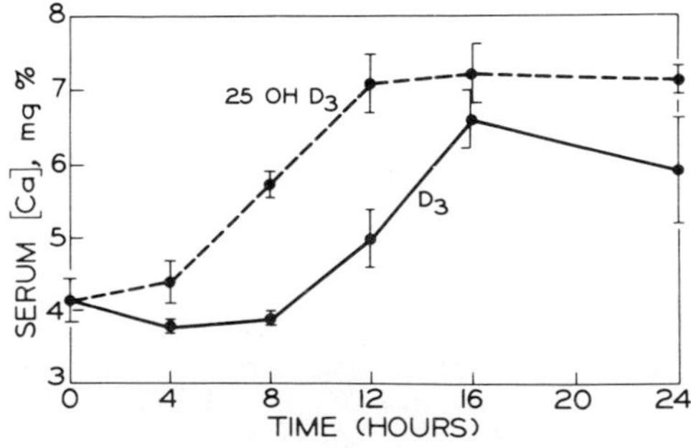

Fig. 5.10. Serum calcium response to 2.5 μg intravenous doses of 25-hydroxycholecalciferol and of vitamin D_3 in vitamin D–deficient rats on a low-calcium diet. (Blunt et al., 1968*c*. Reproduced by permission of the National Academy of Sciences.)

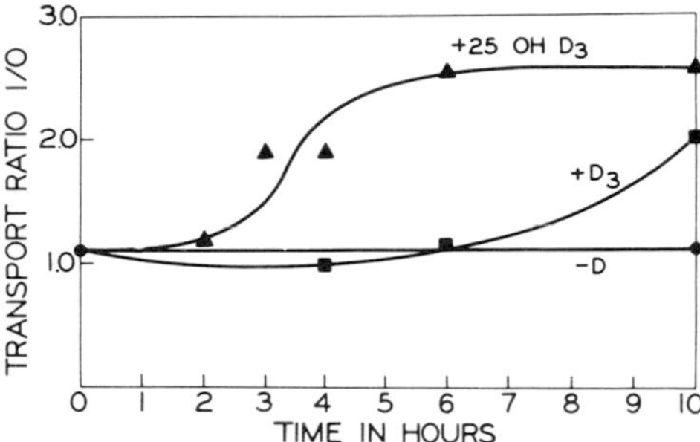

Fig. 5.11. Effect of intrajugular administration of 0.25 μg of 25-hydroxycholecalciferol or vitamin D_3 on calcium transport by everted intestinal sacs, as measured by the ratio (I/O) of ^{45}Ca in the serosal fluid to ^{45}Ca in the mucosal fluid.

to obtain the pure metabolite in sufficient quantities, it was necessary to give each of four pigs 500,000 IU of vitamin D_2 daily for 26 days. The lipid extract from the plasma proteins of these pigs was combined with the extract from the serum of several rats that had previously been given doses of tritiated vitamin D_2 for labeling purposes. More extensive chromatography was necessary to achieve purification, and 310 μg of the 25–OH–D_2 was finally obtained. The identification of the metabolite proceeded along lines similar to those outlined for 25–OH–D_3. The metabolite gave pyro- and isopyrocalciferol derivatives on gas-liquid chromatography, and had an ultraviolet absorption maximum at 265 mμ, thus demonstrating the presence of the calciferol triene system. The mass spectrum showed a molecular ion at m/e 412.3341, corresponding to a molecular formula of $C_{28}H_{44}O_2$, i.e., a hydroxyergocalciferol. The extra

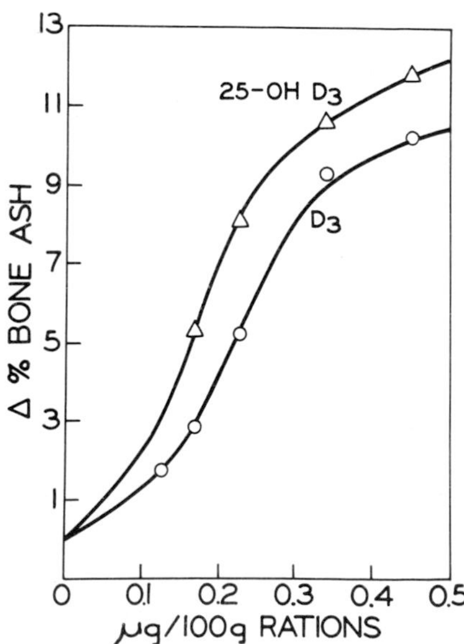

Fig. 5.12. The increase in the percentage of bone ash over the controls for graded doses of 25-hydroxycholecalciferol and vitamin D_3. Each point represents the pooled tibiae of 20 chicks.

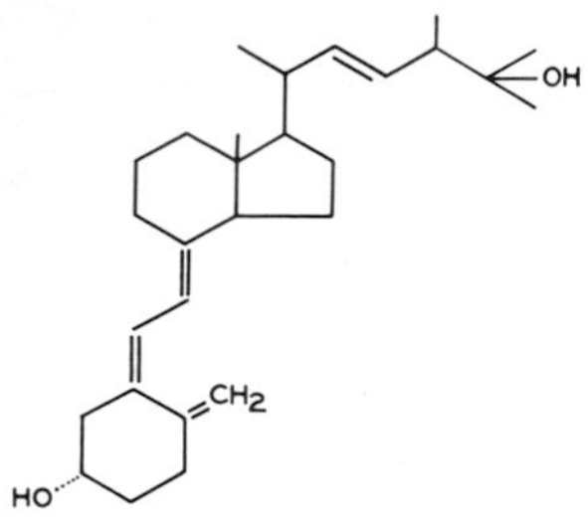

Fig. 5.13. Structure of 25-hydroxyergocalciferol. (Suda et al., 1969*b*. Reproduced by permission of the American Chemical Society.)

hydroxyl was located at C_{25} by an examination of the mass spectrum of the trimethylsilyl ether derivative of the metabolite, which had the molecular ion at *m/e* 556, corresponding to the di-trimethylsilyl ether. The base peak of the spectrum was at *m/e* 131, corresponding to a $C_6H_{15}SiO$ fragment. This peak, which also appears in the spectra of the silyl ether derivatives of 25–hydroxycholesterol and 25–OH–D_3, but not in the spectra of the silyl ethers of vitamin D_2 or D_3, can only have arisen from a C_{25}-trimethylsilyl ether. The nuclear magnetic resonance spectrum of the metabolite provided corroborating evidence for locating the hydroxyl group at C_{25}. Thus the metabolite from vitamin D_2 was identified as 25–hydroxyergocalciferol (25–OH–D_2, Fig. 5.13). 25–OH–D_2 showed an activity of 60 IU/μg when assayed by the rat-line test method.

Synthesis of 25–hydroxycholecalciferol

In order to further investigate the biological properties of 25–OH–D_3, it was necessary to obtain a still larger quantity of the pure material. This was achieved by chemical synthesis of three different starting materials. Each method resulted in the formation of cholesta-5,7-dien-3β,25-diol,

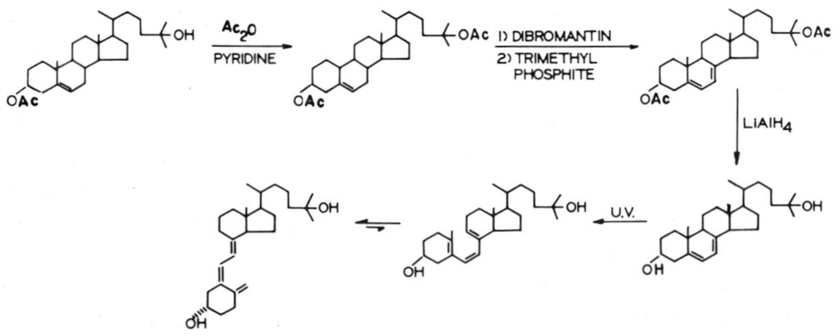

Fig. 5.14. Synthesis of 25-hydroxycholecalciferol from 25-hydroxycholesteryl acetate. (Blunt and DeLuca, 1969. Reproduced by permission of the American Chemical Society.)

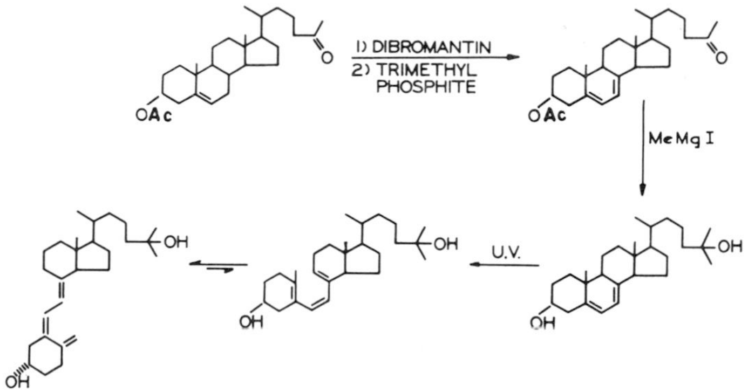

Fig. 5.15. Synthesis of 25-hydroxycholecalciferol from 25-keto-26-norcholesteryl acetate. (Blunt and DeLuca, 1969. Reproduced by permission of the American Chemical Society.)

which was then irradiated with ultraviolet light. The 25–hydroxyprecholecalciferol thus produced underwent thermal rearrangement to 25–OH–D_3. The first method involved bromination-dehydrobromination of the diacetate of 25–hydroxycholesterol (Fig. 5.14). Subsequent hydrolysis of the ester groups gave cholesta-5,7-dien-3β,25-diol. In the second method, 25-keto-26-norcholesteryl acetate was brominated-dehydrobrominated to give 3β-acetoxy-25-keto-26-norcholesta-5,7-diene (Fig. 5.15). Reaction of this with methyl magnesium iodide gave cholesta-5,7-dien-3β,25-diol. The third method utilized the acetate of 5-cholenic acid as a starting material (unpublished; see Fig. 5.16). The cholenic acid was reacted with oxalyl chloride, and the acid chloride produced was then converted to the diazoketone by the addition of diazomethane. The ethyl-3-acetoxy-25-homo-5-cholenate was produced by an Arndt-Eisert reaction with Ag_2O in ethanol. The 25–homoester was reacted with 4 moles of methyl magnesium iodide to yield 25-hydroxycholesterol. The 25–hydroxycholesterol was then converted to the diacetate and reacted sequentially with *N,N*-dibromodimethylhydantoin and trimethyl phosphite to yield the corresponding 5,7 diene. Reduction by lithium aluminum hydride gave cholesta-5,7-dien-3β,25-diol. Another pathway was utilized in which the 25-homoester was first converted to the 5,7 diene homoester. Grignard reaction again yielded the cholesta-5,7-dien-3β,25-diol. The diol from both sources was then irradiated with ultraviolet light, and the 25–hydroxyprecholecalciferol was separated out by chromatography. The 25–hydroxyprecholecalciferol, allowed to stand at room temperature for 2 weeks, converted to the 25–hydroxycholecalciferol, which was purified on silicic acid columns. The pure 25–hydroxycholecalciferol thus produced was identical in all respects to the isolated material from hog plasma.

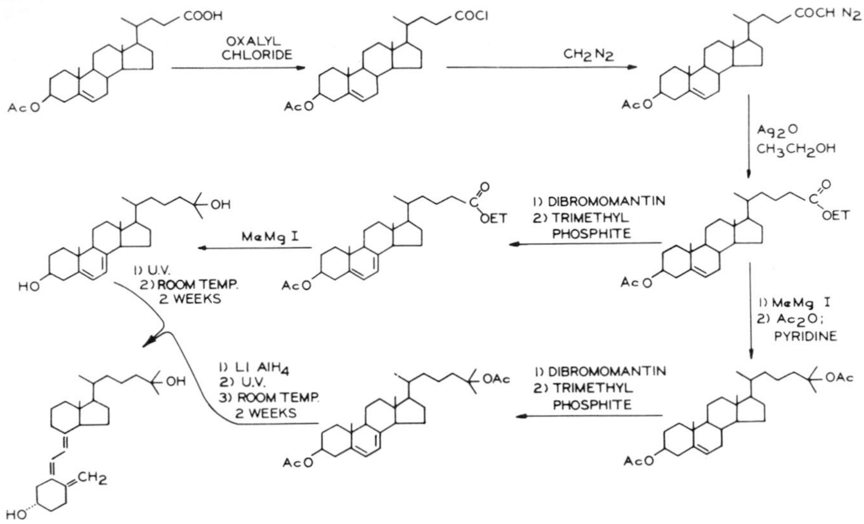

Fig. 5.16. Synthesis of 25-hydroxycholecalciferol from 5-cholenic acid. (DeLuca, Cleveland, and Schroeder, unpublished results.)

Summary

The major biologically active metabolites of vitamins D_3 and D_2 have been isolated from hog plasma and identified as 25–hydroxycholecalciferol and 25–hydroxyergocalciferol, respectively. The 25–hydroxycholecalciferol has been synthesized by three methods. It is 1.5 times more effective than vitamin D_3 in curing rickets in both rats and chicks and it acts more rapidly than vitamin D_3 in stimulating calcium transport in intestine and bone mobilization. These data suggest that, at least at the tissue level, 25–hydroxycholecalciferol represents the metabolically active form of vitamin D_3.

References

Bell, N. H., and P. Bryan. 1965. On the metabolism of C^{14}-vitamin D_3 in the rat. *J. Lab. Clin. Med. 66*:852.

Blunt, J. W., and H. F. DeLuca. 1969. The synthesis of 25–hydroxycholecalciferol. A biologically active metabolite of vitamin D_3. *Biochemistry 8*:671.

Blunt, J. W., H. F. DeLuca, and H. K. Schnoes. 1968. [Blunt et al., 1968*a*.] 25–Hydroxycholecalciferol: A biologically active metabolite of cholecalciferol. *Chem. Commun. 14*:801.

Blunt, J. W., H. F. DeLuca, and H. K. Schnoes. 1968. [Blunt et al., 1968*b*.] 25–Hydroxycholecalciferol: A biologically active metabolite of vitamin D_3. *Biochemistry* 7:3317.

Blunt, J. W., Y. Tanaka, and H. F. DeLuca. 1968. [Blunt et al., 1968*c*.] The biological activity of 25–hydroxycholecalciferol, a metabolite of vitamin D_3. *Proc. Nat. Acad. Sci. U.S.A. 61*:1503.

DeLuca, H. F. 1967. Mechanism of action and metabolic fate of vitamin D. *Vitamins Hormones 25*:315.

Drescher, D. H., H. F. DeLuca, and M. H. Imrie. 1969. Site of discrimination of chicks against vitamin D_2. *Arch. Biochem. Biophys. 130*:657.

Fraser, D. R., and E. Kodicek. 1965. Vitamin D esters: Their isolation and identification in rat tissues. *Biochem. J., 96*:59P.

Fraser, D. R., and E. Kodicek. 1966. The synthesis of vitamin D esters in the rat. *Biochem. J. 100*:67P.

Kodicek, E. 1956. Metabolism of vitamin D, p. 161. *In* G. E. W. Wolstenholme and C. M. O'Connor (eds.), *Ciba Foundation Symposium on Bone Structure and Metabolism.* Little, Brown, Boston.

Lund, J. 1966. Biologically active metabolites of vitamin D. Ph.D. thesis, University of Wisconsin.

Lund, J., and H. F. DeLuca. 1966. Biologically active metabolite of vitamin D_3 from bone, liver, and blood serum. *J. Lipid Res. 7*:739.

Lund, J., H. F. DeLuca, and M. Horsting. 1967. Formation of vitamin D esters *in vivo. Arch. Biochem. Biophys. 120*:513.

Morii, H., J. Lund, P. F. Neville, and H. F. DeLuca. 1967. Biological activity of vitamin D metabolite. *Arch. Biochem. Biophys. 120*:508.

Norman, A. W., J. Lund, and H. F. DeLuca. 1964. Biologically active forms of vitamin D_3 in kidney and intestine. *Arch. Biochem. Biophys. 108*:12.

Stohs, S. J., and H. F. DeLuca. 1967. Subcellular location of vitamin D and its metabolites in intestinal mucosa after a 10 i.u. dose. *Biochemistry 6*:3338.

Suda, T., H. F. DeLuca, H. K. Schnoes, and J. W. Blunt. 1969*a*. 25–Hydroxyergocalciferol: A biologically active metabolite of vitamin D_2. *Biochem. Biophys. Res. Commun. 35*:182.

Suda, T., H. F. DeLuca, H. K. Schnoes, and J. W. Blunt. 1969*b*. The isolation and identification of 25-hydroxyergocalciferol. *Biochemistry 8*:3515.

Trummel, C. L., L. G. Raisz, J. W. Blunt, and H. F. DeLuca. 1969. 25–Hydroxycholecalciferol: Stimulation of bone resorption in tissue culture. *Science 163*:1450.

6

STUDIES ON VITAMIN D METABOLISM

E. Kodicek

Vitamin D esters

Oral doses of 1–^{3}H cholecalciferol given to rachitic and normal young rats result in the appearance of various metabolites. The least polar peak, as revealed by thin-layer chromatography, was shown to consist of a number of long-chain fatty-acid esters of vitamin D. By two-dimensional cochromatography of the ester fraction derived from tissue with synthetic vitamin D esters, the esters were identified as being mainly stearate, palmitate, oleate, and linoleate (Fraser and Kodicek, 1968*a*). While the patterns of liver esters and plasma esters were similar, the fatty-acid esters found in the kidney were less unsaturated (Fig. 6.1). After 24 hr, usually 5%–10% of the vitamin in the tissues was in the form of esters, and occasionally as much as 20% of the ester form of the vitamin was found in the kidncy. The ester concentration in a number of tissues was determined at various times after dosing, and it was noticeable that the small intestine accumulated the highest content of vitamin D esters at the earliest time interval. Indeed, esters were found in the thoracic lymph in a rat given an oral dose of vitamin D while the vitamin was being absorbed (Fraser and Kodicek, 1968*b*). This pointed to the intestine as the tissue where esterification could occur. However, intravenous infusion of vitamin D resulted in the appearance of esters in plasma, liver, and kidney, but not in the small intestine. It was thus obvious that a second site of synthesis had to be postulated.

In order to identify the site and mechanism of esterification, we undertook an in vitro study of various tissues (Fraser and Kodicek, 1968*c*). It was possible that a cholesterol- or retinol-esterifying enzyme was responsible for an unspecific esterification of the vitamin D molecule. While liver and kidney preparations never were able to esterify vitamin D, intestinal preparations gave equivocal results. Since our preparations of this tissue showed a very low cholesterol-esterifying activity, pancreatic juice was used for the in vitro studies. The reaction mechanisms of the

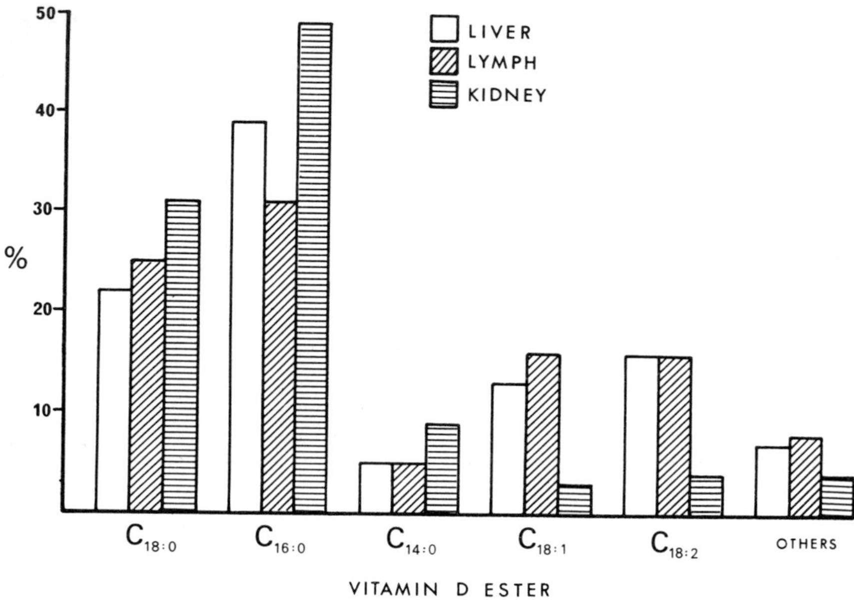

Fig. 6.1. Percentage composition of vitamin D esters in different tissues of the rat.

pancreatic and intestinal enzymes—namely, by using a direct union of free fatty acid and cholesterol without any external energy source—are very similar (Swell et al., 1950; Murthy and Ganguly, 1962). In the presence of pancreatic juice, vitamin D was esterified with oleic acid; specificity studies indicated that it was most likely the cholesterol-esterifying enzyme rather than a retinol-esterifying enzyme that was responsible for this reaction. Thus there was competition when mixed cholesterol and cholecalciferol were used as substrates, but not when retinol instead of cholesterol was the additional substrate. Sodium taurocholate, as a specific cofactor, was required for the esterification of both vitamin D and cholesterol. Furthermore, heavy-metal ions and *p*-choloromercuribenzoic acid had similar inhibitory effects on each reaction rate.

It is of interest that the relative esterification rates of precholecalciferol and cholecalciferol, when compared to that of cholesterol, indicate that the esterification rate of precholecalciferol is about three times that of cholecalciferol and about a quarter that of cholesterol (Fig. 6.2). One can expect that precholecalciferol might be formed also in vivo in skin by irradiation and that its higher affinity might be of importance in conservation of vitamin activity derived from skin irradiation. In contrast to this, U–^{14}C ergocalciferol was esterified at a rate only one fifth that of cholecalciferol.

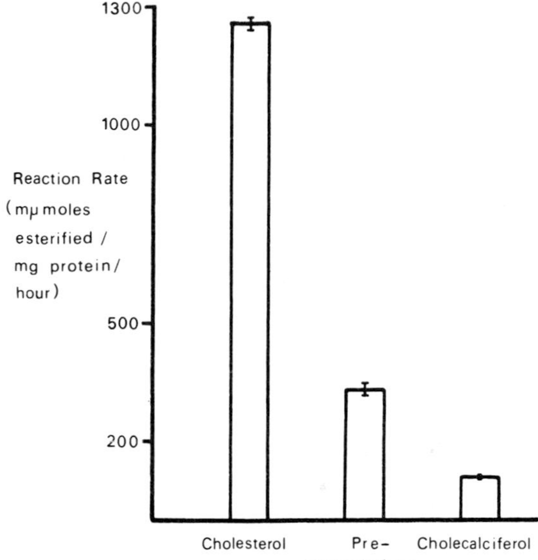

Fig. 6.2. Rates of esterification by pancreatic juice for cholesterol, cholecalciferol, and precholecalciferol. Oleic acid concentration was 0.8 μmole per assay; substrate concentration was 0.4 μmole per assay.

The other site of esterification appears to be plasma, which has a cholesterol-esterifying enzyme that forms cholesterol esters by transferring a fatty acid from phospholipids (Glomset, 1962). Whole plasma from rats esterified vitamin D in vitro; the composition of the fatty acids in the esters formed was similar to that found in cholesterol (Table 6.1).

On the basis of molecular models (Fraser and Kodicek, 1968*d*), it was postulated that the cholesterol-specific enzyme might be expected to act on vitamin D, since the spatial configuration of critical regions such as the hydroxyl group and the C–D rings are very similar for both vitamin D and cholesterol.

It is difficult to speculate on the significance of the esterification of vitamin D. In comparison with the biological activity of orally adminis-

TABLE 6.1. *Fatty-acid composition of 4-^{14}C cholesterol and 1-^{3}H cholecalciferol esters synthesized by rat plasma in vitro*

Degree of fatty acid unsaturation	Fatty acids (%)	
	Cholesterol esters	Cholecalciferol esters
Cx:0	10	14
Cx:1	7	6
Cx:2	29	24
Cx:3	1	4
Cx:4	53	52

tered vitamin D, vitamin D palmitate administered intraperitoneally had almost identical biological activity but its effect was longer lasting (Fraser and Kodicek, 1969); orally administered vitamin D oleate was less active (Bell and Bryan, 1969). It would appear that esters occurring in the animal body might be protected from further metabolism and thus provide the organism with a nutritionally advantageous conservation mechanism.

Conjugated metabolite of cholecalciferol in rat bile

In order to confirm that the biliary route is the main excretory pathway and to separate and characterize the action of the metabolites in bile independently of the action of intestinal bacteria, we gave young, vitamin D–supplemented, bile-duct-cannulated rats 0.34 mg of 1–^{3}H cholecalciferol or 0.54 mg of ^{14}C ergocalciferol by intravenous infusion. The rate of infusion simulated the rate of uptake of a similar oral dose into lymph. About 31% of the dose was excreted into the bile within 24 hr (Bell and Kodicek, 1967, 1969).

Gradient elution chromatography revealed that vitamin D ester, previtamin D, vitamin D, and 25–hydroxyvitamin D were virtually absent. Practically all the radioactivity (92%) was present as highly polar metabolites, which were denoted as A, B, C, D, and E in order of increasing polarity. The three most polar metabolites showed ionic properties; the major component, metabolite D, accounted for one-third of the recovered radioactivity and was further studied in more detail. The ionic nature of metabolite D was confirmed by distribution studies in partitioning solvents. Its mobility on thin-layer plates was increased by methylation and acetylation or by treatment with glycol-splitting agents such as periodate. These properties indicated the presence of a conjugate of glucuronic acid. Incubation with β-glucuronidase produced an increase in lipid-soluble radioactivity, while incubation with the inactivated enzyme or with a specific inhibitor of β-glucuronidase, saccharo-1,4-lactone, gave negative results. When authentic cholecalciferyl-β-D-glucuronide was synthesized and was, together with a sample of metabolite D, converted into the pyridinium salt, column cochromatography with gradient elution revealed that metabolite D was not eluted with the authentic glucuronide but was slightly more polar. That the glucuronide conjugate consisting of metabolite D was not identical with cholecalciferyl glucuronide was further confirmed by cochromatography after the samples were methylated and acetylated; under these conditions, the two glucuronide derivatives were distinctly separated. Only traces of free cholecalciferol could be identified among the products of enzymatic hydrolysis of the metabolite D, in agreement with the results of Avioli and co-workers (1967). The nature of the aglycone fragment of the metabolite is not yet known.

A new tritium-deficient metabolite from 1–^{3}H cholecalciferol in chick intestinal nuclei

Having prepared pure intestinal nuclei of rachitic and normal chicks, the purity of which was checked by enzymatic assays and electron microscopy, we studied the effect of cholecalciferol on the uptake of 5–^{3}H orotic acid into intestinal RNA (Lawson et al., 1969*a*). It could be shown that the incorporation of a 10-min pulse of orotic acid into rapidly labeled nuclear RNA was increased when rachitic chicks were injected at the same time (10 min before being killed) with cholecalciferol (Table 6.2, Exp. 1). These results are in keeping with the effect on RNA synthesis reported by Norman (1966) and Stohs and co-workers (1967). The total intestinal RNA, however, was unaffected by the vitamin D status of the birds.

In view of these results, we investigated DNA-dependent RNA polymerase activities (stimulated by both MG^{++} and Mn^{++}) of isolated intestinal nuclei from chicks (Table 6.3). No stimulation was observed after a dose of 2.5 μg or 125 μg of cholecalciferol after 5 hr and 1 hr, respectively.

TABLE 6.2. *5-^{3}H orotic acid incorporation into intestinal nuclear RNA from rachitic chicks given cholecalciferol*

Experimental conditions	Specific radioactivity of total RNA (dpm/mg)[a]		
	10 min	20 min	60 min
Rachitic chicks			
Total intestinal RNA	230[b]	—	—
RNA from isolated intestinal nuclei	—	—	6,000[c]
Treated chicks			
Total intestinal RNA	410[b]	620[b]	—
RNA from isolated intestinal nuclei	—	—	30,100[c]

Note: Rachitic chicks were given ^{3}H orotic acid before being killed. The treated chicks were each given 125 μg of cholecalciferol intracardially in propylene glycol at the time stated.

[a] Time after cholecalciferol injection.

[b] Exp. 1. Orotic acid was injected intracardially 10 min before the chicks were killed.

[c] Exp. 2. Orotic acid was injected intraperitoneally 20 min before the chicks were killed.

TABLE 6.3. *Effect of cholecalciferol on DNA-dependent RNA polymerase activity*

Dose of cholecalciferol	RNA activity[a] 1 hr	5 hr
Mn^{++}-stimulated activity		
Rachitic control	1090	–
125 μg cholecalciferol	920	–
Mg^{++}-stimulated activity		
Rachitic control	1230	1920
2.5 μg cholecalciferol	1130	1530

Note: RNA polymerase activity (as $\mu\mu$ moles of total ATP incorporated per milligram of DNA) was measured in the isolated intestinal nuclei of chicks that had received cholecalciferol.

[a] Time after cholecalciferol injection.

There were two possible explanations for the absence of any effect of vitamin D. It was possible that, due to changes of nuclear membrane permeability, the precursor pool was highly labeled by the pulse of the radioactive orotic acid; but that would imply change in only one component of the precursor pools, since no increase in the total acid-soluble substances could be noted. An alternative explanation focused our attention on the other factor of the RNA polymerase system, namely, chromatin.

By simultaneously administering 0.25 μg of 4–^{14}C cholecalciferol and 0.25 μg of 1α–^{3}H cholecalciferol (^{3}H:^{14}C = 4.7) to rachitic chicks, we found that the radioactivity of the nuclear-debris fraction and of the remaining supernatant fraction of the intestinal mucosa was lowered after 16 hr, suggestive of a biological loss of tritium (Fig. 6.3) (Lawson et al., 1969*b*). When the lipid extracts of intestinal mucosa (separated into the nuclear debris fraction and supernatant fraction), and of blood, of liver, and of kidney were chromatographed on a silicic acid column, four peaks could be separated; in increasing order of polarity, cholecalciferol ester, cholecalciferol, 25–hydroxycholecalciferol (25–HCC) (Blunt et al., 1968), and a fourth polar peak, P. In the chromatogram of the liver extract, a fifth peak, U, was also observed (Table 6.4). While the first three substances in all tissues showed a ^{3}H:^{14}C ratio close to that of the original double-labeled cholecalciferol, the radioactivity of the peak P varied depending from which tissue extract it originated. In the peak P obtained from blood, little or no change of ^{3}H:^{14}C ratio was observed except that in some instances up to about 5% of the total blood radioactivity may have been due to the tritium-deficient polar metabolite P–^{3}H. Peak P from the intestinal supernatant fraction, the liver, and the kidney, however, showed

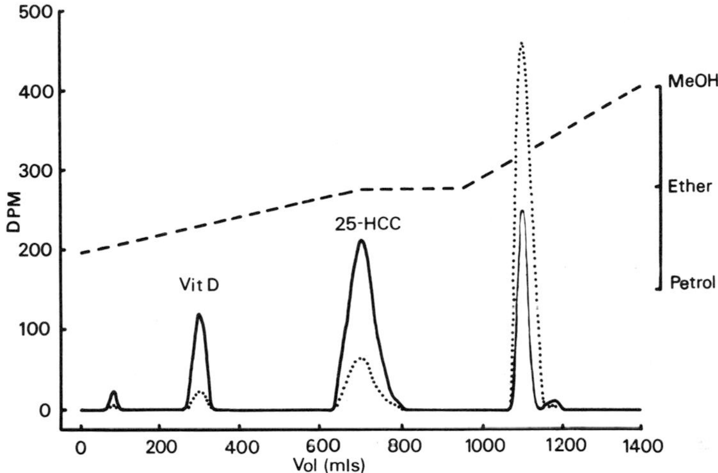

Fig. 6.3. Chromatographic pattern of the lipid extract of the intestinal supernatant fraction from rachitic chicks given simultaneously ^{14}C cholecalciferol (dotted line) and 1-^{3}H cholecalciferol (solid line). (Lawson et al., 1969*b*. Reproduced by permission of *Nature*.)

TABLE 6.4. *^{14}C radioactivity and ^{3}H:^{14}C ratios in the chromatograms of various tissue extracts*

Tissue extract	^{14}C radioactivity [a]					^{3}H:^{14}C ratio [b]				
	Cholecal-ciferol ester	Cholecal-ciferol	25–HCC	Peak P	Peak U	Cholecal-ciferol ester	Cholecal-ciferol	25–HCC	Peak P	Peak U
Liver	1.9	14.5	46.3	27.4	9.8	[c]	4.4	3.8	1.1	2.6
Kidney	3.5	16.6	43.4	35.7	0	5.6	4.7	4.4	1.5	—
Blood	0.5	4.1	78.9	14.2	0	4.0	4.3	4.5	4.7	—
Intestinal supernatant	0.8	6.1	20.7	68.0	0	4.0	4.4	4.5	0.5	—
Intestinal nuclei	0	2.7	0	97.3	0	—	[c]	—	0.2	—

Source: Lawson et al. (1969*b*).

Note: Rachitic chicks were administered simultaneously with 0.25 μg of 4-^{14}C cholecalciferol and 0.25 μg of 1α-^{3}H cholecalciferol (^{3}H:^{14}C = 4.7). The lipid extracts of the various tissues were then chromatographed on a silicic acid column.

[a] As the percentage of the radioactivity recovered from each chromatographic column.

[b] Calculated from the total dpm of ^{3}H and ^{14}C in the sample from each chromatographic fraction.

[c] Not calculated, since a statistically insignificant amount of radioactivity was present in the fraction.

a greatly reduced ratio, which also was observed in lipid extracts of bone. With pure intestinal nuclei, more than 97% of the radioactivity was in the form of the substance P–^{3}H, which had lost practically all its tritium at C–1. When chromatin was prepared from chick intestinal mucosa by the method of Haussler et al. (1968), over 95% of the ^{14}C radioactivity was eluted in the peak P area of the chromatogram with the very low ratio of less than 0.2 (Lawson et al., 1969*c*).

The proportion of the vitamin D metabolites at different times after administration of the double-labeled vitamin was investigated. In blood extracts, the cholecalciferol decreased rapidly; the 25–HCC increased rapidly for 4 hr and then increased more slowly up to 16 hr, at which time it amounted to about 70% of total radioactivity; the substance P rose slightly for 16 hr, at which time it constituted about 10% of total radioactivity recovered in blood. The ^{3}H:^{14}C ratio in blood extracts, however, was not significantly changed in any of these substances. In contrast, (Table 6.5) the nuclear debris fraction of chick intestinal mucosa showed a rapid decline of cholecalciferol, a lesser decrease of ester, but only a small concentration of 25–HCC; the concentration of 25–HCC reached a maximum of 6.5% at 2 hr and then declined to 3.7% after 16 hr. The peak P rose for 2 hr, reached a maximum at 8 hr of 54% of total recovered radioactivity, and remained at this level even at 16 hr. Most of the peak P area could be accounted for by the tritium-deficient substance P–^{3}H.

TABLE 6.5. *Time curve of ^{14}C radioactivity and ^{3}H:^{14}C ratios mucosal nuclear-debris fraction*

Time after vitamin D administration	^{14}C radioactivity [a]				^{3}H:^{14}C ratio [b]			
	Cholecalciferol ester	Cholecalciferol	25–HCC	Peak P	Cholecalciferol ester	Cholecalciferol	25–HCC	Peak P
0.5 hr	26.9	73.1	0	0	2.7	4.8	—	—
2 hr	12.4	56.3	6.5	14.5	5.2	4.5	[c]	0.9
4 hr	12.6	52.1	4.6	20.8	4.4	4.4	[c]	0.8
8 hr	11.8	22.6	4.8	54.0	5.5	4.4	[c]	0.4
16 hr	16.5	17.4	3.7	51.4	2.8	3.6	[c]	0.5

Source: Lawson et al. (1969*b*).

Note: Rachitic chicks were administered simultaneously with 0.25 μg of 4-^{14}C cholecalciferol and 0.25 μg of 1α-^{3}H cholecalciferol (^{3}H:^{14}C = 4.7). ^{14}C radioactivity and ^{3}H:^{14}C ratios for the nuclear-debris fraction were determined at various times.

[a] As the percentage of the radioactivity recovered from each chromatographic column.

[b] Calculated from the total dpm of ^{3}H and ^{14}C in the sample from each chromatographic fraction.

[c] Not calculated, since a statistically insignificant amount of radioactivity was present in the fraction.

The concentration of the substance P–^{3}H appears to be limited, since it was impossible to raise its concentration above 1 ng per gram of intestinal tissue. Furthermore, it was not possible to detect with certainty the tritium-deficient substance P–^{3}H in chicks that had been supplemented previously with adequate vitamin D (Lawson et al., 1969*c*). Similar results have been obtained with the rat and pig.

FORMATION OF PEAK P FROM 25–HCC

A biologically prepared double-labeled 25–HCC, with a ^{3}H:^{14}C ratio of 4.4, was injected into rachitic chicks; 8 hr later, a number of tissues were examined for radioactivity and the ^{3}H:^{14}C ratio was determined (Table 6.6) (Lawson et al., 1969*c*). In the blood extract, about 10% of recovered radioactivity was present in peak P, but no detectable lowering of the radioactivity ratio was observed. The intestinal debris fraction and the rest of intestinal mucosa (the supernatant fraction) contained 81% and 49.5% of radioactivity, respectively, in peak P with significantly lowered ratios of 0.2 and 0.5. Similar results were obtained with lipid extracts of bone, kidney, striated muscle and heart; however, 86% of the radioactivity recovered from adipose tissue extracts was in the form of 25–HCC and the radioactivity ratio was unchanged.

What is the significance of these findings? The increased polarity of the tritium-deficient metabolite P–^{3}H, which is found localized to a great

TABLE 6.6. *^{14}C radioactivity and ^{3}H:^{14}C ratios after 25-hydroxycholecalciferol administration*

Tissue extract	^{14}C radioactivity [a]		^{3}H:^{14}C ratio [b]	
	25–HCC	Peak P	25–HCC	Peak P
Blood	89.9	10.1	4.0	4.7
Intestine				
Nuclear debris	13.6	81.0	[d]	0.2
S.F. fraction [c]	41.5	49.5	3.5	0.5
Bone	80.6	19.4	4.5	2.3

Note: Rachitic chicks were intracardially injected with 0.4 μg of 4-^{14}C,1-^{3}H 25-hydroxycholecalciferol (^{3}H:^{14}C = 4.4). ^{14}C radioactivity and ^{3}H:^{14}C ratios of the various tissues were determined 8 hours later.

[a] As the percentage of the radioactivity recovered from each chromatographic column.

[b] Calculated from the total dpm of ^{3}H and ^{14}C in the sample from each chromatographic fraction.

[c] The S.F. fraction consisted of the rest of the intestinal mucosa after the nuclear-debris fraction was removed.

[d] Not calculated, since a statistically insignificant amount of radioactivity was present in the fraction.

extent in chick intestinal nuclei on chromatin, and its formation from both cholecalciferol and 25–HCC suggest the presence of one additional oxygen function. Although there are other possible interpretations, the simplest one is that the oxygen function is localized on C–1 of the A ring. The 1–^{3}H cholecalciferol has 85% of the tritium in position 1α and 15% in position 1β, as determined by recent degradation studies of the parent molecule (Bell and Kodicek, unpublished); also, practically all the tritium had been lost from the C–1 position. So one is compelled to conclude that a ketone formation at C–1 has occurred. This then would require a hydroxylated intermediate between 25–HCC and the tritium-deficient polar metabolite P–^{3}H.

The biological significance of this metabolite P–^{3}H has still to be evaluated. Haussler and co-workers (Haussler et al., 1968; Haussler and Norman, 1969) have described the existence of a metabolite, designated 4B, which appears to be similar to or identical with our polar metabolite P–^{3}H; they were also able to isolate this metabolite from chick intestinal chromatin. Despite the small quantities available, it has been shown that this metabolite had a greater biological activity than cholecalciferol or 25–HCC (Norman, private communication). It thus appears that the substance P–^{3}H is of importance for the understanding of the metabolic role of vitamin D. The binding of all the nuclear P–^{3}H substance to the chick intestinal chromatin would explain how the vitamin D stimulated the uptake of 5–^{3}H orotic acid into nuclear RNA without increasing either the pool size of RNA and its precursors or the RNA polymerase activity. It is possible that the metabolite of vitamin D functions by affecting (possibly as an allosteric factor) the template capacity of the chromatin as does estradiol (Barker and Warren, 1966).

References

Avioli, L. W., S. W. Lee, J. E. McDonald, J. Lund, and H. F. DeLuca. 1967. Metabolism of vitamin D_3–^{3}H in human subjects: Distribution in blood, bile, feces and urine. *J. Clin. Invest. 46*:983.

Barker, K. L., and J. C. Warren. 1966. Template capacity of uterine chomatin: Control by estradiol. *Proc. Nat. Acad. Sci. U.S.A. 56*:1298.

Bell, N. H., and P. Bryan. 1969. Absorption of vitamin D_3 oleate in the rat. *Amer. J. Clin Nutr. 22*:425.

Bell, P. A. and E. Kodicek. 1967. A conjugated metabolite of vitamin D_3 in rat bile and faeces. *Biochem. J. 105*:34P.

Bell, P. A., and E. Kodicek. 1969. Investigations on metabolites of vitamin D in rat bile. Separation and partial identification of a major metabolite. *Biochem. J. 115*:663.

Blunt, J. W., H. F. DeLuca, and H. K. Schnoes. 1968. 25–Hydroxycholecalciferol. A biologically active metabolite of vitamin D_3. *Biochemistry* 7:3317.

Fraser D. R. and E. Kodicek. 1968*a*. Investigations on vitamin D esters synthesized in rats. Detection and identification. *Biochem. J. 106*:485.

Fraser D. R. and E. Kodicek. 1968*b*. Investigations on vitamin D esters synthesized in rats. Turnover and sites of synthesis. *Biochem. J. 106*:491.

Fraser D. R., and E. Kodicek. 1968*c*. Enzyme studies on the esterification of vitamin D in rat tissues. *Biochem. J. 109*:457.

Fraser, D. R., and E. Kodicek. 1968*d*. Conformational similarities of vitamin D and cholesterol as enzyme substrates. *Nature 220*:1031.

Fraser, D. R., and E. Kodicek. 1969. The metabolism and biological activity of esterified vitamin D in the rat. *Brit. J. Nutr. 23*:135.

Glomset, J. A. 1962. The mechanism of the plasma cholesterol esterification reaction: Plasma fatty acid transferase. *Biochim. Biophys. Acta. 65*:128.

Haussler, M. R., J. F. Myrtle, and A. W. Norman. 1968. The association of a metabolite of vitamin D_3 with intestinal mucosa chromatin *in vivo*. *J. Biol. Chem. 243*:4055.

Haussler, M. R., and A. W. Norman. 1969. Chromosomal receptor for a vitamin D metabolite. *Proc. Nat. Acad. Sci. U.S.A. 62*:155.

Lawson, D. E. M., P. W. Wilson, D. C. Barker, and E. Kodicek. 1969. [Lawson et al, 1969*a*.] Isolation of chick intestinal nuclei: Effect of vitamin D_3 on nuclear metabolism. *Biochem. J. 115*:263.

Lawson, D. E. M., P. W. Wilson, and E. Kodicek. 1969. [Lawson et al., 1969*b*.] New vitamin D metabolite localized in intestinal cell nuclei. *Nature 222*:171.

Lawson, D. E. M., P. W. Wilson, and E. Kodicek. 1969. [Lawson et al, 1969*c*.] Metabolism of vitamin D: A new cholecalciferol metabolite, involving loss of hydrogen at C–1, in chick intestinal nuclei. *Biochem. J. 115*:269.

Murthy, S. K., and J. Ganguly. 1962. Studies on cholesterol esterases of the small intestine and pancreas of rats. *Biochem. J. 83*:460.

Norman, A. W. 1966. Vitamin D mediated synthesis of rapidly labelled RNA from intestinal mucosa. *Biochem. Biophys. Res. Commun. 23*:335.

Stohs, S. J., J. E. Zull, and H. F. DeLuca. 1967. Vitamin D stimulation of [^{3}H] orotic acid incorporation into ribonucleic acid of rat intestinal mucosa. *Biochemistry 6*:1304.

Swell, L., J. E. Byron, and C. R. Treadwell. 1950. Cholesterol esterases. IV. Cholesterol esterase of rat intestinal mucosa. *J. Biol. Chem. 186*:543.

7

ROLE OF VITAMIN D IN BONE METABOLISM

Lawrence G. Raisz and Clarence L. Trummel

The remarkable sensitivity of the gastrointestinal calcium transport system to vitamin D has drawn attention away from the effects of the vitamin on other calcium transport systems. Nevertheless, it is clear that vitamin D has a direct effect on bone. Pharmacologic doses of the vitamin cause hypercalcemia and changes in bone morphology (Chen and Bosmann, 1965). In vitamin D deficiency, bone resorption is impaired and serum calcium concentration decreases (Rasmussen et al., 1963), despite severe secondary hyperparathyroidism (Au and Raisz, 1965). It has been postulated that the vitamin is a necessary cofactor for parathyroid hormone response in bone. This concept may require modification, since it is possible to restore responsiveness to parathyroid hormone in the absence of vitamin D by giving multiple injections of calcium or by feeding lactose, which increases calcium absorption from the gut (Au and Raisz, 1967). More likely, the effect of vitamin D on bone resorption is a separate, direct effect that is synergistic with the effect of parathyroid hormone: when one agent is absent, the tissue is relatively unresponsive to the other.

Bone resorption in culture and 25–HCC and PTH

Several years ago we found that the response of bone to parathyroid extract in tissue culture was less in a medium containing serum from vitamin D–deficient animals than in a medium containing serum from vitamin D–fed animals (Raisz, 1965). We could not show a direct response to large doses of vitamin D in this system, although Goldhaber had shown that

This research was supported in part by grants AM–O6205 and 5–TO1–DE–00003–13 from the United States Public Health Service.

The authors wish to thank Dr. Hector DeLuca and Dr. John W. Blunt for their generous supply of pure 25–hydroxycholecalciferol and of partially purified peak IV metabolite containing 25–HCC used in these studies.

large doses of vitamin D or of dihydrotachysterol could stimulate resorption in mouse calvaria in long-term cultures (Goldhaber, 1963). Recently we re-examined this problem by testing a variety of vitamin D preparations for their ability to increase the release of previously incorporated radioactive calcium from bone shafts of 19-day fetal rats that were maintained in a chemically defined medium in organ culture (Trummel et al., 1969). Unaltered vitamin D_3 or vitamin D_2 added directly to the cultures in several different ways was ineffective during the first three days and caused only partial and inconsistent increases in bone resorption thereafter. However, 25–hydroxycholecalciferol (25–HCC), an active metabolite of vitamin D_3 (Blunt et al., 1968), constantly caused an early stimulation of bone resorption (Table 7.1). In subsequent studies, the effects of 25–HCC were compared with those of parathyroid hormone (PTH). Both agents stimulated bone resorption rapidly, so nearly all the calcium and matrix in the bone shafts of 19-day fetal rats was removed in 3–4 days. The maximally effective dose for PTH was about 1 μg/ml (a concentration of 10^{-7} M) and for 25–HCC, 0.5–1.5 μg/ml (a concentration of 1.3–4 $\times$ 10^{-6} M). These are much larger than the concentrations in normal blood, but the maximally effective concentration of PTH is only ten times greater than the highest values observed in chronically hypocalcemic cows (Sherwood et al.,1968); a similar relation probably holds for the concentration of 25–HCC present in the blood after toxic doses of vitamin D_3. When

TABLE 7.1. *Effect of crystalline vitamin D_3 and 25–HCC on bone resorption*

Treatment	Cumulative ^{45}Ca release (treated/control ratio) 0–3 days	0–6 days
Vitamin D_3		
40 IU/ml	0.91 ± 0.06	0.93 ± 0.06
320 IU/ml	0.99 ± 0.07	1.24 ± 0.17
25–HCC		
9 IU/ml	1.31 ± 0.10[a]	1.43 ± 0.10[a]
18 IU/ml	1.33 ± 0.12[a]	1.65 ± 0.21[a]

Notes: The shafts of the radius and of the ulna were dissected from 19-day fetal rats taken from mothers that had been injected with 0.5 mc of ^{45}Ca on the previous day. The bones were cultured at 37° C in a chemically defined medium (BGJ with 1 mg/ml bovine-serum albumin (fraction V)) and gassed with 5% CO_2, 20% O_2, and 75% N_2. 25–HCC and crystalline vitamin D_3 were added in ethanol, and test and control media were adjusted to contain 1% ethanol.

Values are given as mean ± SE for 4 pairs of cultures.

[a] Significantly different from 1.0, $P < 0.05$.

the two agents are added together in tissue culture, effects are observed at much lower concentrations (Table 7.2). The response is termed synergistic because the two agents together produce an increase in resorption at doses which are ineffective when either is given alone. Ten times these concentrations of either 25–HCC or PTH alone would be required to give an equivalent response. This result indicates that the two agents act at different sites in the cell, but are related in such a fashion that the effect of one can multiply, rather than just add to, the effect of the other.

TABLE 7.2. *Synergistic effect of low doses of PTH and 25-HCC on bone resorption*

	Cumulative ^{45}Ca release (treated/control ratio)	
Treatment	0–2 days	0–4 days
PTH (0.03 μg/ml)	1.03 ± 0.13	1.04 ± 0.05
25–HCC (0.015 μg/ml)	0.96 ± 0.04	0.96 ± 0.07
PTH (0.03 μg/ml) + 25HCC (0.015 μg/ml)	1.45 ± 0.16[a]	1.75 ± 0.28[a]

Notes: For procedure, see note to Table 7.1.
Values are given as mean ± SE for 4 pairs of cultures.
[a] Significantly different from 1.0, $P < 0.05$.

Brief periods of treatment with PTH or with 25–HCC can cause prolonged stimulation of bone resorption in tissue culture (Table 7.3). Presumably these agents induce a subsequent morphologic response that is characterized by osteoclastic and fibroblastic proliferation. The response to maximal doses of PTH and of 25–HCC is not significantly different

TABLE 7.3. *Effect of brief vs. continuous exposure to submaximal and maximal doses of PTH and 25–HCC on bone resorption*

	48-hr ^{45}Ca release (treated/control ratio)	
Treatment	6-hr exposure	Continuous exposure
Submaximal doses		
PTH (0.3 μg/ml)	1.14 ± 0.09	1.50 ± 0.15[a]
25–HCC (0.5 μg/ml)	1.16 ± 0.04[a]	1.55 ± 0.07[a]
Maximal doses		
PTH (1.0 μg/ml)	1.79 ± 0.07[a]	1.88 ± 0.09[a]
25–HCC (1.5 μg/ml)	1.70 ± 0.20[a]	1.98 ± 0.14[a]

Notes: For procedure, see note to Table 7.1.
Values are given as mean ± SE for 4 pairs of cultures.
[a] Significantly different from 1.0, $P < 0.05$.

when the agents are given for only 6 hr or are present in the culture continuously. With submaximal doses, shorter exposure decreases the response. The effect of dose and duration of exposure on the response is a complex relation and may depend on variations in the cell population. Since both agents can induce a similar cell transformation, yet may act at different sites, it is possible that some common secondary effect is responsible for the changes in nuclear transcription and the subsequent new RNA synthesis required for bone resorption (Raisz et al., 1968). This common effect, or "second messenger," could be cyclic 3′,5′-adenosine monophosphate, the production of which is stimulated by PTH (Chase et al., 1969). It is also possible that induction could be mediated by the similar effects of the two agents on ion translocation. This possibility is supported by the observation that the induction of resorption by either PTH or 25–HCC is dependent on the concentration of calcium in the medium (Table 7.4). If the calcium concentration of the medium is de-

TABLE 7.4. *Effect of changing calcium concentration during induction on the response of bone resorption to PTH and 25–HCC*

	48-hr ^{45}Ca release (treated/control ratio)	
Treatment	Normal calcium	Low calcium
25–HCC (1.5 μg/ml)	1.60 ± 0.06	1.31 ± 0.07 [a]
PTH (1 μg/ml)	1.88 ± 0.28	1.15 ± 0.15 [a]

Notes: Procedure was as described in note to Table 7.1 except that cultures were treated for 6 hr in a medium with either 25–HCC or PTH and with either normal (5 mg/100 ml) or low (2 mg/100 ml) concentrations of calcium. Cultures were then transferred to a medium without PTH or 25–HCC and at normal calcium concentration for the subsequent 42 hr.

Values are given as mean ± SE for 4 pairs of cultures.

[a] Significantly different from response in normal concentration of calcium, $P < 0.05$.

creased during the initial 6-hr exposure to either agent and the bones are transferred to a medium of normal calcium concentration, the subsequent resorptive response is decreased. The hypothesis that calcium translocation initiates nuclear transcription has been suggested previously (Zull et al., 1966) and would explain how such different molecules as 25–HCC and PTH produce such similar responses.

The response to 25–HCC can be inhibited by the agents that inhibit the PTH response. Just as with PTH, calcitonin blocks the initial increase in release of ^{45}Ca stimulated by 25–HCC but there is a subsequent escape from the inhibition (Trummel et al., 1969; Friedman et al., 1968). Increasing the phosphate concentration in the medium can also inhibit

TABLE 7.5. *Effect of albumin on the response of bone resorption to PTH and 25–HCC*

Treatment	48-hr ^{45}Ca release (treated/control ratio)	
	BGJ and albumin	BGJ alone
25–HCC (1.5μg/ml)	1.64 $\pm$ 0.11 [a]	1.51 $\pm$ 0.11 [a]
PTH (1.5 μg/ml)	1.57 $\pm$ 0.08 [a]	1.02 $\pm$ 0.04

Notes: For procedure, see note to Table 7.1. Albumin used was 1 mg/ml of bovine fraction V.

Values are given as mean $\pm$ SE for 4 pairs of cultures.

[a] Significantly different from 1.0, $P < 0.05$.

bone resorption stimulated by 25–HCC (Trummel and Raisz, unpublished observation). Some differences in inhibitory effects have been noted. When albumin is absent from the medium, the PTH response is lost but the response to 25–HCC persists (Table 7.5). This may be simply because PTH is adsorbed on glass surfaces when albumin is not present. The availability of an agent that can stimulate resorption in a protein-free medium may aid in the identification of enzymes and other macromolecules released from bone during the resorptive process. A surprising difference between 25–HCC and PTH has been shown by the effects of hydrocortisone. Relatively low concentrations of hydrocortisone can inhibit PTH-stimulated bone resorption (Stern, 1969) but cannot inhibit the response to a maximal dose (4×10^{-6} M) of 25–HCC (Fig. 7.1). These data do not rule out the possibility that hydrocortisone can inhibit the effects of lower concentrations of 25–HCC.

While it is clear that 25–HCC can be formed by enzymatic conversion of vitamin D in the liver, the late and variable responses to large doses of vitamin D_3 in our culture system could mean that bone also makes an

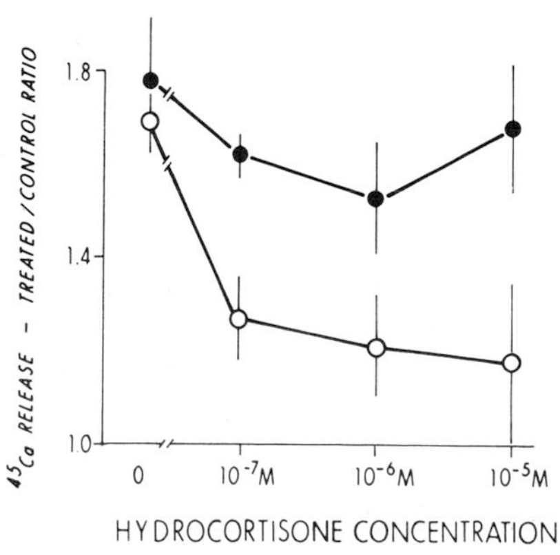

Fig. 7.1. Effect of hydrocortisone on the stimulation of bone resorption by 1.5 μg/ml of 25–HCC (upper curve) or by 1 μg/ml of parathyroid hormone (lower curve) during 48 hr in tissue culture. Values are given as the mean $\pm$ SE for 4 pairs of cultures. Hydrocortisone was added to both treated and control cultures in the indicated concentrations.

active metabolic product. To test this we incubated bones for 2 days with 150 IU/ml of vitamin D_3. The media were subsequently assayed and showed no ability to stimulate resorption of fresh bone cultures. Hence if any 25–HCC was made, it either was subsequently destroyed or was present in such a low concentration (i.e., less than 2 IU/ml) that it was undetectable by this assay (Trummel and Raisz, unpublished observation).

We do not know whether vitamin D or its metabolites have any important direct effects on bone formation. In vitamin D deficiency, the development of osteomalacia or rickets is accompanied by decreased bone formation and growth. In deficient chicks, a marked increase in the incorporation of labeled proline into hydroxyproline in bone is observed 12 hr after treatment with vitamin D, at a time when serum calcium concentration has not yet returned to normal (Canas et al., 1969). The possibility that vitamin D directly stimulates the synthesis of bone matrix was suggested but remains unproven. It is possible that the effect of vitamin D on bone matrix requires that vitamin D be transformed to some metabolite other than 25–HCC.

Conclusion

The active metabolite of vitamin D_3, 25–hydroxycholecalciferol, can directly stimulate bone resorption in tissue culture. Its effects are generally similar to those of parathyroid hormone. However, at low doses the two agents are synergistic, suggesting that they do not act at the same site in bone. Since bone can become less responsive to parathyroid hormone in vitamin D deficiency, it is likely that the amount of 25–hydroxycholecalciferol normally present is important in the physiologic regulation of bone resorption in vivo.

References

Au, W. Y. W., and L. G. Raisz. 1965. Effect of vitamin D and dietary calcium on parathyroid activity. *Amer. J. Physiol. 209*:637–42.

Au, W. Y. W., and L. G. Raisz. 1967. Restoration of parathyroid responsiveness in vitamin D–deficient rats by parenteral calcium or dietary lactose. *J. Clin. Invest. 46*:1572–78.

Blunt, J. W., Y. Tanaka, and H. F. DeLuca. 1968. The biological activity of 25–hydroxycholecalciferol, a metabolite of vitamin D_3. *Proc. Nat. Acad. Sci. U.S.A. 61*:1503–06.

Canas, F., J. S. Brand, W. F. Neuman, and A. R. Terepka. 1969. Some effects of vitamin D_3 on collagen synthesis in rachitic chick cortical bone. *Amer. J. Physiol. 216*:1092–96.

Chase, L. R., S. A. Fedak, and G. D. Aurbach. 1969. Activation of skeletal adenyl cyclase by parathyroid hormone *in vitro*. *Endocrinology 84*:761–68.

Chen, P. S., Jr., and H. B. Bosmann. 1965. Comparison of the hypercalcemic action of vitamins D_2 and D_3 in chicks and the effect on tetracycline fixation by bone. *J. Nutr. 87*:148–54.

Friedman, J., W. Y. W. Au, and L. G. Raisz. 1968. Responses of fetal rat bone to thyrocalcitonin in tissue culture. *Endrocinology 82*:149–56.

Goldhaber, P. 1963. Some chemical factors influencing bone resorption in tissue culture, pp. 609–36. *In* R. F. Sognnaes (ed.), *Mechanisms of Hard Tissue Destruction*. AAAS, No. 75, Washington, D.C.

Raisz, L. G. 1965. Bone resorption in tissue culture. Factors influencing the response to parathyroid hormone. *J. Clin. Invest. 44*:103–16.

Raisz, L. G., J. S. Brand, W. Y. W. Au, and I. Niemann. 1968. Interactions of parathyroid hormone and thyrocalcitonin on bone resorption in tissue culture, pp. 370–80. *In* R. V. Talmage and L. F. Belanger (eds.), *Parathyroid Hormone and Thyrocalcitonin (Calcitonin)*. Excerpta Medica Foundation, New York.

Rasmussen, H., H. DeLuca, C. Arnaud, C. Hawker, and M. Von Stedingk. 1963. The relationship between vitamin D and parathyroid hormone. *J. Clin.Invest. 42*:1940–46.

Sherwood, L. M., G. P. Mayer, C. F. Ramberg, Jr., D. S. Kronfeld, G. D. Aurbach, and J. T. Potts, Jr. 1968. Regulation of parathyroid hormone secretion: proportional control by calcium, lack of effect of phosphate. *Endocrinology 83*:1043–51.

Stern, P. H. 1969. Inhibition by steroids of parathyroid hormone-induced Ca-45 release from embryonic rat bone *in vitro*. *J. Pharmacol. Exp. Ther.* 168:211–17.

Trummel, C. L., L. G. Raisz, J. W. Blunt, and H. F. DeLuca. 1969. 25–Hydroxycholecalciferol: Stimulation of bone resorption in tissue culture. *Science 163*:1450–51.

Zull, J. E., E. Czarnowska-Misztal, and H. F. DeLuca. 1966. On the relationship between vitamin D action and actinomycin-sensitive processes. *Proc. Nat. Acad. Sci. U.S.A. 55*:177–84.

8

RENAL EFFECTS OF VITAMIN D

Charles Y. C. Pak and Frederic C. Bartter

The exact functional role of vitamin D in the regulation of renal tubular transport of calcium and of phosphorus has been difficult to define (Bartter, 1970). The major problem has been to separate the direct effects of vitamin D from the indirect ones that appear as sequelae after vitamin D is administered. For instance, vitamin D characteristically produces an elevation in the concentration of circulating calcium ions; this in turn may suppress the secretion of parathyroid hormone and stimulate the secretion of calcitonin. Each of these factors – changes in serum calcium concentration and in the secretion of parathyroid hormone and of calcitonin – may affect the renal tubular transport of calcium and of phosphorus independently of vitamin D. The failure to recognize the functional role of these factors could therefore lead to erroneous conclusions about the renal action of vitamin D.

We shall first review and discuss the known effects of changes in serum calcium concentration, of parathyroid hormone, and of calcitonin on the renal transport of calcium and of phosphorus. We shall then consider the effects of vitamin D that are independent of these factors.

Effect of increasing serum calcium concentration

Elevation of serum calcium concentration by calcium infusion usually leads to an increase in urinary phosphorus excretion independently of the effect of an indirectly stimulated parathyroid hormone (Howard et al., 1952, 1953; Nordin and Fraser, 1954; Eisenberg, 1965). The effect of a short-term calcium infusion in a thyroparathyroidectomized dog is shown in Figure 8.1. An elevation of serum calcium from approximately 8mg/100 ml to 12 mg/100 ml was achieved with a 4-hr infusion of 15 mg of calcium per kilogram of body weight. Serum phosphorus concentration rose slightly, as shown by others (Crawford et al., 1955). However, tubular reabsorption of phosphorus (TRP) decreased to produce a marked increase in urinary phosphorus excretion.

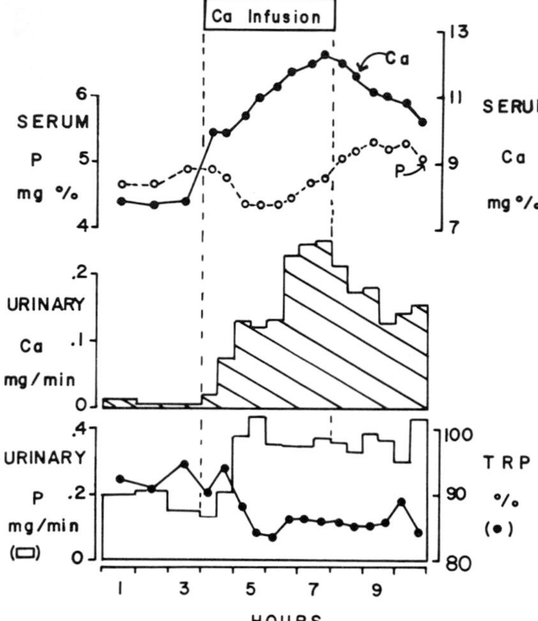

Fig. 8.1. Effect of a short-term (4 hr) calcium infusion on serum calcium concentration, urinary excretion of phosphorus, and the tubular reabsorption of phosphorus in a thyroparathyroidectomized dog.

With sustained calcium infusion, a marked fall in tubular reabsorption of phosphorus causes phosphaturia to persist despite a fall in serum phosphorus concentration and a lack of any consistent change in glomerular filtration rate (Eisenberg, 1965). A characteristic response is illustrated in Figure 8.2. In a patient with post-surgical hypoparathyroidism, serum calcium concentration was raised from approximately 8 mg/100 ml to as high as 14.3 mg/100 ml with sustained (4 days) calcium infusions. Urinary phosphorus excretion rose significantly despite a progressive fall in serum phosphorus concentration. However, a marked elevation of serum calcium concentration may decrease, rather than increase, urinary phosphorus excretion (Chambers, et al., 1956; Lavender and Pullman, 1963). In such cases, a decrease in glomerular filtration rate and an increase in tubular reabsorption of phosphorus are usually observed.

The elevation of serum calcium concentration by calcium infusion also affects directly the renal tubular transport of calcium (Bernstein et al., 1963). Renal clearance of calcium increases with the rise in diffusible or ultrafilterable serum calcium concentration. A characteristic response is shown in Figure 8.3. In 3 thyroparathyroidectomized dogs, one-half-hour renal clearances of calcium were obtained at various concentrations of serum calcium achieved with calcium infusion. The calcium clearance ratio, i.e., the percentage of filtered calcium which was excreted, increased with the ultrafilterable serum calcium concentration. The exact mechanism by which calcium infusion modifies the renal tubular transport of cal-

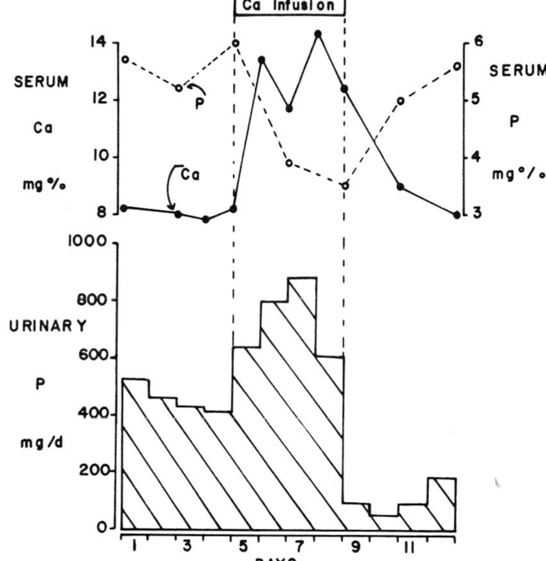

Fig. 8.2. Effect of a long-term (4 days) calcium infusion on serum calcium concentration, urinary phosphorus excretion, and serum phosphorus concentration in a patient with post-operative, hypoparathyroidism.

cium and of phosphorus is not known and is currently being explored in our laboratory.

Effect of parathyroid hormone

The effect of parathyroid hormone on the renal tubular transport of phosphorus and of calcium is widely recognized and will be briefly described here. Parathyroidectomy decreases urinary phosphorus excretion, and the administration of parathyroid extract increases it (Greenwald, 1911; Albright and Ellsworth, 1929; Albright, et al., 1929; Ellsworth and Howard, 1934). These effects preceded, and were not caused by, changes in serum calcium concentration. The increase in urinary phosphorus resulting from the administration of parathyroid hormone far exceeds that resulting from the increase in serum calcium concentration (Ney et al., 1965). Furthermore, when parathyroid hormone is infused into one renal artery

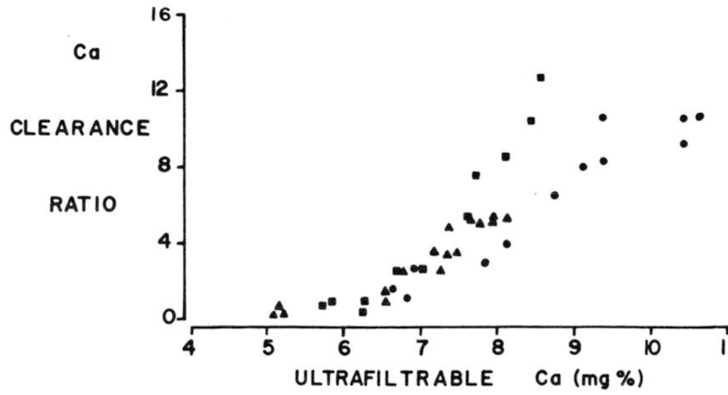

Fig. 8.3. Effect of calcium infusion on renal clearance of calcium in 3 thyroparathyroidectomized dogs. Each dog is designated by a different symbol.

in a dog, that kidney excretes more urinary phosphorus than the control kidney, even though the concentration of calcium in the renal arterial blood is the same for both kidneys (Lavender et al., 1961).

Parathyroid hormone also directly affects the renal tubular transport of calcium: it decreases renal excretion of calcium and increases renal tubular reabsorption of calcium (Talmage and Kraintz, 1954; Buchanan et al., 1959; Kleeman et al., 1961; Bernstein et al., 1963). This effect persists in the absence of any significant change in serum calcium concentration (Eisenberg, 1968). When the serum calcium concentration in patients with hypoparathyroidism was maintained in the normal range by infusion of calcium, the administration of parathyroid hormone markedly decreased the urinary excretion of calcium.

Effect of calcitonin

There is considerable disagreement regarding the role of calcitonin in the renal tubular transport of calcium and phosphorus (Kenny and Heiskell, 1965; Milhaud and Moukhtar, 1966; Rasmussen et al., 1967; Russell and Fleisch, 1967; Higgins et al., 1969; Clark and Kenny, 1969). However, recent studies in our laboratory suggest that this hormone does not have a significant effect on the renal tubular reabsorption of phosphorus (Pak et al., 1969), as shown in Figure 8.4. Eight thyroparathy-

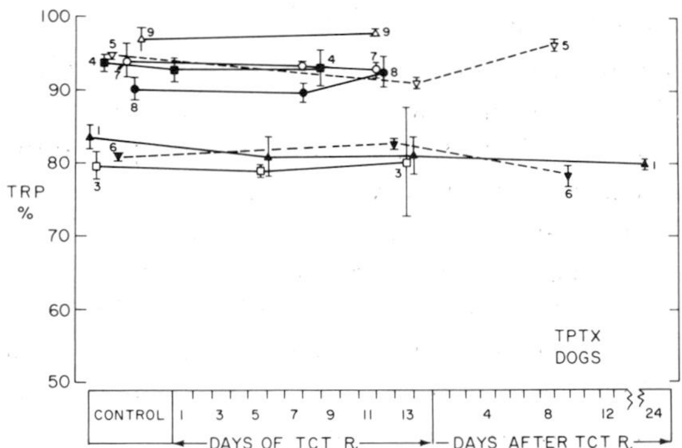

Fig. 8.4. Effect of calcitonin (TCT) on tubular reabsorption of phosphorus in 8 thyroparathyroidectomized (TPTX) dogs. One-hour renal clearances were determined three times during the control period and again at various times during TCT administration (R_x). In three dogs, the renal clearances were repeated after treatment with TCT was stopped. Each dog is designated by a different symbol and number. Values are given as mean ± SE.

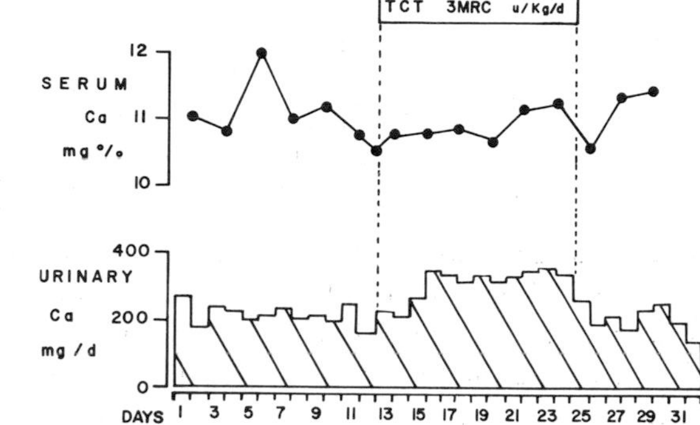

Fig. 8.5. Effect of calcitonin (TCT) on renal tubular transport of calcium in a patient with parathyroid hyperplasia. Dose of calcitonin, given intramuscularly, was 1 MRC unit per kilogram of body weight every 8 hr for 12 days.

roidectomized dogs were maintained on a constant diet of balanced dog food. Each dog received, intramuscularly, 4 MRC units of calcitonin (Armour) per kilogram of body weight, twice a day for 14 days. Renal clearance studies, consisting of 3 one-hour clearances, were performed during the control period and again at various times during and after treatment with calcitonin. There was no significant change in renal tubular transport of phosphorus in any of the 8 dogs. In contrast, in intact dogs, calcitonin caused a significant decrease in tubular reabsorption of phosphorus, presumably through stimulation of parathyroid function.

The effect of calcitonin on the renal tubular transport of calcium is less certain. However, our preliminary evidence suggests that this hormone increases calcium clearance. A daily dose of 3 MRC units of calcitonin per kilogram of body weight was given, intramuscularly, for 12 days to a patient with parathyroid hyperplasia (Fig. 8.5). Despite a slight decrease in serum calcium concentration, urinary calcium excretion nearly doubled during treatment. Since there was no significant change in endogenous creatinine clearance, the fraction of filtered calcium which was excreted and the calcium clearance probably rose with treatment.

Effect of vitamin D

The role of vitamin D in the renal tubular transport of calcium and phosphorus will now be considered in the light of the known effects of changes in serum calcium concentration, of parathyroid hormone, and of calcitonin.

The effect of vitamin D in the renal tubular transport of phosphorus was evaluated in rachitic dogs that were thyroparathyroidectomized (Ney et al., 1968). Thus the influences of parathyroid hormone and of calcitonin were removed. Renal clearance studies were performed 2 hr after the intravenous administration of vitamin D_3, 24 hr after intramuscular administration of vitamin D_2 (100,000 IU), and after 6 or more days of

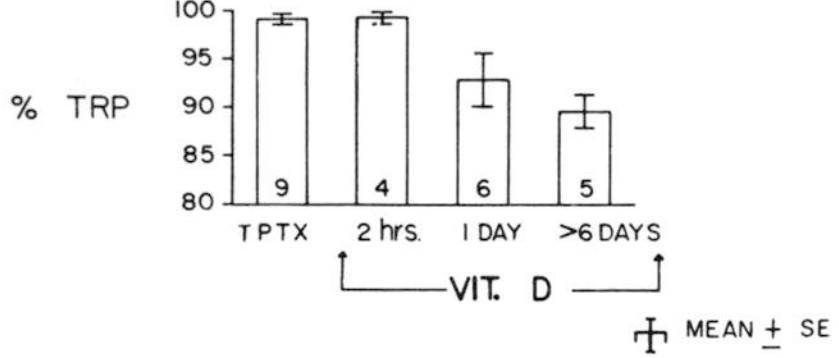

Fig. 8.6. Effect of vitamin D on tubular reabsorption of phosphorus in thyroparathyroidectomized (TPTX) rachitic pups. Numbers within the blocks give the number of dogs studied.

oral administration of vitamin D_2 (30,000 IU per day) (Figure 8.6). Renal tubular reabsorption of phosphorus did not change significantly after 2 hr, but it decreased considerably 1 day after vitamin D was administered. These effects cannot be ascribed entirely to an increase in serum calcium concentration: in 4 of the dogs, vitamin D produced phosphaturia before there was an increase in serum calcium concentration (Fig. 8.7). In these dogs, tubular reabsorption of phosphorus fell despite a decrease or no change in the serum calcium concentration. Figure 8.8 shows the relationship between tubular reabsorption of phosphorus and serum calcium concentration. In these rachitic pups, the tubular reabsorption of phosphorus did not change significantly with increases in serum calcium concentration. However, at a similar concentration of serum calcium, the tubular reabsorption of phosphorus was generally lower during vitamin D administration than prior to it. These conclusions support a hypothesis

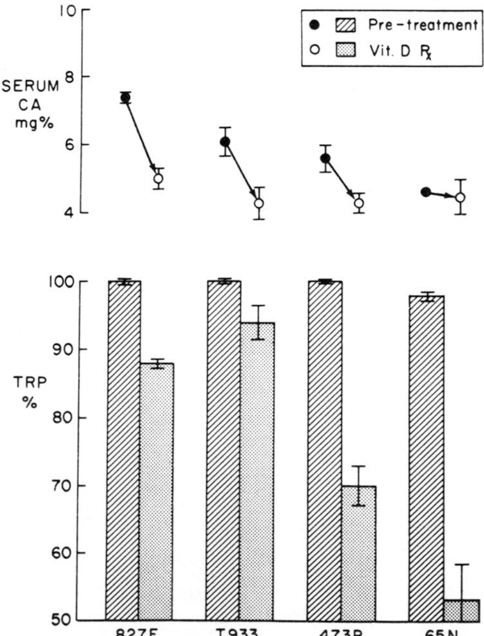

Fig. 8.7. Effect of vitamin D on tubular reabsorption of phosphorus in 4 thyroparathyroidectomized rachitic pups, before serum calcium concentration increased. Values are given as mean ± SE.

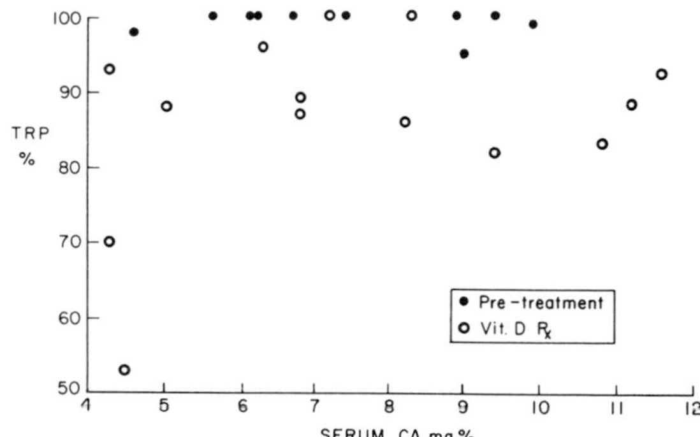

Fig. 8.8. Effect of vitamin D on tubular reabsorption of phosphorus in 10 thyroparathyroidectomized rachitic pups.

suggested by renal clearance studies of thyroparathyroidectomized rats (Crawford et al., 1955), and by studies of thyroparathyroidectomized, nonrachitic, fully grown dogs.

In the thyroparathyroidectomized, nonrachitic, fully grown dogs, the tubular reabsorption of phosphorus was determined at various concentrations of serum calcium achieved by calcium infusion. Unlike the rachitic pups, the tubular reabsorption of phosphorus in these dogs decreased with increases in serum calcium concentration. After 50,000 IU of vitamin D_2 was administered intramuscularly daily for 3 days, the tubular reabsorption of phosphorus at similar concentrations of serum calcium was considerably lower than before administration of vitamin D (Fig. 8.9).

In contrast to the phosphaturic response to vitamin D, the renal clearance of calcium is probably not directly influenced by this vitamin. In patients with hypoparathyroidism, the fraction of filtered calcium which is excreted is essentially the same at the same concentration of serum

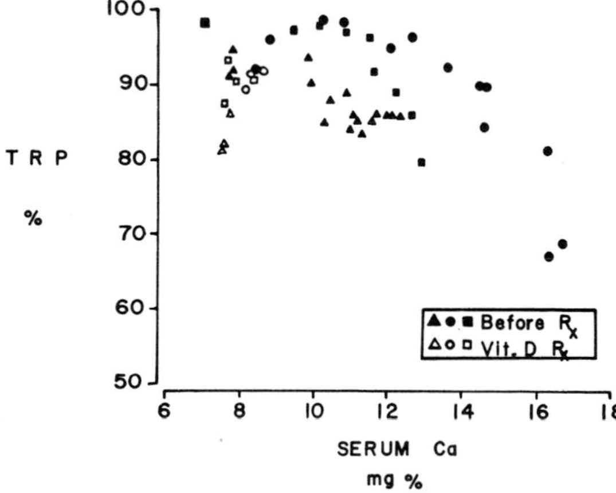

Fig. 8.9. Effect of vitamin D on tubular reabsorption of phosphorus in 3 thyroparathyroidectomized nonrachitic dogs. Each dog is designated by a different symbol.

calcium, whether it is produced by calcium infusion or by vitamin D (Bernstein et al., 1963).

In summary, the role of vitamin D in the renal tubular transport of calcium and of phosphorus was examined by separating the effects of vitamin D alone from those caused by changes in serum calcium concentration and secretion of parathyroid hormone and calcitonin which may follow the administration of vitamin D. An elevation in serum calcium concentration increases the renal clearance of calcium and phosphorus independently of parathyroid hormone and of calcitonin. Parathyroid hormone increases the clearance of phosphorus and decreases that of calcium. Calcitonin does not affect phosphorus clearance in the dog, but it appears to increase calcium clearance in man.

In evaluating the renal effects of vitamin D, the influences of parathyroid hormone and calcitonin were removed by evaluating the action of the vitamin in patients or dogs that had been thyroparathyroidectomized. The effect of changes in serum calcium concentration was studied by examining the renal clearances of calcium and phosphorus at similar serum calcium concentrations before and during administration of vitamin D. Under these circumstances, vitamin D was shown to increase renal clearance of phosphorus in the dog and not to affect the clearance of calcium in man.

References

Albright, F., W. Bauer, M. Ropes, and J. C. Aub. 1929. Studies of calcium and phosphorus metabolism. IV. The effect of the parathyroid hormone. *J. Clin. Invest.* 7:139.

Albright, F., and R. Ellsworth. 1929. Studies on the physiology of the parathyroid glands. I. Calcium and phosphorus studies on a case of idiopathic hypoparathyroidism. *J. Clin. Invest.* 7:183.

Bartter, F. C. 1970. Vitamin D, parathyroid hormone and the kidney. *In* C. Rouiller and A. F. Muller (eds.), *The Kidney.* Academic Press, New York. (In press.)

Bernstein, D., C. R. Kleeman, and M. H. Maxwell. 1963. The effect of calcium infusions, parathyroid hormone, and vitamin D on renal clearance of calcium. *Proc. Soc. Exp. Biol. Med.* 112:253.

Buchanan, G. D., F. W. Kraintz, and R. V. Talmage. 1959. Renal excretion of calcium and phosphate in the mouse as influenced by parathyroids. *Proc. Soc. Exp. Biol. Med.* 101:306.

Chambers, E. L., Jr., G. T. Gordan, L. Goldman, and E. C. Reifenstein, Jr. 1956. Tests for hyperparathyroidism: tubular reabsorption of phosphate, phosphate deprivation, and calcium infusion. *J. Clin. Endocrinol.* 16:1507.

Clark, J. D., and A. D. Kenny. 1969. Hog thyrocalcitonin in the dog: urinary calcium, phosphorus, magnesium and sodium responses. *Endocrinology 84*:1199.

Crawford, J. D., D. Bribety, N. B. Talbot, M. Terry, E. A. Maclachlon, K. Van Loon, and M. F. Morrill. 1955. Mechanism of renal tubular phosphate reabsorption and the influence thereon of vitamin D in completely parathyroidectomized rats. *Amer. J. Physiol. 180*:156.

Eisenberg, E. 1965. Effects of serum calcium level and parathyroid extracts on phosphate and calcium excretion in hypoparathyroid patients. *J. Clin. Invest. 44*:942.

Eisenberg, E. 1968. Renal effects of parathyroid hormone, p. 465. *In* R. V. Talmage, and L. F. Belanger (eds.), *Parathyroid Hormone and Thyrocalcitonin (Calcitonin)*. Excerpta Medica Foundation, New York.

Ellsworth, R., and J. E. Howard. 1934. Studies on the physiology of parathyroid glands. VII. Some responses of normal human kidneys and blood to intravenous parathyroid extract. *Bull. Johns Hopkins Hosp. 55*:296.

Greenwald, I. 1911. The effect of parathyroidectomy upon metabolism. *Amer. J. Physiol. 28*:103.

Higgins, J. T., Jr., D. M. Smith, and C. C. Johnston, Jr. 1969. Unilateral renal arterial infusion of thyrocalcitonin in the dog. *Clin. Res. 17*:286.

Howard, J. E., T. R. Hopkins, and T. B. Connor. 1952. The use of intravenous calcium as a measure of activity of the parathyroid glands. *Trans. Ass. Amer. Physicians 65*:351.

Howard, J. E., T. R. Hopkins, and T. B. Connor. 1953. On certain physiologic responses to intravenous injection of calcium salts into normal hyperparathyroid and hypoparathyroid persons. *J. Clin. Endocrinol. 13*:1.

Kenny, A. D., and C. A. Heiskell. 1965. Effect of crude thyrocalcitonin on calcium and phosphorous metabolism in rats. *Proc. Soc. Exp. Biol. Med. 120*:269.

Kleeman, C. R., D. Bernstein, R. Rockney, J. T. Dowling, and M. H. Maxwell. 1961. Studies on the renal clearance of diffusible calcium and the role of the parathyroid glands in its regulation, p. 353. *In* R. O. Greep and R. V. Talmage (eds.), *The Parathyroids*. Charles C Thomas, Springfield, Ill.

Lavender, A. R., and T. N. Pullman. 1963. Changes in inorganic phosphate excretion induced by renal arterial infusion of calcium. *Amer. J. Physiol. 205*:1025.

Lavender, A. R., T. N. Pullman, H. Rasmussen, and I. Aho. 1961. Studies on the intrarenal effects of parathyroid hormone, p. 406. *In* R. O. Greep and R. V. Talmage (eds.), *The Parathyroids*. Charles C Thomas, Springfield, Ill.

Milhaud, G., and M. S. Moukhtar. 1966. Antagonistic and synergistic actions of thyrocalcitonin and parathyroid hormone on the levels of calcium and phosphate in the rat. *Nature 211*:1186.

Ney, R. L., W. Au, G. Kelly, I. Radde, and F. C. Bartter. 1965. Actions of parathyroid hormone in the vitamin D–deficient dog. *J. Clin. Invest. 44*:2003.

Ney, R. L., G. Kelly, and F. C. Bartter. 1968. Actions of vitamin D independent of the parathyroid glands. *Endocrinology 82*:760.

Nordin, B. E. C., and R. Fraser. 1954. The effects of intravenous calcium on phosphate excretion. *Clin. Sci. 13*:477.

Pak, C. Y. C., B. Ruskin, and A. Casper. 1969. Renal effects of thyrocalcitonin, p. 154. *In* S. Taylor (ed.), *Proceedings of the Second International Symposium on Calcitonin and the C Cells.* Heinemann Medical Books, London.

Rasmussen, H., C. Anast, and C. Arnaud. 1967. Thyrocalcitonin, EGTA, and urinary electrolyte excretion. *J. Clin. Invest. 46*:746.

Russell, R. G. G., and H. Fleisch. 1967. The renal effects of thyrocalcitonin in the pig and dog, p. 297. *In* M. Selwin Taylor (ed.), *Calcitonin. Proceedings of the Symposium on Thyrocalcitonin and the C Cells.* Springer-Verlag, New York.

Talmage, R. V., and F. W. Kraintz. 1954. Progressive changes in renal phosphate and calcium excretion in rats following parathyroidectomy or parathyroid administration. *Proc. Soc. Exp. Biol. Med. 87*:263.

9

PHYSIOLOGIC EFFECTS OF VITAMIN D, PARATHYROID HORMONE, AND CALCITONIN

Mark J. Melancon, Jr., H. Morii, and H. F. DeLuca

In discussing the interrelation between vitamin D, parathyroid hormone (PTH), and calcitonin (CT), a good starting point is the enumeration of the well established effects of these three calcium homeostatic agents (Table 9.1). A consideration of the time course of their responses

TABLE 9.1. *Physiological effects of vitamin D, PTH, and CT*

Vitamin D	Increases bone resorption Increases intestinal absorption of calcium and secondarily of phosphate
Parathyroid hormone	Increases bone resorption Increases calcium absorption by kidney Increases phosphate excretion by kidney
Calcitonin	Decreases bone resorption

immediately points to similarities and differences in their modes of action. When vitamin D is injected into vitamin D–deficient rats, there is an 8–12 hr lag before intestinal transport of calcium is significantly increased and a 12–16 hr delay before bone mobilization sufficient to raise serum calcium occurs. Even when 25–hydroxycholecalciferol, the probable metabolically active form of vitamin D_3, is administered, a number of hours is required for these effects to be exhibited (Blunt et al., 1968). As has been well established, this time is required for a sequence of RNA and protein synthetic events required to manifest the action of vitamin D.

These studies were supported by a contract from the United States Atomic Energy Commission, AT (11-1)–1668.

On the other hand, the effects of PTH on phosphate excretion by the kidney are discernible in 5–10 min (Beutner and Munson, 1960). The substantial effects of both PTH and CT on bone, as monitored by urinary hydroxyproline, are presently measurable at 1 hr (Pechet et al., 1967; Rasmussen et al., 1968), but might well be as rapid as the kidney effect. In either case, it is obvious that there is no lag nor any evidence of protein synthesis occurring before the actions of PTH or CT are manifested (DeLuca et al., 1968).

Dependence of PTH–induced bone mobilization but not phosphate diuresis on vitamin D

One of the questions studied recently concerning the interrelation between vitamin D and PTH is whether or not PTH can function without the presence of vitamin D. On the basis of data obtained from studies utilizing isolated mitochondria (DeLuca et al., 1962; Sallis et al., 1963), it was suggested by Rasmussen and co-workers (1963) that PTH might be able to exert its usual effects in causing phosphate excretion in the absence of vitamin D but that vitamin D was required for PTH to mediate calcium mobilization from bone. To examine this possibility, weanling rats were fed a purified vitamin D–free diet (DeLuca et al., 1961), with or without a normal vitamin D supplement. After three to four weeks of this dietary regimen, the vitamin D–deficient rats exhibited low serum calcium values and retarded growth. At this time the rats were injected with PTH. The data in Table 9.2 show that the serum calcium levels of the vitamin D–deficient rats were almost completely unaffected by PTH, requiring a massive dose of 2000 U.S.P. units of hormone to obtain an elevation in serum calcium. Serum phosphate rose rapidly after parathyroidectomy (Fig. 9.1). Thus, although endogenous PTH had a substantial effect on phosphate diuresis in the vitamin D–deficient rat, doses of 25–500 U.S.P. units of the hormone, sufficient to give large elevations of serum calcium in rats possessing normal amounts of the vitamin, were without effect in vitamin D–deficient rats. It appeared, therefore, that PTH could affect phosphate excretion by the kidney but could not affect bone mobilization in vitamin D–deficient rats.

Harrison and associates (1958) reported that vitamin D–deficient rats showed no serum calcium rise after being injected with 200 U.S.P. units of parathyroid extract (PTE). If 100 IU of vitamin D was given 48 hr before the PTE, there was a normal response to the hormone. Thus PTE was unable to induce bone mobilization in vitamin D deficiency. In addition, although PTE had little if any effect in lowering serum phosphate in the vitamin D–deficient rats, it did in fact lower serum phosphate when the

TABLE 9.2. *Effect of PTH on plasma calcium in vitamin D–fed and vitamin D–deficient rats*

Treatment	Plasma calcium (mg/100 ml)
Vitamin D–fed rats	
Control	10.6 ± 0.8
25 U.S.P. units PTH	11.6 ± 0.6[a]
100 U.S.P. units PTH	12.1 ± 0.8[b]
2000 U.S.P. units PTH	17.5 ± 0.9[b]
Vitamin D–deficient rats	
Control	6.9 ± 0.3
100 U.S.P. units PTH	6.8 ± 0.4
500 U.S.P. units PTH	7.1 ± 0.4
2000 U.S.P. units PTH	10.7 ± 0.2[b]

Source: Rasmussen et al. (1963).

Notes: The plasma was obtained 6 hr after PTH was injected. There were 8 animals in each group.

Values are given as mean ± SE.

[a] $P < 0.05$ when compared with controls.

[b] $P < 0.01$ when compared with controls.

rats were pretreated with vitamin D. Thus it appeared that the kidney was also refractory to PTH in vitamin D deficiency. To corroborate this, Harrison and Harrison (1964) later reported measurements of urinary phosphate in similar experiments. PTH or vitamin D alone had little effect on urinary phosphate, but when the rats were pretreated with vitamin D, PTH caused about a three-fold increase in urinary phosphate during the 6-hr period after PTH was injected. The two sets of experiments were in agreement that bone is not responsive to PTH in vitamin D deficiency,

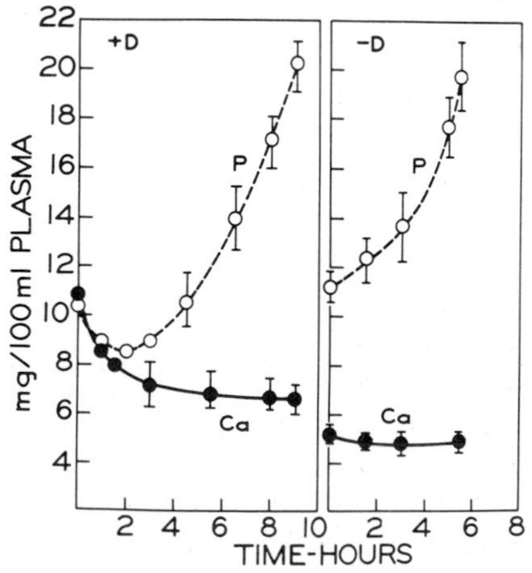

Fig. 9.1. Effect of PTX by electric cautery on serum calcium and phosphate of vitamin D-fed rats receiving a low-calcium diet (left) and of vitamin D–deficient rats receiving a normal-calcium diet (right). (Rasmussen et al., 1963. Reproduced by permission of the *Journal of Clinical Investigation.*)

but were not in agreement as to whether or not the kidney was refractory to PTH under these conditions.

Arnaud and associates (1966), in a series of perfusion studies in thyroparathyroidectomized vitamin D–deficient rats, showed that PTH was able to increase urinary phosphate and to decrease urinary calcium. It did appear, however, that there was a trend toward decreased responsiveness of the kidney to PTH in vitamin D deficiency. Evidently, parathyroidectomized vitamin D–deficient rats exhibit PTH-induced phosphate diuresis, whereas intact animals do not. The difference is probably due to a high level of circulating endogenous PTH in the intact vitamin D–deficient rats already affecting this system to near-maximal levels. An additional factor is the decreased ability of the kidney to excrete phosphate during hypocalcemia, a matter which has been discussed recently by Eisenberg (1968).

There have been reports of PTH inducing bone mobilization in vitamin D–deficient mice (Nichols et al., 1963), dogs (Ney et al., 1965), and rats (Toverud, 1964). These observations of PTH effects in vitamin D–deficient mice and dogs may be due to species differences, and the results in rats have been questioned in regard to the degree of vitamin D deficiency achieved. Rasmussen and associates (1963) showed that as little as 0.3 IU of vitamin D restored PTH responsiveness to vitamin D–deficient rats (Table 9.3). These results indicate the extreme degree of vitamin D depletion required to eliminate responsiveness to PTH.

Thus it appears that, in a truly vitamin D–deficient rat, PTH cannot mobilize bone but can affect the handling of calcium and phosphate by the kidney. This is not unreasonable in view of the fact that bone is a

TABLE 9.3. *Effect of small amounts of vitamin D on PTH responsiveness in vitamin D–deficient rats*

	Plasma calcium (mg/100 ml)	
Treatment	Mock surgery	Parathyroidectomy
Control	4.9	4.8
0.05 IU × 6[a]	7.4	4.6
0.5 IU × 6[a]	10.5	8.7
1000 IU[b]	10.6	8.6

Source: Rasmussen et al. (1963).

Note: Vitamin D–deficient rats were fed a 0.47% Ca^{++}, 0.3% P diet for 3–4 weeks. Rats were parathyroidectomized by electric cautery or were given mock surgery; rats were killed 6 hr later for serum calcium analysis.

[a] Indicated dosage of vitamin D given daily for 6 days.

[b] Dosage of vitamin D given 48 hr before surgery.

target tissue of vitamin D, while such has not been demonstrated for the kidney.

Lack of vitamin D dependence on calcitonin inhibition of bone mobilization

A few years ago we made a study of the action of CT and PTH alone and together in vitamin D–deficient rats (Morii and DeLuca, 1967). Weanling rats were made vitamin D deficient as described earlier (DeLuca et al., 1961) and used 4–5 weeks later. The data presented in Table 9.4 show that, as expected, thyroparathyroidectomy (TPTX) had no effect on serum calcium. However, CT was able to reduce even further the low serum calcium of vitamin D deficiency. Of great interest was the observation that this hypocalcemia was transient in the intact rats but was maintained indefinitely in the TPTX rats. This result suggested that endogenous PTH was somehow counteracting the effect of CT, even in vitamin D–deficient animals. The lack of effect of PTH on serum calcium in TPTX vitamin D–deficient rats is shown in Table 9.5. The table shows that exogenous PTH was able to prevent the hypocalcemic action of CT. The ability of CT to lower the serum phosphate under these conditions is shown in Table 9.6, in which data are presented showing that the phosphatemia after TPTX in both vitamin D–deficient and vitamin D–repleted rats is similarly reduced by CT. Thus, although PTH does not affect serum calcium unless either vitamin D or CT is present, CT can lower serum calcium and phosphate in the complete absence of vitamin D and PTH. PTH can, however, prevent the hypocalcemic action of CT in vitamin D–deficient rats. In other words, CT can reduce bone mobilization even

TABLE 9.4. *Effect of CT on serum calcium in vitamin D–deficient rats*

	Serum calcium (mg/100 ml)[a]			
Treatment	Before	After 1 hr	After 2 hr	After 4 hr
CT[b]	4.5 ± 0.3[c,d] (6)	3.4 ± 0.1[c] (6)	3.5 ± 0.2[d] (5)	4.5 ± 0.3 (7)
TPTX	—	4.1 ± 0.2 (5)	4.3 ± 0.3[c] (4)	4.3 ± 0.3[e] (4)
TPTX + CT[b]	—	3.7 ± 0.3 (6)	2.9 ± 0.2[c] (6)	2.8 ± 0.2[e] (6)

Source: Morii and DeLuca (1967).

Note: Values are given as mean ± SE. Numbers in parentheses are the number of rats in each group.

[a] By time after surgery and/or injection.

[b] 5.5 units of CT per 180 g of body weight injected subcutaneously.

[c] $P < 0.005$.

[d] $P < 0.025$.

[e] $P < 0.01$.

TABLE 9.5. *Effect of CT and/or PTH on serum calcium in vitamin D–deficient thyroparathyroidectomized rats*

Treatment	Serum calcium (mg/100 ml)[a]			
	Before	After 2 hr	After 4 hr	After 6 hr
Control	4.2 ± 0.2 (9)	3.7 ± 0.1[d] (8)	3.5 ± 0.2[e] (5)	3.6 ± 0.2[e] (5)
CT[b]	4.1 ± 0.1 (5)	2.7 ± 0.1[d] (4)	2.8 ± 0.1[e] (5)	2.9 ± 0.1[e] (5)
PTH[c]	4.2 ± 0.2 (5)	4.1 ± 0.2 (5)	4.1 ± 0.3 (5)	4.0 ± 0.5 (5)
CT[b] + PTH[c]	4.1 ± 0.2 (7)	3.5 ± 0.3 (6)	3.7 ± 0.3 (4)	3.9 ± 0.3 (4)

Source: Morii and DeLuca (1967).

Notes: Vitamin D–deficient rats were thyroparathyroidectomized and immediately given the indicated injection.

Values are given as mean ± SE. Numbers in parentheses are the number of rats in each group.

[a] By time after injection or (for control rats) after thyroparathyroidectomy.

[b] 5.5 units of CT per 180 g of body weight injected subcutaneously.

[c] 50 units of PTH (Eli Lilly) per 180 g of body weight injected subcutaneously.

[d] $P < 0.005$.

[e] $P < 0.025$.

in vitamin D deficiency, while PTH can only act to prevent this reduction by CT.

Summary of interrelationships between vitamin D, PTH, and CT

These observations led to the formulation of a model of bone mobilization which we have proposed (DeLuca et al., 1968) to explain the effects of vitamin D, of PTH, and of CT (Fig. 9.2). Vitamin D gives rise to a system that mobilizes, or transports, calcium. Further movement out of the cell of calcium mobilized by vitamin D is mediated by PTH and CT. PTH increases "calcium permeability" of the cell membrane, and CT decreases calcium permeability. Under normal circumstances – i.e., PTH and CT both absent in a vitamin D–sufficient animal – the permeability of this cell membrane would be the limiting factor in the transfer of calcium from bone to blood. However, in vitamin D deficiency, the reduced amount

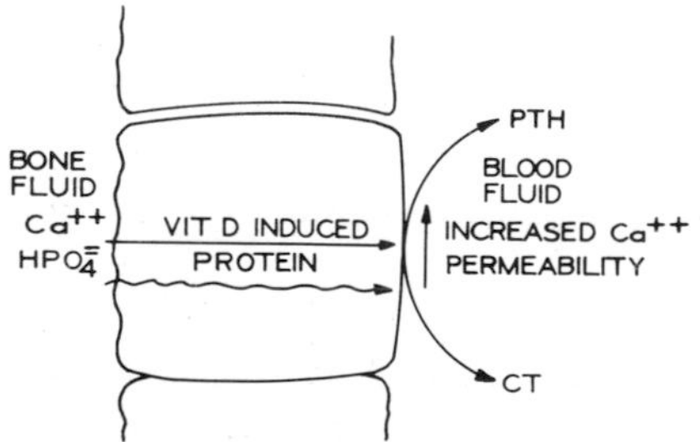

Fig. 9.2. Proposed model of actions of vitamin D, PTH, and CT on bone mobilization. (DeLuca et al., 1968. Reproduced by permission of the Excerpta Medica Foundation.)

TABLE 9.6. *Effect of CT on serum phosphate in thyroparathyroidectomized rats*

Experimental conditions	Serum phosphate (mg/100 ml)[a] Before	After 4 hr	After 5 hr[b]	After 7 hr[c]
Vitamin D–deficient rats				
Control	10.6 ± 0.9 (5)	12.0 ± 1.0 (4)	13.4 ± 0.8 (3)	14.0 ± 0.2 (2)
CT[d]	11.2 ± 0.5 (8)	13.7 ± 0.5[e] (8)	12.2 ± 0.3[e] (5)	14.9 ± 0.5 (7)
Vitamin D–fed rats				
Control	11.0 ± 0.3 (6)	13.1 ± 0.2 (6)	13.4 ± 0.7 (6)	14.1 ± 0.4 (5)
CT[d]	10.3 ± 0.2 (7)	13.3 ± 0.4[f] (7)	11.1 ± 0.7[f] (5)	12.4 ± 0.4 (5)

Source: Morii and DeLuca (1967).

Notes: 7 Hirsch units of vitamin D_3 was given *per os* three times every week.

Values are given as mean ± SE. Numbers in parentheses are the number of rats in each group.

[a] By time after thyroparathyroidectomy.

[b] 1 hr after CT injection.

[c] 3 hr after CT injection.

[d] 5.5 units of CT per 180 g of body weight injected subcutaneously.

[e] $P < 0.05$.

[f] $P < 0.025$.

of bone mobilization is the limiting factor. The addition of CT to the deficient animal sufficiently reduces the permeability of the cell membrane to calcium, and again makes it the limiting factor. It is this effect of CT that PTH can counteract even in the vitamin D–deficient animal.

Other reports on the interrelation of vitamin D, PTH, and CT

Another report of interest concerning the interrelation of vitamin D, PTH, and CT is the report of Au and Raisz (1967) which indicates that dietary lactose or calcium injections can restore PTH responsiveness in vitamin D–deficient rats. They found that dietary lactose or calcium injections can raise the serum calcium levels of vitamin D–deficient rats, that these levels fall after parathyroidectomy (PTX), and that PTH can restore them to pre-PTX levels. In our laboratory the effects of dietary lactose and calcium injections on the serum calcium levels in vitamin D–deficient rats have been duplicated, but as yet we cannot comment on the PTH responsiveness of the rats. In their perfusion studies, Arnaud and associates (1966) were unable to obtain an increase in serum calcium induced by PTH in vitamin D–deficient rats that were perfused to elevate their serum calcium to normal levels. As an explanation of their observations of PTH responsiveness, Au and Raisz have suggested that an early step in PTH action may involve its causing calcium to enter the cell and that, in vitamin D–deficient rats, with uncalcified osteoid and low serum calcium, this step may not be possible. It would seem advisable to reserve judgment on this hypothesis until it is determined whether the elevation in serum calcium elevation caused by PTH is due to increased intestinal absorption of calcium or is due to release of cellular calcium, or whether it is indeed an indication of bone mobilization.

Action of physiologic and pharmacologic amounts of vitamin D in the absence of PTH

Although very small amounts of vitamin D enable PTH to maintain normal serum calcium, physiological levels of vitamin D alone cannot do so. Obviously then, physiologic amounts of the vitamin also require the presence of PTH for the manifestation of its action on bone mobilization. This is well known from the fact that lowered serum calcium occurs after PTX of normal rats. However, the ability of large amounts of vitamin D to maintain reasonable serum calcium levels in the presence of little or no PTH has been demonstrated by the use of vitamin D in hypoparathyroidism, whether surgical or otherwise. We have shown in surgically thyroparathyroidectomized rats that 20,000 IU of vitamin D per day can maintain normal serum calcium levels even without calcium in the diet, although the serum calcium level drops rapidly when the high dosage of vitamin D is stopped (DeLuca et al., 1968) (Fig. 9.3). The ability of vitamin D to act alone in this manner probably depends upon a pharmacological action of the vitamin that is distinct from its physiological effects. Zull and associates (1966) have shown that actinomycin did not block the effect of 40,000 IU of vitamin D on calcium permeability in everted duodenal sacs or the release of calcium by isolated mitochondria, although actinomycin was fully able to block physiologic responses to the vitamin. It thus appears that possibly a pharmacological action of vitamin D enables the vitamin to bind directly to membranes and thus increase calcium permeability. Serum phosphate (Fig. 9.4) was reduced by the vitamin D treat-

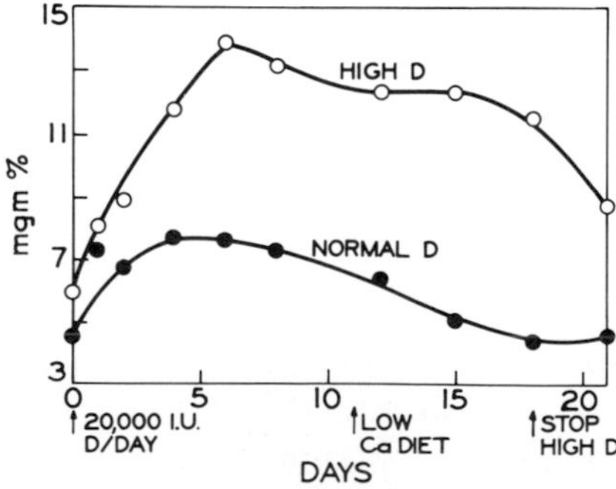

Fig. 9.3. Serum calcium of TPTX rats given normal and high levels of vitamin D. Rats fed a diet containing normal amounts of vitamin D, calcium, and phosphate. Three days after TPTX, some rats received 20,000 IU of vitamin D per day orally. Where indicated, all rats were placed on a low-calcium diet. (DeLuca et al., 1968. Reproduced by permission of Excerpta Medica Foundation.)

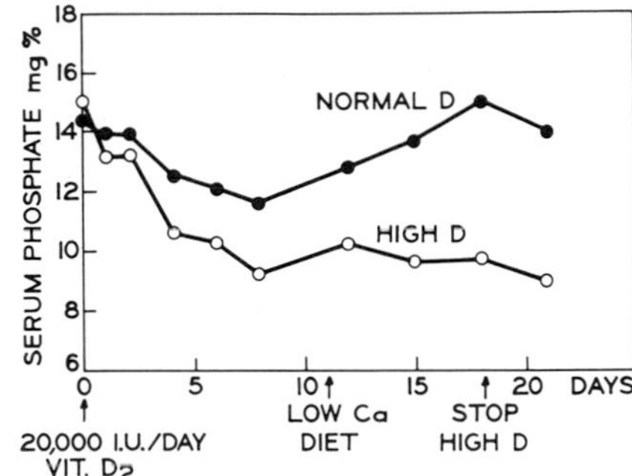

Fig. 9.4. Serum phosphate of TPTX rats given normal and high levels of vitamin D. Conditions were as described in the legend to Figure 9.3.

ment and remained at this more reasonable level even when the vitamin D intake was reduced to normal levels for 3 or more days.

Control of vitamin D–induced hypercalcemia by endogenous calcitonin

Of greater interest, however, was the result obtained when vitamin D was given before surgery. In such a case, a daily dose of 40,000 IU of vitamin D for 3–4 days caused a slight elevation of serum calcium in rats. After TPTX, there was an additional, transient elevation of serum calcium in these animals (Fig. 9.5), and serum phosphate also increased. Because of the negative feedback mechanism of PTH secretion, one might expect that levels of circulating PTH would be very low and therefore that there would be no change in serum calcium after PTX. This result, however, suggests that thyroid removal and thus the action of endogenous CT might be important. There was, in fact, no change in serum calcium and only a small increase in serum phosphate 8 hr after surgical PTX in the rats with a high vitamin D content (Table 9.7) (Melancon and DeLuca, 1969). Thyroidectomy subsequent to PTX produced a result similar to TPTX. It had been reported that CT could reduce the hypercalcemia of hypervitaminosis D (Gudmundsson et al., 1965; Mittleman et al., 1967).

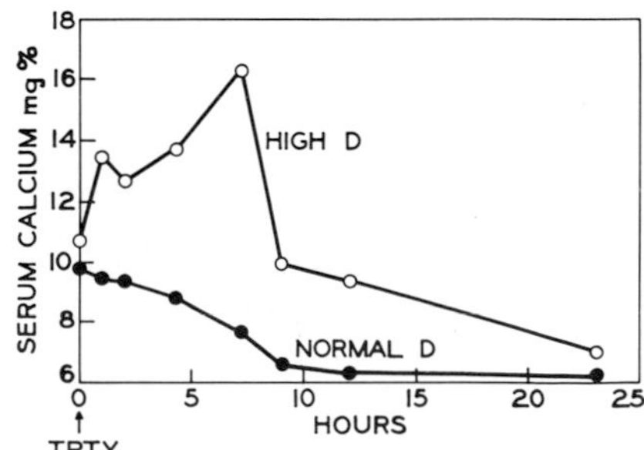

Fig. 9.5. Serum calcium in calcium-depleted rats given normal levels (lower curve) or high levels (upper curve) of vitamin D. All rats were fed a low-calcium diet for 4–5 days, some were then given 40,000 IU of vitamin D_3 daily for 3 days, and then all rats were TPTX. (DeLuca et al., 1968. Reproduced by permission of Excerpta Medica Foundation.)

TABLE 9.7. *Serum calcium and phosphate levels after thyroparathyroidectomy or parathyroidectomy ± thyroidectomy of rats given high levels of vitamin D*

	Serum calcium (mg/100 ml)[a]			Serum prosphate (mg/100 ml)[a]		
Treatment	At 0 hr	After 3½ hr	After 7 hr	At 0 hr	After 3½ hr	After 7 hr
Initially intact rats						
Control ($n = 5$)	9.7 ± 0.4	9.3 ± 0.3	9.9 ± 0.5	9.3 ± 0.3	9.9 ± 0.4	8.9 ± 0.4
Mock surgery ($n = 4$)	9.8 ± 0.8	9.7 ± 0.4	9.4 ± 0.2	9.2 ± 0.4	9.5 ± 0.3	9.4 ± 0.3
TPTX ($n = 4$)	9.4 ± 0.6	11.1 ± 0.5[c]	11.9 ± 0.6[c]	10.3 ± 0.5	10.0 ± 0.7[c]	16.4 ± 1.0[c]
Parathyroidectomized rats[b]						
+ THYRX ($n = 5$)	9.9 ± 0.4	9.4 ± 0.6	12.0 ± 0.8[d]	10.7 ± 0.6	11.9 ± 0.9	16.9 ± 3.1[d]
+ Mock surgery ($n = 5$)	10.5 ± 0.3	9.3 ± 0.3	9.3 ± 0.2	10.6 ± 0.3	11.7 ± 0.5	11.1 ± 0.3

Notes: Normal rats were given a daily dose of 40,000 IU of vitamin D for 3–4 days before the experiments. Rats that had been parathyroidectomized 8 hr previously were either thyroidectomized (THYRX) or given mock surgery. Intact rats were either thyroparathyroidectomized, given mock surgery, or given no treatment.

Values are given as mean ± SE.

[a] By time after surgery or (for control rats) after initial blood sample.

[b] Rats had been parathyroidectomized 8 hr previously.

[c] On the basis of 3 rats.

[d] On the basis of 4 rats.

In this case (Table 9.8) exogenous CT also prevented hypercalcemia in addition to preventing hyperphosphatemia. PTH caused an additional hypercalcemia while preventing the rise in serum phosphate. When both hormones were given, the serum calcium was the same as when neither was used; however, not only was the rise in serum phosphate prevented, but its level was actually reduced. These observations, coupled with data on urinary calcium and phosphate, give a clear picture. CT, by reducing the effects of TPTX on serum calcium and phosphate, caused a slight reduction in their excretion. PTH elevated serum calcium levels, but

TABLE 9.8. *Effect of CT and PTH in thyroparathyroidectomized rats given high levels of Vitamin D*

	Serum calcium (mg/100 ml)[a]		Serum phosphate (mg/100 ml)[a]		Total urine calcium	Total urine phosphate
Injection	At 0 hr	After 6 hr	At 0 hr	After 6 hr	(mg)	(mg)
Vehicle	9.7 ± 0.2	13.3 ± 0.3	11.6 ± 0.2	13.5 ± 0.2	1.1	6.0
CT[b]	9.8 ± 0.5	8.8 ± 0.8	12.1 ± 0.3	11.6 ± 0.4	0.8	4.2
PTH[c]	10.1 ± 0.4	15.3 ± 0.4	12.5 ± 0.8	11.3 ± 1.4	1.0	10.1
CT + PTH[d]	9.2 ± 0.5	12.9 ± 0.2	10.9 ± 1.0	8.1 ± 0.5	0.3	13.4

Source: Some of this data has appeared in Melancon and DeLuca (1969).

Notes: Normal rats that had been given a daily dose of 40,000 IU of vitamin D for 3 days were thyroparathyroidectomized. Immediately after, and at 1½ hr, 3 hr, and 4½ hr after surgery, they received 1 ml of water by stomach tube and were injected with vehicle (dilute acetic acid) alone or the appropriate hormone solution.

Values are given by mean ± SE. All values represent the results of 3 rats.

[a] By time after thyroparathyroidectomy.

[b] 110 μg (26 mMRC units) of CT given in each of the three injections.

[c] 180 μg (about 20 U.S.P. units) of PTH given in each of the three injections.

[d] 115 μg of CT and 184 μg of PTH given in each of the three injections.

did not significantly affect urinary calcium because it also increased calcium resorption by the kidney. The PTH-induced phosphate diuretic effect is also obvious. When both hormones were given together, their effects on bone offset each other, whereas the effects of PTH on the handling of calcium and phosphate by the kidney are again obvious. Thus these hormones appear to be working normally in the animals with a high vitamin D content. It also appears from these data that PTH is not being secreted in the rats with a high vitamin D content and that a balance between the action of high levels of vitamin D and of endogenous CT is responsible for maintaining serum calcium under these conditions.

Cyclic adenosine monophosphate and PTH action

A recent development which bears on this discussion of PTH action is the relation of cyclic 3′,5′-adenosine monophosphate (CAMP) to the actions of PTH and CT. A number of relationships between PTH and CAMP, both in vivo and in vitro, have been demonstrated by Chase and Aurbach (1967, 1968*a*, 1968*b*), while Wells and Lloyd (1967, 1968*a*, 1968*b*) have shown that agents which mediate CAMP cause changes in serum calcium. The agreement between PTH and CAMP in these studies seems too precise to be merely fortuitous. The data of Rasmussen and associates (1968), which show that urinary responses to PTH and to dibutyryl-CAMP are different, and the data of Raisz and Klein (1969), which show that tissue culture responses to PTH and CAMP differ, indicate that mediating CAMP levels may only be one of the cellular effects of these hormones.

Summary

Vitamin D is required for PTH-dependent bone resorption. Likewise, the effect of physiologic amounts of vitamin D on bone resorption requires that PTH also be present. At high levels of vitamin D, however, PTH is not required for vitamin D–induced bone mobilization. It is likely that vitamin D exerts a direct pharmacologic effect on membranes and therefore permits high levels of bone mobilization without PTH.

CT can decrease bone mobilization induced by vitamin D or by PTH and, in addition, can depress bone mobilization even when these two agents are absent.

PTH can increase bone mobilization in the presence of normal or large amounts of vitamin D. It can also counteract the effect of CT to depress bone mobilization, whether or not vitamin D is present. PTH can increase calcium resorption by the kidney and decrease phosphate resorption by the kidney, whether or not vitamin D is present. However, in intact vitamin D–deficient rats, which have low serum calcium and high levels of circulating PTH, these effects may not be readily observable. A cellular model of bone mobilization has been suggested to take into account the action of all three homeostatic agents.

References

Arnaud, C., H. Rasmussen, and C. Anast. 1966. Further studies on the interrelationship between parathyroid hormone and vitamin D. *J. Clin. Invest. 45*:1955.

Au, W. Y. W., and L. G. Raisz. 1967. Restoration of parathyroid responsiveness in vitamin D–deficient rats by parental calcium or dietary lactose. *J. Clin. Invest. 46*:1572.

Beutner, E. H., and P. L. Munson. 1960. Time course of urinary excretion of inorganic phosphate by rats after parathyroidectomy and after injection of parathyroid extract. *Endocrinology 66*:610.

Blunt, J. W., Y. Tanaka, and H. F. DeLuca. 1968. The biological activity of 25–hydroxycholecalciferol, a metabolite of vitamin D_3. *Proc. Nat. Acad. Sci. U.S.A. 61*:1503.

Chase, L. R., and G. D. Aurbach. 1967. Parathyroid function and the renal excretion of 3′5′-adenylic acid. *Proc. Nat. Acad. Sci. U.S.A. 58*:518.

Chase, L. R., and G. D. Aurbach. 1968*a*. Renal adenyl cyclase: anatomically separate sites for parathyroid hormone and vasopressin. *Science 159*:545.

Chase, L. R., and G. D. Aurbach. 1968*b*. Cyclic AMP and the mechanism of action of parathyroid hormone. *In* R. V. Talmage and L. F. Bélanger (eds.), *Parathyroid Hormone and Thyrocalcitonin (Calcitonin)*. Excerpta Medica Foundation, New York.

DeLuca, H. F., G. Guroff, H. Steenbock, S. Reiser, and M. R. Mannatt. 1961. Effect of various vitamin deficiencies on citric acid metabolism in the rat. *J. Nutr. 75*:175.

DeLuca, H. F., G. W. Engstrom, and H. Rasmussen. 1962. The action of vitamin D and parathyroid hormone *in vitro* on calcium uptake and release by kidney mitochondria. *Proc. Nat. Acad. Sci. U.S.A. 48*:1604.

DeLuca, H. F., H. Morii, and M. J. Melancon, Jr. 1968. The interaction of vitamin D, parathyroid hormone, and thyrocalcitonin. *In* R. V. Talmage and L. F. Bélanger (eds.), *Parathyroid Hormone and Thyrocalcitonin (Calcitonin)*. Excerpta Medica Foundation, New York.

Eisenberg, E. 1968. Renal effects of parathyroid hormone. *In* R. V. Talmage and L. F. Bélanger (eds.), *Parathyroid Hormone and Thyrocalcitonin (Calcitonin)*. Excerpta Medica Foundation, New York.

Gudmundsson, T. V., I. MacIntyre, and H. A. Soliman. 1965. The isolation of thyrocalcitonin and a study of its effect in the rat. *Proc. Roy. Soc.* [*Biol.*] *164*:460.

Harrison, H. E., and H. C. Harrison. 1964. The interaction of vitamin D and parathyroid hormone on calcium, phosphorous and magnesium homeostasis in the rat. *Metabolism 13*:952.

Harrison, H. E., H. C. Harrison, and E. A. Park. 1958. Vitamin D and citrate metabolism. Effect of vitamin D in rats fed diets adequate in both calcium and phosphorous. *Amer. J. Physiol. 192*:432.

Melancon, M. J., Jr., and H. F. DeLuca. 1969. Interrelationships between thyrocalcitonin, parathyroid hormone, and vitamin D: Control of serum calcium in hypervitaminosis D. *Endocrinology 85*:704.

Mittleman, R., A. Chausmer, J. Bellavia, and S. Wallach. 1967. Thyrocalcitonin activity in hypercalcemia produced by calcium salts, parathyroid hormone and vitamin D. *Endocrinology 81*:599.

Morii, H., and H. F. DeLuca. 1967. Relationship between vitamin D deficiency, thyrocalcitonin, and parathyroid hormone. *Amer. J. Physiol. 213*:358.

Ney, R. L., W. Y. W. Au, G. Kelly, I. Radde, and F. C. Bartter. 1965. Actions of parathyroid hormone in the vitamin D–deficient dog. *J. Clin. Invest. 44*:2003.

Nichols, G., Jr., S. Schartum, and G. M. Vaes. 1963. Some effects of vitamin D and parathyroid hormone on the calcium and phosphorus metabolism of bone *in vitro*. *Acta Physiol. Scand. 57*:51.

Pechet, M. M., E. Bobadilla, E. L. Carroll, and R. H. Hesse. 1967. Regulation of bone resorption and formation: Influences of thyrocalcitonin, parathyroid hormone, neutral phosphate, and vitamin D_3. *Amer. J. Med. 43*:696.

Raisz, L. G., and D. C. Klein. 1969. Stimulation of bone resorption by dibutyryl cyclic 3′,5′-adenosine monophosphate *in vitro*. *Fed. Proc. 28*:320.

Rasmussen, H., H. F. DeLuca, C. Arnaud, C. Hawker, and M. Von Stedingk. 1963. The relationship between vitamin D and parathyroid hormone. *J. Clin. Invest. 42*:1940.

Rasmussen, H., N. Nagata, J. Feinblatt, and D. Fast. 1968. Parathyroid hormone, membranes, ions, and enzymes. *In* R. V. Talmage and L. F. Bélanger (eds.), *Parathyroid Hormone and Thyrocalcitonin (Calcitonin)*. Excerpta Medica Foundation, New York.

Sallis, J. D., H. F. DeLuca, and H. Rasmussen. 1963. Parathyroid hormone-dependent uptake of inorganic phosphate by mitochondria. *J. Clin. Invest. 238*:4098.

Toverud, S. U. 1964. The effect of parathyroid hormone and vitamin D on serum calcium in rats. *Acta Physiol. Scand. 62*:391.

Wells, H., and W. Lloyd. 1967. Effects of theophylline on the serum calcium of rats after parathyroidectomy and administration of parathyroid hormone. *Endocrinology 81*:139.

Wells, H., and W. Lloyd. 1968*a*. Inhibition of the hypocalcemic action of thyrocalcitonin by theophylline and isoproterenol. *Endocrinology 82*:468.

Wells, H., and W. Lloyd. 1968*b*. Possible involvement of cyclic AMP in the actions of thyrocalcitonin and parathyroid hormone. *In* R. V. Talmage and L. F. Bélanger (eds.), *Parathyroid Hormone and Thyrocalcitonin (Calcitonin)*. Excerpta Medica Foundation, New York.

Zull, J. E., E. Czarnowska-Misztal, and H. F. DeLuca. 1966. On the relationship between vitamin D action and actinomycin-sensitive processes. *Proc. Nat. Acad. Sci U.S.A. 55*:177.

10

CLINICAL ASPECTS OF VITAMIN D

Edmund R. Yendt, H. F. DeLuca,

Diosdado A. Garcia, and Moussa Cohanim

Vitamin D deficiency

It is distressing to report that although rickets has been eliminated as a major medical problem in many countries of the world, a significant number of cases still occur today, fifty years after Mellanby (1919*a*, 1919*b*) demonstrated that the disease could be prevented and cured with cod-liver oil. There has been a marked decline in incidence in the United States, undoubtedly due to the long-established practice of fortifying fresh and evaporated milk and almost all commercial infant formulas with vitamin D. A recent survey in the United States indicated that the incidence of rickets was only one case in 2,791 pediatric admissions. Over a 5-year period only 853 cases were admitted to the 226 hospitals participating in the survey (American Academy of Pediatrics, 1962). Not a single case was discovered in the city of Pittsburgh during the decade ending in 1960 (Danowski, 1962). In Canada, however, where the fortification of dairy milk was prohibited by federal regulation until recently, the incidence of rickets has been higher. More than 100 cases were admitted to the Montreal Children's Hospital and the Hospital for Sick Children, Toronto, during a 12-month period in 1965–66 (Canadian Pediatric Society, unpublished data). In Great Britain, a survey carried out by the British Paediatric Association (1964) over a 17-month period in 1960–61 indicated that an average of 3 cases per month was being reported. Most of the affected infants were breast-fed or given fresh dairy milk, which is unfortified in Great Britain, and were not given vitamin supplements. Many of them were dark-skinned children of recent immigrants (Benson et al., 1963; Arneil and Crosbie, 1963; Stewart et al., 1964). Recent statistics from Glasgow indicate that the incidence of rickets is higher there

This work is supported by the Medical Research Council of Canada, Grant MT681.

now than in 1961 (Richards et al., 1968). A dietary survey conducted in Canada in 1963 and 1964 indicated that 30% of the infants and children surveyed received less than the recommended daily intake of 400 IU of vitamin D (Broadfoot et al., 1966), and in two surveys recently conducted in Scotland it was estimated that 25%–33% of the infants received less than 100 IU daily from all sources except sunshine (Richards et al., 1968).

In adults, vitamin D deficiency due to inadequate dietary intake is now uncommon but it definitely occurs (Dent, 1957; van Buchem, 1959; Gough et al., 1964; Chalmers et al., 1967; Anderson et al., 1966) even in North America (Connor, personal communication). Vitamin D deficiency in adults is usually secondary to intestinal malabsorption due to idiopathic steatorrhoea (Linder and Harris, 1929; Badenoch and Fourman, 1954), disease of the small intestine (Volwiler, 1957), prolonged biliary obstruction (Ahrens et al., 1950; Atkinson et al., 1956), and pancreatic insufficiency (Bauer and Marble, 1932). Absorption of tritiated vitamin D_3 is impaired in all of these conditions, and the degree of malabsorption of the vitamin is related to the fat excretion in the feces (Thompson et al., 1966*a*).

A most interesting cause of vitamin D deficiency in the adult is that resulting from gastrectomy. Osteomalacia is not an uncommon complication of gastrectomy (Deller et al., 1963; Jones et al., 1963; Clark, 1964), even in the absence of steatorrhoea (Thompson et al., 1966*a*), and is clearly due to vitamin D deficiency, since the patients have no detectable vitamin D–like activity in plasma (Thompson et al., 1966*b*) and respond to physiologic doses of vitamin D (Morgan et al., 1965). In some of these patients, dietary intake of vitamin D or exposure to sunlight did not differ significantly from the normal, suggesting that impaired intestinal absorption was responsible for the vitamin deficiency (Morgan et al., 1965). Absorption of tritium-labeled vitamin D_3 has been found to be either within or just below the normal range in patients with postgastrectomy osteomalacia but normal in 4 postgastrectomy patients without osteomalacia, even though 2 of the latter group had steatorrhoea (Thompson et al., 1966*a*). The same workers suggest, however, that, after tritiated vitamin D has been administered orally, plasma radioactivity may be a less sensitive criterion of absorption than the fecal excretion of radioactivity (Thompson et al., 1967).

The time has certainly come for a re-examination of the pathogenesis of rickets and osteomalacia due to vitamin D deficiency. The classic concept is that in vitamin D deficiency the Ca × P product of the blood (Howland and Kramer, 1921), and hence in the extracellular fluids, falls below the critical level necessary for mineralization of epiphyseal cartilage and bone matrix. This simple concept has recently been questioned, particularly by Stanbury (1964), who points out that in the osteomalacia associated with chronic renal insufficiency (which admittedly is a somewhat different situation), pharmacologic doses of vitamin D may promote healing without any measurable change in the Ca × P products. However, in a recent re-appraisal of this concept, Nordin and Smith (1967) point out that, with the possible exception of renal failure, a reduced Ca × P product is associated with all types of rickets and osteomalacia, and that elevation of the product by whatever means cures the disease.

It would appear that osteoid as initially produced by the osteoblast is noncalcifiable and that, before mineralization can take place, there occurs a variety of biochemical changes, a process referred to as maturation (Harris and Heaney, 1969; Johnson, 1966), which is thought to be under osteoblastic control (Harris and Heaney, 1969). In osteomalacia, the characteristic histochemical changes which normally precede mineralization are absent, but return with effective treatment even before the plasma mineral levels change (Johnson, 1966). Identical histochemical abnormalities have been observed in the matrix of both vitamin D–deficient and vitamin D–resistant osteomalacia (Johnson, 1966). It has been suggested that, in osteomalacia, hypophosphatemia might be the common factor responsible for the osteoblastic dysfunction resulting in defective maturation (Harris and Heaney, 1969). In this regard, however, the recent report of Bordier and his associates (1968) is particularly pertinent because it suggests that in vitamin D deficiency the normal pre-mineralization changes in bone matrix may be absent even though serum calcium and phosphorus levels are normal. Specifically, Bordier and co-workers stained undecalcified bone with toluidine blue and solochrome-cyanine-R. These stains differentiate calcified bone from unmineralized osteoid, but in addition they show up a darkly staining zone at the junction of osteoid and trabecular bone. This zone, known as the calcification front, is said to be visible in normal subjects at over 80% of the interfaces between osteoid and trabecular bone, but is virtually absent in osteomalacia although it reappears after vitamin D therapy (Matrajt et al., 1967). In a group of postgastrectomy patients with normal levels of serum calcium and phosphorus, the proportion of osteoid with a calcification front was reduced even though the absolute amount of osteoid was not increased (Bordier et al., 1968). This abnormality was corrected by the administration of a single intravenous dose of 1 mg of D_3 without necessarily being accompanied by changes in the levels of serum calcium or phosphorus. On the basis of their studies, Bordier and associates conclude that vitamin D promotes the formation of the calcification front by a direct effect on bone. If confirmed, this concept will necessitate a radical revision of our ideas concerning the pathogenesis of rickets and osteomalacia in vitamin D deficiency.

The use of pharmacologic doses of vitamin D in the treatment of hypoparathyroidism

The effects of pharmacologic doses of vitamin D are best illustrated in hypoparathyroidism, where the action of the vitamin is not modified by changing parathyroid function. These effects were classically depicted in a study performed by the late Dr. R. F. Farquharson in 1941 and 1942 (Fig. 10.1). A patient with post-thyroidectomy hypoparathyroidism was given 2.5 mg of ergocalciferol daily for 5½ weeks in 1941. The characteristic rise in serum calcium levels is seen here, and it is now generally

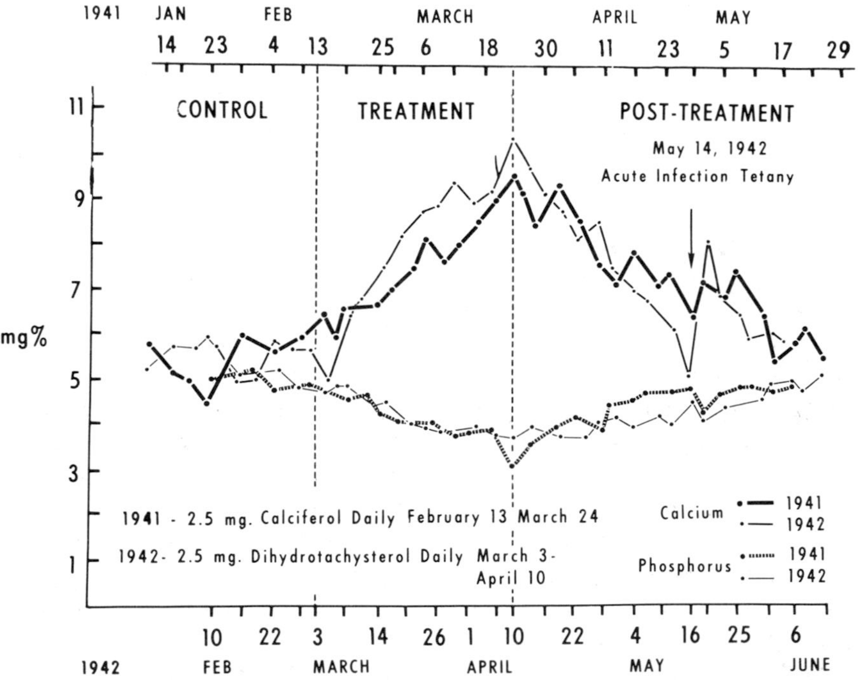

Fig. 10.1. Effects of ergocalciferol and Hytakerol on serum calcium and phosphorus levels in a patient with post-thyroidectomy hypoparathyroidism. In 1941 (from February 13 to March 24) the patient received 2.5 mg of ergocalciferol daily. In 1942 (from March 3 to April 10) the patient received 2 ml of Hytakerol daily. (At that time it was thought that Hytakerol contained 1.25 mg of dihydrotachysterol per milliliter.) (R. F. Farquharson, unpublished observations. Figure reproduced from the *International Encyclopedia of Pharmacology and Therapeutics* by permission of Pergamon Press Ltd.)

recognized that this effect is largely due to a direct resorptive effect of the vitamin upon bone, since it can be produced experimentally in animals on calcium-free diets (Hess et al., 1931). The point which we wish to emphasize, however, is that the maximum effect of the daily administration of 100,000 IU of vitamin D_2 to this patient was not achieved for 5 weeks after beginning treatment, and it is possible that its peak effect would have been observed at a later date had not the vitamin been discontinued at that time. There is a widespread lack of awareness of this fundamental fact among physicians, who often express concern when their patients are still hypocalcemic and possibly symptomatic after only 1–2 weeks of starting vitamin D. As a result, frequent increases in dosage may be made during the first few weeks of treatment. At best, this practice lengthens the time necessary to establish maintenance requirements and, at worst, increases the danger of vitamin D intoxication. After the vitamin D was discontinued in this patient, some evidence of its effects persisted for at least 7 weeks and, in hypervitaminosis D, evidence of toxicity may persist for well over 1 year (Howard and Meyer, 1948).

The characteristic fall in serum phosphorus levels associated with vitamin D administration in hypoparathyroidism is secondary to phosphaturia. Albright and Reifenstein (1948) attributed this to a "phosphaturic effect" of vitamin D and suggested that the vitamin, like parathyroid hormone, directly inhibited the renal tubular conservation of phosphate. However, it has been recently demonstrated in hypoparathyroidism (Eisenberg, 1968) and in pseudohypoparathyroidism (Mautalen et al., 1967) that the restoration of normal serum calcium levels by prolonged calcium infusions produces phosphaturia and restores serum phosphorus levels to normal as a result of diminished renal tubular reabsorption of phosphorus. At the present time there is no good evidence that vitamin D has a direct effect upon the renal tubular handling of phosphate, either in promoting or diminishing phosphaturia.

In 1942 (as indicated in the legend to Figure 10.1), it was generally believed that Hytakerol was dihydrotachysterol. It is now known, of course, that Hytakerol (AT_{10} in Europe) is a mixture of steroids and that its biologic activity is largely attributable to dihydrovitamin D_2 II, an isomer of dihydrotachysterol with similar effects but less potency (Terepka et al, 1961). The study demonstrates, however, that Hytakerol offered no particular therapeutic advantages over ergocalciferol even though numerous statements to the contrary were being made at the time—an important observation in view of the fact that Hytakerol was much more expensive than vitamin D_2. Great variation in the potency of Hytakerol and AT_{10} has also been reported (Butler, 1954; Terepka et al., 1961; Dent and Friedman, 1964*a*).

Since pure crystalline dihydrotachysterol has become available, it would appear that its use offers certain theoretic advantages over ergocalciferol in patients requiring pharmacologic doses of vitamin D. Harrison and co-workers (1967) have shown that it is more potent on a weight basis, 1 mg of dihydrotachysterol being approximately equivalent to 3 mg of ergocalciferol. Furthermore, the hypercalcemic and hypercalciuric effects of dihydrotachysterol were evident sooner and subsided more quickly than was the case with ergocalciferol, which is an advantage in the event of overdosage. At the present time, however, pure dihydrotachysterol is not available on a prescription basis in Canada or the United States.

Before leaving the question of choice of compounds for patients requiring pharmacologic doses of vitamin D, it should be pointed out that although vitamin D_3 (cholecalciferol) was once considered more efficacious than vitamin D_2 (ergocalciferol) in the prophylaxis and treatment of human rickets (Bicknell and Prescott, 1953), both forms of the vitamin are now thought to be of approximately equal potency in humans (Drake, 1937; Harris, 1956; Harrison, 1963). Since ergocalciferol is less expensive than cholecalciferol, its use has been much more widespread. However, the form in which ergocalciferol is administered may be of real and practical significance (Dent et al., 1953; Parfitt, 1968). In both Britain and Australia, the popular preparation has been a sugar-coated tablet normally containing 1.25 mg (50,000 IU) of ergocalciferol. These tablets may be inadequately absorbed in some patients (Himsworth and Maisels, 1940; Dent et al., 1953) and may lose their strength if not stored under ideal conditions, particularly if they are made with calcium salts as incipient (Dent et al., 1953). For this reason it is common to include an excess or "overage." As a result of these various factors, the true ergocalciferol content of these tablets may vary widely. The administration of ergocalciferol in the form of an oily solution containing an antioxidant put up in opaque gelatin capsules has proven to be a much more satisfactory way of administering the vitamin. It has been suggested (Parfitt, 1968) that the possibility of marked variation in the absorption and potency of commercial vitamin D preparations may account for certain cases of vitamin D "resistance," for the variability in the maintenance dosage of vitamin D found to be satisfactory by different authors, and for the need to adjust dosage once a satisfactory regimen is worked out. It is abundantly clear that steps should be taken to correct some of these inconsistencies now associated with the use of pharmacologic doses of vitamin D.

We would like to add one final word about the management of hypoparathyroidism. We prefer to maintain serum calcium levels in the low normal range to minimize the degree of hypercalciuria. Some patients are quite comfortable even when slightly hypocalcemic (8.5–9.0 mg / ml) and, if this is the case, there seems to be no particular harm in allowing this situation to continue.

Vitamin D resistance in hypoparathyroidism

Clinically, resistance to pharmacologic doses of vitamin D is encountered in resistant rickets, renal insufficiency, and the occasional patient with hypoparathyroidism. In the first two conditions, the demonstration of abnormal metabolism of vitamin D by Avioli and his associates (1967, 1968*b*, 1969) has shed considerable light on the problem. The nature of vitamin D resistance in hypoparathyroidism is still unclear, and the somewhat confused state of the literature at the present time warrants a brief review of the problem. Perhaps one of the most unusual cases in the literature is a patient with idiopathic hypoparathyroidism associated with porphyria (Howard and Connor, 1954). This patient had persistent hypocalcemia and tetany despite the daily administration of 500,000 IU of ergocalciferol and 160 g of calcium lactate. When cortisone was administered there was a prompt return of serum calcium to normal, and it was postulated that the patient had some sort of an absorptive defect for vitamin D which was corrected by cortisone. We are unaware of any other reports in which the vitamin D–resistant state was corrected in this fashion. Ordinarily, the administration of cortisone is more apt to have an adverse clinical effect on hypoparathyroidism (Moehlig and Steinbach, 1954; Papadatos and Klein, 1954; Kahn et al., 1968).

Another aspect of vitamin D resistance in hypoparathyroidism which should be taken into consideration is the reports which indicate that some patients who are resistant to ergocalciferol may respond to AT_{10} or dihydrotachysterol and that the reverse may also be true (Dent et al., 1955; Dent and Friedman, 1964*a*; Harrison et al., 1967), whereas others are resistant to both vitamin D_2 and D_3 as well as to dihydrotachysterol (Pak et al., 1969). The question arises as to whether or not dihydrotachysterol is itself active or whether, as is the case with vitamin D_3, its effect is dependent upon conversion to an active metabolite.

Finally, there are at least three reports that vitamin D refractoriness in hypoparathyroidism was corrected by the administration of magnesium supplements (Homer, 1961; Jones and Fourman, 1966; Harrison et al., 1967). We have also had experience with a similar unreported case which demonstrated this phenomenon in a dramatic fashion.

In our patient, an adult female with idiopathic hypoparathyroidism, we had been unable to maintain consistent normocalcemia despite large doses of ergocalciferol administered by both the oral and parenteral routes (Fig. 10.2). The addition of cortisone and AT_{10} had been without benefit.

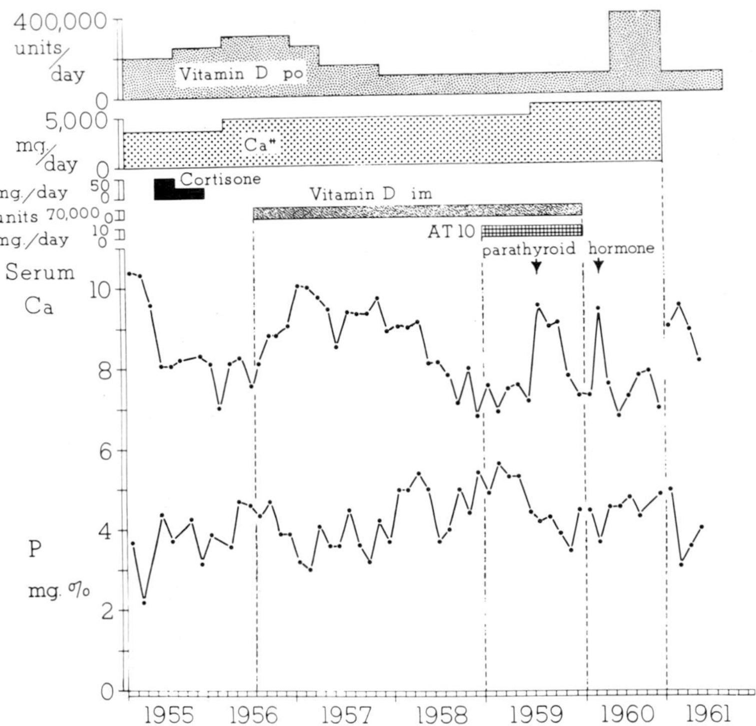

Fig. 10.2. E. M. Idiopathic hypoparathyroidism: Clinical course, 1955–61, showing intermittent hypocalcemia (accompanied by severe tetany) despite large amounts of vitamin D_2 (administered orally and intramuscularly), AT_{10}, and supplementary calcium (chart indicates mg elemental calcium). There was a normal response to Parathormone (Lilly) on two separate occasions.

The interruption in the serum calcium and phosphorus lines in the latter part of 1960 is coincidental with a period of hypercalcemia which followed the administration of magnesium salts (see Fig. 10.3).

The patient was normally sensitive, however, to the administration of parathyroid extract, given on two separate occasions. A surprising observation was that, on both these occasions, the serum calcium remained within the normal range for the ensuing 4–6 weeks despite the fact that no other change had been made in her treatment. At this point, September 1960, it was noted that serum magnesium was persistently below our normal range, and we began to give her magnesium, at first in the form of sulfate and then as citrate. Not only did the serum calcium and phosphorus levels return to normal but she became seriously hypercalcemic, and both the vitamin D and supplementary calcium had to be temporarily discontinued (Fig. 10.3). Magnesium supplements were also discontinued.

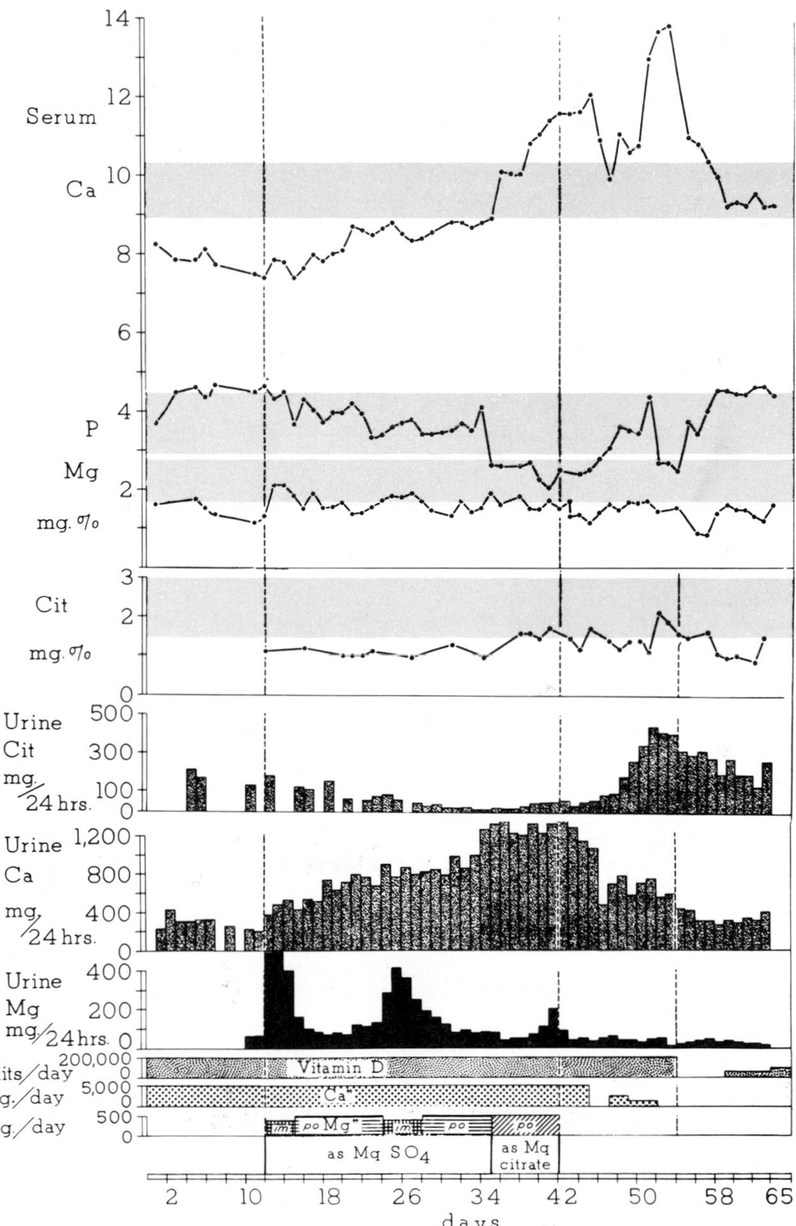

Fig. 10.3. E. M. Idiopathic hypoparathyroidism: Response to magnesium supplements. The charts were begun October 1960.

For approximately 6 weeks she remained in clinical and biochemical remission, but then she developed symptoms of tetany again as well as hypocalcemia and hypomagnesemia. As before, there was little or no response to the usually effective doses of vitamin D and calcium, but with the administration of magnesium salts she once again experienced rapid clinical improvement, a rapid fall in serum phosphorus levels, and a slower rise in serum calcium levels (Fig. 10.4). Since then, with the use of daily magnesium supplements, it has not been difficult to maintain normocalcemia with the usual doses of vitamin D and calcium.

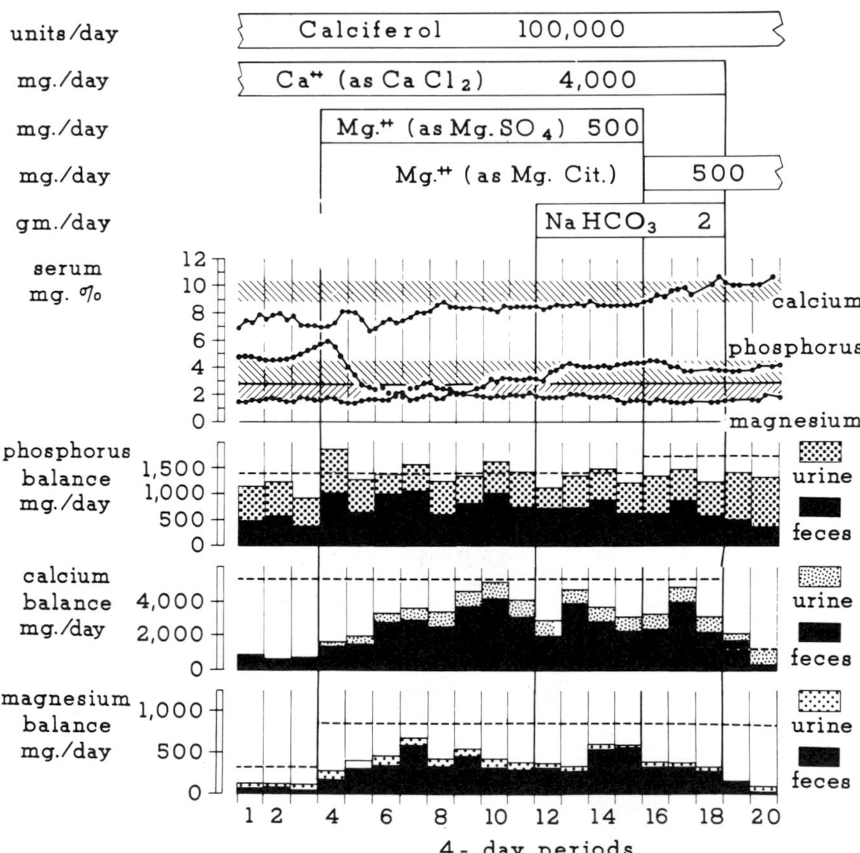

Fig. 10.4. E. M. Idiopathic hypoparathyroidism: Response of phosphorus, calcium, and magnesium balance to magnesium supplements. Balance studies were begun March 27, 1961. The patient had been taking 100,000 IU of ergocalciferol daily since December 1960.

This is all very puzzling. The administration of magnesium sulfate was without effect on serum calcium and phosphorus levels in patients with mild post-thyroidectomy hypoparathyroidism who had not been treated with vitamin D or calcium supplements (Fig. 10.5). We have also carried out a series of experiments in magnesium-deficient rats and have found that the degree of hypercalcemia resulting from toxic doses of vitamin D in no way differed from the responses observed in control animals (E. R. Yendt, unpublished observations).

Is the vitamin D resistance in this type of patient related to altered metabolism of vitamin D or to end organ (i.e., skeleton) resistance? If altered metabolism is the explanation, it is interesting to speculate as to the mechanism by which magnesium corrects this defect. Defective synthesis of 25–OH–D has been reported in a hypoparathyroid patient who was markedly hypocalcemic despite the administration of large doses of vitamin D_2, vitamin D_3, dihydrotachysterol, and supplementary calcium.

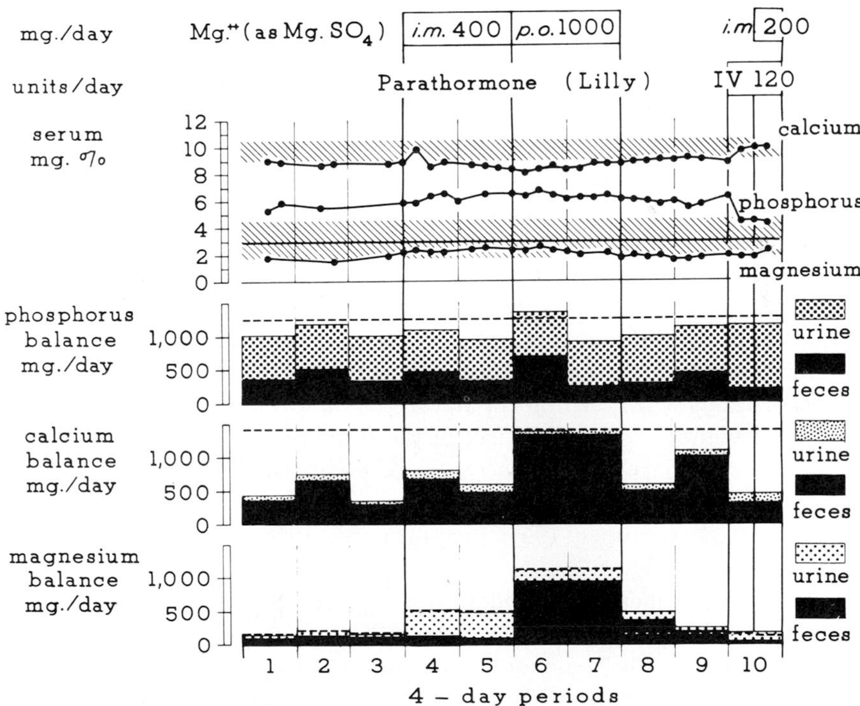

Fig. 10.5. M. G. Mild hypoparathyroidism (post-thyroidectomy): Effect of magnesium sulfate on serum calcium, phosphorus, and magnesium levels and on phosphorus, calcium, and magnesium balance.

In this patient there was a prompt rise in serum calcium with doses of 25–hydroxycholecalciferol in the range of 1200–2000 units per day (Pak et al., 1969). Serum calcium levels did not rise completely to normal in this patient but might have done so had larger doses of 25–hydroxycholecalciferol been given. If altered metabolism of vitamin D is the explanation for the refractory state in our patient and others like her, it is clear that the administration of magnesium must have corrected this disturbance in some fashion which as yet is not clearly understood. Although patients with magnesium deficiency are frequently unresponsive to parathyroid hormone, our patient was quite sensitive to the hormone, and this would constitute some evidence against extreme deficiency of 25–hydroxycholecalciferol.

Vitamin D–refractory (hypophosphatemic) rickets and osteomalacia

This disorder, which is in many areas the commonest cause of juvenile rickets (Dent and Harris, 1956; Stewart et al., 1964), originally derived its name from the failure of therapeutic doses of vitamin D to heal the skeletal lesions. But the term "vitamin D–resistant" or "vitamin D–refractory" rickets was considered by some to be inappropriate because it implies that the disorder resulted from some inherent resistance to the action of vitamin D. The contention was that, if the pathogenesis of the disorder were unrelated to vitamin D, the failure to respond to therapeutic doses of the vitamin should engender little surprise, and it was not necessary to conclude that there was an inherent resistance to the vitamin. Until recently, the fundamental biochemical defect leading to the failure of mineralization of osteoid and cartilage was thought to be hypophosphatemia due to impaired renal tubular conservation of phosphate. There were two schools of thought concerning the nature of the tubular dysfunction, one that it represented a primary defect in phosphate transport, and the other that it was secondary to hypersecretion of parathyroid hormone induced by failure of the intestine to absorb sufficient quantities of calcium (Winters et al., 1958; Stanbury, 1958; Jackson et al., 1958; Wilson et al., 1965; Williams et al., 1966).

Although an element of secondary hyperparathyroidism probably exists in many of these patients (Fraser et al., 1959; Field and Reiss, 1960), we have always been unhappy about assigning the primary pathogenetic role to intestinal malabsorption of calcium with secondary hyperparathyroidism. Intestinal malabsorption of calcium occurs in all types of osteomalacia, including that associated with the Fanconi syndrome and renal tubular acidosis (E. R. Yendt, unpublished observations), and may simply reflect the inability of the rachitic or osteomalacic skeleton to utilize calcium, possibly due to the absence of some unrecognized hormonal factor or triggering mechanism, as suggested by Nicolaysen (1943). We have carried out experiments which demonstrate that in vitamin D–refractory osteomalacia the gut is capable of absorbing calcium if the skeleton is able to utilize it (Wilson et al., 1965). The object of the experiment was to promote skeletal mineralization by the continuous intravenous infusion of phosphate (Fraser et al., 1957) and to observe the effect on fecal calcium excretion. In the first experiment, fecal calcium approximated intake and the patient was in negative calcium balance during the control periods (Fig. 10.6). Phosphate infusion led to a sharp fall in fecal calcium and a strongly positive calcium balance.

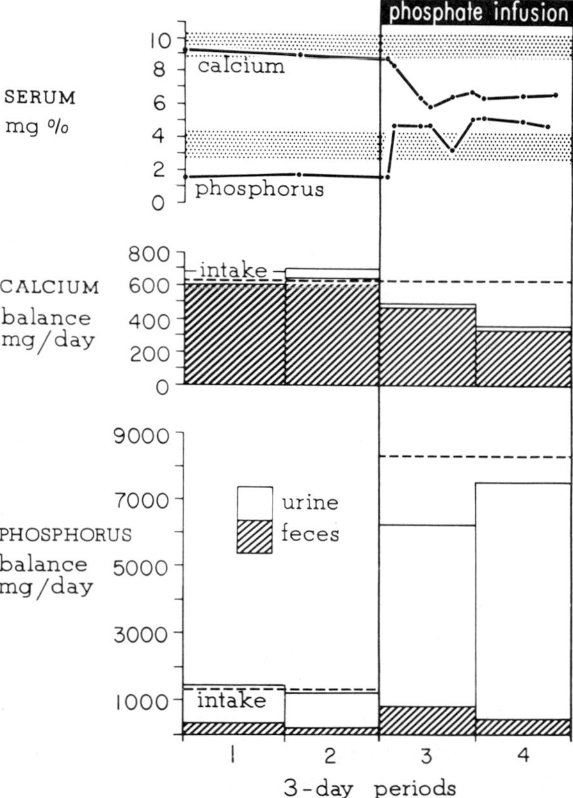

Fig. 10.6. J. B. Hypophosphatemic osteomalacia (adult onset): Effect of continuous 6-day phosphate infusion on calcium and phosphorus balance. The shaded areas indicate the normal ranges for serum calcium and phosphorus levels in our laboratory. (For further details, see case 2, Wilson et al., 1965. Figure reproduced by permission of *Medicine*.)

In the second experiment, phosphate was infused after a 16-day control period during which fecal calcium was high, and the calcium balance of the patient was neither significantly negative or positive (Fig. 10.7). However, during and after an 8-day continuous infusion of phosphate, the fecal calcium fell and the patient retained significant quantities of calcium. The administration of phosphate by mouth has also been shown to result in enhanced intestinal calcium absorption and positive calcium balance (Saville et al., 1955). Our studies have also demonstrated that the renal tubular handling of phosphate in patients with this disorder is clearly different from that observed in primary hyperparathyroidism (Wilson et al., 1965).

With the recent demonstration of abnormal vitamin D metabolism in refractory rickets (Avioli et al., 1967), the designation "vitamin D–resistant rickets" gains new respectability. However, the question must still be asked whether the impaired or absent conversion of vitamin D to its active metabolite 25–hydroxycholecalciferol provides an adequate explanation for all aspects of refractory rickets. Certain difficulties are immediately apparent. Why does the intestine absorb calcium after phosphate is administered if the patients are truly vitamin D–deficient? Why do these patients not develop hypocalcemia (Nordin and Smith, 1967) and / or hypocalciuria as do patients with simple vitamin D–deficient rickets? Why do they not develop a pattern of amino-aciduria similar to that seen in simple vitamin D–deficient rickets? (Harrison and Harrison, 1967).

The development of hypophosphatemia also requires explanation. If vitamin D does not primarily promote renal tubular conservation of phosphate – and this has never been convincingly demonstrated – some other mechanism such as secondary hyperparathyroidism must be invoked to explain the renal phosphate leak. I have already referred to the dissimilarities in the renal handling of phosphate which exist between patients with refractory rickets and those with primary hyperparathyroidism (Wilson et al., 1965). Further, if hypophosphatemia is due to secondary hyperparathyroidism, some explanation is necessary for the fact that it so often persists when patients are made hypercalcemic by pharmacologic doses of vitamin D. That phenomenon may be akin to the persistent hypophosphatemia sometimes observed in primary hyperparathyroidism after a parathyroid adenoma is removed; the hypophosphatemia in this case is probably related to the extreme avidity of the healing skeleton for calcium and phosphate. In this regard it should be recalled that, in simple vitamin D–deficient rickets, serum calcium and phosphorus levels generally rise to normal within a few weeks of beginning vitamin D. A third, intriguing explanation for the hypophosphatemia is that some of the abnormal metabolites of vitamin D which have been demonstrated in this disorder

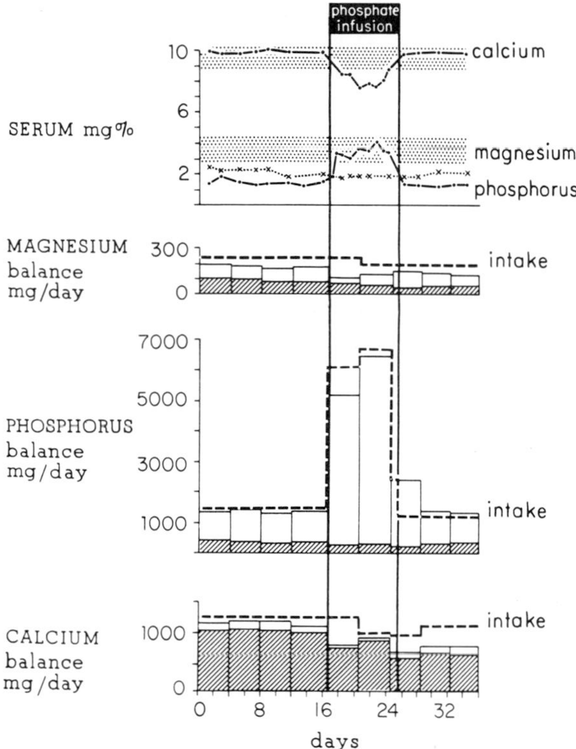

Fig. 10.7. L. R. Hypophosphatemic (vitamin D–refractory) osteomalacia: Effects of a continuous 8-day phosphate infusion on calcium, phosphorus, and magnesium balance. (For further details, see case 5, Wilson et al., 1965. Figure reproduced by permission of *Medicine*.)

(Avioli et al., 1967) may themselves be phosphaturic. The isolation of these metabolites and the elucidation of their metabolic effects, if any, will be awaited with great interest. Finally, it is still possible that these patients may have a fundamental defect in phosphate transport as well as altered metabolism of vitamin D.

The aim of therapy in resistant rickets and osteomalacia is to raise serum phosphorus levels sufficiently to allow skeletal mineralization to proceed. It is not necessary that the serum phosphorus be restored completely to normal. Indeed it has rarely been possible to do so. The classic form of therapy has been the use of massive doses (50,000–1,500,000 IU) of vitamin D daily (Albright et al., 1937), as a result of which a smaller proportion of the filtered phosphate load is excreted in the urine and serum phosphorus levels rise to a variable degree, but rarely to normal. The likely explanation for this effect of vitamin D is that the vitamin D–induced release of bone mineral into extracellular fluid suppresses parathyroid activity.

Unfortunately, treatment with vitamin D alone has been far from satisfactory. The response is highly variable. Some patients respond reasonably well to 50,000–75,000 IU per day (Harrison, 1964), but sometimes healing does not occur even with much larger doses (Frame and Smith, 1958; Harrison, 1964). Serum phosphorus levels may not rise significantly until the patient is hypercalcemic, and even then normophosphatemia is usually not achieved. Even when hypercalcemia has not been an obvious clinical problem, patients treated with vitamin D have been shown by renal biopsy to have intratubular deposits of calcium (Nigrin et al., 1962). With vitamin D therapy, fecal calcium may fall, but calcium balance does not necessarily become more positive because there is a marked concomitant increase in urine calcium (Rose, 1964). A further major defect of vitamin D therapy has been that the growth of affected children is not normal, resulting in dwarfism (West et al., 1964; Dent and Friedman, 1964*b*).

The use of smaller amounts (e.g., 12,500–50,000 IU per day) of vitamin D, along with oral phosphate supplements, has in certain quarters been thought to be superior to the use of vitamin D alone (West et al., 1964; Wilson et al., 1965). Healing may occur more rapidly than with a dose of vitamin D four to eight times as great given alone (West et al., 1964). Higher serum phosphorus levels are achieved, greater calcium retention is produced as a result of diminished urinary calcium (Frame and Smith, 1958; West et al., 1964), and sometimes fecal calcium also falls (Saville et al., 1955). As yet it is not known whether combined therapy with vitamin D and phosphate will prevent dwarfism. Phosphate therapy without vitamin D has produced healing in some adults with vitamin D–refractory osteomalacia (Wilson et al., 1965; Nagant de Deuxchaisnes and Krane, 1967), but in other cases was without benefit either in producing initial healing or in preventing recurrence (Rose, 1964; West et al., 1964). Phosphate treatment results in stimulation of initially low-normal rates of bone turnover so that both bone formation and resorption is increased, and it has been suggested that the stimulation of bone resorption may result in part from secondary hyperparathyroidism (Nagant de Deuxchaisnes and Krane, 1967).

In view of the possibility that phosphate therapy might well result in secondary hyperparathyroidism, our recent experience with two patients treated with both vitamin D and large oral phosphate supplements is of considerable interest. Both these patients were classical cases of vitamin

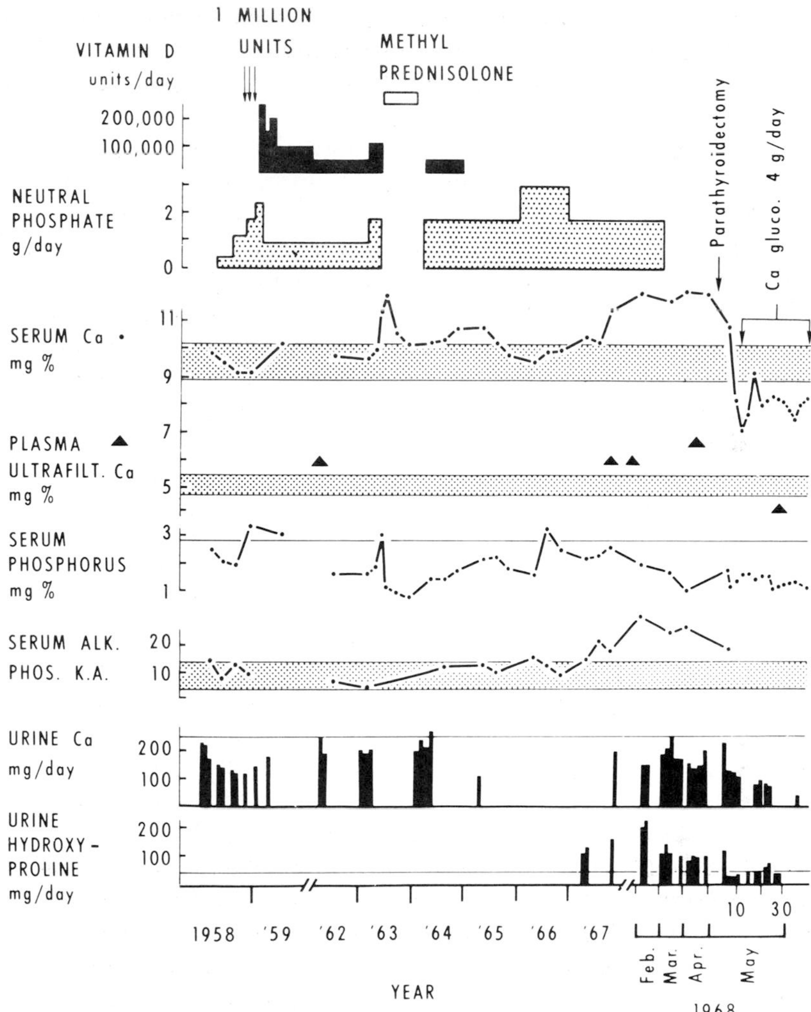

Fig. 10.8. H. K. Hypophosphatemic (vitamin D–refractory) osteomalacia: Development of hyperparathyroidism while on oral phosphate therapy. (For detailed case report to 1963, see case 1, Wilson et al., 1965.)

D–refractory rickets beginning in infancy. In the first (Fig. 10.8), a female aged 33, combined therapy with vitamin D and phosphate was begun 10 years ago, and her response was excellent as judged clinically, radiologically, and by bone biopsy. In 1965 she was noted to have mild hypercalcemia, and the vitamin D was discontinued. Her serum calcium subsequently returned to normal, but in 1967 she developed persistent hypercalcemia accompanied by elevated serum alkaline phosphate levels, urinary hydroxyproline excretion, and increasing bone pain. Calcium kinetic studies showed increased bone turnover. Neck exploration performed in April 1968 revealed three markedly enlarged and hyperplastic parathyroid glands, which were removed. A fourth gland, which was only slightly enlarged, was allowed to remain. Postoperatively, skeletal pain gradually lessened and disappeared and serum alkaline phosphatase levels and urinary hydroxyproline excretion fell to normal. The patient was hypocalcemic for a while, but this was corrected with oral calcium supplements. Fasting serum phosphorus levels have remained well below normal, but oral phosphate supplements now result in much greater increments in serum phosphorus levels than at any time in the past.

The history of the second patient, a male aged 33, was essentially similar to that of the first (Fig. 10.9). He, too, had a good response to combined therapy with vitamin D and phosphate supplements, begun in 1963, although serum alkaline phosphatase levels never fell completely to normal. It should be noted that, in this patient, serum calcium levels even initially were at the very upper limit of the normal range and by the end of 1966 were definitely elevated, as were serum alkaline phosphatase levels and urinary hydroxyproline excretion. At this time, bone pain was also becoming a problem. Hypercalcemia persisted for well over one year after vitamin D had been discontinued, and parathyroid exploration was performed in February 1968. Only two parathyroid glands were discovered: one was markedly enlarged and hyperplastic, measuring 4 cm in length; the other was slightly, but definitely, enlarged. Both glands were removed. Postoperatively, the response was similar to that seen in the first patient: There has been a dramatic disappearance of bone pain. Urinary hydroxyproline excretion fell to normal, but serum alkaline phosphatase levels remained slightly elevated (13–15 King-Armstrong units). There was mild hypocalcemia for 7 months after the operation. Fasting serum phosphorus levels have been persistently below normal but once again higher serum phosphorus levels were achieved with phosphate supplements than at any previous time.

Was the overt hyperparathyroidism in these patients related to phosphate therapy? It is difficult to reach a final conclusion at this time. The development of hypercalcemia due to parathyroid hyperfunction has been documented in at least two previous cases of vitamin D–resistant rickets where large phosphate supplements were not given (Henneman et al.,

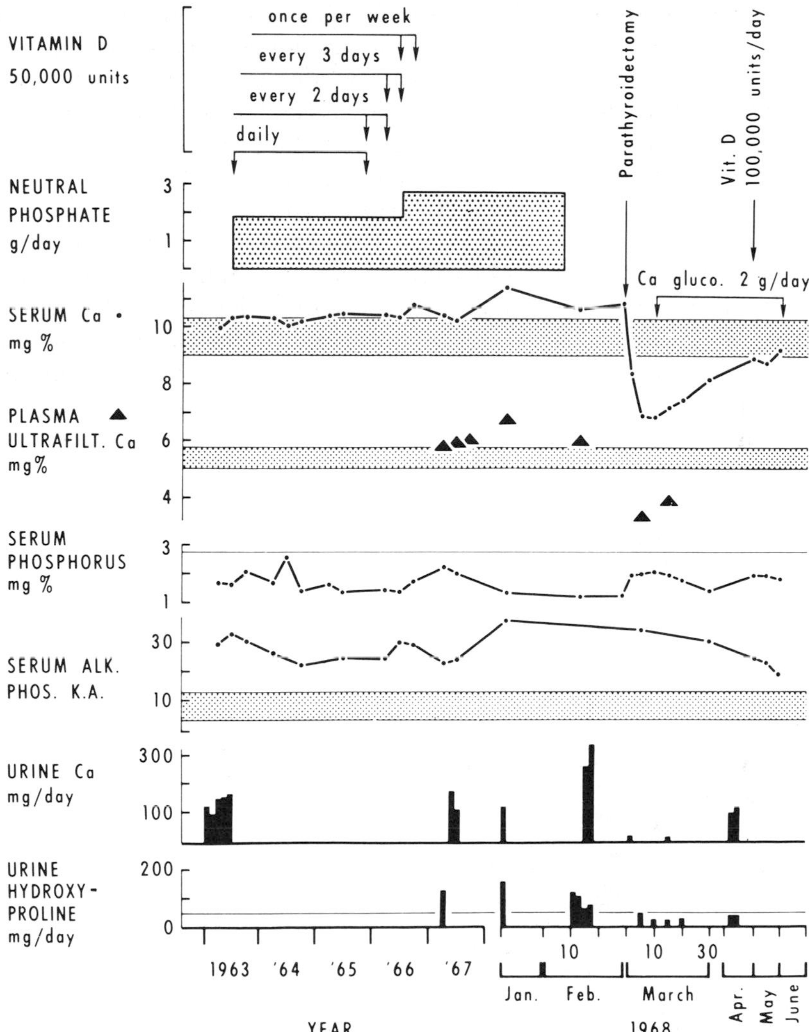

Fig. 10.9. L. R. Hypophosphatemic (vitamin D–refractory) osteomalacia: Development of hyperparathyroidism while on oral phosphate therapy. (For detailed case report to 1963, see case 5, Wilson et al., 1965.)

1962; Glanville and Bloom, 1965). It has also been shown that phosphate infusion stimulates the parathyroid glands only secondarily by lowering serum calcium concentration (Sherwood et al., 1968) and at no time prior to parathyroidectomy was hypocalcemia observed in our patients. On the other hand Reiss (1968), using standard radioimmunoassay techniques, has found elevated blood levels of parathyroid hormone in patients with early renal insufficiency without hypocalcemia and, in such patients, parathyroid hormone levels have fallen to normal following correction of the hyperphosphatemia with aluminum gels.

The recent isolation and synthesis of the active metabolite of vitamin D, 25–hydroxycholecalciferol, gives rise to the hope that a more effective therapy for resistant rickets is in sight. With this in mind we are studying, in collaboration with Dr. DeLuca, the effects of 25–hydroxycholecalciferol in a classical case of D–resistant rickets (Fig. 10.10). Despite long-term therapy with pharmacologic doses of vitamin D, this 13-year-old boy (patient E. Q.) has marked bone deformities and is stunted. His subnormal pattern of growth is shown in Figure 10.11. His serum phosphorus levels

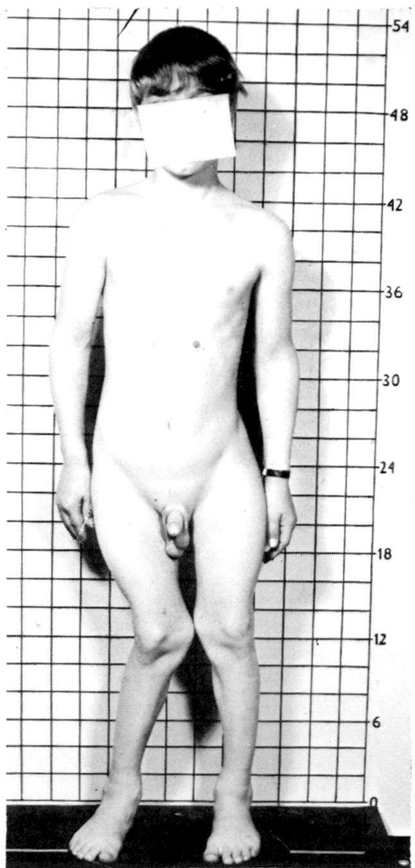

Fig. 10.10. E. Q. (Age 13). Hypophosphatemic (vitamin D–refractory) rickets. The patient has marked skeletal deformities despite ergocalciferol therapy.

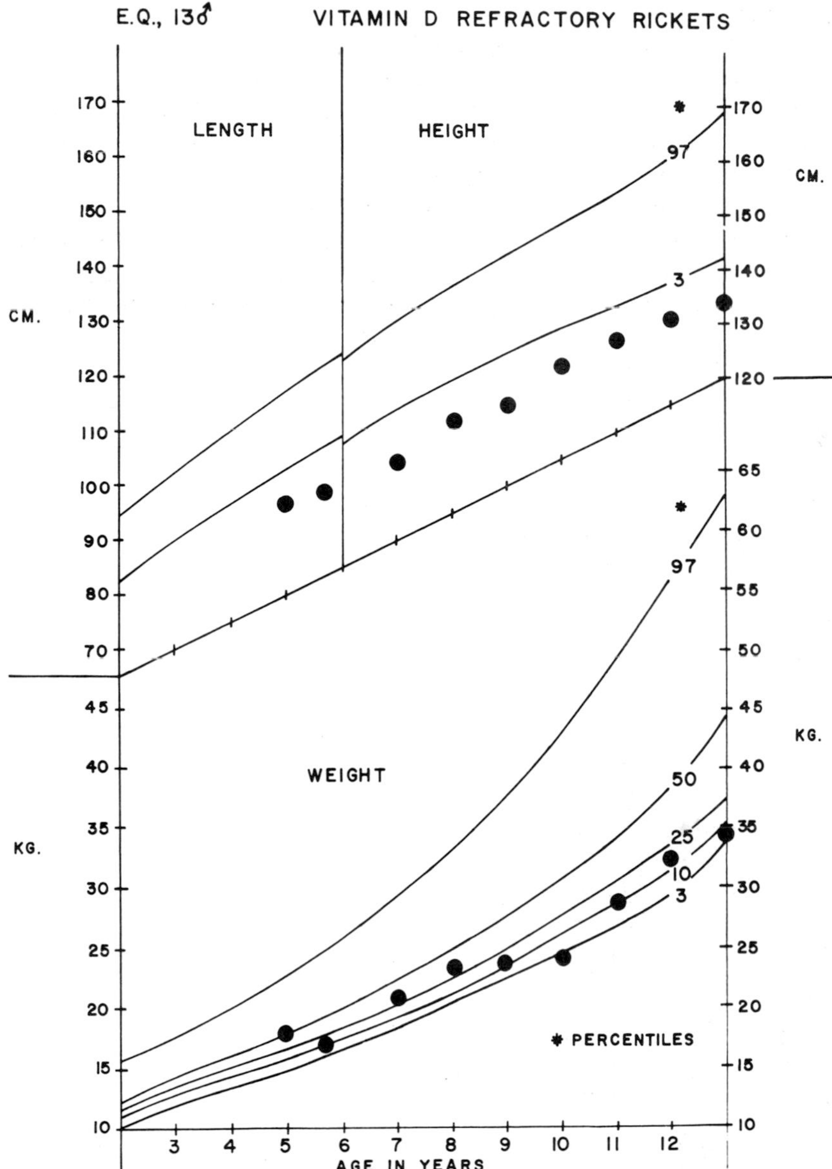

Fig. 10.11. E. Q. Hypophosphatemic (vitamin D–refractory) rickets: Growth chart. Heavy dots indicate patient's values, showing the failure to achieve normal height on ergocalciferol therapy. (Stuart Anthropometric Chart reproduced by permission of the Children's Hospital Medical Center.)

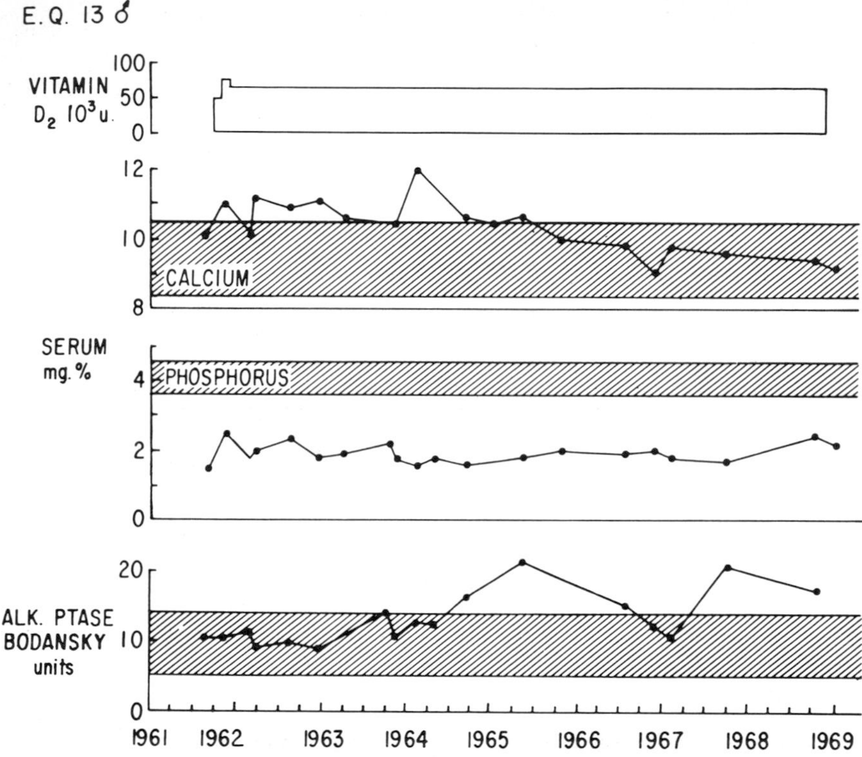

Fig. 10.12. E. Q. Hypophosphatemic (vitamin D–refractory) rickets: Course, 1961–69, showing persistent hypophosphatemia and elevated alkaline phosphatase levels despite ergocalciferol therapy.

have always been consistently below normal and, for the past several years, the serum alkaline phosphatase levels have been elevated (Fig. 10.12). Urinary hydroxyproline excretion is also elevated. Studies of vitamin D metabolism in this patient performed by Dr. DeLuca indicated that no 25–hydroxycholecalciferol appeared in the plasma after the injection of tritiated vitamin D_3.

At the present time metabolic balance studies are being carried out on the patient in the Special Investigation Unit of Kingston General Hospital (Fig. 10.13). Vitamin D_2 was discontinued 6 months ago with no particular changes in any of the parameters being studied. Following a 28-day control period, 25–hydroxycholecalciferol administration was begun in a dosage of 800 units daily. As of 20 days after beginning treatment, there had been no change in any of the parameters we are measuring,

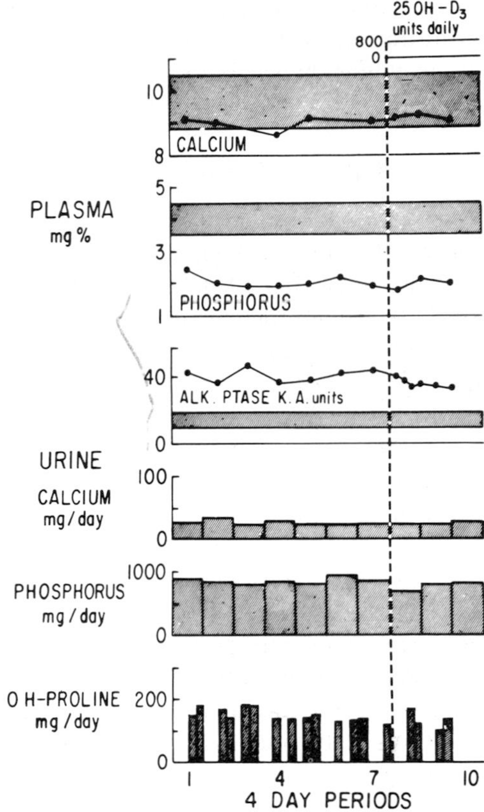

Fig. 10.13. E. Q. Metabolic studies before and during administration of 25-hydroxycholecalciferol.

which include serum calcium, phosphorus, alkaline phosphatase and citrate levels, urinary calcium, phosphorus, citrate, and hydroxyproline.*

It is too early to derive definite conclusions from the apparent failure of response to 25–hydroxycholecalciferol after only 3 weeks of treatment. However, if this had been a case of simple D–deficiency rickets, the serum values would probably have begun to return to normal by now. If on the other hand secondary hyperparathyroidism is a major factor in this particular patient, the persistent hypophosphatemia is perhaps not surprising, for we have seen in the two previous cases that the degree of hyperplasia may be so great that the glands escape from normal regulatory mechanisms and function in an autonomous fashion. The result of long-term therapy

* Over the succeeding 11 months, the dose of 25–OH–D was gradually increased to 6000 units daily without significant clinical, biochemical; or radiologic evidence of improvement.

in this and similar patients will be most interesting to observe. The administration of 25–hydroxycholecalciferol to patients with resistant rickets in whom hyperplastic parathyroid glands have been removed is another approach to the problem which should be explored.

Vitamin D toxicity

The various manifestations of vitamin D intoxication have been described repeatedly since the condition was first reported in the experimental animal (Pfannenstiel, 1928; Kreitmair and Moll, 1928) and in man (Reed, 1938). Although the dangers of the vitamin have been known for 40 years, cases of hypervitaminosis D in humans still occur with distressing frequency. On one occasion within the past two years, there were on my service at the Toronto General Hospital three patients suffering from this condition. All of them had sustained serious and probably irreversible renal damage before the condition was recognized. Most patients with this condition nowadays have been given pharmacologic doses of vitamin D for the treatment of hypoparathyroidism, although the use of large doses of vitamin D or dihydrotachysterol in the treatment of resistant rickets and the osteodystrophy associated with chronic renal failure also gives rise to this complication.

Serious toxicity resulting from the use of vitamin D should be a preventable disorder, and most cases would not occur if proper precautions were routinely taken when pharmacologic doses are prescribed. The following points are worthy of emphasis:

1. Patients for whom pharmacologic doses of vitamin D are prescribed should be warned of its dangers, and emphasis should be placed upon the need for close medical supervision for the entire time they are receiving this agent, whether it be days, months, years, or decades, as well as on the importance of reporting unusual symptoms promptly.

2. All patients receiving pharmacologic doses of vitamin D should have their blood calcium levels checked repeatedly for the entire period of treatment. This should be done at least 3–4 times a year and more often if dosage is being adjusted. The practice of adjusting vitamin D dosage by assessing urinary calcium excretion by the Sulkowitch's test is dangerous and has no place in modern practice.

3. Vitamin D intoxication may develop suddenly in patients who have been seemingly well controlled for years on a constant dose of vitamin D.

4. Even slight degrees of hypercalcemia due to vitamin D overdosage may be associated with serious toxicity and irreversible renal damage. In this regard, it should be pointed out that the normal range for serum calcium levels is considerably narrower than the often quoted 9–11 mg/100

ml. In one of our patients who experienced severe irreversible renal damage, the serum calcium level never exceeded 11 mg/100 ml.

5. Patients recovering from a bout of vitamin D intoxication may be acutely sensitive to vitamin D for a period of many months even though their serum calcium levels have returned to normal or, in the case of hypoparathyroid patients, to below normal. In the latter group of patients it may be preferable to maintain normocalcemia by the use of calcium supplements rather than by reinstituting treatment with vitamin D at an early date. They may also be quite sensitive to supplementary calcium at this stage (Leeson and Fourman, 1966, and E. R. Yendt, unpublished observations).

The toxic effects of hypervitaminosis D are generally ascribed to hypercalcemia, and we have found no clinical evidence of vitamin D toxicity in the absence of elevated serum calcium levels. Over the years, however, there has been a series of papers describing the occurrence of metastatic calcification due to the administration of vitamin D in the absence of hypercalcemia (Smith and Elvore, 1929; Shelling, 1930; Ham and Portuondo, 1933; Cowdry and Scott, 1936; Reed et al., 1939; Mathieu et al., 1964; Friedman and Roberts, 1966), and some workers have concluded that metastatic calcification produced by vitamin D results not from hypercalcemia but from a direct effect of the vitamin on tissues (Fourman et al., 1968). Although some of these reports do not stand up to close scrutiny, it is probably premature to regard the matter as closed.

Another interesting and puzzling observation related to experimental hypervitaminosis D is that massive doses of vitamin A decrease the mortality as well as the soft tissue calcification and skeletal resorption produced by vitamin D in the rat (Gross-Selbeck, 1935; Morgan et al., 1937; Hendricks et al., 1947; Clark and Bassett, 1962). This is an unexpected finding, since hypervitaminosis A by itself stimulates bone resorption with extraordinary rarefaction of bones and spontaneous fractures in the experimental animal (Fell, 1964) and in man (Gerber et al., 1954; Coffey, 1950; Knudson and Rothman, 1953; Jowsey and Riggs, 1968).

The treatment of hypervitaminosis D varies with the degree of hypercalcemia and the gravity of the clinical situation. If hypercalcemia is mild and asymptomatic, withdrawal of the vitamin D and calcium supplements may be all that is necessary. In more severe cases the administration of glucocorticoids is generally the treatment of choice. In most cases, the administration of 150–200 mg cortisone or its equivalent daily in three or four divided doses restores blood calcium levels to normal within two weeks (Connor et al., 1956; Dent, 1956; Winberg and Zetterstrom, 1956; Verner et al., 1958), although failure to respond to cortisone has occasionally been described (Henkin et al., 1966).

Although the exact mechanism by which cortisone corrects hypercalcemia in vitamin D intoxication is unknown, there is abundant evidence that the adrenal glucocorticoids significantly alter the absorption, metabolism, and action of vitamin D. Hydrocortisone opposes the action of vitamin D on calcium transfer across the intestinal wall in the rat (Harrison, 1961) and in the chick (Sallis and Holdsworth, 1962), and blocks the vitamin D–induced elevation of bone and serum citrate (Harrison et al., 1958; Guroff et al., 1963). Glucocorticoids and vitamin D also have opposing effects on the binding of calcium to isolated mitochondria in the rat liver (Kimberg and Goldstein, 1967). In the human, prednisone leads to a derangement in vitamin D metabolism resulting in the diminished accumulation in plasma of its biologically active metabolites (Avioli et al., 1968*a*).

When calcitonin becomes available for clinical use, it may prove to be the treatment of choice for hypervitaminosis D. In a 3-year-old child whose plasma calcium was 20 mg/100 ml following the ingestion of 3,000,000 units of vitamin D_2, the administration of 0.4 MRC units of calcitonin for 6 days resulted in the return of blood calcium levels to normal (Milhaud, 1968).

Before leaving this topic, it should be pointed out that although the administration of orthophosphates is an effective means of treating many hypercalcemic states (Goldsmith and Ingbar, 1966), its use in hypervitaminosis D is potentially hazardous. In 1930 Shelling showed that, in experimental ergocalciferol toxicity, metastatic calcification was increased with high phosphorus diets. This finding has been recently confirmed by Spaulding and Walser (1969), who have shown that mortality as well as metastatic calcification is greatly increased by the administration of phosphate to rats receiving toxic doses of ergocalciferol.

Vitamin D hypersensitivity

Perhaps the best example of a clinical state associated with vitamin D hypersensitivity is sarcoidosis. Although some patients with this disease are able to tolerate doses of vitamin D as high as 150,000–200,000 IU daily without apparent ill effect (Scadding, 1950; Larsson et al., 1952; Jackson and Dancaster, 1959), intolerance to doses of this magnitude is encountered with much greater frequency than in the general population (Curtis et al., 1947; Robertson, 1948; Nelson, 1949; Scadding, 1950; Larsson et al., 1952; Jackson and Dancaster, 1959; Ballard, 1960). Toxicity has resulted from as little as 10,000 IU daily (Scadding, 1950; Anderson et al., 1954; Cantwell, 1954; Mather, 1957; Bell et al., 1964), and a marked rise in serum calcium was noted in one patient who ingested one pint of cod-liver oil monthly (approximately 1000 IU per day) (Harrell and Fisher, 1939). Intestinal absorption of calcium is frequently excessive in sarcoidosis (Anderson et al., 1954; Henneman et al., 1956; Bell et al., 1964), and may be further increased by administering 10,000 IU of vitamin D daily, a dose which has little effect on intestinal calcium absorption in normal subjects (Bell et al., 1964). The frequent occurrence of hypercalcemia in sarcoid patients who are not taking extra vitamin D has been attributed to hypersensitivity to the small amounts of vitamin D obtained from diet and exposure to ultraviolet irradiation (Anderson et al., 1954; Bell et al., 1964). Calcium and phosphorus balance in these patients resembles that seen in hypervitaminosis D, and there is generally an excellent response to cortisone treatment as in hypervitaminosis D (Anderson et al., 1954). Furthermore, the incidence of hypercalcemia in patients with sarcoidosis is greater during the summer months (Taylor et al., 1963).

The cause of the increased sensitivity to vitamin D in sarcoidosis has not been established. Serum antirachitic activity has been found to be normal (Thomas et al., 1959; Bell et al., 1964). There appears to be no additional published data which shed light on the nature of this disturbance, although the reported observation that the response to parathyroid extract is also exaggerated in sarcoidosis suggests that in this disorder the bone may be more sensitive to factors promoting bone resorption (Rhodes et al., 1963).

References

Ahrens, E. H., Jr., M. A. Payne, H. G. Kunkel, W. J. Eisenmenger, and S. H. Blondhein. 1950. Primary biliary cirrhosis. *Medicine 29*:299.

Albright, F., A. M. Butler, and E. Bloomberg. 1937. Rickets resistant to vitamin D therapy. *Amer. J. Dis. Child. 54*:529.

Albright, F., and E. C. Reifenstein, Jr. 1948. *The Parathyroid Glands and Metabolic Bone Disease: Selected Studies.* Williams & Wilkins, Baltimore.

American Academy of Pediatrics, Report of the Committee on Nutrition. 1962. Infantile scurvy and nutritional rickets in the United States. *Pediatrics 29*:646.

Anderson, I., A. E. R. Campbell, A. Dunn, and J. B. M. Runciman. 1966. Osteomalacia in elderly women. *Scot. Med. J. 11*:429.

Anderson, J., C. E. Dent, C. Harper, and G. R. Philpot. 1954. Effect of cortisone on calcium metabolism in sarcoidosis with hypercalcemia. Possible antagonistic actions of cortisone and vitamin D. *Lancet 1954(2)*:720.

Arneil, G. C., and J. C. Crosbie. 1963. Infantile rickets returns to Glasgow. *Lancet 1963(2)*:423.

Atkinson, M., B. E. C. Nordin, and S. Sherlock. 1956. Malabsorption and bone disease in prolonged obstructive jaundice. *Quart. J. Med. 25*:299.

Avioli, L. V., S. J. Birge, and S. W. Lee. 1968*a*. [Avioli et al., 1968*a*.] Effects of prednisone in vitamin D metabolism in man. *J. Clin. Endocrinol. 28*:1341.

Avioli, L. V., S. Birge, S. W. Lee, and E. Slatopolsky. 1968*b*. [Avioli et al., 1968*b*.] The metabolic fate of vitamin D_3–^{3}H in chronic renal failure. *J. Clin. Invest. 47*:2239.

Avioli, L. V., S. J. Birge, and E. Slatopolsky. 1969. The nature of vitamin D resistance of patients with chronic renal disease. *Arch. Intern. Med. 124*:451.

Avioli, L. V., T. F. Williams, J. Lund, and H. F. DeLuca. 1967. Metabolism of vitamin D_3–^{3}H in vitamin D–resistant rickets and familial hypophosphatemia. *J. Clin. Invest. 46*:1907.

Badenoch, J., and P. Fourman. 1954. Osteomalacia in steatorrhoea. *Quart. J. Med. 23*:165.

Ballard, H. S. 1960. Irreversible renal failure following short term therapy in sarcoidosis. *Arch. Intern. Med. 106*:112.

Bauer, W., and A. Marble. 1932. Studies on the mode of action of irradiated ergosterol. II. Its effect on the calcium and phosphorus metabolism of individuals with calcium deficiency diseases. *J. Clin. Invest. 11*:21.

Bell, N. H., J. R. Gill, and F. C. Bartter. 1964. On the abnormal calcium absorption in sarcoidosis. Evidence for increased sensitivity to vitamin D. *Amer. J. Med. 36(4)*:500.

Benson, P. F., C. E. Stround, N. J. Mitchell, and A. Nicolaides. 1963. Rickets in immigrant children in London. *Brit. Med. J. 1963(1)*:1054.

Bicknell F., and F. Prescott. 1953. *The Vitamins in Medicine*, p. 517. Heinemann, London.

Bordier, P. H., H. Matrajt, D. Hioco, G. W. Hepner, G. R. Thompson, and C. C. Booth. 1968. Subclinical vitamin D deficiency following gastric surgery. *Lancet 1968(1)*: No. 7540, p. 437.

British Paediatric Association Report. 1964. Infantile hypercalcemia, nutritional rickets and infantile scurvy in Great Britain. *Brit. Med. J. 1964(1)*:1659.

Broadfoot, B. V. R., M. L. Trenholme, E. P. McClinton, S. H. Thompson, and E. J. Cowan. 1966. Vitamin D intakes of Ontario children. *Can. Med. Ass. J. 94*:332.

Butler, A. M. 1954. *In* E. C. Reifenstein, Jr. (ed.), *Metabolic Interrelations. Transactions of the Fifth Conference*, p. 338. The Josiah Macy Jr. Foundation, New York.

Cantwell, D. F. 1954. Sarcoidosis with renal involvement. *Irish. J. Med. Sci. 6*:223.

Chalmers, J., W. D. H. Conacher, D. L. Gardner, and P. J. Scott. 1967. Osteomalacia — a common disease in elderly women. *J. Bone Joint Surg. 49B*:403.

Clark, C. G. 1964. Late post-gastrectomy syndromes. Post-gastrectomy bone disease. *Proc. Roy. Soc. Med. 57*:580.

Clark, I., and C. A. L. Bassett. 1962. The amelioration of hypervitaminosis D in rats with vitamin A. *J. Exp. Med. 115*:147.

Coffey, J. 1950. Chronic poisoning due to excess of vitamin A. Description of the clinical and Roentgen manifestations in seven infants and young children. *Pediatrics 5*:672.

Connor, T. B., T. R. Hopkins, W. C. Thomas, Jr., R. A. Carey, and J. E. Howard. 1956. Use of cortisone and ACTH in hypercalcemic states. *J. Clin. Endocrinol. 16*:945.

Cowry, E. V., and G. H. Scott. 1936. Effect on monkeys of small doses of a concentrated preparation of Viosterol. *Arch. Pathol.* 22:1.

Curtis, A. C., H. Taylor, and R. H. Grekin. 1947. Sarcoidosis: Results of treatment with varying amounts of calciferol and dihydrotachysterol. *J. Invest. Dermatol. 9*:131.

Danowski, T. S. 1962. *Clinical Endocrinology*. Vol. 3, *Calcium, Phosphorus, Parathyroids and Bone*. Williams and Wilkins, Baltimore.

Deller, D. J., R. G. Edwards, and M. Addison. 1963. Calcium metabolism and the bones after partial gastrectomy. II. The nature and cause of the bone disorder. *Australas. Ann. Med. 12*:295.

Dent, C. E. 1956. Cortisone test for hyperparathyroidism. *Brit Med. J. 1956(1)*:230.

Dent, C. E. 1957. Pain in some metabolic bone diseases not due to steatorrhoea or renal failure. *Proc. Roy. Soc. Med. 50*:377.

Dent, C. E., and M. Friedman. 1964*a*. A comparison between AT–10 and pure dihydrotachysterol in controlling hypoparathyroidism. *Lancet 1964*(2):164.

Dent, C. E., and M. Friedman. 1964*b*. Hypercalciuric rickets associated with renal tubular damage. *Arch. Dis. Child. 39*:240.

Dent, C. E., and H. Harris. 1956. Hereditary forms of rickets and osteomalacia. *J. Bone Joint Surg. 38B*:204.

Dent, C. E., C. M. Harper, M. E. Morgans, G. R. Philpot, and W. R. Trotter. 1955. Insensitivity to vitamin D developing during the treatment of postoperative tetany. Its specificity as regards the form of vitamin D taken. *Lancet 1955(2)*:687.

Dent, C. E., W. R. Trotter, and T. A. Whittet. 1953. Calciferol tablets. *Pharm. J. 170*:124.

Drake, T. G. H. 1937. Comparison of the antirachitic effects on human beings of vitamin D from different sources. *Amer. J. Dis. Child. 53*:754.

Eisenberg, E. 1968. Renal effects of parathyroid hormone p. 465. *In* R. V. Talmage and L. F. Belanger (eds.), *Parathyroid Hormone and Thyrocalcitonin (Calcitonin)*. Proceedings of the Third Parathyroid Conference. Excerpta Medica Foundation, New York.

Fell, H. B. 1964. Some factors in the regulation of cell physiology in skeletal tissues p. 189. *In* H. M. Frost, M.D. (ed.), *Henry Ford Hospital International Symposium*. Little, Brown, Boston.

Field, M. H., and E. Reiss. 1960. Vitamin D resistant rickets: the effect of calcium infusion on phosphate reabsorption. *J. Clin. Invest. 39*:1807.

Fourman, P., D. Roger, M. J. Levell, and D. B. Morgan. 1968. *Calcium Metabolism and the Bone* (2nd ed.), p. 305. Blackwell Scientific Publications, Oxford and Edinburgh.

Frame, B., and R. W. Smith. 1958. Phosphate diabetes. *Amer. J. Med. 25*:771.

Fraser, D., N. T. Jaco, E. R. Yendt, J. Mann, and E. Liu. 1957. The induction of in vitro and in vivo calcification in bones of children suffering from vitamin

D resistant rickets without recourse to large doses of vitamin D. *Amer J. Dis. Child. 93*:84.

Fraser, D., J. M. Leeming, E. A. Cerwenka, and K. Kenyeres. 1959. Studies of the pathogenesis in the high renal clearance of phosphate in hypophosphatemic vitamin D refractory rickets of the simple type. *Amer. J. Dis. Child. 98*:586.

Friedman, W. F., and W. C. Roberts. 1966. Vitamin D and the supravalvular aortic stenosis syndrome. The transplacental effects of vitamin D on the aorta of the rabbit. *Circulation 34*:77.

Gerber, A., A. P. Raab, and A. E. Sobel. 1954. Vitamin A poisoning in adults. *Amer J. Med. 16*:729.

Glanville, H. J., and R. Bloom. 1965. Case of renal tubular osteomalacia (Dent Type II) with later development of autonomous parathyroid tumours. *Brit. Med. J. 1965(2)*:26.

Goldsmith, R. S., and S. H. Ingbar. 1966. Inorganic phosphate treatment of hypercalcemia of diverse etiologies. *New Engl. J. Med. 274*:1.

Gough, K. R., O. C. Lloyd, and M. R. Wilb. 1964. Nutritional osteomalacia. *Lancet 1964(2)*:1261.

Gross-Selbeck, C. 1935. Uber die Verhutung von Vitamin D–Schaden Durch Vitamin A Zufutterung. *Klin. Wochensch. 14*:61.

Guroff, G., H. F. DeLuca, and H. Steenbock. 1963. Citrate and action of vitamin D on calcium and phosphorus metabolism. *Amer. J. Physiol. 204*:833.

Ham, A., and B. C. Portuondo. 1933. Relation of serum calcium to pathologic calcifications of hypervitaminosis D. *Arch. Pathol. 16*:1.

Harrell, G. T., and S. Fisher. 1939. Blood chemical changes in Boeck's Sarcoid with particular references to protein, calcium and phosphatase values. *J. Clin. Invest. 18*:687.

Harris, L. J. 1956. Vitamin D and bone p. 617. *In* G. H. Bourne (ed.), *The Biochemistry and Physiology of Bone.* Academic Press, New York.

Harris, W. H., and R. P. Heaney. 1969. Skeletal Renewal and bone disease. *New Engl. J. Med. 280*: No. 4, p. 193; No. 5, p. 253; No. 6, p. 303.

Harrison, H. E. 1961. Vitamin D and calcium and phosphate transport. *Pediatrics 28*:531.

Harrison, H. E. 1963. Rickets, pp. 1–63. *In* J. Brenneman (ed.), *Practice of Pediatrics.* W. F. Prior Co. Inc., Hagerstown, Maryland.

Harrison, H. E. 1964. Primary vitamin D resistant rickets. *J. Pediat. 64*:618.

Harrison, H. E., and H. C. Harrison. 1967. Vitamin D resistant rickets, pp. 343–54. *In* D. J. Hioco (ed.), *L'Osteomalacie.* Masson et Cie, Paris.

Harrison, H. C., H. E. Harrison, and E. A. Park. 1958. Vitamin D and citrate metabolism; effect of vitamin D in rats fed diets adequate in both calcium and phosphorus. *Amer. J. Physiol. 192*:432.

Harrison, H. E., F. Lifshitz, and R. M. Blizzard. 1967. Dihydrotachysterol and calciferol in vitamin D therapy. *New Engl. J. Med. 276*:894.

Hendricks, J. B., A. F. Morgan, and R. M. Freytag. 1947. Chronic moderate hypervitaminosis D in young dogs. *Amer. J. Physiol. 149*:319.

Henkin, R. I., M. Lotz, and F. C. Bartter. 1966. Treatment of hypervitaminosis D by peritoneal dialysis. The removal of calcium and vitamin D by peritoneal dialysis. Third International Congress of Nephrology, Washington, D.C. Published extracts *2*:209.

Henneman, P. H., E. F. Dempsey, E. L. Carroll, and F. Albright. 1956. The cause of hypercalciuria in sarcoid and its treatment with cortisone and sodium phytate. *J. Clin. Invest. 35*:1229.

Henneman, P. H., E. F. Dempsey, E. L. Carroll, and D. H. Henneman. 1962. Acquired vitamin D resistant osteomalacia; a new variety characterized by hypercalcemia, low serum bicarbonate and hyperglucinuria. *Metabolism 11*:103.

Hess, A. F., H. R. Benjamin, and J. Gross. 1931. The source of excess calcium in hypercalcemia induced by irradiated ergosterol. *J. Biol. Chem. 94*:1.

Himsworth, H. P., and M. Maisels. 1940. Vitamins D_2 and D_3 and AT–10 in congenital thyroid and parathyroid deficiency. *Lancet 1940(1)*:959.

Homer, L. 1961. Hypoparathyroidism requiring massive amounts of medication with apparent response to magnesium sulphate. *J. Clin. Endocrinol. 21*:219.

Howard, J. E., and R. J. Meyer. 1948. Intoxication with vitamin D. *J. Clin. Endocrinol. 8*:895.

Howard, J. E., and T. B. Connor. 1954. Some experiences with the use of vitamin D in the treatment of hypoparathyroidism. *Trans. Ass. Amer. Physicians 67*:199.

Howland, J., and B. Kramer. 1921. Calcium and phosphorus in the serum in relation to rickets. *Amer. J. Dis. Child. 22*:105.

Jackson, W. P., and C. Dancaster. 1959. A consideration of the hypercalciuria in sarcoidosis, idiopathic hypercalciuria and that produced by vitamin D. A new suggestion regarding calcium metabolism. *J. Clin. Endocrinol. 19*:658.

Jackson, W. P., E. Dowdle, and G. C. Linder. 1958. Vitamin D resistant osteomalacia. *Brit. Med. J. 1958(1)*:1269.

Johnson, L. C. 1966. Kinetics of skeletal remodelling. A further consideration of the theoretical biology of bone, p. 66. *In* D. Bergsma (ed.), *Structural Organization of the Skeleton: A Symposium.* Birth Defects Original Article Series *2(1)*. National Foundation, New York.

Jones, C. T., J. A. Williams, and G. Nicholson. 1963. *In* F. A. R. Stammers and J. A. Williams (eds.), *Partial Gastrectomy*, p. 190. Butterworth, London.

Jones, K. H., and P. Fourman. 1966. Effects of infusions of magnesium and of calcium in parathyroid insufficiency. *Clin. Sci. 20*:139.

Jowsey, J., and B. L. Riggs. 1968. Bone changes in a patient with hypervitaminosis A. *J. Clin. Endocrinol. 28*:1833.

Kahn, A., I. Snapper, and A. Drucker. 1968. Corticosteroid-induced tetany in latent hypoparathyroidism. *Arch. Intern. Med. 114*:434.

Kimberg, D. V., and S. A. Goldstein. 1967. Binding of calcium by liver mitochondria: an effect of steroid hormones in vitamin D–depleted and parathyroidectomized rats. *Endocrinology 80*:89.

Knudson, A. G., Jr., and P. E. Rothman. 1953. Hypervitaminosis A. A review with a discussion of Vitamin A. *Amer. J. Dis. Child. 85*:316.

Kreitmair, H., and T. Moll. 1928. Hypervitaminose Durch Grosse Dosen Vitamin D. *Munchen Med. Wochensch. 75*:637.

Larsson, L. G., A. Liljestrand, and H. Wahlund. 1952. Treatment of sarcoidosis with calciferol. *Acta Med. Scand. 143*:280.

Leeson, P. M., and P. Fourman. 1966. Increased sensitivity to vitamin D after vitamin D poisoning. *Lancet 1966(1)*:1182.

Linder, G. C., and C. F. Harris. 1929. Calcium and phosphorus metabolism in chronic diarrhoea. *Quart. J. Med. 23*:195.

Mather, G. 1957. Calcium metabolism and bone changes in sarcoidosis. *Brit. Med. J. 1957(1)*:248.

Mathieu, H., P. Cuisinier-Gleizes, R. Habib, H. Dulac, M. Lacoste, E. Gyrard, and P. Roger. Action toxique de la vitamine A sans hypercalcemie chez le rat parathyroidectomise I Etude des lesions anatomiques. *Pathol. Biol. (Paris) 12*:674.

Matrajt, H., P. Bordier, and D. Hioco. 1967. Mesures histologiques semi-quantitative dans 17 observations d'osteomalacies nutritionelle et renales. Influence de la vitamine D p. 101. *In* D. J. Hioco (ed.), *L'Osteomalacie*. Masson & Cie, Paris.

Mautalen, C. A., J. F. Dymling, and M. Horwith. 1967. Pseudohypoparathyroidism. 1942–1966. A negative progress report. *Amer. J. Med. 42*:977.

Mellanby, E. 1919*a*. The part played by accessory food factors in the etiology of rickets. *J. Physiol. 52*:lili.

Mellanby, E. 1919*b*. An experimental investigation on rickets. *Lancet 196*:407.

Milhaud, G. 1968. Utilization of thyrocalcitonin in man in normal and pathological conditions p. 86. *In* R. V. Talmage and L. F. Belanger (eds.), *Parathyroid Hormone and Thyrocalcitonin (Calcitonin)*. Proceedings of the Third Parathyroid Conference. Excerpta Medica Foundation, New York.

Moehlig, R. C., and A. L. Steinbach. 1954. Cortisone interference with calcium therapy in hypoparathyroidism. *J. Amer. Med. Ass. 154*:42.

Morgan, A. F., L. Kimmel, and N. C. Hawkins. 1937. A comparison of the hypervitaminoses induced by irradiated ergosterol and fish liver oil concentrates. *J. Biol. Chem. 120*:85.

Morgan, D. B., C. R. Paterson, C. G. Woods, C. N. Pulvertaft, and P. Fourman. 1965. Osteomalacia after gastrectomy. A response to very small doses of Vitamin D. *Lancet 1965(2)*:1089.

Nagant de Deuxchaisnes, C. N., and S. M. Krane. 1967. The treatment of adult phosphate diabetes and Fanconi syndrome with neutral sodium phosphate. *Amer. J. Med. 43*:508.

Nelson, C. T. 1949. Calciferol in treatment of sarcoidosis. *J. Invest. Dermatol. 13*:81.

Nicolaysen, R. 1943. The absorption of calcium as a function of body saturation with calcium. *Acta Physiol. Scand. 5*:200.

Nigrin, G., W. A. Cochrane, D. Jannigan, and A. Ernst. 1962. Results of calcium infusion and renal biopsy studies in refractory rickets. *Amer. J. Dis. Child. 104*:478 (Abstr.)

Nordin, B. E. C., and D. A. Smith. 1967. Pathogenesis and treatment of osteomalacia p. 379. *In* D. J. Hioco (ed.), *L'Osteomalacie*. Masson & Cie, Paris.

Pak, C. Y. C., H. F. DeLuca, J. M. Chavez de los Rios and T. Suda. 1969. Treatment of vitamin D resistance with 25–hydroxycholecalciferol. *Clin. Res. 17*:291.

Papadatos, C., and R. Klein. 1954. Addison's disease in a boy with hypoparathyroidism. *J. Clin. Endocrinol. 14*:653.

Parfitt, A. M. 1968. A clinical comparison of two preparations of calciferol. *Australas. Ann. Med. 17*:56.

Pfannenstiel, W. 1928. Weitere Beobachtungen uber Wirkungen Bestrahten Ergosterins im Tierversuch. *Munchen Med. Wochensch. 75*:1113.

Reed, C. I. 1938. On the nature of the toxic action of vitamin D. *Proc. Soc. Exp. Biol. Med. 38*:791.

Reed, C. I., H. G. Struck, and I. E. Steck. 1939. Vitamin D; chemistry, physiology, pharmacology, pathology, experimental and clinical investigations. Univ. of Chicago Press, Chicago.

Reiss, E., J. M. Canterbury, and R. T. Belinsky. 1968. Measurement of serum parathyroid hormone in renal insufficiency. Conference on Divalent Ion Metabolism and Osteodystrophy in Chronic Renal Failure, Santa Barbara, California, 1968.

Rhodes, J., E. H. Reynolds, J. D. Fitzgerald, and P. Fourman. 1963. Exaggerated response to parathyroid extract in sarcoidosis. *Lancet 1963(2)*:598.

Richards, I. D. G., E. M. Sweet, and G. C. Arneil. 1968. Infantile rickets persists in Glasgow. *Lancet 1968(1)*:803.

Robertson, R. F. 1948. Vitamin D in treatment of Boeck's Sarcoidosis. *Brit Med. J. 1948(2)*:1059.

Rose, G. A. 1964. Role of phosphate in treatment of renal tubular (hypophosphatemic) rickets and osteomalacia. *Br. Med. J. 1964(2)*:857.

Sallis, J. D., and E. S. Holdsworth. 1962. Calcium metabolism in relation to vitamin D_3 and adrenal function in the chick. *Amer. J. Physiol. 203*:506.

Saville, P. D., J. R. Nassim, H. Stevenson, L. Mulligan, and N. Carey. 1955. The effect of AT–10 on calcium and phosphorus metabolism in resistant rickets. *Clin. Sci. 14*:489.

Scadding, J. G. 1950. Sarcoidosis with special reference to lung changes. *Brit. Med. J. 1950(1)*:745.

Shelling, D. H. 1930. Relation of calcium and phosphorus of diet to toxicity of viosterol. *Proc. Soc. Exp. Biol. Med. 28*:298.

Sherwood, L. M., G. P. Mayer, C. F. Ramberg, Jr., D. S. Kronfeld, G. D. Aurback, and J. T. Potts, Jr. 1968. Regulation of parathyroid hormone secretion: proportional control by calcium, lack of effect of phosphate. *Endocrinology 83*:1043.

Smith, M. I., and E. Elvore. 1929. The action of irradiated ergosterol in the rabbit. *Public Health Rep. 44*:1245.

Spaulding, S. W., and M. Walser. 1969. Oral phosphate therapy in experimental hypercalcemia. *Clin. Res. 17*:395.

Stanbury, S. W. 1958. Some aspects of disordered renal tubular function. *Advances. Intern. Med. 9*:231.

Stanbury, S. W. 1964. Calcium and phosphorus metabolism in chronic renal failure. *In* J. de Graeff and B. Leijnse (eds.), *Water and Electrolyte Metabolism*. Vol. 2. American Elsevier, New York.

Stanbury, S. W. 1968. Bone disease in uremia. *Am. J. Med. 44*:714.

Stewart, W. K., R. G. Mitchell, H. G. Morgan, K. G. Lowe, and J. Thompson. 1964. The changing incidence of rickets and infantile hypercalcemia as seen in Dundee. *Lancet 1964(1)*:679.

Taylor, R. L., H. J. Lynch, and W. G. Wysor, Jr. 1963. Seasonal influence of sunlight on the hypercalcemia of sarcoidosis. *Amer. J. Med. 34*:221.

Terepka, A. R., P. S. Chen, Jr., and B. Jorgensen. 1961. Nature of hytakerol (AT–10) and its comparison with crystalline dihydrotachysterol. *Endocrinology 68*:996.

Thomas, W. C., Jr., H. G. Morgan, T. B. Connor, L. Haddock, C. E. Bills, and J. E. Howard. 1959. Studies of antiricketic activity in sera from patients with disorders of calcium metabolism and preliminary observations on the mode of transport of vitamin D in human serum. *J. Clin. Invest. 38*:1078.

Thompson, G. R., B. Lewis, and C. C. Booth. 1966 [Thompson et al., 1966*a*.] Vitamin D absorption after partial gastrectomy. *Lancet 1966(1)*:457.

Thompson, G. R., G. Neale, B. Lewis, M. Watts, and C. C. Booth. 1967. Plasma vitamin D-like activity and vitamin D absorption in man p. 337. *In* D. J. Hioco (ed.), *L'Osteomalacie*. Masson & Cie, Paris.

Thompson, G. R., G. Neale, J. M. Watts, and C. C. Booth. 1966. [Thompson et al., 1966*b*.] Detection of vitamin D deficiency after partial gastrectomy. *Lancet 1966(1)*:623.

Van Buchem, F. S. P. 1959. Osteomalacia: pathogenesis and treatment. *Brit. Med. J. 1959(1)*:933.

Verner, J. V., Jr., F. L. Engel, and H. T. McPherson. 1958. Vitamin D intoxication: Report of two cases treated with cortisone. *Ann. Intern. Med. 48*:765.

Volwiler, W. 1957. Gastrointestinal malabsorptive syndromes. *Amer. J. Med. 23*:250.

West, C. D., J. C. Blanton, F. N. Silverman, and N. H. Holland. 1964. Use of phosphate salts as an adjunct to vitamin D in the treatment of hypophosphatemic vitamin D refractory rickets. *J. Pediat. 64*:469.

Williams, T. F., R. W. Winters, and C. H. Burnett. 1966 Familial (hereditary) vitamin D–resistant rickets with hypophosphatemia pp. 1179–1204. *In* J. B. Stanbury, J. B. Wyngaarden, and D. S. Fredrickson (eds.), *The Metabolic Basis of Inherited Disease*. 2nd ed. McGraw-Hill, New York.

Wilson, D. R., S. E. York, Z. F. Jaworski, and E. R. Yendt. 1965. Studies in hypophosphatemic vitamin D refractory osteomalacia in adults. *Medicine 44*:99.

Winberg, J., and R. Zetterstrom. 1956. Cortisone treatment in vitamin D intoxication. *Acta Paediat. 45*:96.

Winters, R. W., J. B. Graham, T. F. Williams, V. W. McFalls, and C. H. Burnett. 1958. A genetic study of familial hypophosphatemia and vitamin D resistant rickets with a review of the literature. *Medicine 37*:97.

11

CURRENT CONCEPTS OF VITAMIN D_3 METABOLISM IN MAN

Louis V. Avioli

Introduction

Since its isolation and identification as an antirachitic factor by Askew and co-workers (1931) and Windaus and co-workers (1932), vitamin D has been recognized as one of the most important factors in the regulation of calcium absorption and bone metabolism. Loomis (1967) has noted that the term "vitamin D" is a misnomer, since its endogenous production by the skin and distribution by the blood stream for action on bone and intestine all resemble hormonal rather than dietary vitamin activity.

During the forty years subsequent to its discovery, relatively little was known about the synthesis and metabolic fate of vitamin D in man despite an adequate antirachitic biological assay, intensive clinical investigation, and observed therapeutic success with crystalline preparations. This ignorance has led to accumulated reports and reviews of certain clinical syndromes, all of which have been characterized by either an exaggerated or blunted response to vitamin D. Thus one is confronted with an abnormal sensitivity to vitamin D in patients with sarcoidosis (Bell and Bartter, 1964; Henneman et al., 1956; Bell et al., 1964), and idiopathic hypercalcemia of infancy (Taussig, 1966; Anita et al., 1967). There is resistance to vitamin D in certain forms of familial hypophosphatemic rickets (Winters et al., 1958; Burnett et al., 1964), renal osteodystrophy (Dent et al., 1961; Stanbury and Lumb, 1962), acquired gluten-sensitive enteropathies (Nassim et al., 1959), primary biliary cirrhosis (Kehayoglou et al., 1968), and fibrogenesis imperfecta ossium (Baker et al., 1966). The last represents a unique generalized bone disorder with a highly specific matrix abnor-

These researches were supported in part by Grant AM–11674 from the National Institute of Arthritis and Metabolic Diseases and by United States Atomic Energy Commission Contract AT(11–1)–1742.

mality which responds to dihydrotachysterol but not to vitamin D_2. The reported antagonism between vitamin D and glucocorticoids (Papadatos and Klein, 1954; Verner et al., 1958) affords another example of the cliches which have been used to disguise our ignorance of vitamin D metabolism in man. An evaluation of vitamin D metabolism in these aforementioned clinical disorders of calcium and bone metabolism as well as in normal man has been hampered by the lack of sophisticated quantitative-analytical methods for the isolation and measurement of vitamin D in biological specimens, as well as by the unavailability of purified radioactive vitamin D preparations suitable for investigation in human subjects.

In 1955 Kodicek reported a biosynthetic yeast preparation of ^{14}C ergosterol with specific activities in the range of 5–63 dpm/IU and, in 1956, described for the first time the metabolic fate of vitamin D in the rat. He and his collaborators subsequently (1960) administered this vitamin D preparation orally to infants ranging in age from 3 days to 15 months with inoperable brain deformities. The results of these preliminary investigations, which appear to represent the first radioactive vitamin D studies in humans, suggested that the metabolism of vitamin D in infants is similar to that in the rat. Radioactivity was found in the blood, liver, and kidneys of these infants, and only an insignificant portion of the administered radioactivity could be accounted for in cumulative urine and fecal collections. Whereas earlier, breakdown products of vitamin D had been reported in animal experimentation, no reported attempt was made by Kodicek at that time to isolate and identify metabolites of vitamin D_2 in any biological specimens.

After these preliminary observations were made, continued interest in the biochemistry and metabolism of vitamin D led to refinements in isotopic labeling and methods of purification, and chemical synthesis of biologically active preparations of 1,2–^{3}H vitamin D_3 which were finally obtained from 1,2–^{3}H cholesterol with specific activities of 5,000–26,000 dpm/IU (Neville and DeLuca, 1966). These radiochemically pure vitamin D preparations with sufficiently high specific radioactivity for the detection of metabolic intermediates were subsequently incorporated by investigators into a series of superb animal experiments, which led to a detailed analysis of the subcellular location and mechanism of vitamin D action as well as the isolation of a biologically active vitamin D_3 metabolite, finally realized in porcine plasma as 25–hydroxycholecalciferol (Blunt et al., 1968).

Despite the current availability of and continued experimentation with vitamin D preparations of high specific activity in man, the vicissitudes and limitations necessarily imposed by human experimentation coupled with the renewed acceleration of vitamin D research in animals has resulted in a "vitamin D information gap," which still precludes direct correlation of the results obtained in animals with a knowledge of vitamin D activity in man. However, with the advent of the radioactive preparations, considerable knowledge of the absorption and metabolic fate of vitamin D has been recently accumulated in normal human volunteers and in subjects with various disorders of calcium and bone metabolism.

Intestinal absorption of vitamin D

Since Kodicek's original observations (1960) that between 13% and 23% of an oral dose of ^{14}C vitamin D_2 was recoverable from the feces of infants within 3 days, additional information on the absorption of vitamin D in man was nonexistent until 1966. At that time, Thompson and associates reported on the concentrations of plasma, stool, and urine radioactivity after the oral administration of tritium-labeled vitamin D_3 (^3H vitamin D_3) to normal subjects and to patients with intestinal malabsorption. The absorption of ^3H vitamin D_3 was calculated in these studies on the assumption that the radioactivity not recovered in the feces during the subsequent 6-day cumulative period had been absorbed. Net absorption of doses of either 0.5 mg or 1.0 mg of ^3H vitamin D_3 in seven control subjects was reported to range from 62.4% to 91.3% (with a mean of 78.6%). Most of the recoverable nonabsorbed fecal radioactivity (68.4%–85.8%) was concluded to be unaltered vitamin D_3 on the basis of thin layer chromatography. Two to three hours following the oral dose, 45%–100% of the plasma radioactivity was present in a chylomicron fraction. The association of ^3H vitamin D_3 with plasma chylomicrons led these investigators to postulate that vitamin D_3 in man, as in the rat (Schachter et al., 1964), is normally absorbed primarily through lymphatic channels. Blomstrand and Forsgren (1967) subsequently reported on studies concerning the intestinal absorption and esterification of ^3H vitamin D_3 in man after the common thoracic duct was cannulated. They confirmed the absorption of the vitamin through the lymphatic pathway in man and noted that only a minor portion of the absorbed ^3H vitamin D_3 was esterified. Their results, although preliminary, also established the obligatory role of bile for the absorption of vitamin D_3 in man. These observations were confirmed in studies of thoracic-duct-cannulated patients of two groups: those with normal biliary intestinal drainage and others with either biliary fistulae or common bile duct obstruction (Avioli and Lee, 1968). Moreover, a biologically potent metabolite of vitamin D_3 was also recovered from lymph. Although bile was deemed essential for the intestinal absorption of vitamin D, it appeared to play an insignificant role in the intestinal conversion of vitamin D_3 to its biologically active metabolite.

Considerable disagreement still exists regarding the site of vitamin D absorption in the intestine of animals. Data derived from the experiments of Norman and DeLuca (1963) and of Callow and associates (1966) suggest that the ileum is the primary site of absorption, but Schachter and coworkers (1964) conclude that the jejunum has a greater capacity for absorbing vitamin D than does the ileum. The results of human experimentation are still inconclusive, but a recent report on a patient with a small jejunal remnant following intestinal resection demonstrated that this segment is capable of efficient vitamin D absorption (Thompson et al., 1965). Since there is ample evidence for multipotential function of different parts of the intestine so that one segment can assume the function normally performed by another, it is still premature to assume that the jejunum is the site of optimum vitamin D absorption in man simply because absorption is documented in cases of extensive ileal resection.

Transport and metabolic fate of vitamin D in man

The transport of vitamin D in blood has been studied in considerable detail in animals (Chalk and Kodicek, 1961; Rikkers and DeLuca, 1967), and there is general agreement that the vitamin is bound to α_2-globulin and lipoproteins in stable and non-ultrafiltrable forms. Recently, Rikkers and DeLuca (1967), using physiologic doses of ^{3}H vitamin D_3 preparations and polyacrylamide-disc electrophoretic techniques, have conclusively demonstrated that, in the rat, vitamin D_3 as well as its biologically active metabolite is bound primarily to a circulating α_2-globulin. Studies on vitamin D transport in man, limited in the past to incorporating large nonphysiologic doses of vitamin D and biological assays (Thomas et al., 1959; DeCrousaz et al., 1965), have demonstrated vitamin D activity in α_1- and α_2-globulin plasma fractions. Avioli and associates (1968*b*), utilizing polyvinyl block and immunoelectrophoretic techniques, have demonstrated that in human subjects vitamin D_3 and its biologically active metabolite are associated with circulating albumin, α_1- and α_2-globulin protein fractions. The biological significance of this relationship is still uncertain. DeLuca (1967) has suggested the possibility that the normal plasma vitamin D protein carriers may play an essential role in the transfer of vitamin D and its metabolites to specific metabolic receptor sites in bone and the gastrointestinal tract.

Considerable knowledge has been gained recently concerning the metabolic fate of oral or intravenous vitamin D preparations in man. As noted in Figure 11.1, after ^{3}H vitamin D_3 is injected into human subjects, the plasma disappearance curve is characteristically biphasic with the half-life of plasma ^{3}H vitamin D_3 ranging between 20 and 30 hr (Avioli et al., 1967*a*).

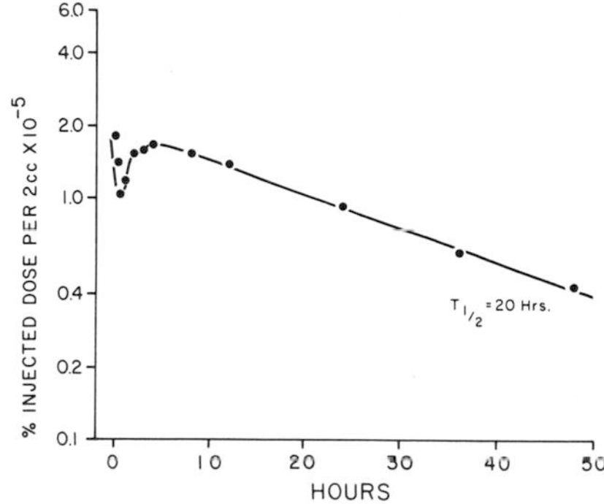

Fig. 11.1. Plasma ^{3}H vitamin D_3 of a normal human subject after the injection of ^{3}H vitamin D_3.

Since a 4–6 hr lag usually occurs between the administration of vitamin D and the appearance of its earliest physiological effect, the biphasic plasma curve may represent either different metabolic pools with varied rates of turnover or certain physiological processes essential for the transport and localization of the vitamin at its functional sites. By means of methanol and chloroform extraction of serial plasma samples, followed by silicic acid column chromatography, the metabolic transformation of vitamin D is reflected in the plasma by the gradual emergence of at least three vitamin D metabolites over a 72 hr period (Fig. 11.2). Peak II, as yet unidentified, has never been found in significant quantities in man and is probably of limited biological significance; peak III has been identified as biologically unaltered vitamin D_3; peak IV, although structurally unidentified in man to date, has been shown to possess antirachitic activity (Avioli et al., 1967*a*), as measured by the line test assay described in *U.S. Pharmacopoeia*, as well as a remarkable ability to restore calcium uptake in the duodenal slices of rachitic rats, surpassing that of the parent compound (Fig. 11.3). Peak IV does not appear to be homogenous in man and, as reported by DeLuca (1967) for the rat, is composed of at least three components, only one of which is biologically active. As noted previously, the structure of a similar biologically potent vitamin D metabolite has been identified in porcine plasma as 25-hydroxycholecalciferol (Blunt et al., 1968). Peak V (Fig. 11.2) is also still unidentified in man, but as shown in Table 11.1, it is biologically inert. To date, it represents the only vitamin D metabolite which has been recovered from urine (Avioli et al., 1968*a*). In some studies with human volunteers, a substance less polar than vitamin D_3 has been identified in plasma and, in accordance with the nomenclature established in animal experimentation, designated peak I. In animal studies with ^{3}H vitamin D_3, peak I has been conclusively demonstrated to contain esters of vitamin D and long-chain fatty acids (Fraser and Kodicek, 1968). Such seems to be the case in humans as well, since saponification of chloroform

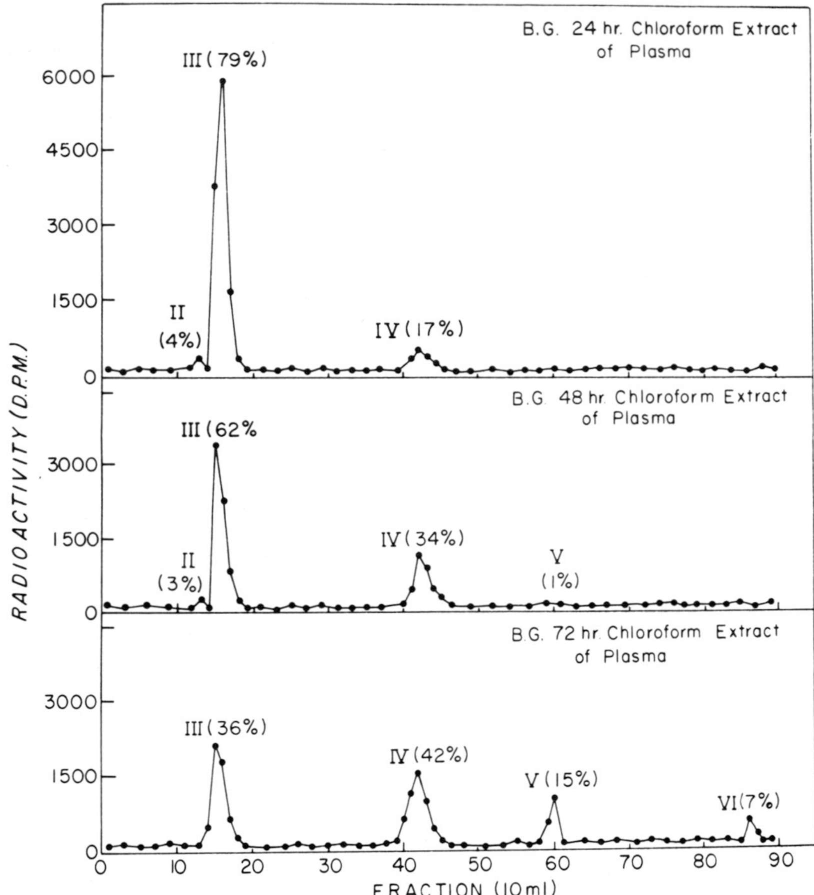

Fig. 11.2. Silicic acid column profile of plasma chloroform extracts of plasma obtained in a normal human subject 24 hr, 48 hr, and 72 hr after an oral dose of ^{3}H vitamin D_3. (Avioli et al., 1968*b*. Reproduced by permission of the *Journal of Clinical Investigation.*)

plasma extracts obtained following ^{3}H vitamin D_3 injection results in the disappearance of peak I and accumulation of free ^{3}H vitamin D_3 (Fig. 11.4). To date, the lack of sufficient assayable quantities of peak I in humans precludes any knowledge of its biological activity. The tentative identification of vitamin D_3 esters in the lymph of humans (Blomstrand and Forsgren, 1967) is, however, consistent with in vivo vitamin esterification during absorption from the gastrointestinal tract.

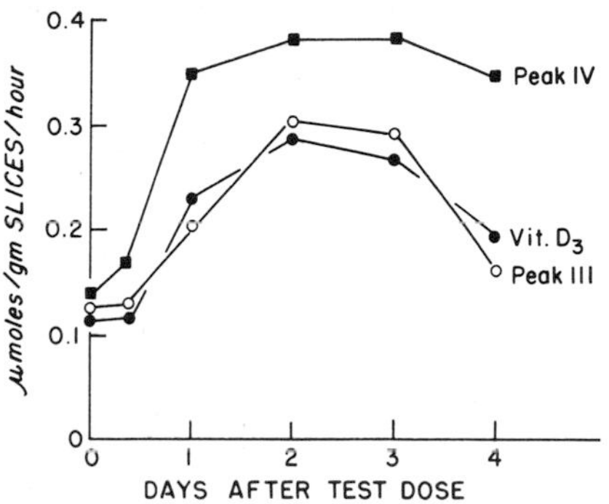

Fig. 11.3. Oxygen-dependent accumulation of calcium by rat duodenal slices at various intervals following 0.25 IU of crystalline vitamin D_3 and amounts of peak III and peak IV isolated from normal human plasma corresponding to 0.25 IU of vitamin D_3. The amount of each compound tested was estimated on the basis of the specific activity of the injected ^3H vitamin D_3.

TABLE 11.1. *Biological activity of fractions from normal serum 25 hr after intravenous administration of ^3H vitamin D_3*

Fraction	Number of rats in assay	Calcification score
Peak III	8	5 ± 1.0
Peak IV	8	6 ± 1.0
Peak V	8	0
Vitamin D standard[a]	8	5 ± 0.5

Note: All substances were bioassayed by line-test technique as published in *U.S. Pharmacopoeia* (15th ed., Easton, Pa., 1955, p. 889). Amount of each compound was estimated on the basis of the specific activity of the parent vitamin ^3H vitamin D_3 (160,000 dpm = 1 μg).

[a] Each rat was given 4.0 IU of vitamin D.

Recent studies of patients with complete biliary fistulae (Avioli et al., 1967*a*) or cirrhosis establish the importance of the liver in the regulation and metabolism of circulating vitamin D and its metabolites in man (Scott et al., 1965; Avioli et al., 1967*a*). They also reveal that the major biliary metabolite of vitamin D in man, as in the rat (Bell and Kodicek, 1967), is a glucuronide conjugate (Fig. 11.5). The data derived from studies on patients with biliary fistulae and given intravenous injections of ^3H vitamin D_3 indicate that the passage of vitamin D and its metabolites through the bile and into the intestine represents an obligatory stage for the enterohepatic circulation and fecal excretion of vitamin D metabolites by man.

For the 48–72 hr period following either oral or intravenous ^3H vitamin D_3 administration, less than 3% of the dose (Fig. 11.6) is recoverable in urine, primarily as biologically inactive, water-soluble metabolites (Avioli et al., 1967*a*). As illustrated in Figure 11.5, glucuronide and acid ^3H vitamin D_3 conjugates also account for over 25% of the water-soluble urinary radioactivity.

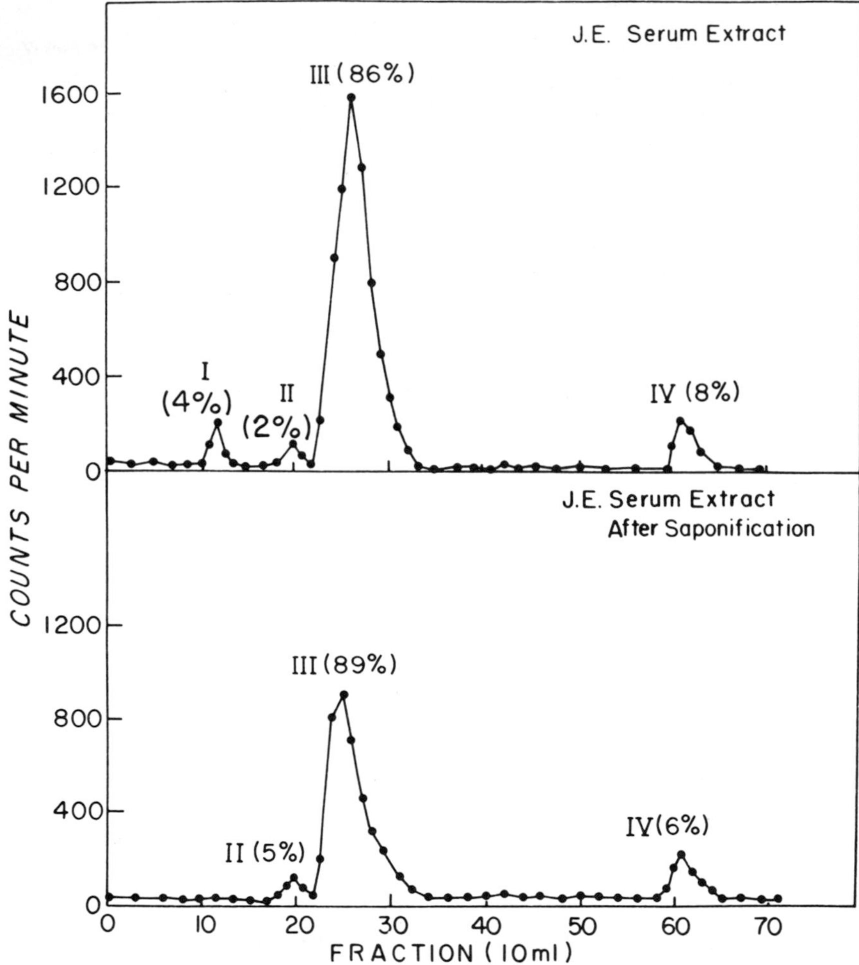

Fig. 11.4. Silicic acid column chromatography of a chloroform extract of human plasma obtained 24 hr after an injection of ^{3}H vitamin D_3. The lower panel represents chromatographic separation of an ether extract of the saponified material. Note the disappearance of peak I. (Avioli et al., 1967*b*. Reproduced by permission of the *Journal of Clinical Investigation.*)

Since by definition bioassay techniques are essentially end-point determinants of nonspecific biological activity, the presence of active vitamin D metabolites from human plasma precludes an adequate biological appraisal of circulating levels of unaltered vitamin D_3. Methods such as infrared, ultraviolet, and fluorescent analysis, heretofore proposed for the chemical determination of vitamin D, suffer primarily from lack of speci-

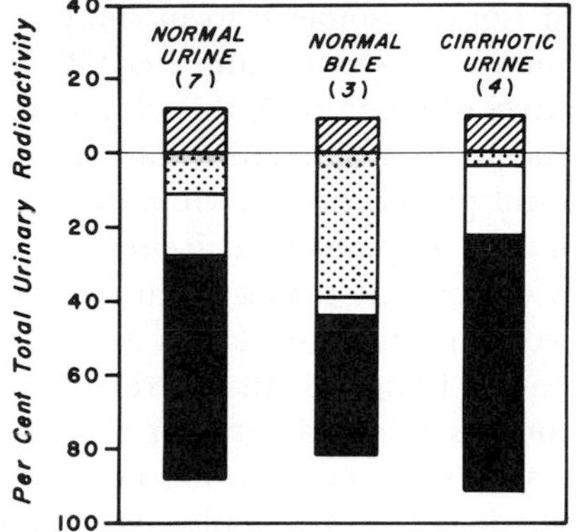

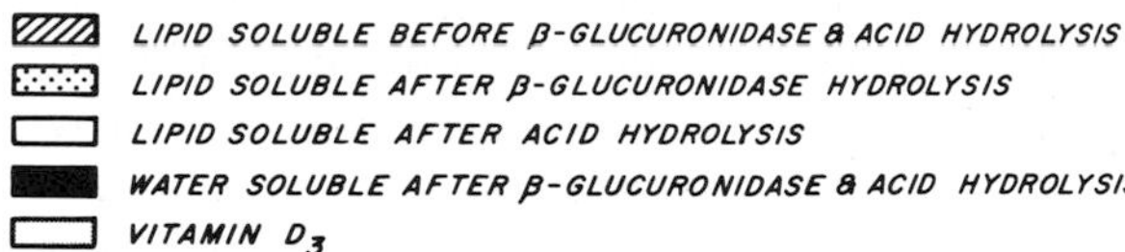

Fig. 11.5. Activity of urine in 7 normal subjects, of bile in 3 normal subjects, and of urine in 4 cirrhotic patients, after an injection of ^{3}H vitamin D_3. The height of the bar in each case represents the mean value for the group. Note the identification of free ^{3}H vitamin D_3 in the glucuronide fraction of normal urine and bile. (Avioli et al., 1967*a*. Reproduced by permission of the *Journal of Clinical Investigation*.)

ficity and sensitivity (Passannante and Avioli, 1966), and are usually applicable only to high-potency biological preparations free from other interfering substances such as β-carotene and vitamin A. Naturally occurring vitamin D_3 has a 6-*cis* configuration and appears as a double peak in a gas chromatograph as a result of thermal cyclization (Ziffer et al., 1960). Since

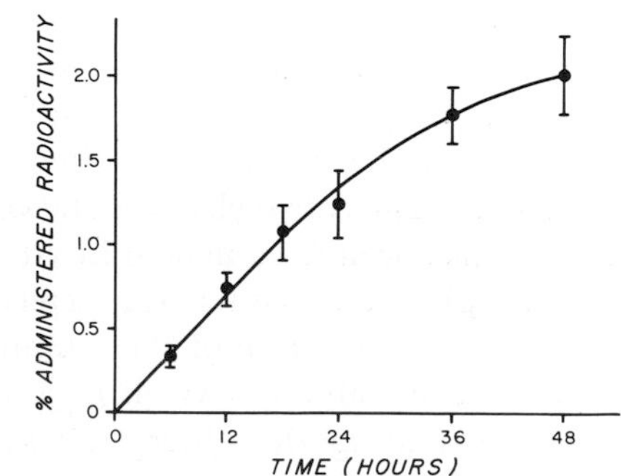

Fig. 11.6. Cumulative excretion of total urinary radioactivity after an injection of ^{3}H vitamin D_3. Each point represents the mean ± 2 SE in 10 subjects.

the resulting pyro and isopyro isomeric forms may be quantitatively related to the original compound (Avioli and Lee, 1966), and because they are not natural derivatives of vitamin D, this chromatographic technique, combined with the principles of isotope dilution and previously published methods for isolation and purification of vitamin D from plasma (Avioli et al., 1967*a*), has been used to quantitate circulating levels of vitamin D_3 in man. In 50 normal out-patient subjects, ranging in age from 6 to 85 years, the vitamin D_3 concentration in plasma after overnight fasting was 8–45 ng/ml, with a mean of 19 ng/ml. In this relatively small population, no significant correlation was observed between age and plasma vitamin D_3 content and no seasonal differences were found. These values are to be compared with those obtained by routine bioassay techniques by Warkany and Mabon (1940), who, while commenting on the results of 155 assays, found vitamin D activity levels similar in adults and children, with values ranging from 0.6–1.7 IU/ml and averaging 1.1 IU/ml of serum. Their values are approximately 50% higher (1 IU = 25 ng) than those obtained with the gas chromatographic–isotope dilution procedure cited above and may reflect combined biological estimates of vitamin D_3 and its active metabolite.

Abnormal metabolism of vitamin D

The recent availability of chemically pure vitamin D preparations with high specific activity has prompted what may be an unprecedented analysis of vitamin D absorption and metabolism in certain clinical disorders of calcium and bone metabolism. Accordingly, malabsorption of ^3H vitamin D_3 has been demonstrated in patients with celiac disease, chronic pancreatitis, and biliary obstruction (Thompson et al, 1966), and an alteration in the metabolic fate of ^3H vitamin D_3 has been found in patients with cirrhosis (Scott et al., 1965; Avioli et al., 1967*a*) and osteoporosis (Scott et al., 1965). The defect in vitamin D metabolism observed in patients with long-standing liver disease is characterized by a prolonged D_3 biological half-life in plasma and by decreased excretion of vitamin D_3–glucuronide metabolites (Fig. 11.7). These observations are consistent with the recent findings of Horsting and DeLuca (1969) which document the presence of an hepatic enzyme system capable of hydroxylating vitamin D_3 to its active 25–hydroxylated metabolic form. Abnormal vitamin D_3 metabolism has been documented in vitamin D–resistant rickets and familial hypophosphatemia, and is characterized primarily by a decrease in the fractional turnover rate of the vitamin and its conversion to the biologically active metabolite (Avioli et al., 1967*b*). Thompson and co-workers (1965), evaluating the absorption of vitamin D in patients with post-

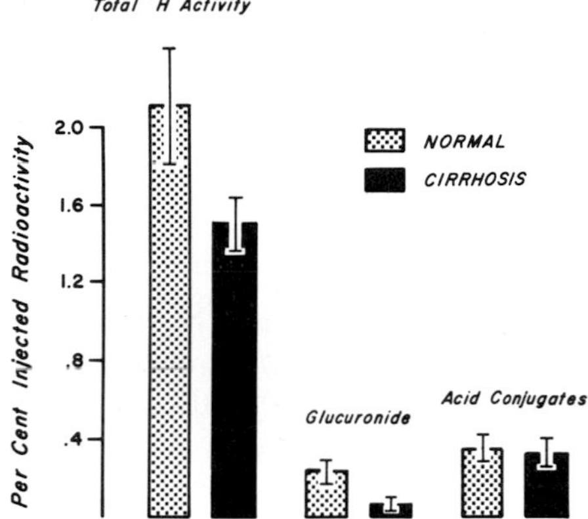

Fig. 11.7. Total ^{3}H, ^{3}H glucuronide, and ^{3}H acid conjugated in normal and cirrhotic subjects excreted in urine for the 48-hr period following an intravenous dose of ^{3}H vitamin D_3. The height of each vertical bar represents the mean $\pm$ 2 SE in 8 patients.

gastrectomy osteomalacia by means of tritium-labeled vitamin D_3, have concluded that defective diet and inadequate exposure to sunlight, rather than malabsorption of vitamin D_3, are primarily responsible for the osteomalacia. Recently, Avioli and co-workers (1968*b*) have also defined the abnormal metabolic fate of orally administered ^{3}H vitamin D_3 in patients with chronic renal failure and associated renal osteodystrophy. Since the metabolic abnormalities were reversed by renal homotransplantation, but not by chronic hemodialysis, it was tentatively concluded that the vitamin D resistance often observed in patients with uremia and renal osteodystrophy stems from circulating, abnormal, ultrafiltrable substances (or substance) which alter vitamin D metabolism in such a way as to accelerate its degradation and the formation of biologically inactive metabolites. Finally, current observations on the effect of glucocorticoids on the absorption and metabolic fate of ^{3}H vitamin D_3 relate the observed vitamin D–glucocorticoids antagonism to a rapid vitamin D_3 turnover, a diminished production of the active vitamin D_3 metabolite, and subsequent decrease in the intestinal absorption of calcium (Avioli et al., 1968*a*).

Conclusion

Five decades after the recognition of the antirachitic properties of sunlight, renewed interest in the metabolism of vitamin D in man is proceeding at an accelerated pace. Incited by provocative demonstrations in laboratory animals, and assisted by refinements in both biochemical methodology and radioisotopic synthetic techniques, the clinical investigator has proceeded to define in rapid succession the manner by which vitamin D is normally absorbed from the intestine, its metabolic conversion to a potent biologically active metabolite, and the deranged absorptive as well as altered metabolic patterns in some disorders of calcium and bone metabolism. Despite these achievements, many lines of investigation may still be profitably followed since present concepts of vitamin D secretion, metabolism, and biological action in man are still inadequately defined.

References

Anita, A. J., H. E. Wiltse, R. D. Rowe, E. L. Pitt, S. Levin, O. E. Ottesen, and R. E. Cooke. 1967. Pathogenesis of the supravalvular aortic stenosis syndrome. *J. Pediat. 71*:431.

Askew, F. A., H. M. Bruce, R. K. Callow, J. St. L. Philpot, and T. A. Webster. 1931. Crystalline vitamin D. *Nature 128*:758.

Avioli, L. V., S. J. Birge, and S. W. Lee. 1968. [Avioli et al., 1968*a*.] Effects of prednisone on vitamin D metabolism in man. *J. Clin. Endocrinol. 28*:1341.

Avioli, L. V., S. J. Birge, S. W. Lee, and E. Slatopolsky. 1968. [Avioli et al., 1968*b*.] The metabolic fate of vitamin D_3–^3H in chronic renal failure. *J. Clin. Invest. 47*:2239.

Avioli, L. V., and S. W. Lee. 1966. Detection of nanogram quantities of vitamin D by gas-liquid chromatography. *Anal. Biochem. 16*:193.

Avioli, L. V., and S. W. Lee. 1968. Intestinal absorption and metabolism of vitamin D_3 in man, p. 101. In *Third International Congress of Endocrinology, Abstracts of Brief Communications.* Excerpta Medica Foundation, Int. Congress Series, No. 157. (Abstr.)

Avioli, L. V., S. W. Lee, J. E. McDonald, J. Lund, and H. F. DeLuca. 1967. [Avioli et al., 1967*a*.] Metabolism of vitamin D_3–^3H in human subjects: distribution in blood, bile, feces and urine. *J. Clin. Invest. 46*:983.

Avioli, L. V., T. F. Williams, J. Lund, and H. F. DeLuca. 1967. [Avioli et al., 1967*b*.] Metabolism of vitamin D_3–^3H in vitamin D–resistant rickets and familial hypophosphatemia. *J. Clin. Invest. 46*:1907.

Baker, S. L., C. E. Dent, M. Friedman, and L. Watson. 1966. Fibrogenesis imperfecta ossium. *J. Bone Joint Surg. 48B*:804.

Bell, N. H., and F. C. Bartter. 1964. Transient reversal of hyperabsorption of calcium and of abnormal sensitivity to vitamin D in a patient with sarcoidosis during episode of nephritis. *Ann. Intern. Med. 61*:702.

Bell, N. H., J. R. Gill, Jr., and F. C. Bartter. 1964. On the abnormal calcium absorption in sarcoidosis. Evidence for increased sensitivity to vitamin D. *Amer. J. Med. 36*:500.

Bell, P. A., and E. Kodicek. 1967. A conjugated metabolite of vitamin D_3 in rat bile and faeces. *Biochem. J. 105*:34P.

Blomstrand, R., and L. Forsgren. 1967. Intestinal absorption and esterification of vitamin D_3–1,2–^3H in man. *Acta Chem. Scand. 21*:1662.

Blunt, J. W., H. F. DeLuca, and H. K. Schnoes. 1968. 25–hydroxycholecalciferol; a biologically active metabolite of cholecalciferol. *Chem. Commun.* No. 14:p.801.

Burnett, C. H., C. E. Dent, C. Harper, and B. J. Warland. 1964. Vitamin D–resistant rickets: analysis of twenty-four pedigrees with hereditary and sporadic cases. *Amer. J. Med. 36*:222.

Callow, R. R., E. Kodicek, and G. A. Thompson. 1966. Metabolism of tritiated vitamin D. *Proc. Roy. Soc.* [*Biol.*] *164*:1.

Chalk, E. J., and E. Kodicek. 1961. The association of ^{14}C-labeled vitamin D_2 with rat serum proteins. *Biochem. J. 79*:1.

DeCrousaz, P., B. Blanc, and I. Antener. 1965. Vitamin D activity in normal human serum and serum proteins. *Helv. Odont. Acta. 9*:151.

DeLuca, H. J. 1967. Mechanism of action and metabolic fate of vitamin D. *Vitamins Hormones 25*:315.

Dent, C. E., C. M. Harper, and G. R. Philpot. 1961. Treatment of renal-glomerular osteodystrophy. *Quart. J. Med. 30*:1.

Fraser, D. R., and E. Kodicek. 1968. Investigations on vitamin D esters synthesized in rats: Turnover and sites of synthesis. *Biochem. J. 106*:485.

Henneman, P. H., E. F. Dempsy, E. L. Carroll, and F. Albright. 1956. The cause of hypercalciuria in sarcoid and its treatment with cortisone and sodium phytate. *J. Clin. Invest. 35*:1229.

Horsting, M., and H. F. DeLuca. 1969. *In vitro* production of 25–hydroxycholecalciferol. *Biochem. Biophys. Res. Commun. 36*:251.

Kehayoglou, A. K., C. D. Holdsworth, J. E. Agnew, M. J. Whelton, and S. Sherlock. 1968. Bone disease and calcium absorption in primary biliary cirrhosis. *Lancet 1*:715.

Kodicek, E. 1955. The biosynthesis of ^{14}C-labelled ergocalciferol. *Biochem. J. 60*:xxv.

Kodicek, E. 1956. Metabolic studies on vitamin D, p. 161. *In* G. E. W. Wolstenholme and C. M. O'Connor (eds.), *Ciba Foundation Symposium on Bone Structure and Metabolism.* Little, Brown, Boston.

Kodicek, E. 1960. The fate of ^{14}C-labeled vitamin D_2 in rats and infants, p. 515. *In* S. Garattini and G. Paoletti (eds.), *Drugs Affecting Lipid Metabolism.* Elsevier Press, Amsterdam.

Loomis, W. F. 1967. Skin-pigment regulation of vitamin D biosynthesis in man. *Science 157*:501.

Nassim, J. R., P. D. Saville, P. B. Cook, and L. Mulligan. 1959. The effects of vitamin D and gluten-free diet in idiopathic steatorrhoea. *Quart. J. Med. 28*:141.

Neville, P. F., and H. F. DeLuca. 1966. The synthesis of [1,2–^{3}H] vitamin D_3 and the tissue localization of a 0.25 μg (10 IU) dose per rat. *Biochemistry 5*:2201.

Norman, A. W., and H. F. DeLuca. 1963. The preparation of H^3–vitamins D_2 and D_3 and their localization in the rat. *Biochemistry. 2*:1160.

Papadatos, C., and R. Klein. 1954. Addison's disease in boy with hypoparathyroidism. *J. Clin. Endocrinol. 14*:653.

Passannante, A. J., and L. V. Avioli. 1966. Studies on the ultraviolet fluorescence of vitamin D and related compounds in acid-alcohol solutions. *Anal. Biochem. 15*:287.

Rikkers, H., and H. F. DeLuca. 1967. An *in vivo* study of the carrier proteins of ^{3}H–vitamin D_3 and D_4 in rat serum. *Amer. J. Physiol. 213*:380.

Schachter, D., J. D. Finkelstein, and S. Kowarski. 1964. Metabolism of vitamin D. I. Preparation of radioactive vitamin D and its intestinal absorption in the rat. *J. Clin. Invest. 43*:787.

Scott, K. G., F. S. Smyth, C. T. Peng, W. A. Reilly, E. A. Stevenson, and J. N. Castle. 1965. Measurements of the plasma levels of tritiated vitamin D_3 in control and rachitic, cirrhotic and osteoporotic patients. *Strahlentherapy* Suppl. 60:317.

Stanbury, S. W., and G. A. Lumb. 1962. Metabolic studies of renal osteodystrophy. I. Calcium, phosphorus and nitrogen metabolism in rickets, osteomalacia and hyperparathyroidism complicating chronic uremia and in the osteomalacia of the adult Fanconi syndrome. *Medicine 41*:1.

Taussig, H. B. 1966. Possible injury to the cardiovascular system from vitamin D. *Ann. Intern. Med. 65*:1195.

Thomas, W. C., Jr., H. G. Morgan, T. B. Connor, L. Haddock, C. E. Bells, and J. E. Howard. 1959. Studies of antiricketic activity in sera from patients with disorders of calcium metabolism and preliminary observations on the mode of transport of vitamin D in human serum. *J. Clin. Invest. 38*:1078.

Thompson, G. R., B. Lewis, and C. C. Booth. 1966. Absorption of vitamin D_3–^{3}H in control subjects and patients with intestinal malabsorption. *J. Clin. Invest. 45*:94.

Thompson, G. R., B. Lewis, G. Neale, and C. C. Booth. 1965. Mechanisms of vitamin D deficiency in patients with lesions of the gastrointestinal tract. *Quart. J. Med. 34*:486.

Verner, J. V., Jr., F. L. Engel, and H. T. McPherson. 1958. Vitamin D intoxication: report of two cases treated with cortisone. *Ann. Intern. Med. 48*:765.

Warkany, J., and H. E. Mabon. 1940. Estimation of vitamin D in blood serum. *Amer. J. Dis. Child. 60*:606.

Windaus, A., O. Linsert, A. Luttringhaus, and G. Weidlich. 1932. Uber das krystallisierte VitaminD_2. *Ann. Chem. 492*:226.

Winters, R. W., J. B. Graham, T. F. Williams, V. W. McFalls, and C. H. Burnett. 1958. A genetic study of familial hypophosphatemia and vitamin D–resistant rickets with a review of the literature. *Medicine 37*:97.

Ziffer, H., W. J. A. Vanden Heuvel, E. O. A. Haahti, and E. C. Horning. 1960. Gas chromatographic behavior of vitamins D_2 and D_3. *J. Amer. Chem. Soc. 82*:6411.

A

TREATMENT OF HYPOPARATHYROIDISM WITH 25-HYDROXYCHOLECALCIFEROL

Charles Y. C. Pak and H. F. DeLuca

It has long been assumed that unaltered vitamin D_3 is responsible for its metabolic and physiologic manifestations. However, largely through the work of DeLuca and associates, it is now known that vitamin D_3 is converted in vivo into a number of metabolites (Lund and DeLuca, 1966). One of these, recently identified as 25–hydroxycholecalciferol (25–OH–D_3) (Blunt et al., 1968), is believed to be the metabolically active form of the vitamin. Recent studies indicate that the biological activity of vitamin D_3 on gut and bone can be ascribed to 25–OH–D_3 (Trummel et al., 1969). This compound may be clinically useful in patients with vitamin D resistance, especially in cases of defective 25–hydroxylation of vitamin D_3.

We have so far treated two patients with postsurgical hypoparathyroidism and vitamin D resistance, and two patients with idiopathic hypoparathyroidism. Three of the four patients responded satisfactorily to 5000 IU per day (0.091 mg per day), or less, of 25–OH–D_3. (For 25–OH–D_3, 1 IU = 0.018 μg.)

A study of one of the four patients will be described in detail (Pak et al., 1969). The patient (A. S.) is a 44-year-old housewife who has been resistant to treatment with large doses of crystalline dihydrotachysterol (DHT) (4 mg per day), Hytakerol (up to 7.5 mg per day), and vitamin D_2 and vitamin D_3 (each up to 600,000 IU per day) for 13 years. She was persistently hypocalcemic with a serum calcium concentration of approximately 7 mg/100 ml, seldom exceeding 8 mg/100 ml.

The effect of 25–OH–D_3 was evaluated while the patient, on metabolic regimen, was taking orally 4 g per day of calcium, 135 ml per day of Amphojel, and 4 mg per day of crystalline dihydrotachysterol (Fig. A.1). During the first 12 days, when she was not taking 25–OH–D_3, serum calcium concentration averaged 6.6 mg/100 ml, and the average urinary calcium excretion was 42 mg per day. She was therefore markedly resistant to 4 mg per day of crystalline dihydrotachysterol. Oral administration of 400–800 IU per day

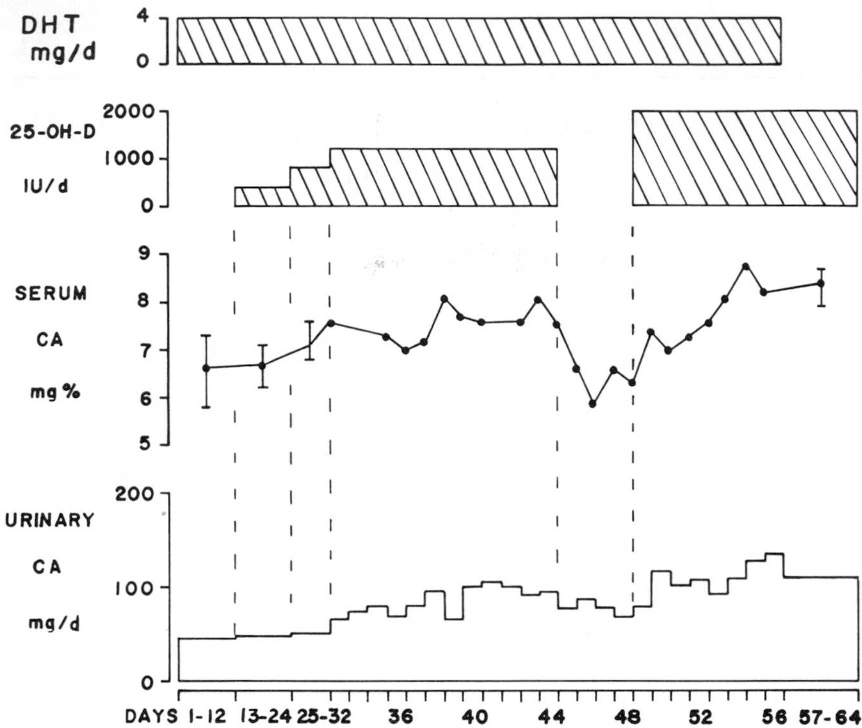

Fig. A.1. Response to the first course of 25–OH–D_3 administration in patient A. S. Results of the first 32 days have been combined into two 12-day periods and one 8-day period; the mean and the range of the serum calcium concentration and the mean of the urinary calcium excretion are presented for each period.

of 25–OH–D_3 did not significantly change either serum or urinary calcium. On 1200 IU per day of 25–OH–D_3 there was an increase in both serum and urinary calcium. Serum calcium concentration rose to a high of 8.1 mg/100 ml and urinary calcium excretion approximately doubled. When 25–OH–D_3 treatment was stopped for four days, serum calcium concentration fell rapidly to a low of 5.9 mg/100 ml and urinary calcium excretion decreased from 95 mg per day to 69 mg per day. Reinstitution of treatment at 2000 IU per day resulted in a prompt rise in serum and urinary calcium. On this regimen, mean serum calcium concentration was 8.3 mg/100 ml and mean urinary calcium excretion was 108 mg per day. These changes were accompanied by a marked subjective improvement. Chvostek's sign turned from positive to negative, and there was a marked alleviation of carpopedal spasm.

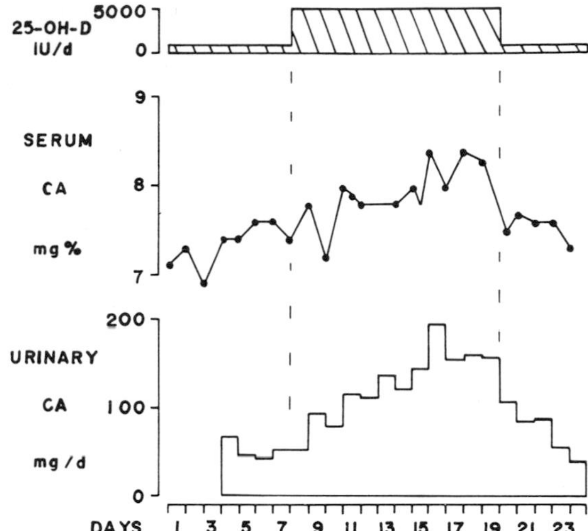

Fig. A.2. Response to the second course of 25–OH–D_3 administration in patient A. S.

Three months later, the patient received another course of treatment with 25–OH–D_3 (Fig. A.2). She received a higher dose of 25–OH–D_3 than before (5000 IU per day), and crystalline dihydrotachysterol was withdrawn. She again responded by increases in both serum and urinary calcium. When the dose of 25–OH–D_3 was lowered to 800 IU per day, serum and urinary calcium fell rapidly. In this patient, 25–OH–D_3 therapy was accompanied by a significant increase in the gastrointestinal absorption of calcium and an increase in total urinary hydroxyproline excretion.

Two patients with idiopathic hypoparathyroidism also responded to 5000 IU per day of 25–OH–D_3 with an increase in serum concentration. One patient was resistant to 10 mg per day of Hytakerol and was allegedly resistant to vitamin D_2 before he was referred to us. The second patient was responsive to 0.5 mg per day of crystalline dihydrotachysterol. However, he has shown varying sensitivity to crystalline dihydrotachysterol, often developing hypercalcemia. The only patient who did not respond to 25–OH–D_3 had moderate renal impairment secondary to vitamin D intoxication four years before.

We feel that 25–OH–D_3 is clinically useful in the treatment of some patients with vitamin D resistance as well as in subjects who show varying sensitivity to commercial preparations of vitamin D.

References

Blunt, J. W., H. F. DeLuca, and H. K. Schnoes. 1968. 25–Hydroxycholecalciferol: A biologically active metabolite of vitamin D_3. *Biochemistry* 7:3317.

Lund, J., and H. F. DeLuca. 1966. Biologically active metabolite of vitamin D_3 from bone, liver and blood serum. *J. Lipid Res.* *7*:739.

Pak, C. Y. C., H. F. DeLuca, J. M. Chavez de los Rios, and T. Suda. 1969. Treatment of vitamin D resistance with 25–hydroxycholecalciferol. *Clin. Res.* *17*:291.

Trummel, C. L., L. G. Raisz, J. W. Blunt, and H. F. DeLuca. 1969. 25–Hydroxycholecalciferol: stimulation of bone resorption in tissue culture. *Science* *163*:1450.

B

STUDIES ON VITAMIN D METABOLISM

Anthony W. Norman

Introduction

One of the hallmarks of vitamin D action is that there is a limited time lag between the administration of vitamin D and the initiation of every one of its physiological responses (Norman, 1968). In view of this it seemed appropriate to initiate a study of the mechanism of vitamin D action that would place heavy emphasis on elucidating the nature of the biochemical and physiological events that occur between administration of the vitamin and the initiation of the physiological response. Of necessity this implies studying the biochemical fate of vitamin D.

Initial studies on the metabolism of ^3H vitamin D_3 in rat intestinal mucosa by Norman and associates (1964) indicated that after the rats received an oral dose of 500 IU, the majority of the radioactivity existed as unmetabolized vitamin D_3 and there was also a significant amount of a more polar metabolite, designated peak 4. This metabolite was found to have significant biological activity as measured by the line test for rats.

Subsequent studies carried out independently by DeLuca and associates and by Norman and associates indicated two shortcomings in the earlier work of Norman, Lund, and DeLuca (1964): First, it was essential to administer physiologic doses (i.e., 10–50 IU) of ^3H vitamin D_3* rather than 500–1000 IU; and it was also necessary to utilize gradient elution systems during silicic acid chromatography that only gradually, rather than rapidly, increased in polarity. Accordingly, Neville and DeLuca (1966) and Lund and DeLuca (1966) found that after rats received a dose of 10 IU of vita-

* For Vitamin D_3 1 IU (0.065 nmole) = 0.25 μg. The minimum daily physiologic requirement for vitamin D_3 in the chick is 10 IU (Hibberd and Norman, 1969).

This research was supported in part by United States Public Health Service Grant AM–09012.

The extensive collaboration of Dr. Mark R. Haussler, Dr. Thomas H. Adams, and Mr. James F. Myrtle and the technical assistance of Miss Patricia Roberts throughout the course of these studies are gratefully acknowledged.

min D_3, metabolite peak 4 was the predominant form present in rat serum. They also reported that peak 4 was able to act more rapidly than the parent vitamin in stimulating calcium transport. Haussler and co-workers (1968) found that the peak 4 produced under the conditions of Norman and co-workers (1964) was in reality composed of at least three metabolites. It was also apparent that, in chick intestinal mucosa, only one of these metabolites was localized in the nucleus (Haussler and Norman, 1967) and its chromatin fraction (Haussler et al., 1968). Since these reports, the metabolism of vitamin D has received attention in a number of laboratories (Avioli, 1969; Blunt et al., 1968*a*, 1968*b*; Lawson et al., 1969; Mawer et al., 1969; Norman et al., 1969).

Metabolism of small doses of vitamin D_3

Some typical results concerning both the pattern of metabolites present after a physiological dose of vitamin D_3 and the subcellular localization of the metabolites in the chick intestinal mucosa are shown in Fig. B.1. We were able to compare the relative rates of migration of all metabolites that may be present by extensive use of a double labeling technique. Ten chicks were each given intracardial injections of 10 IU (0.65 nmole) of labeled vitamin D_3 15 hr before being killed. The entire mucosa was isolated from the five chicks which had received 1,2–^{3}H vitamin D_3; intestinal chromatin was prepared from the five chicks which had received 4–^{14}C vitamin D_3. The samples were extracted for total lipids by the procedure of Bligh and Dyer (1959). The combined extracts were chromatographed on a silicic acid column by the more extensive elution system of Haussler and associates (1968). Unmetabolized vitamin D_3 was located by adding non-radioactive vitamin D_3.

The results were that peak 4 was resolved into three subpeaks, denoted 4A, 4B, and 4C. The majority of the radioactivity was present in peak 4B.

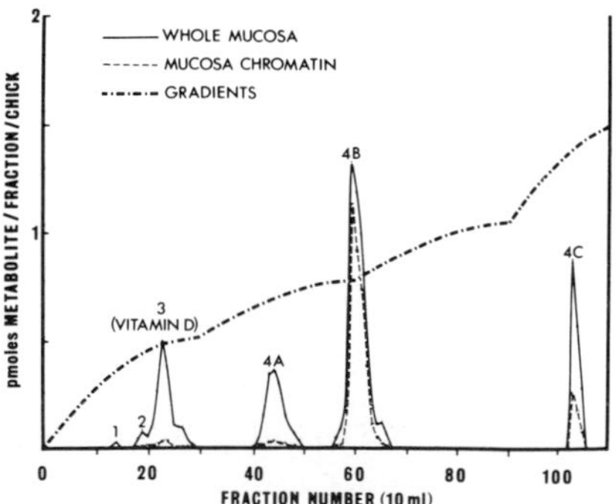

Fig. B.1. Silicic acid column chromatography of the radioactivity from both whole intestinal mucosa and mucosa in chicks given 10 IU (0.65 nmole) of labeled vitamin D_3. The successive gradients were 100% diethyl ether, 50% dichloroethane, 100% dichloroethane, and 100% methanol.

Peak 3 represents unaltered vitamin D_3, whereas peak 1 has been identified as an ester of vitamin D_3 (Lund et al., 1967). It is clear that approximately 70% of the peak 4B present in the intestinal mucosa is localized in the mucosal chromatin fraction. When corrected for DNA loss incurred during preparation of the chromatin, the localization of peak 4B in the chromatin fraction approaches 100%. Lawson and associates (1969) have recently confirmed that the major metabolite of vitamin D_3 present in the intestine is associated with the chromatin fraction. We have also found (Haussler et al., 1968) that peaks 4A and 4B are radiochemically homogeneous when chromatographed in two additional systems.

With the development of the new, more extensive chromatographic system, we were able to study the relative amounts of vitamin D_3 and the two predominant metabolites, 4A and 4B, in chick liver, plasma, and intestine as functions of the administered dose. The chicks were given intracardial injections of 10 IU, 20 IU, 50 IU, 100 IU, 500 IU, and 1000 IU of radioactive vitamin D_3. The lipid extraction of the tissues and silicic acid chromatography were as described by Haussler and co-workers (1968). As shown in Figure B.2, metabolite 4A is found primarily in the blood, while metabolite 4B is present in highest concentrations in the intestine. This distribution is particularly evident at the physiological dose levels of 1–50 IU. In the liver the amount of metabolite 4A present was slightly greater than 4B at all dose levels examined. In view of these results, caution should be exercised in comparing various tissue metabolic patterns (Avioli, 1969; Lund et al., 1967; Lund and DeLuca, 1966; Neville and DeLuca, 1966; Norman et al., 1964), found with the old chromatography system of Norman and co-workers (1964). Although each tissue has similar amounts of composite peak 4, the relative amounts of metabolites 4A, 4B, and 4C vary for each tissue.

When DeLuca and associates (Blunt et al., 1968*a*, 1968*b*) characterized a metabolite of vitamin D_3 (isolated from porcine blood) as being 25–OH–cholecalciferol (25–HCC), it was crucial for us to ascertain whether

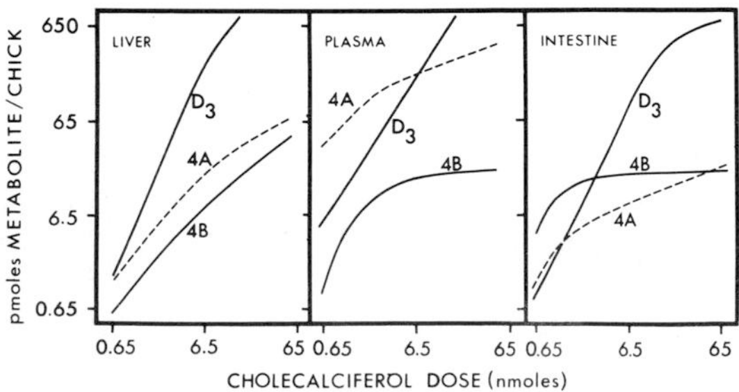

Fig. B.2. Comparative localization of vitamin D_3 and its metabolites as a function of dose in chick liver, plasma, and intestine. The results are presented in log-log fashion.

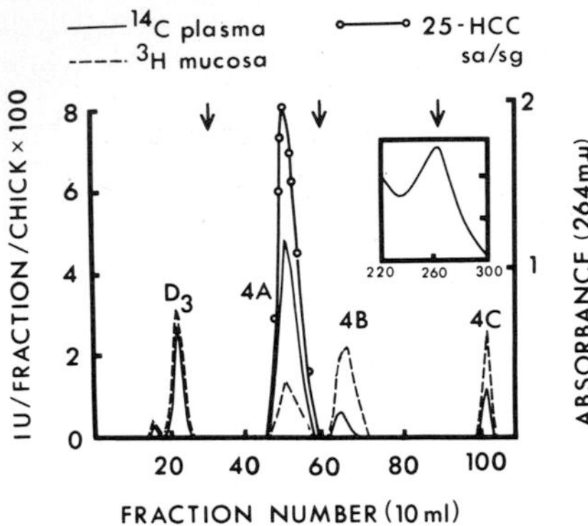

Fig. B.3. Cochromatography of metabolite 4A from intestine and plasma with 25–HCC. The characteristic ultraviolet spectrum of 25–HCC is given in the insert.

this was identical with either of our metabolites 4A and 4B. We cochromatographed both metabolites 4A and 4B from intestine and plasma with 25–HCC. The intestinal and plasma lipids were obtained from two groups of 2–3 chicks each, where the chicks had received 25 IU (1.62 nmole) of 1,2–^{3}H vitamin D_3 and 25 IU of 4–^{14}C vitamin D_3, respectively, 15 hr before being killed. Authentic 25–OH–cholecalciferol, 0.5 mg, was added to the combined lipid extract immediately before it was chromatographed on a silicic acid column by the procedure of Haussler and co-workers (1968). The 25–HCC was located by measuring the absorbance at 264 mμ and the characteristic spectrum in all 110 fractions. The results for metabolite 4A are given in Figure B.3. Fractions containing absorbance at 264 mμ and the characteristic spectrum of 25–HCC were found only in tubes 48–59, the exact region of migration of metabolite 4A, so metabolite 4A from either chick plasma or intestinal mucosa migrates identically with authentic 25–HCC.

It was also important to examine the possible biological activity of metabolites 4A and 4B relative to the parent vitamin D. The results of a typical experiment are shown in Figure B.4. The lipid extracts of 110

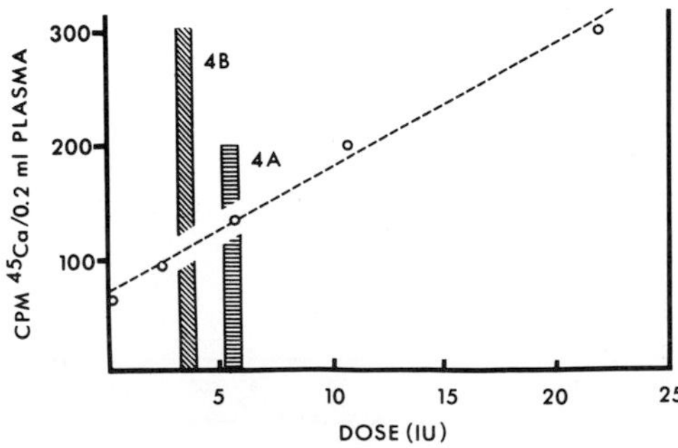

Fig. B.4. Biological assay of metabolites 4A (25–HCC) and 4B. The response to standard amounts of vitamin D_3 is shown by the dashed line. Metabolites 4A and 4B were fed at levels of 5.5 IU and 4.0 IU respectively.

chicks were chromatographed with the more extensive silicic acid system to isolate the radioactive metabolite 4A from the blood or the radioactive metabolite 4B from the mucosa. Standard amounts of vitamin D_3 and the metabolites were then fed orally to different groups of rachitic chicks; 24 hr later 2.0 mg of $^{40}Ca^{++}$ + $^{45}Ca^{++}$ were placed in each duodenum; 30 min later the appearance of $^{45}Ca^{++}$ in the blood was determined. This biological assay measures the appearance of a vitamin D–induced calcium absorption system in the rachitic chick (Norman, 1966*a*). Clearly, both metabolites 4A and 4B are able to increase intestinal absorption of a dose of $^{45}Ca^{++}$ to an extent equivalent to that obtained by vitamin D_3. It is important to note that the data presented in the figure have not been corrected for possible tritium loss. In view of the recent reports by Lawson and associates (1969) concerning tritium loss from the 1–α position of vitamin D_3, no definite statement may be made at this time concerning the absolute biological activity of these metabolites.

Further studies on the physiological significance of metabolite 4B are shown in Figure B.5. These results were obtained after rachitic chicks were administered 10 IU of 1,2–^{3}H vitamin D_3 intracardially. The amount of each metabolite was determined by silicic acid chromatography of the

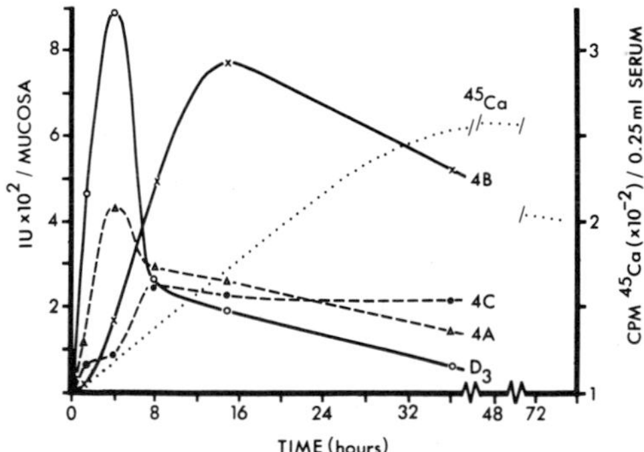

Fig. B.5. Time course and biological response of vitamin D_3 and its metabolites in the intestine of rachitic chicks after an intracardial dose of 10 IU (0.65 nmole) radioactive vitamin D_3. The biological response of increased intestinal calcium absorption is shown as a dotted line. The curve showing the location of metabolite 4B in the chromatin fraction has been omitted, but would trail the metabolite 4B of the total mucosal extract by approximately 30 min and would plateau at 14 hr at a value of approximately 0.06 IU/chick mucosa.

total lipid extracts by the procedure of Haussler and co-workers (1968). The biological response was determined in the manner described for the preceding studies (Norman, 1966*a*). Maximal concentrations were attained at 4 hr for vitamin D_3 and metabolite 4A, at 8 hr for 4C, and at 14 hr for 4B, whereas it took 45–50 hr to generate the maximum biological response. These kinetic data suggest that vitamin D_3 is rapidly converted into metabolite 4A (25–HCC), which, in turn, is probably converted into 4B. The site of the latter conversion is unknown at the present time. Metabolite 4B then becomes selectively localized in the intestinal chromatin where it possibly initiates the biological response. This response is relatively slow and may involve the synthesis of several enzymes or proteins necessary for calcium transport, e.g., calcium binding protein (Wasserman et al., 1968), or it may involve extensive alteration of the mucosal brush border membrane (Adams et al., 1969).

In recent years a new working hypothesis has been advanced for the mechanism of action of vitamin D (Norman 1965, 1966*a*, 1968; Zull et al., 1965; DeLuca, 1967; Haussler and Norman, 1969). It states that the vitamin may be acting analogously to other steroids such as the hormones ecdysone (Karlson, 1961), estrogen (Hamilton et al., 1968), hydrocortisone (Kenney and Albritton, 1965), testosterone (Bruchovsky and Wilson, 1968), and aldosterone (Edelman et al., 1963) in terms of its ability to activate or stimulate the biochemical expression of genetic information. This hypothesis was based primarily upon the fact that actinomycin D, an inhibitor of DNA-directed RNA synthesis, can block the response to vitamin D (Norman, 1965, 1966*a*; Zull et al., 1965) and that vitamin D administration will stimulate *de novo* RNA synthesis (Norman, 1966*b*; Stohs et al., 1967; Zull et al., 1966).

In view of the results reported here and also those from the laboratories of DeLuca (Lund and DeLuca, 1966) and Kodicek (Lawson et al., 1969), it would seem that a metabolite of vitamin D, rather than the parent vitamin, is the "active form" which initiates the physiologic response. In this respect metabolite 4B satisfies a number of important criteria characteristic of the series of biochemical and physiologic events normally attributed to vitamin D: (a) Metabolite 4B is found in the intestinal mucosa, a known target organ for vitamin D; (b) The majority of the radioactivity present in the intestine after a physiologic dose of radioactive vitamin D is metabolite 4B; (c) Its biological activity is at least equivalent to that of vitamin D; (d) It is found in close association with the site of actinomycin D–sensitive events, the intestinal nucleus and its chromatin fraction; (e) It appears in the intestinal chromatin in a temporal sequence consistent with the appearance of the physiologic response. It remains to the later chapters of the vitamin D story, however, to ascertain whether the active form of vitamin D is metabolite 4B, 25–OH–cholecalciferol, or some other compound.

References

Adams, T. H., R. G. Wong, and A. W. Norman. 1969. Vitamin D mediated calcium transport. *Fed. Proc. 28*:759. (Abstr.)

Avioli, L. 1969. Absorption and metabolism of vitamin D_3 in man. *J. Clin. Nutr. 22*:437.

Bligh, E. G., and W. J. Dyer, 1959. A rapid method of total lipid extraction and purification. *Can. J. Biochem. Physiol. 37*:911.

Blunt, J. W., H. F. DeLuca, and H. K. Schnoes. 1968*a*. 25–hydroxycholecalciferol: a biological active metabolite of vitamin D_3. *Biochemistry 7*:3317.

Blunt, J. W., Y. Tanaka, and H. F. DeLuca. 1968*b*. Biological activity of 25–hydroxycholecalciferol. A metabolite of vitamin D_3. *Proc. Nat. Acad. Sci. U.S.A. 61*:1503.

Bruchovsky, N., and J. D. Wilson. 1968. The intranuclear binding of testosterone and 5α-androstan-17β-ol-3-one by rat prostrate. *J. Biol. Chem. 243*:5953.

DeLuca, H. F. 1967. Mechanism of action and metabolic fate of vitamin D. *Vitamins Hormones 25*:315.

Edelman, I. S., R. Bogoroch, and G. A. Porter. 1963. On the mechanism of action of aldosterone on sodium transport: the role of protein synthesis. *Proc. Nat. Acad. Sci. U.S.A. 50*:1169.

Hamilton, T. H., C. C. Widnell, and J. R. Tata. 1968. Synthesis of RNA during early estrogen action. *J. Biol. Chem. 243*:408.

Haussler M. R., J. F. Myrtle, and A. W. Norman. 1968. The association of a metabolite of vitamin D_3 with intestinal mucosa chromatin, *in vivo*. *J. Biol. Chem. 243*:4055.

Haussler, M. R., and A. W. Norman. 1967. The subcellular distribution of physiological doses of vitamin D_3. *Arch. Biochem. Biophys. 118*:145.

Haussler, M. R., and A. W. Norman. 1969. Chromosomal receptor for a vitamin D metabolite. *Proc. Nat. Acad. Sci U.S.A. 62*:155.

Hibberd, K. A., and A. W. Norman. 1969. Comparative biological effects of vitamin D_2 and D_3 and dihydrotachysterol$_2$ and dihydrotachysterol$_3$ in the chick. *Biochem. Pharmacol. 18*:000.

Karlson, P. 1961. Biochemische Wirkungsweise der Hormone. *Deut. Med. J. 86*:668.

Kenney, F. T., and W. L. Albritton. 1965. Repression of enzyme synthesis at the translational level and its hormonal control. *Proc. Nat. Acad. Sci. U.S.A. 45*:1693.

Lawson, D. E. M., P. W. Wilson, and F. Kodicek. 1969. Metabolism of vitamin D. A new cholecalciferol metabolite, involving loss of hydrogen at C–1, in chick intestinal nuclei. *Biochem. J. 115*:269.

Lund, J., and H. F. DeLuca. 1966. Biologically active metabolite of vitamin D_3 from bone, liver, and blood serum. *J. Lipid Res.* *7*:739.

Lund, J., H. F. DeLuca, and M. Horsting. 1967. The formation of vitamin D esters *in vivo. Arch. Biochem. Biophys. 120*:513.

Mawer, E. B., G. A. Lumb, and S. W. Stanbury. 1969. Long biological half-life of vitamin D_3 and its polar metabolites in human serum. *Nature 222*:482.

Neville, P. F., and H. F. DeLuca. 1966. The synthesis of 1,2–^{3}H–vitamin D_3 and the tissue localization of a 0.25 μg (10 IU) dose per rat. *Biochemistry 5*:2201.

Norman, A. W. 1965. Actinomycin D and the response to vitamin D. *Science 149*:184.

Norman, A. W. 1966*a*. Actinomycin D effect on lag in vitamin D–mediated calcium absorption in the chick. *Amer. J. Physiol. 211*:829.

Norman, A. W. 1966*b*. Vitamin D–mediated synthesis of rapidly labeled RNA from intestinal mucosa. *Biochem. Biophys. Res. Commun. 23*:335.

Norman, A. W. 1968. The mode of action of vitamin D. *Biol. Rev. 43*:97.

Norman, A. W., M. R. Haussler, T. H. Adams, J. F. Myrtle, P. Roberts, and K. A. Hibberd. 1969. Basic studies on the mechanism of action of vitamin D. *Nutrition 22*:396.

Norman, A. W., J. Lund, and H. F. DeLuca. 1964. Biologically active forms of vitamin D_3 in kidney and intestine. *Arch. Biochem. Biophys. 108*:12.

Stohs, S. J., J. E. Zull, and H. F. DeLuca. 1967. Vitamin D stimulation of [^{3}H]–orotic acid incorporation into ribonucleic acid of rat intestinal mucosa. *Biochemistry 6*:1304.

Wasserman, R. H., R. A. Corradino, and A. N. Taylor. 1968. Vitamin D–dependent calcium binding protein. Purification and some properties. *J. Biol. Chem. 243*:3978.

Zull, J. E., E. Czarnowska-Misztal, and H. F. DeLuca. 1965. Actinomycin D inhibition of vitamin D action. *Science 149*:182.

Zull, J. E., S. J. Stohs, and H. F. DeLuca. 1966. The relationship between vitamin D action and actinomycin sensitive processes. *Fed. Proc. 25*:545. (Abstr.)

VITAMIN A

THE DIRECT ACTION OF VITAMIN A ON SKELETAL TISSUE IN VITRO

Honor B. Fell

This report is intended to summarize some aspects of the work that my colleagues and I have done at the Strangeways Laboratory on the direct action of vitamin A on tissues in vitro. Recently we have made further progress in studies on the action of hypervitaminosis A on bone and cartilage, so I propose to restrict my report to the effects of the vitamin on skeletal tissue.

Morphological changes

Our research on the biological action of vitamin A began in 1951, when the late Sir Edward Mellanby first aroused my interest in the subject, about which, at that time, I knew nothing. He thought that the organ culture technique that we had developed at the Strangeways Laboratory might provide a new approach to the problem. It had long been known that, at least in some species, excess of vitamin A in the diet caused resorption of bone, often leading to spontaneous fractures. But in 1951 it was uncertain whether the vitamin acted directly on the skeletal tissue or whether its effect was mediated through some other organ, possibly the parathyroid. It seemed to us that it should be possible to answer this question by cultivating bone and cartilage in a medium to which an excess of vitamin A had been added. In an organ culture all systemic effects are automatically excluded, so if the explanted bone underwent resorption under these conditions, that could only be due to a direct action of the vitamin on the skeletal cells. We therefore decided to undertake the experiments (Fell and Mellanby, 1952).

We used the well ossified limb bones of fetal mice near term and the cartilaginous limb-bone rudiments from 6-day embryonic chicks. The bones

The author is indebted to the Royal Society and to the editors of the *Biochemical Journal*, the *Journal of Physiology*, and *Nature* for permission to reproduce figures. The figures were prepared and the photographs taken by Mr. M. Applin.

from one side of each embryo were explanted in a medium (a plasma and embryo extract clot) to which we had added retinol or retinyl acetate, and those from the opposite side in a control medium without vitamin A. The result was unequivocal and dramatic: in a few days the matrix of the bone and cartilage disappeared in the presence of the vitamin (Figs. 12.1, 12.2). It was interesting that this breakdown of intercellular material was not associated with cellular necrosis; on the contrary, the healthier the cells, the more rapid was the disintegration of the tissue, and a high toxic dose of the vitamin was less effective than a much lower concentration. So it was clear that, in our system, vitamin A acted directly on the tissue and its maximum effect was produced by cells that were physiologically active but in some way physiologically abnormal.

When these experiments were made, the only way to obtain a clue to the biochemical action of the vitamin on these tiny explants was by radioautography. In collaboration with S. R. Pelc (Fell et al., 1956) we investigated the effect of the vitamin on the uptake and release of $^{35}SO_4$ as indicated by radioautography, using the cartilaginous limb-bone rudiments of 6-day embryonic chicks. When sections of such explants are examined by ordinary histological methods, the first visible change produced in the cartilage matrix by the vitamin is loss of metachromasia, so the intercellular material appears colorless after such stains as toluidine blue (Fig. 12.3). Radioautographs of explants prelabeled with $^{35}SO_4$ showed

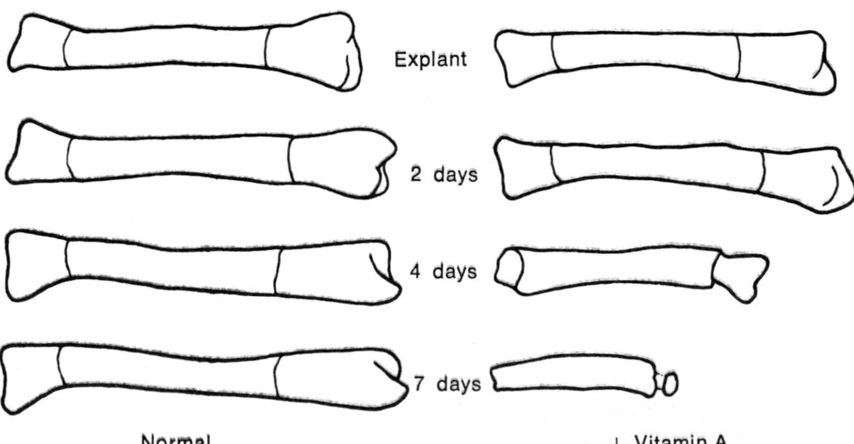

Fig. 12.1. *Camera lucida* drawings of living radii from a late mouse fetus. During 7 days' cultivation, the control explant (left) enlarged and remained intact, but after the first 2 days in medium containing excess vitamin A (right), the terminal cartilage began to shrink and the bone to be resorbed. (Fell and Mellanby, 1952. Reproduced by permission of the *Journal of Physiology*.)

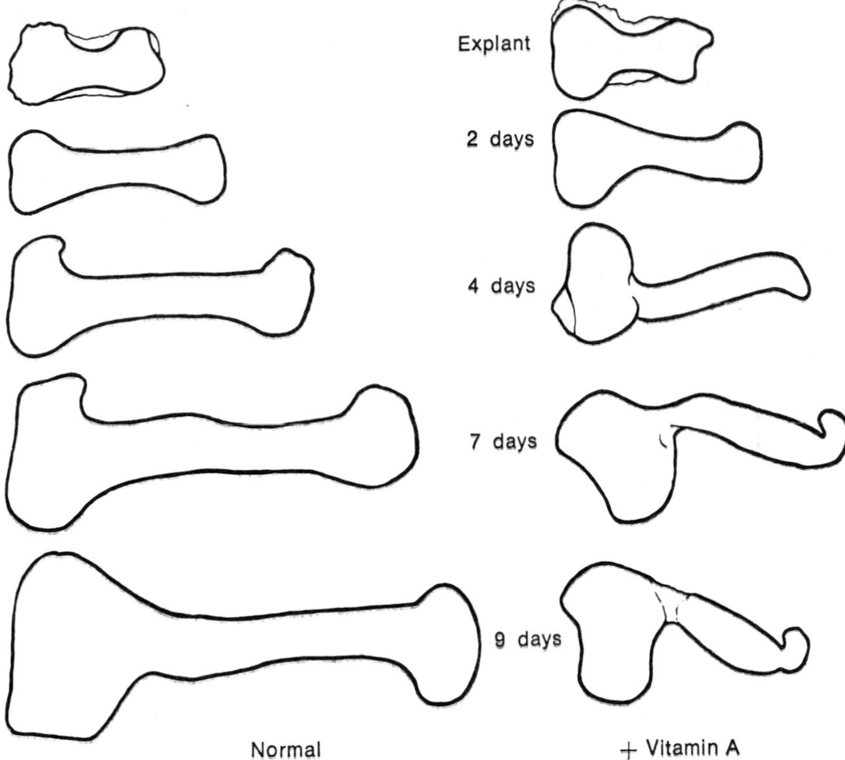

Fig. 12.2. Camera lucida drawings of a pair of living (cartilaginous) femora from a 6-day chick embryo. The control (left) enlarged to several times its original size, but in the vitamin A–treated explant (right), growth was arrested after 2 days, and the shape became distorted. (Fell and Mellanby, 1952. Reproduced by permission of the *Journal of Physiology*.)

that this loss of staining capacity was always correlated with loss of radioactive label. In other experiments, explants were grown in the presence of vitamin A for 6 days, by which time most of the metachromatic material had disappeared; they were then treated with $^{35}SO_4$. The cartilage failed to incorporate sulfate. To explain these results, we suggested the following hypothesis: (a) excess vitamin A causes cells either to elaborate a new enzyme which converts chondroitin sulfate to a more soluble form, or to produce excessive amounts of an enzyme which is already present in the tissue; (b) this enzyme diffuses into the matrix; and (c) once cells have begun to produce this enzyme, they continue to do so. As we shall see, this hypothesis, though not correct, was not very far from the truth. Sadly enough, Sir Edward died before this paper was published, so he never saw the later developments of the research that he had initiated.

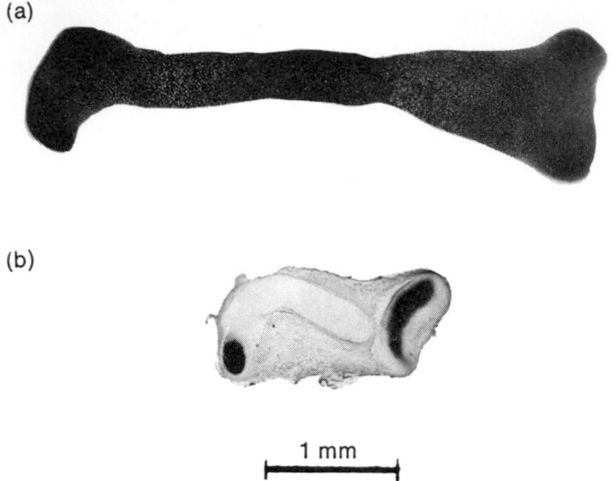

Fig. 12.3. Pair of femora from a 7-day chick embryo grown in culture for 8 days. Sections were stained with toluidine blue. (a) Control; note intense metachromasia of the cartilage matrix. (b) Rudiment grown in medium containing 9.6 IU retinol/ml; the explant has shrunk, and lost its metachromasia except in the center of the epiphysial region. (Fell et al., 1962. Reproduced by permission of the *Biochemical Journal*.)

Biochemical changes induced by vitamin A in cartilage

ENZYMIC ACTIVITY

I had often noticed that explants grown on a plasma and embryo extract clot containing added vitamin A liquefied the clot much more extensively than their controls. This suggested that the vitamin had somehow increased the proteolytic activity of the tissue. For no good reason that I can recall, I suspected that the protease responsible was a cathepsin.

In 1959, I encountered some research of which I had been unaware, which reawakened my interest in this apparent increase in proteolytic activity of bone and cartilage exposed to vitamin A. Lewis Thomas, who was spending a sabbatical year in Cambridge, told me of his experiments on the effect of injecting the vegetable protease papain into rabbits (Thomas, 1956). This treatment depleted cartilage matrix throughout the body, causing it to lose its metachromatic material and rigidity, but did no serious damage to the chondrocytes. The rabbit was none the worse for the treatment, except that its ears drooped like a spaniel's; when the administration of papain ceased, the cartilage rapidly regenerated the missing material and the ears became stiff again. In view of Thomas's results, it seemed possible that the breakdown of matrix in the vitamin A–treated explants of embryonic cartilage might indeed be due to the increased proteolytic activity indicated by the extensive liquefaction of the culture medium in the presence of the vitamin.

We therefore compared the effects of papain and vitamin A on limb-bone rudiments in culture (Fell and Thomas, 1960). When added to the medium, the two agents had a very similar effect on cartilage matrix; bone matrix, however, appeared unaffected by papain, whereas it was rapidly resorbed under the influence of vitamin A. We tentatively concluded that the changes in cartilage seen in experimental hypervitaminosis A may be the result of activation of a proteolytic enzyme or enzymes with properties similar to those of papain.

Here the matter might have rested, but for my biochemical colleagues John Dingle and Jack Lucy. Microchemical methods had greatly improved since Mellanby and I had begun our studies in 1951, and Dingle and Lucy thought that the changes we had observed in our vitamin A–treated explants could now be investigated at the biochemical level.

Our first biochemical experiments (Dingle et al., 1961) were made to see whether the increased liquefaction of the clot in the vitamin A–treated cultures was in fact due to an increased proteolytic activity. Cartilaginous limb-bone rudiments from 6–7 day embryonic chicks were grown on a plasma and embryo extract clot with or without the addition of retinol (10 IU/ml). Examination of the used culture medium showed that there was twice as much acid-soluble nitrogen in the medium of the vitamin A–treated explants as in that of their paired controls; this provided some support for the view that the vitamin had increased the proteolytic activity of the explants, as originally suspected.

In the same study, Dingle and Lucy investigated certain effects of vitamin A on the composition and metabolism of the explant. After 6 days, in the presence of retinol, the wet and dry weights and amino sugar content of the treated rudiments were about half those of the controls, the ribonucleic acid was 40% and deoxyribonucleic acid 80% of the control values. The vitamin depressed the rate of oxygen consumption but increased that of lactic acid formation.

Having got so far, we were not sure what to do next. For lack of a better idea, we decided to study the extraction of intercellular components from normal embryonic cartilage, using standard biochemical methods (Lucy et al., 1961), in the hope that it might shed light on the process by which the matrix was degraded in the vitamin A–treated explants. We placed the cartilaginous limb bones of normal 8–9 day chick embryos in various salt solutions commonly used for the extraction of chondroitin sulfate, and kept them at 4 C for various periods; as controls, we immersed similar bones in distilled water. When we examined the treated bones histologically, we were rather disconcerted to find that only the controls in distilled water showed any change in the matrix, as indicated by loss of metachromasia. On reflection, however, we became rather excited about this unexpected result, because it seemed possible that breakdown of the intercellular material in the water-treated controls might be due to enzymes released from the cells by hypotonicity. We designed some experiments to test this hypothesis.

For this investigation the rudiments were pretreated with distilled water for 1 hr at 4C to disrupt the cells and their organelles and so release any intracellular enzymes into the matrix. They were then incubated for 1–24 hr in buffer solutions of *p*H 1–8. We found that between *pH* 3 and 5 the metachromasia of the matrix was greatly reduced, half the hexosamine content was lost as polysaccharide of high molecular weight, and protein components also were liberated into the buffer. Above and below *p*H 3–5 there was little effect on the matrix. My colleagues then made an extract of the bone rudiments and tested its proteolytic activity. The extract was found to contain a protease with a *p*H optimum of 3.0 with a hemoglobin substrate. Further experiments showed that the activity was located in cytoplasmic particles from which it could be liberated by water, and it was destroyed at a temperature of 100 C.

From these results it seemed clear that normal chondrocytes contained an enzyme or enzymes capable of producing an effect on cartilage matrix that resembled the change induced in the explants by vitamin A. Since the protease had an acid *p*H optimum and was located in cytoplasmic particles, it seemed probable that it was a cathepsin, and, in view of its properties, Dingle suspected that it was cathepsin D. This has recently been confirmed by Alan Barrett (unpublished). In addition, Peter Weston (1969) has demonstrated that the embryonic cartilage contains an antigen that by immunological methods is indistinguishable from the purified cathepsin D isolated from chicken liver by Barrett (unpublished).

It seemed reasonable to expect that the protease we had found in normal embryonic cartilage would prove to be identical with that produced by the vitamin A–treated explants. We therefore investigated further the effect of retinol on the proteolytic activity of limb-bone rudiments in organ culture.

We cultivated the humerus, femur, and tibia of 7-day embryos on a plasma and embryo extract clot with or without added retinol (10 IU/ml) for 4–8 days. The explants were then transferred to a synthetic fluid medium for an additional 30 hr. During this latter period the release of proteolytic activity into the medium was estimated at various intervals. At the end of the experiment the amount of proteolytic activity remaining in the tissue was measured. The results (Fig. 12.4) showed that in 24 hr the vitamin A–treated explants released far more (up to 7 times more) proteolytic activity than their paired controls. When Dingle estimated the activity remaining in the explants at the end of the culture period, he found that it was at least as high as, and sometimes higher than, that in the controls. Thus the vitamin had caused an increased synthesis of the enzyme as well as an increased release. The protease had the same *p*H optimum as that isolated from normal cartilage. We have since confirmed these early results, using a fluid medium instead of a plasma and embryo extract clot;

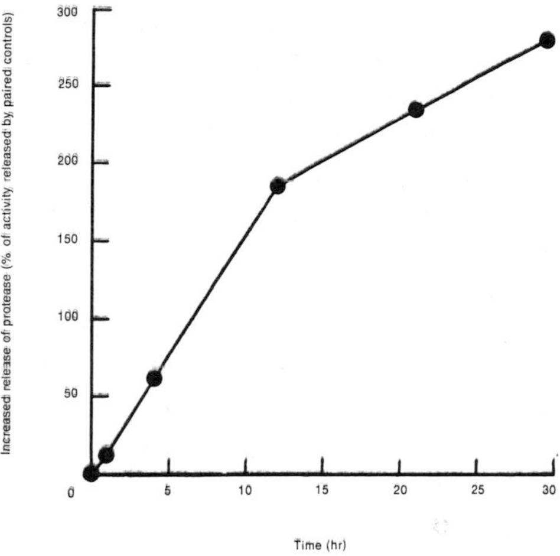

Fig. 12.4. Release of protease from vitamin A–treated limb-bone rudiments from 7-day embryonic chicks. Sixteen rudiments were grown in the presence of 10 IU retinol/ml medium (plasma and embryo extract clot) for 6 days, then transferred to synthetic medium without vitamin A for 30 hr; paired control rudiments without added retinol were treated in a similar way. Samples of the synthetic medium were removed at intervals and their proteolytic activity was measured. The effect of the vitamin is expressed as a percentage of the enzyme activity released by the controls at each time. (Fell and Dingle, 1963.)

this enables us to measure the amount of proteolytic activity released by the explants throughout the 6–8 day culture period.

THE EFFECT ON BIOLOGICAL MEMBRANES

Very early in our research, my colleagues and I wondered how the effect of hypervitaminosis A was mediated at the cellular level. The essential clue was provided by Dingle (1961). Since the protease of the embryonic cartilage appeared to be a cathepsin, and since it was associated with cytoplasmic particles, he suggested that it might be of lysosomal origin and that possibly vitamin A released the hydrolases by altering the physicochemical properties of the lysosomal membranes.

To test this hypothesis, Dingle isolated the lysosome-rich fraction of rat liver (Gianetto and de Duve, 1955) and then treated it with retinol. The vitamin rapidly released a cathepsin with a *p*H optimum of 3.0 which closely resembled the acid protease liberated from embryonic chicken cartilage by hypo-osmotic treatment. The vitamin did not disrupt the organelles, which appeared intact when examined in the electron microscope by Audrey Glauert. This effect had a high degree of molecular specificity (Fell et al., 1962); many compounds related to retinol were tested on this system, but, at a concentration of 0.7 μmole, only retinoic acid had an effect comparable to that of retinol, which at this concentration released about two-thirds of the bound protease.

Dingle thought that this increased permeability of the lysosomes, with consequent release of bound enzymes induced by vitamin A, might be due to a direct effect of the vitamin on the lysosomal membranes, and that retinol might be a membrane-active compound. Subsequently work by

Lucy, Dingle, and other members of the Laboratory (for review, see Dingle and Lucy, 1965) showed this hypothesis to be correct. Retinol caused hemolysis of red cells and swelling of isolated mitochondria, and altered all the membrane systems of intact tissue cells in suspension.

In studies on the chemical properties of retinol, Lucy and Lichti (1969) found that the active forms of vitamin A (retinol and retinoic acid) behave as electron donors. They suggest that the chemical properties of the vitamin responsible for its biological activity may become apparent only when the vitamin is at an interface between lipid and water, as in a biological membrane.

DEGRADATION OF CARTILAGE MATRIX

The experiments quoted above (Lucy et al., 1961), on the autolytic degradation of matrix in normal bone rudiments pretreated with water and then incubated at low *p*H, indicated that the acid protease of the cartilage digested the protein moiety of the mucoprotein complex and so liberated polmeric chondroitin sulfate and amino acid residues into the medium. This process would be unlikely to have much biological significance, however, unless the acid protease would digest cartilage matrix at physiological as well as acid *p*H.

To investigate this question (Fell and Dingle, 1963) normal limb-bone rudiments from 9–day chick embryos were incubated for 6 hr in a crude lysosomal extract prepared from rat liver and buffered at different *p*H values; unfortunately it was not possible to obtain sufficient enzyme for these experiments from the small cartilaginous rudiments. Controls were incubated in the same buffers without extract. The results showed that the lysosomal extract was very effective in degrading the matrix at neutral *p*H (Fig. 12.5). Recently Barrett (unpublished) has demonstrated that purified cathepsin D from chicken liver can also digest chondromucoprotein at neutral *p*H.

We have now begun to examine in detail the breakdown of cartilage matrix in limb-bone rudiments in culture, using a micro-analytical method developed by A. J. Barrett, J. T. Dingle, and R. I. G. Morrison (unpublished). For these experiments 8–day (chick) limb-bone rudiments are cultivated for 24 hr in a control medium containing $^{35}SO_4$; this is then replaced by a nonradioactive control medium. After 24 hr of incubation in the unlabeled medium to remove unfixed isotope from the tissue, the explants are thoroughly rinsed in Tyrode's solution and transferred to a medium with or without the addition of vitamin A. The used medium is collected for analysis at 2-day intervals and replaced by fresh; at the end of the experiments the explants also are harvested for analysis. In the presence of the vitamin far more labeled material is shed into the medium

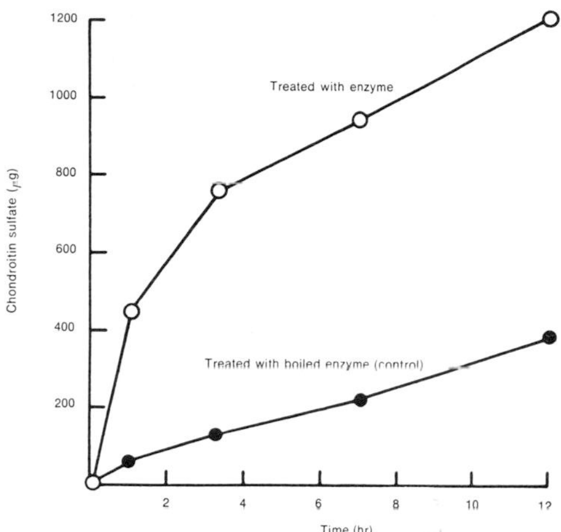

Fig. 12.5. Release of chondroitin sulfate by lysosomal extract at physiological *p*H from limb-bone rudiments from 10-day chick embryos. Normal rudiments ex vivo were incubated at 37 C in 0.1 M phosphate buffer, *p*H 7.0, containing lysosomal extract. Controls were incubated in medium containing extract that had been heated at 100 C for 3 min. The liberation of polysaccharide was measured in samples taken at intervals. (Fell and Dingle, 1963.)

than in the control cultures (Fig. 12.6). Preliminary results (Morrison, Barrett, Dingle, and Fell, unpublished) have shown that the breakdown products produced under the influence of vitamin A are virtually the same as those formed by the action of pure cathespin D on isolated chondromucoprotein of high molecular weight.

THE SYNTHESIS OF INTERCELLULAR COMPONENTS

We wished to know (Dingle et al., 1966) how vitamin A affected the synthesis of the components of cartilage matrix: whether synthesis would

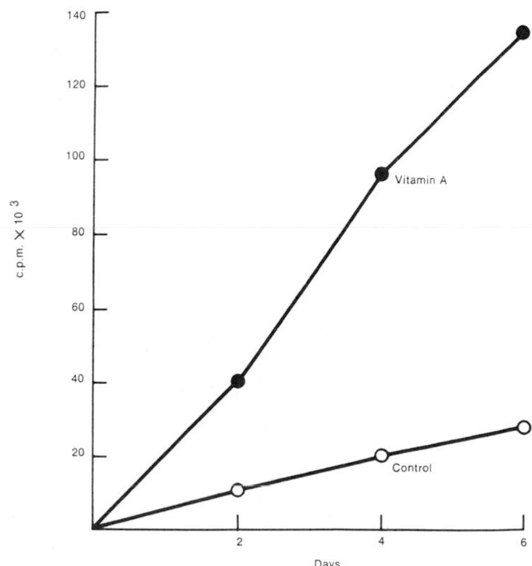

Fig. 12.6. The effect of vitamin A (7.5 IU/ml) on the release of $^{35}SO_4$ from 8-day (chick) limb-bone rudiments during 6 days' cultivation. (Dingle and Fell, unpublished.)

be inhibited, or whether the components would be formed but shed into the medium instead of being incorporated into intercellular material. The latter alternative proved to be correct.

Limb-bone rudiments from 7-day embryonic chicks were cultivated in a fluid medium with or without the addition of retinol. The amounts of hexosamine and hydroxyproline liberated into the culture medium and remaining in the explants at the end of the experiment were measured. Both compounds were found to be actively synthesized in the presence of vitamin A, but most of the material was shed into the medium instead of being incorporated in matrix as in the paired controls. If the effect of the vitamin was not too drastic, the total amount of hexosamine and hydroxyproline produced (i.e., the amount in the medium plus that remaining in the explant) was almost the same as in the controls.

SPECIFICITY OF EFFECT

Vitamin A has a high degree of molecular specificity (Fell et al., 1962) in its action on cartilaginous limb-bone rudiments in culture. The effects on the explants of hydrogenated vitamin A, vitamin A epoxide, anhydrovitamin A, retinoic acid, β-ionone, citral, and phytol were examined. Of these compounds, only retinoic acid was active.

INHIBITION OF EFFECT

Three substances are known to inhibit the effect of vitamin A on cartilaginous limb-bone rudiments in culture. These are amino-caproic acid (EAC), cortisol, and a specific antiserum to cathepsin D.

Ali (1964) showed that EAC at high concentrations inhibits the action of lysosomal acid protease in rabbit ear cartilage. In our experiments, when added to the culture medium, it partially inhibited the breakdown of cartilage matrix in response to vitamin A (Fell and Dingle, unpublished).

Cortisol stabilizes lysosomal membranes (Weissmann and Dingle, 1961) and so inhibits the release of the enzymes. In a fairly high concentration (7.5 μg/ml of medium; Fell and Thomas, 1961), but not at physiological levels (Dingle et al., 1966), it retarded the dissolution of cartilage matrix in retinol-treated explants.

Experiments now in progress are of greater interest. Weston and associates (1969) raised, in rabbits, a specific precipitating antiserum to Barrett's pure chicken cathepsin D, and this is being used to examine the role of the enzyme in the breakdown of cartilage matrix. In experiments on the autolysis of normal cartilage in the system described by Lucy et al. (1961), fresh antiserum added to the buffer (*p*H 6.0) in a concentration of 10% inhibited the loss of polysaccharide by 82% during 9 hr of incubation (Fig. 12.7). Pure γ-globulin prepared from the antiserum inhibited both the autolytic degradation of cartilage matrix and the action of pure cathepsin D on iso-

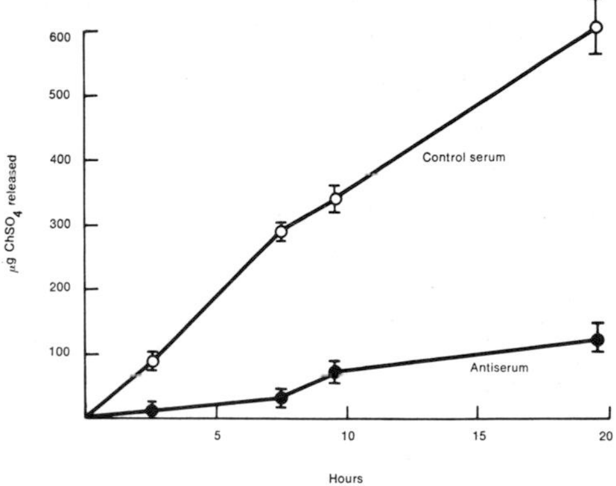

Fig. 12.7. The inhibitory effect of antiserum against cathepsin D on the release of polysaccharide during autolysis of normal 10-day (chick) limb-bone rudiments ex vivo. The rudiments were incubated for 19 hr in buffer at *p*H 6.0 in the presence of 10% of either normal rabbit serum or antiserum against pure cathepsin D; the polysaccharide released was measured at intervals. The results are the mean of 7 experiments. (Weston et al., 1969. Reproduced by permission of *Nature.*)

lated chondromucoprotein. Preliminary experiments with several batches of antiserum (Weston, Barrett, Dingle, and Fell, unpublished) have shown that the antiserum inhibits the breakdown of cartilage matrix in explanted limb-bone rudiments treated with vitamin A (Table 12.1).

Changes induced in bone by vitamin A

We have done much more work on the action of vitamin A on cartilage than on its effect on bone. This is because the response of cartilage is simpler and more easily studied.

TABLE 12.1. *Effect of antiserum against cathepsin D on retinol-treated limb-bone rudiments*

Serum	Effect on weight: Wet weight (mg)	Effect on weight: Dry weight (mg)	Effect on release of $^{35}SO_4$ (count/min per culture): Uptake	Release	% Inhibition
R2	27.8	4.45	93,450	12,730	33
NS	20.2	2.76	92,740	18,900	

Source: Dingle, Weston, Barrett, and Fell (unpublished data).

Note: Limb-bone rudiments from 8-day (chick) embryos were cultivated for 24 hr in synthetic medium + 15% heat-inactivated normal rabbit serum + 1 μCi $^{35}SO_4$/ml, then washed and incubated for a further 24 hr in the same medium without $^{35}SO_4$. They were again washed and transferred to fresh culture dishes containing synthetic medium + retinol (7.5 IU vitamin A/ml) + 36% heat-inactivated normal rabbit serum (NS) (controls) or 36% heat-inactivated rabbit antiserum against chicken cathepsin D (R2). After 6 days' cultivation in these media, the explants were weighed; both wet and dry weights were considerably higher in the R2-treated rudiments. The release of $^{35}SO_4$ into the medium during the first 2 days after transfer to medium containing retinol was measured; R2 had inhibited the release of the isotope by 33%.

That explanted bone reacts to vitamin A was shown by the original experiments of Fell and Mellanby (1952), already cited, in which the well ossified limb bones of fetal mice near term were rapidly resorbed in the presence of retinol.

Recently, John Reynolds (1968) has investigated some of the biochemical changes induced by retinol in calvariae from late fetal rats. Paired explants were obtained by cutting each calvaria in half along the median suture. These half calvariae underwent extensive resorption in a medium containing retinol (22 IU/ml) (Fig. 12.8) and, as compared with their untreated paired controls, lost hexosamine, hydroxyproline and calcium (Reynolds, 1968; Reynolds et al., 1968). They also showed increased synthesis and release of lysosomal acid protease (Reynolds, 1968). Recently, Reynolds, Minkin, and Evanson (unpublished) have found that, in addition, the calvariae secreted into the medium a collagenase which was active at *p*H 7.4 on collagen gels made from ^{14}C-labeled collagen obtained from rat skin. Bones treated with retinol released about three times as much collagenolytic activity as their paired controls. Like the collagenolytic factor liberated from explants of metaphyseal bone from rats pretreated with parathyroid hormone (Walker et al., 1964), the enzyme could not be detected in the tissue itself, but only in the culture medium.

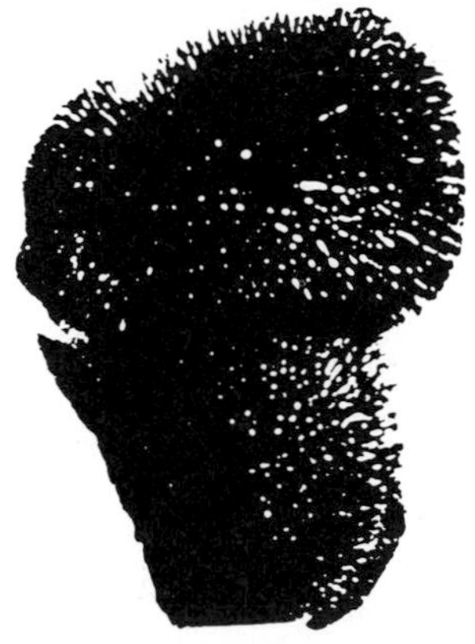

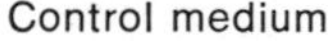

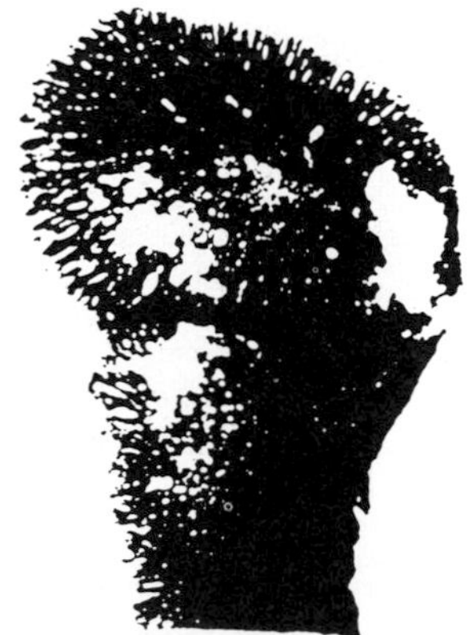

Fig. 12.8. Effect of retinol on half calvariae from a 19-day fetal rat grown for 6 days in vitro in synthetic medium + 0.5% crystalline bovine plasma albumin. Explants were stained for calcium by von Kossa's method and mounted whole. Note extensive resorption of bone in the retinol-treated explant (right). (Reynolds, unpublished.)

Reynolds and his co-workers have studied the effect of calcitonin on bone resorption induced in culture by vitamin A. (Calcitonin is a recently discovered peptide hormone secreted by special cells in the thyroid gland; in vivo it inhibits the release of calcium from the skeleton.) The hormone completely inhibited the loss of calcium from the vitamin A–treated explants (Fig. 12.9), but not that of hexosamine or hydroxyproline; nor did it inhibit the increased synthesis and release of the lysosomal protease (Fig. 12.10). On the other hand, preliminary results indicate that calcitonin significantly reduced the amount of collagenolytic factor present in the medium.

Conclusions

These experiments on hypervitaminosis A showed for the first time that under certain conditions the intact living cells of connective tissue may secrete lysosomal enzymes into their environment, and that at least one of these enzymes, cathepsin D, then participates in the breakdown of connective tissue matrix by degrading intercellular mucoprotein of high molecular weight. The enzymic and cytological mechanisms responsible for the digestion of collagen are not yet understood. Whether lysosomal enzymes are concerned in this process, perhaps by unmasking the collagen

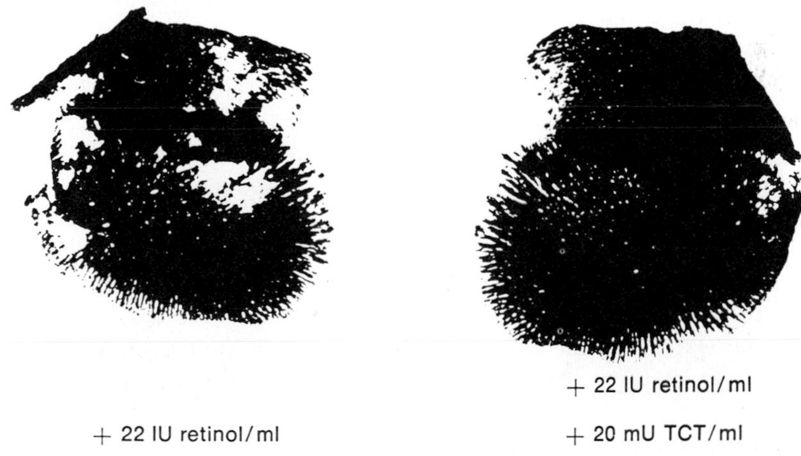

Fig. 12.9. Inhibitory effect of calcitonin (TCT) on bone resorption induced by retinol in half calvariae in culture. The explants were obtained from a 19-day fetal rat and were grown for 6 days in synthetic medium + 0.5% crystalline bovine serum albumin. Explants were stained for calcium by von Kossa's method and mounted whole. Calcitonin (right) has completely inhibited the loss of calcium in response to retinol. (Reynolds, 1968. Reproduced by permission of the Royal Society.)

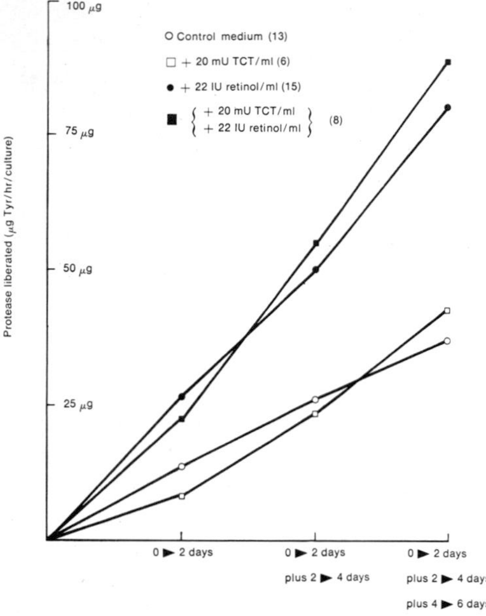

Fig. 12.10. Acid protease activity liberated at each subculture by half calvariae exposed to various agents. The explants were obtained from 19-day fetal rats and were grown for 6 days in synthetic medium + 0.5% crystalline bovine serum albumin with different additions. The points on the curves represent the average values for each treatment (number of samples assayed shown in parentheses). Retinol greatly increased the secretion of the protease, but calcitonin (TCT) had no effect. (Reynolds, 1968. Reproduced by permission of the Royal Society.)

fibers and so rendering them accessible to a collagenase of nonlysosomal origin, remains to be seen. The use of antiserum against cathepsin D may help to elucidate the problem.

Our current hypothesis concerning the action of hypervitaminosis A on the lysosomal system of skeletal cells is that the vitamin enters the membranes of the primary lysosomes and the plasmalemma, and alters their physical properties in such a way as to promote fusion between the two; this would increase the secretion of lysosomal enzymes into the environment. We do not believe that the vitamin causes a release of lysosomal enzymes into the cytoplasm, except possibly with very toxic doses of retinol. This is emphasized, because our views on this point have sometimes been misunderstood and misquoted. Since vitamin A appears to alter all the membrane systems of the cell, the lysosomal action that we have studied is probably only one of many effects, most of which have not yet been identified.

At present the physiological action of vitamin A is unknown, but the demonstration that retinol is a membrane-active substance may provide a clue to the vitamin's normal site of action in the cell.

References

Ali, S. Y. 1964. The degradation of cartilage matrix by intracellular protease. *Biochem. J. 93*:611.

Dingle, J. T. 1961. Studies on the mode of action of excess of vitamin A. III. Release of a bound protease by the action of vitamin A. *Biochem. J. 79*:509.

Dingle, J. T., H. B. Fell, and J. A. Lucy. 1966. Synthesis of connective-tissue components: The effect of retinol and hydrocortisone on cultured limb-bone rudiments. *Biochem. J. 98*:173.

Dingle, J. T., and J. A. Lucy. 1965. Vitamin A, carotenoids and cell function. *Biol. Rev. 40*:422.

Dingle, J. T., J. A. Lucy, and H. B. Fell. 1961. Studies on the mode of action of excess of vitamin A. I. Effect of excess of vitamin A on the metabolism and composition of embryonic chick limb cartilage grown in organ culture. *Biochem. J. 79*:497.

Fell, H. B., and J. T. Dingle. 1963. Studies on the mode of action of excess of vitamin A. VI. Lysosomal protease and the degradation of cartilage matrix. *Biochem. J. 87*:403.

Fell, H. B., J. T. Dingle, and M. Webb. 1962. Studies on the mode of action of excess of vitamin A. IV. The specificity of the effect on embryonic chick-limb cartilage in culture and on isolated rat-liver lysosomes. *Biochem. J. 83*:63.

Fell, H. B., and E. Mellanby. 1952. The effect of hypervitaminosis A on embryonic limb-bones cultivated *in vitro*. *J. Physiol. 116*:320.

Fell, H. B., E. Mellanby, and S. R. Pelc. 1956. Influence of excess vitamin A on the sulphate metabolism of bone rudiments grown in vitro. *J. Physiol. 134*:179.

Fell, H. B., and L. Thomas. 1960. Comparison of the effects of papain and vitamin A on cartilage. II. The effects on organ cultures of embryonic skeletal tissue. *J. Exp. Med. 111*:719.

Fell, H. B., and L. Thomas. 1961. The influence of hydrocortisone on the action of excess vitamin A on limb bone rudiments in culture. *J. Exp. Med. 114*:343.

Gianetto, R., and C. de Duve. 1955. Tissue fractionation studies. IV. Comparative study of the binding of acid phosphatase and cathepsin by rat liver particles. *Biochem. J. 59*:433.

Lucy, J. A., J. T. Dingle, and H. B. Fell. 1961. Studies on the mode of action of excess of vitamin A. II. A possible role of intracellular proteases in the degradation of cartilage matrix. *Biochem. J. 79*:500.

Lucy, J. A., and U. Lichti. 1969. Reactions of vitamin A with acceptors of electrons: Formation of radical anions from 7,7,8,8-tetracyanoquinodimethane and tetrachloro-1,4-benzoquinone. *Biochem. J. 112*:221.

Reynolds, J. J. 1968. Inhibition by calcitonin of bone resorption induced *in vitro* by vitamin A. *Proc. Roy. Soc.* [*Biol.*] *170*:61.

Reynolds, J. J., J. T. Dingle, T. V. Gudmundsson, and I. MacIntyre. 1968. Bone resorption *in vitro* and its inhibition by calcitonin, p. 223. *In* S. Taylor (ed.), *Calcitonin. Proceedings of the Symposium on Thyrocalcitonin and the C Cells*. Heinemann, London.

Thomas, L. 1956. Reversible collapse of rabbit ears after intravenous papain, and prevention of recovery by cortisone. *J. Exp. Med. 104*:245.

Walker, D. G., C. M. Lapiere, and J. A. Gross. 1964. A collagenolytic factor in rat bone promoted by parathyroid extract. *Biochem. Biophys. Res. Commun. 15*:397.

Weissmann, G., and J. T. Dingle. 1961. Release of lysosomal protease by ultraviolet irradiation and its inhibition by hydrocortisone. *Exp. Cell. Res.* *25*:207.

Weston, P. D. 1969. A specific antiserum of lysosomal cathepsin D. *Immunology* *17*:421.

Weston, P. D., A. J. Barrett, and J. T. Dingle. 1969. Specific inhibition of cartilage breakdown. *Nature* *222*:285.

13

RETINOL TRANSPORT IN HUMAN PLASMA

DeWitt S. Goodman

Our laboratory's interest in the metabolism and plasma transport of vitamin A developed out of a long-standing and continuing interest in the metabolism of cholesterol (Goodman, 1965). Retinol is a 20-carbon alcohol which resembles cholesterol in many of its physicochemical properties. Cholesterol and other lipids, except for free fatty acids (Fredrickson and Gordon, 1958) and lysolecithin (Switzer and Eder, 1965), circulate in plasma mainly in the form of plasma lipoprotein molecules with hydrated densities of less than 1.21 (Fredrickson et al., 1967). On a priori grounds, one might therefore expect the lipid alcohol retinol also to circulate in plasma in association with one or more of the known plasma lipoproteins. It has been known for several years, however, that vitamin A mainly circulates in plasma as retinol associated with the proteins of hydrated density greater than 1.21 (Krinsky et al., 1958; Garbers et al., 1960). In our laboratory, for example, more than 90% of the plasma retinol is usually found in the bottom portion of the ultracentrifuge tube when plasma is adjusted to a density of 1.21 and ultracentrifuged at $104{,}000 \times g$ for 36 hr. These findings suggested that retinol circulates in plasma in association with a specific transport protein. This protein has been reported to differ from serum albumin in man (Krinsky et al., 1958) and to have α_1- (Garbers et al., 1960) or α_2-mobility (Glover and Walker, 1964) in the rat. It has also been suggested that this protein might be identical with the tryptophan-rich prealbumin in human serum (Alvsaker et al., 1967).

Isolation of human retinol-binding protein

It is now clear that retinol does indeed circulate in human plasma bound to a specific transport protein, retinol-binding protein (RBP). We have

The studies summarized here were carried out in collaboration with Dr. M. Kanai, Dr. A. Raz, Dr. F. R. Smith, and Mr. T. Shiratori. This work was supported by grant No. AM–05968 from the National Institutes of Health. DeW. S. Goodman is a Career Scientist of the Health Research Council of the City of New York under Contract I–399.

recently reported the purification and partial characterization of RBP (Kanai et al., 1968). In order to study this protein, we injected normal human volunteers intravenously with ^{14}C retinol dispersed in their own plasma. Plasma was collected 1–3 days later, and the purification of RBP was quantitatively monitored by assaying for ^{14}C. Purification was also monitored by spectrophotometrically assaying for retinol in total lipid extracts of plasma fractions and by observing the characteristic fluorescence of the protein-bound retinol.

By the use of these assays, a purification scheme for RBP was developed, which now consists of the sequence: chromatography on DEAE-Sephadex (Fig. 13.1), gel filtration on Sephadex G–200, re-chromatography on a smaller column of DEAE-Sephadex, preparative polyacrylamide gel electrophoresis, and, finally, chromatography on Sephadex G–100 (Kanai et al., 1968; Raz and Goodman, 1969). These procedures result in preparations of RBP which are more than 99% pure, having been purified 1,500- to 2,000-fold.

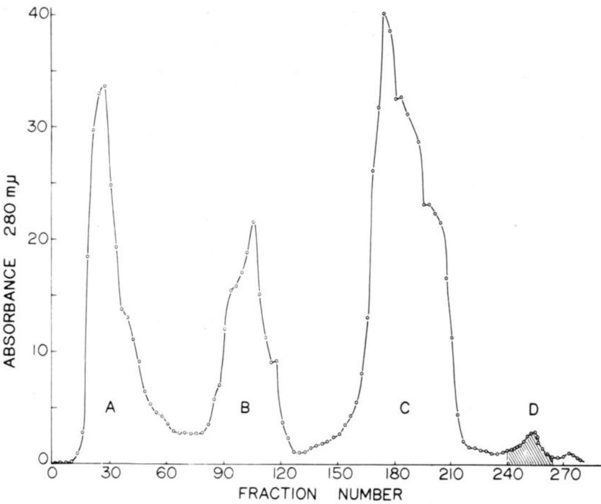

Fig. 13.1. Chromatography of plasma on a column of DEAE-Sephadex. One liter of plasma was concentrated and subjected to chromatography with 0.05 M phosphate buffer (*p*H 7.5) and a linear gradient of NaCl from 0 M to 1.0 M as eluting solvent. Three major peaks of protein were obtained. Peak A consisted mainly of γ-globulins; peak C, of serum albumin. The fractions comprising the small peak D (shaded area) were strongly fluorescent and contained prealbumin and RBP as their major components. (Raz and Goodman, 1969. Reproduced by permission of the American Society of Biological Chemists.)

Physical characteristics of RBP

Purified RBP has an α_1-mobility on electrophoresis and has a molecular weight of approximately 21,000. The molecular weight was estimated by analytical ultracentrifuge studies and by gel filtration on a standardized column of Sephadex G–100. RBP appeared homogenous in the analytical ultracentrifuge, with a sedimentation velocity ($S_{20,w}$) of about 2.2 *S*. Despite this apparent homogeneity, purified RBP displays microheterogeneity on polyacrylamide disc gel electrophoresis, and usually contains three close bands with α_1-mobility. The fastest-moving band is not fluorescent under ultraviolet light, does not contain bound retinol, and appears to consist of apo-RBP (that is, RBP without bound retinol). The other two bands are both fluorescent and contain bound retinol. The relative amounts of these three bands in a given isolated RBP preparation depend on the relative freshness of the plasma sample used, and on the rapidity of the purification and the extent of handling during the purification procedures. When RBP is isolated by rapid purification from freshly drawn plasma, the preparation consists mainly of the slower of the two fluorescent bands. Our findings suggest that during the processes of purification and analysis the naturally occurring holo-RBP (RBP containing bound retinol) is gradually converted to a more rapidly migrating form of the holoprotein (perhaps by loss of a labile amide group), which is in turn converted to the retinol-free apoprotein. The 3 RBP bands are immunologically indistinguishable and were found to react identically with an antiserum prepared against purified RBP (Smith and Goodman, unpublished).

In solution, RBP has an ultraviolet absorption spectrum with two peaks: at 330 mμ (resulting from the protein-bound retinol) and at 280 mμ. The molar extinction and the absorption peak position of retinol when bound to RBP and in aqueous solution appear to be the same as for retinol itself in solution in benzene. Solutions of RBP are strongly fluorescent with maximum uncorrected excitation frequency at 332 mμ and maximum uncorrected emission frequency at 463 mμ. The relative fluorescence intensity of retinol bound to RBP (in aqueous solution) is an order of magnitude greater than that of retinol in solution in any one of a variety of organic solvents. In addition, for retinol bound to RBP, the emission peak due to fluorescence shows a "blue shift" of about 15–20 mμ, compared with retinol itself in solution in organic solvents. These data are consistent with the interpretation that retinol is tightly bound to RBP in a fixed position with restricted mobility.

A molecule of RBP appears to possess one binding site for one molecule of retinol. There are no fatty acid or fatty acyl chains present in purified

RBP. The amino acid composition of RBP differs from that of any previously reported plasma protein, including protein moieties of the plasma lipoproteins. The ratio of polar to nonpolar amino acids in RBP is not particularly unusual for a globular protein. RBP is unusual, however, in containing a very high content of aromatic amino acids, with an estimated 8 residues per molecule (6.1% by weight) of tyrosine and 4 residues per molecule (3.5% by weight) of tryptophan; the protein also contains 10–11 residues per molecule of phenylalanine. The usual concentration of RBP in plasma is approximately 4–5 mg/100 ml.

Association of RBP with prealbumin

In plasma, RBP circulates as a complex, together with another, larger protein that has prealbumin mobility on electrophoresis. The formation of the complex is demonstrated by the experiment summarized in Figure 13.2. Purified prealbumin and RBP, both obtained after preparative gel electrophoresis (Kanai et al., 1968; Raz and Goodman, 1969), were mixed together to form three different solutions with different ratios of prealbumin to RBP. The three solutions were then serially chromatographed on the same column of Sephadex G–100. As shown in the top panel of Figure 13.2, when the ratio of prealbumin to RBP was relatively high, all of the RBP (as indicated by the broken line for 330 mμ absorption) chromatographed together with the prealbumin as a single peak. The effluent volume of this peak corresponded to that expected for a protein of molecu-

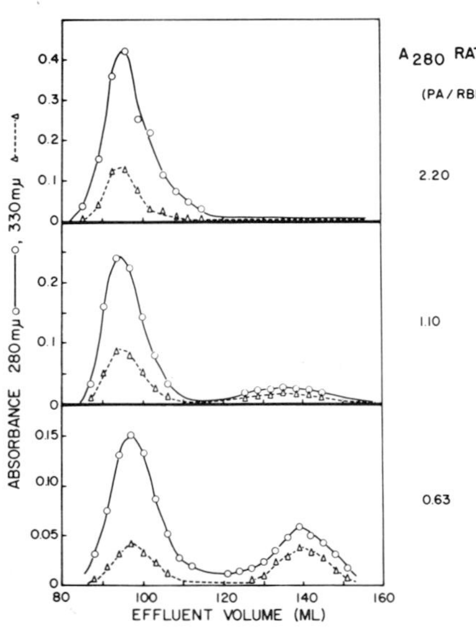

Fig. 13.2. Formation of complex between prealbumin and RBP. Three mixtures of identical volumes but with different ratios of prealbumin to RBP were chromatographed serially on a single column of Sephadex G–100. The relative amounts of the two proteins were estimated from the ratio of the absorbance at 280 mμ due to each in the final mixture (indicated on the right). The absorbance ratio, 330 mμ/280 mμ, for the purified RBP used in this experiment was 0.8. (Kanai et al., 1968. Reproduced by permission of the *Journal of Clinical Investigation.*)

lar weight of roughly 70,000 to 80,000. In contrast, if RBP had been chromatographed alone on this column it would have been eluted much later, at an effluent volume corresponding to its molecular weight of about 21,000. This experiment demonstrates the formation of a complex between prealbumin and RBP.

The capacity of prealbumin for forming a complex with RBP is limited. Thus, when the relative amount of RBP in the mixture was increased progressively, as shown in the middle and bottom panels of Figure 13.2, the prealbumin became saturated with RBP and the excess, uncomplexed RBP was then eluted as a second peak at an effluent volume characteristic of purified RBP alone.

As a control to this experiment, purified RBP was mixed with a large amount of human serum albumin, and the mixture was chromatographed on a column of Sephadex G–100. No complex was formed between the RBP and serum albumin. Similar results were obtained with other serum proteins.

The formation of a complex between RBP and prealbumin has also been demonstrated by the analytical ultracentrifuge studies summarized in Table 13.1. In these studies, pure RBP sedimented with a velocity of 2.1 *S*, whereas pure prealbumin had an $S_{20,w}$ value of 3.7 *S*. When the two proteins were mixed in nearly stoichiometric proportion they formed a complex which sedimented as a single homogeneous component with a velocity of 4.6 *S*. Moreover, the molecular weight of the complex was estimated to be very close to the sum of the molecular weights of RBP and of prealbumin. These studies conclusively establish the formation of a complex between the two proteins in a molar ratio of 1:1. Further analytical ultracentrifuge studies, in which RBP-prealbumin mixtures containing either RBP or prealbumin in excess of a 1:1 molar ratio were employed, demonstrated in every case the presence of the RBP-prealbumin complex

TABLE 13.1. *Analytical ultracentrifugation of RBP, prealbumin, and a 1:1 molar mixture of the two proteins*

Protein analyzed	$S_{20,w}$	Molecular weight
RBP	2.13	21,400
Prealbumin	3.70	49,400
RBP-prealbumin	4.57	70,200

Note: Protein solutions were of the following concentrations: 0.1 M phosphate buffer, *p*H 7.0; sedimentation velocity, 0.43–0.68 mg/ml; sedimentation equilibrium, 0.054–0.085 mg/ml. Molecular weights were calculated as described by Yphantis (1964). These analyses were carried out by Dr. W. Poillon and Dr. P. Feigelson.

in 1:1 molar ratio, together with the free, uncomplexed protein present in excess of this molar ratio.

The RBP-prealbumin complex which circulates in plasma remains intact during chromatography on columns of Sephadex or of DEAE-Sephadex, but dissociates during gel electrophoresis, so the separated RBP and prealbumin can be isolated. The complex is again formed when solutions of the purified RBP and prealbumin are mixed together. On the basis of studies of gel filtration at different *p*H values, we estimate that the association constant for the interaction of RBP with prealbumin is of the order of 10^8; this estimate may, however, be incorrect by an order of magnitude or more. Retinol transport in plasma thus involves both a lipid-protein (retinol-RBP) interaction and a protein-protein (RBP-prealbumin) interaction.

Interaction of retinol with RBP

In order to study the interaction of retinol with RBP, we have developed a method for the removal of retinol from RBP without denaturation of the protein, that is, for the formation of apo-RBP from holo-RBP. In this method, an aqueous solution of RBP and an equal volume of heptane are shaken together in an amber flask under nitrogen, under controlled conditions. During the shaking, retinol is gradually extracted from the RBP and into the heptane phase. The results of a typical extraction experiment are illustrated in Figure 13.3. Before extraction, the aqueous RBP solution had the absorption spectrum shown in the upper right-hand panel, whereas the heptane phase was devoid of ultraviolet absorption. After the mixture had been shaken for 6 hr, 75%–80% of the retinol was extracted into the heptane phase, which showed a retinol absorption peak with absorbance

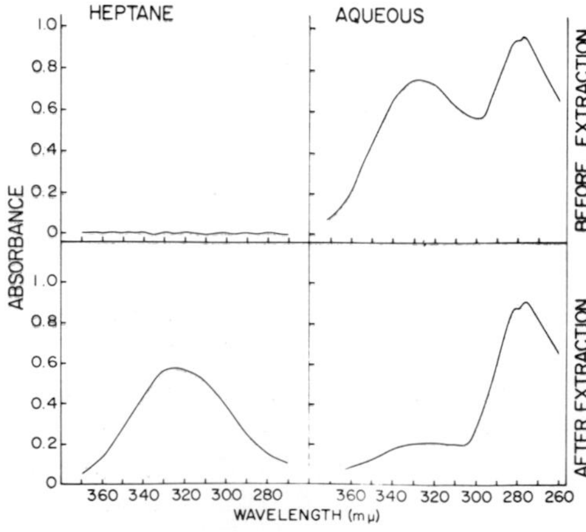

Fig. 13.3. Production of apo-RBP from holo-RBP by extraction of retinol from RBP with heptane.

0.6 (lower left-hand panel). The 330 mμ absorption peak of RBP was decreased by a comparable amount (lower right-hand panel). This experiment illustrates the method of extracting retinol from RBP and directly establishes the fact that the RBP absorption peak at 330 mμ is due to the retinol bound to the protein. The experiment also confirms the conclusion that the molar extinction of retinol bound to RBP is about the same as that of retinol in solution in organic solvents, since the sum of the two lower spectra closely approximates the initial RBP spectrum shown in the upper right-hand panel.

Using this procedure, we conducted experiments to examine the effect of the formation of the RBP-prealbumin complex on the interaction of retinol with RBP (Goodman and Raz, unpublished). Solutions of RBP alone and solutions of the RBP-prealbumin complex were extracted with heptane simultaneously, under several different conditions. The rate of removal of retinol from the RBP-prealbumin complex was markedly less than the rate of removal from RBP alone. These findings suggest that the interaction of retinol with RBP is stabilized by the formation of the RBP-prealbumin complex. This conclusion is also supported by the results of recent studies, in which fluorescence spectroscopy was employed, of the thermal stability of RBP (Goodman and Leslie, unpublished). In these studies it was found that the retinol-RBP complex has greater thermal stability when prealbumin is present than when it is not. The protein-protein interaction may hence serve to stabilize and protect the retinol bound to RBP. In addition, the protein-protein interaction clearly protects the RBP molecule by preventing the glomerular filtration of the relatively small RBP molecule and hence the loss of RBP in the urine.

Interaction of thyroxine with prealbumin

The plasma prealbumin which forms a complex with RBP is the same protein which binds thyroxine and which has been previously studied as one of the transport proteins for plasma thyroxine (Purdy et al., 1965; Oppenheimer et al., 1965). Since the interaction of RBP with prealbumin appears to affect the interaction of retinol with RPB, a study was conducted to examine the effects of the interaction of prealbumin with RBP on the binding of thyroxine by prealbumin (Raz and Goodman, 1969). The thyroxine-prealbumin interaction was quantitatively studied by the method of equilibrium dialysis, with ^{131}I–labeled thyroxine. Prealbumin was found to possess a single binding site for one molecule of thyroxine. The apparent association constant for the thyroxine-prealbumin interaction was approximately 1.6×10^7. The binding capacity and affinity of prealbumin for thyroxine were not affected by the presence or absence of RBP. Moreover, the binding of thyroxine to prealbumin did not interfere with the interaction of prealbumin with RBP. The interaction of prealbumin with thyroxine thus appears to be independent of the prealbumin-RBP interaction.

Model of RBP, retinol, and prealbumin complex

Figure 13.4 shows our working model for the retinol transport system in human plasma. The lower, smaller unit represents RBP; the upper unit, prealbumin. Since retinol is known from crystallographic studies to be a relatively flat, planar molecular, we presume that RBP contains a thin cleft in its tertiary structure and that the retinol molecule resides within the hydrophobic interior of this cleft. Furthermore, since retinol is more difficult to extract from the RBP-prealbumin complex than from RBP alone, we suggest that the opening of the cleft may be blocked in the protein-protein complex; thus the retinol molecule is fully insulated from its environment. Finally, the binding site for thyroxine on prealbumin is considered to be located at a position on the prealbumin molecule quite removed from the RBP-prealbumin binding site.

At the present time our studies of this system are proceeding along two major lines, one chemical and the other clinical and physiological. Along chemical lines we would like to explore further each of the three interactions illustrated in Figure 13.4. Recent studies have suggested that different features are involved in the different interactions (Raz et al., 1970). In the presence of 6 M urea, for example, the RBP-prealbumin complex is completely disrupted, whereas the retinol-RBP complex remains intact. The effect of urea on the protein-protein interaction is fully reversible. In contrast, when the two disulfide bonds of RBP are reduced and alkylated, the binding of retinol by RBP is completely disrupted, whereas the

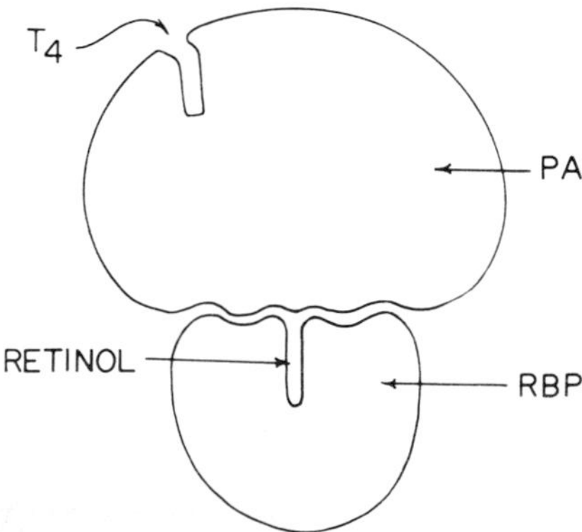

Fig. 13.4. The retinol transport system in human plasma. The two proteins are identified on the right; the binding sites for the ligands which bind to each protein, on the left.

altered RBP retains a slight (although drastically reduced) affinity for prealbumin.

In order to carry out clinical and physiological studies involving RBP, we have prepared ^{131}I-labeled RBP and an antiserum in rabbits against pure, unlabeled RBP. RBP is immunologically different from all other plasma proteins, including plasma prealbumin. With these preparations, we have developed a radioimmunoassay for the level of RBP in plasma (Smith and Goodman, unpublished). Further studies are now planned to examine the level and the turnover of RBP in normal and diseased humans in order to explore the metabolism and the role of this protein in human health and disease.

References

Alvsaker, J. O., F. B. Haugli, and S. G. Laland. 1967. The presence of vitamin A in human tryptophane-rich prealbumin. *Biochem. J. 102*:362.

Fredrickson, D. S., and R. S. Gordon, Jr. 1958. Transport of fatty acids. *Physiol. Rev. 38*:585.

Fredrickson, D. S., R. I. Levy, and R. S. Lees. 1967. Fat transport in lipoproteins: An integrated approach to mechanisms and disorders. *New Engl. J. Med. 276*:34.

Garbers, C. F., J. Gillman, and M. Peisach. 1960. The transport of vitamin A in rat serum with special reference to the occurrence of unidentified metabolites of vitamin A in the rat. *Biochem. J. 75*:124.

Glover, J., and R. J. Walker. 1964. Absorption and transport of vitamin A. *Exp. Eye Res. 3*:374.

Goodman, DeW. S. 1965. Cholesterol ester metabolism. *Physiol. Rev. 45*:747.

Kanai, M., A. Raz, and DeW. S. Goodman. 1968. Retinol-binding protein: the transport protein for vitamin A in human plasma. *J. Clin. Invest. 47*:2025.

Krinsky, N. I., D. G. Cornwell, and J. L. Oncley. 1958. The transport of vitamin A and carotenoids in human plasma. *Arch. Biochem. Biophys. 73*:233.

Oppenheimer, J. H., M. I. Surks, J. S. Smith, and R. Squef. 1965. Isolation and characterization of human thyroxine-binding prealbumin. *J. Biol. Chem. 240*:173.

Purdy, R. H., K. A. Woeber, M. T. Holloway, and S. H. Ingbar. 1965. Preparation of crystalline thyroxine-binding prealbumin from human plasma. *Biochemistry 4*:1888.

Raz, A., and DeW. S. Goodman. 1969. The interaction of thyroxine with human plasma prealbumin and with the prealbumin-retinol binding protein complex. *J. Biol. Chem. 244*:3230.

Raz, A., T. Shiratori, and DeW. S. Goodman. 1970. Studies on the protein-protein and protein-ligand interactions involved in retinol transport in plasma. *J. Biol. Chem. 245*:1903.

Switzer, S., and H. A. Eder. 1965. Transport of lysolecithin by albumin in human and rat plasma. *J. Lipid Res. 6*:506.

Yphantis, D. A. 1964. Equilibrium ultracentrifugation of dilute solutions. *Biochemistry 3*:297.

14

ENZYMATIC TRANSFORMATIONS OF VITAMIN A, WITH PARTICULAR EMPHASIS ON CAROTENOID CLEAVAGE

James Allen Olson and M. R. Lakshmanan

During the dawn of the era of modern nutritional science, Harry Steenbock was one of the first nutritionists to become concerned about biological transformations of vitamin A. It is interesting to recall the exciting events of those early days, distant now by over half a century. McCollum, Osborne, Mendel, and Drummond, to cite the most notable, were finding that some fat-soluble component was required for the growth of experimental animals. In 1915 McCollum and Davis termed this growth-stimulating component "fat-soluble factor A." Not all fats, however, stimulated growth; butter fat and egg yolk extracts were effective, for example, whereas lard was not. Since the most active fats, and particularly those of vegetable origin, were yellow in color, whereas inactive fats were generally colorless, Steenbock (1919) deduced that the yellow-colored substance might be the growth-stimulating compound.

But there were some puzzling exceptions to this broad generalization. Steenbock found that the yellow pigment carotene had biological activity, whereas the yellow pigment xanthophyll did not. Furthermore, some fatty oils such as cod-liver oil, although essentially colorless, nonetheless had very high biological activity. To resolve these seemingly contradictory observations, Steenbock (1919) suggested, with remarkable insight, that biologically active carotenoids might be converted into a yet undefined *leuko* form which retained its biological activity. Steenbock was right, but his brilliant suggestion was not generally accepted for almost a decade.

This research was supported by the Rockefeller Foundation and by Grants-in-Aid from the National Institutes of Arthritis and Metabolic Diseases (5–RO1–AM–11367) and from the Faculty of Graduate Studies, University of Medical Sciences, Bangkok.

The authors acknowledge with great pleasure the excellent secretarial help of Miss Patchari Karnasuta and the drafting skill of Miss Waneda Thongthin.

We must realize, however, that some thorny problems faced nutritionists in the early 1920's. The other fat-soluble vitamins had not yet been discovered, for example, and the effects of various deficiencies tended to be lumped together; the instability of vitamin A and carotenoids in the presence of oxygen and light was not fully recognized; and standard procedures for biological assay were not well defined. Something was known about the metabolism of sugars, but little thought was given to the possible metabolism of these mysterious lipoid growth factors—except, of course, by Steenbock.

Subsequently Steenbock and Boutwell (1920) and Steenbock and Gross (1920) showed that yellow pigmentation was associated closely with vitamin A activity in a large series of plant products. Yellow maize, for example, is biologically active, whereas white maize is not; the yellow sweet potato is active, whereas the common white potato is not.

But what of the *leuko* form postulated by Steenbock? Within two years Takahashi (1922) obtained a highly active concentrate of cod-liver oil possessing many of the characteristic biological and chemical properties of vitamin A. During the latter part of that decade, increasingly successful attempts were made to purify and characterize vitamin A. This work culminated in the determination of the structure of the vitamin by Karrer, Morf, and Schopp in 1931.

But was carotene actually converted into this biologically active *leuko* form, or did it only enhance or activate the vitamin? In 1930 Thomas Moore clearly showed that β-carotene, when given to vitamin A–deficient rats, was indeed converted into vitamin A (measured as blue Lovibond color units), and the latter was stored in the liver. These experiments by Moore gave rise to three significant questions: What kinds of carotenoids or precursors are converted into vitamin A? Where does the conversion take place? And what is the chemical mechanism of the conversion reaction? Although many efforts have been made to answer these queries during the past forty years, unambiguous responses have only been possible in the last few years. In this chapter I will deal with these three queries in some detail, and then will briefly consider the over-all metabolism of vitamin A in the mammal.

Biological activity of the carotenes

After the demonstration that β-carotene was a precursor of vitamin A, a large number of carotene derivatives were isolated or synthesized and their activity in stimulating the growth of rats or chicks was assessed. The structures of some typical carotenoids and of vitamin A are shown in Figure 14.1. Of all carotenoids tested, all-*trans* β-carotene (I, Fig. 14.1) proved

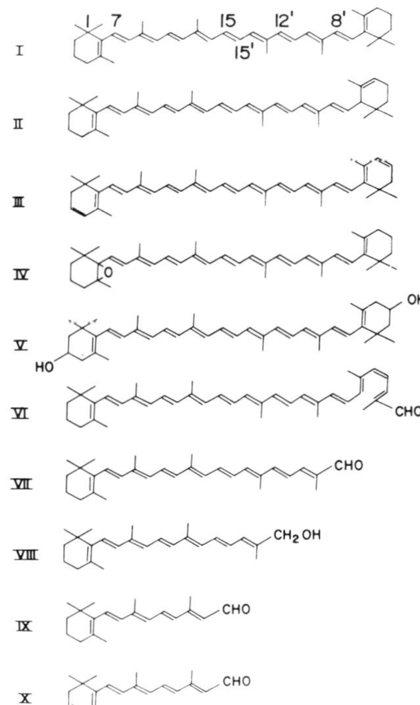

Fig. 14.1. Some typical all-*trans* carotenoid derivatives. I: β-carotene; II: α-carotene; III: Bis-3,3′-dehydro-β-carotene; IV: 5,6-epoxy-β-carotene; V: zeaxanthin; VI: 3′,4′-dehydro-18′-oxo-γ-carotene; VII: β-apo-8′-carotenal; VIII: β-apo-12′-carotenol; IX: all-*trans* retinal; X: all-*trans* 3-dehydroretinal.

to be the best provitamin, although its biological activity was only about 50% that of all-*trans* retinol. A comparison of the relative activities of various carotenoids is given in Table 14.1. The structures of carotenoids in Tables 14.1 and 14.2 have been depicted in the special way, i.e., as analogs of the retinyl moiety. Thus β-carotene is written as a symmetrical compound composed of two retinyl moieties joined head to head with a double bond. Clearly, most carotenoids with vitamin A activity contain the unsubstituted retinyl moiety. The exceptions — canthaxanthin, astaxanthin, and related compounds — however, are converted into vitamin A to an appreciable degree only in fish (Grangaud et al., 1964; Gross and Budowski, 1966), although astaxanthin does produce a slight antixerophthalmic effect in the rat (Grangaud et al., 1964).

Although one-half of the molecule apparently must have the retinyl moiety in order to produce vitamin A activity in the mammal, the other half may vary widely in structure. For example, it may be acyclic as in γ-carotene, it may be rather saturated as in β-zeacarotene, it may be greatly shortened as in the β-apocarotenols, or it may be lengthened as in homo-β-carotene. Furthermore, oxygen may be present in the molecule in various oxidation states.

TABLE 14.1. *All-trans carotenoids with vitamin A activity*

Compound	Moiety structure[a]	Relative biological activity[b]
Retinol	—	200
3-dehydroretinol	—	80
Hydrocarbons		
β-carotene	$(Retinyl:)_2$	100
3-dehydro-β-carotene	Retinyl:3-dehydroretinyl	75
α-carotene	Retinyl:α-retinyl	53
γ-carotene	Retinyl:geranyl-geranyl-4,8-diene	43
β-zeacarotene	Retinyl:geranyl-geranyl-4-ene	40
Homo-β-carotene	Retinyl:retinylvinyl	20
Bis-3,3′-dehydro-β-carotene	$(3\text{-dehydroretinyl:})_2$	38
Oxygenated derivatives		
Cryptoxanthin	Retinyl:3-hydroxyretinyl	57
Echinenone	Retinyl:4-ketoretinyl	44
5,6-epoxy-β-carotene	Retinyl:5,6-epoxyretinyl	21
Torularhodin	Retinyl:geranyl-geranyl-4,8,12-tetraen-16-oic acid	< 50
Dehydrolutein	3-dehydroretinyl:3-hydroxy-retinyl	ca. 40[c]
Canthaxanthin	$(4\text{-ketoretinyl:})_2$	140[c]
Astaxanthin	$(3\text{-hydroxy-4-ketoretinyl:})_2$	ca. 80[c]
Apocarotenol derivatives		
β-apo-14′-carotenol	Retinyl:ethanol	(7)[d]
β-apo-12′-carotenal	Retinyl:α-methylbutenal	(125)
Methyl β-apo-12′-carotenoate	Retinyl:methyl α-methylbutenoate	(200)
β-apo-10′-carotenal	Retinyl:γ-methylhexadienal	(> 100)
β-apo-8′-carotenal	Retinyl:α.ε-dimethyloctatrienal	(40), 72

Note: The approximate biological activities cited in this table are from Moore (1957), Glover (1960), Goodwin (1963), and Subbarayan et al. (1966) for the chick and the rat; and were calculated from liver storage data of Gross and Budowski (1966) for fish.

[a] Colon (:) indicates a double bond joining two moieties head to head.

[b] In reference to activity of β-carotene (= 100).

[c] In fish.

[d] Relative daily requirement.

Some carotenoids that do not produce any vitamin A activity in rats and chicks are listed in Table 14.2. The only derivative listed containing the retinyl moiety is decapopreno-β-carotene, which contains two additional isoprenyl residues in the middle of the symmetrical chain. Carotenoids which are acyclic or which bear hydroxyl groups on both β-ionone rings are inactive. We should also briefly consider *cis-trans* isomers of these compounds. With very few exceptions, various *cis* isomers of both carotenoids and vitamin A derivatives are less biologically active than the all-*trans* isomer. These studies on growth-stimulating effects of various

TABLE 14.2. *Carotenoids without vitamin A activity*

Compound	Moiety structure[a]
Hydrocarbons	
Phytoene	(Geranyl-geranyl:)$_2$
Lycopene	(Geranyl-geranyl-4,8-diene:)$_2$
Decapopreno-β-carotene	(Retinylprenyl:)$_2$
retro-β-carotene	(*retro*-anhydroretinyl:)$_2$
Oxygenated derivatives	
Zeaxanthin	(3-hydroxyretinyl:)$_2$
Isozeaxanthin	(4-hydroxyretinyl:)$_2$
Lutein	3-hydroxyretinyl:3-hydroxy-α-retinyl
5,6:5′,6′-diepoxy-β-carotene	(5,6-epoxyretinyl:)$_2$
5,8:5′,8′-diepoxy-β-carotene	(5,8-epoxyretinyl:)$_2$
Astacin	(3,4-diketoretinyl:)$_2$

[a] Colon (:) indicates a double bond joining two moieties head to head.

carotenoids have clearly defined the minimal structural requirement for vitamin A activity in the mammal: namely, the presence of an unsubstituted retinyl moiety.

The relative biological activity of a compound in stimulating the growth process, however, is the sum of many complex physiological processes within the animal, including the compound's dispersion in a proper micellar form, its stability, its absorption, its conversion into retinol, its storage, and its metabolism by alternate pathways. Carotenoids are probably less active biologically than all-*trans* retinol and retinyl ester because they are generally absorbed less efficiently from the gut and because their cleavage product, retinal, is in part oxidized to retinoic acid, which is less active physiologically and is excreted rapidly from the animal. Various carotenoids may differ in biological activity because of differences in absorption rate or stability and also because of different rates of cleavage into retinal. From an enzymatic standpoint, therefore, two interesting questions may be asked: Is one enzyme or several responsible for the conversion of various carotenoids into vitamin A? And does any correlation exist between the rate of cleavage and the biological activity of a given carotenoid? A profitable approach to these questions necessarily awaited the isolation of an enzyme from tissue extracts, which occurred only several years ago (Goodman and Huang, 1965; Olson and Hayaishi, 1965).

Enzymatic cleavage of carotenes

Although carotene cleavage activity is present in intestinal homogenates of most mammals, the relative activity of the enzyme in different species varies considerably and, for the species we have examined, is highest in the rabbit (Table 14.3). Taking the rabbit as an example, we might briefly consider the relationship between an animal's actual requirement for vitamin A and its ability to cleave β-carotene. In the rabbit, the daily vitamin A requirement for optimal growth and longevity is presumably about 20 μg/kg, about midway between the daily requirement of the rat (30 μg/kg) and that of man (10 μg/kg). From the activity observed in mucosal homogenates, we have calculated that the intestine of an adult rabbit can convert between 750 μg and 2,500 μg of β-carotene into vitamin A per kg of total weight per day. Clearly the rabbit possesses a great excess of carotene cleavage capacity, which might maximally yield between 40 and 130 times the amount of vitamin A required.

TABLE 14.3. *Estimated activity of carotenoid 15,15′-dioxygenase in crude intestinal mucosal homogenates of various species*

Species	Estimated maximal activity[a] (nmole β-carotene cleaved per mg protein per hr at 37 C)
Rabbit	0.40
Rat[b]	0.23–0.29
Chicken	0.09
Guinea pig	0.05
Hog[c]	0.03

[a] For technical reasons most assays were conducted at a β-carotene concentration of 10^{-6} M, and some assays were conducted with 10^{-6} M β-apo-10′-carotenol. By assuming a K_m of 2×10^{-6} M for all carotenoids and a ratio of 20 for relative cleavage rates of β-apocarotenol to β-carotene, we were able to estimate the V_{max}.

[b] Goodman et al. (1967).

[c] Goodman (1969).

PURIFICATION OF THE CLEAVAGE ENZYME

In order to study the specificity of the enzyme more readily, Dr. J. L. Pope purified the enzyme by the following procedure. Rabbits were not fed for at least one day and were killed by a blow on the head. Segments of the intestine were removed, chilled in ice, perfused with cold isotonic sodium chloride and then slit along the mesenteric line. The mucosa was scraped off with a glass microscope slide and then was homogenized in 8 volumes of 0.1 M potassium phosphate buffer *p*H 7.8. The enzyme was sufficiently stable without adding nicotinamide and magnesium chloride to the homogenate. After the homogenate was centrifuged for 90 min at 8000 *g*, the supernatant solution was decanted and heated at 53–55 C for 6 min. Then the solution was brought to 25% saturation with ammonium sulfate, the precipitate was centrifuged off, and additional ammonium sulfate was added to bring the solution to 50% saturation. As for rat intestinal enzyme (Goodman and Huang, 1965), the resulting precipitate contains most of the enzyme activity. After most of the ammonium sulfate was removed from the precipitate by dialysis, the chilled solution was treated with two volumes of cold acetone, and the precipitate was centrifuged off and dissolved in buffer. As shown in Table 14.4, the enzyme

TABLE 14.4. *Purification of carotene 15,15′-dioxygenase from the intestinal mucosa of the rabbit*

Preparation	Total activity (nmole carotene cleaved per hr at 37 C)	Total protein (mg)	Specific activity (nmole carotene cleaved per mg per hr at 37 C)
Mucosal homogenate	72.6	382	0.19
Supernatant solution (48,000 × g, 90 min)	51.9	129	0.40
Heated supernatant solution (53–55 C, 6 min)	45.0	60	0.75
Precipitate (25%–50% sat. $(NH_4)_2SO_4$)	22.5	13	1.73
Precipitate (0%–68% acetone)	12.9	5.3	2.44

was purified about 13-fold by this procedure. The enzyme has also been purified about 75-fold from homogenates of hog intestine (Goodman, 1969), but the initial specific activity of the crude hog enzyme is much lower than that of the rabbit enzyme (Table 14.3). The cleavage enzyme has also been purified about 3-fold from the rat intestine (Goodman et al., 1967).

SPECIFICITY OF THE CLEAVAGE ENZYME

Using this partially purified enzyme from the rabbit intestine, we determined its activity in relation to various carotenoids (Lakshmanan et al., 1968, 1969). The enzyme was assayed by measuring the formation of retinal (Fig. 14.1, IX) as its thiobarbituric acid complex, which has an $E^{1\%}_{1cm}$ value of 2163 at 520 nm (Futterman and Saslaw, 1961). Since we desired to compare the biological activity of various carotenoids with the enzymatic rate of vitamin A synthesis from them, the enzyme activity is expressed as the rate of retinal formation per mg of protein per hr in Table 14.5. This specific activity is the same as the rate of cleavage of most carotenoids, but is twice the rate of β-carotene cleavage. For β-carotene, α-carotene (II, Fig. 14.1), and 3′,4′-dehydro-18′-oxo-γ-carotene (VI, Fig. 14.1), the growth-promoting activity and the enzymatic rate of formation of retinal are roughly comparable (Table 14.5). It is interesting to note that 3′,4′-

TABLE 14.5. *Cleavage of various carotenoids by carotenoid 15,15′-dioxygenase of rabbit intestine*

Compound	Growth-promoting activity[a]	Relative formation rate of retinal derivatives[a]
β-carotene	100	100
α-carotene	53	48
3′,4′-dehydro-18′-oxo-γ-carotene	$<$ 50[b]	100
Bis-3,3′-dehydro-β-carotene	38	54
5,6-epoxy-β-carotene	21	0
5,6:5′,6′-diepoxy-β-carotene	0	0
Zeaxanthin	0	ca. 30[c]

[a] In reference to activity of β-carotene (= 100).
[b] Activity of torularhodin.
[c] Unidentified product.

dehydro-18′-oxo-γ-carotene is the aldehyde derivative of the naturally occurring carotenic acid torularhodin, which is biologically active. Bis-3-3′-dehydro-β-carotene (Fig. 14.1, III) is cleaved at a significant rate to yield two molecules of vitamin A_2 aldehyde (Fig. 14.1, X). To our knowledge this is the first demonstration of the enzymatic formation of vitamin A_2, a prominent photopigment in the eyes of many fresh water and some marine fish. Although zeaxanthin (Fig. 14.1, V), the dihydroxy derivative of β-carotene, is biologically inactive, some aldehyde, possibly 3-hydroxyretinal, is formed at an appreciable rate. This product, however, has not been adequately characterized.

On the other hand, the epoxy derivatives of β-carotene are not cleaved by the enzyme. This is somewhat puzzling, in that the monoepoxy derivative (Fig. 14.1, IV) has appreciable growth-promoting activity, whereas the diepoxy derivative has very little, if any. Since 5,6-epoxy-β-carotene does not inhibit the cleavage of other carotenoids, its inertness is difficult to explain. In the intact animal, of course, the epoxide might possibly be reduced first to a hydroxy derivative, de-epoxidized to unsaturated compounds, or cleaved by a different enzyme at the β-ionone ring before the 15,15′ cleavage enzyme acts.

A particularly interesting group of compounds with high vitamin A activity are the β-apocarotenol derivatives (Fig. 14.1, VII, VIII). These compounds are derivatives of β-carotene with one of the β-ionone rings and part of the side chain removed. In view of the high biological activity of these compounds, Glover and Redfearn (1954) made the interesting suggestion that each molecule of β-carotene and of other carotenoids might be oxidized to one molecule of retinal by a stepwise process through a series of β-apocarotenals. Glover (1960) showed that several radioactive β-apocarotenals were converted into vitamin A ester with the concomitant release of small radioactive fragments. Although some β-apocarotenals have been identified in the horse intestine, the conversion of carotenoids to β-apocarotenals has never been demonstrated in mammals.

When several β-apocarotenal derivatives were incubated with the rabbit intestinal cleavage enzyme, however, we noted a rapid formation of retinal (Table 14.6). Indeed, all of the β-apocarotenals were cleaved more rapidly than β-carotene. The most active carotenal was β-apo-10′-carotenal, which was cleaved about 11 times more rapidly than β-carotene and which yielded about 5½ times as much retinal per unit time. When the terminal aldehyde group was reduced, the resulting β-apocarotenols were cleaved about twice as rapidly as the aldehydes. The β-apocarotenoic acids, on the other hand, were somewhat less active than the aldehydes. Possibly the lower biological activity of some of the β-apocarotenals may be due to their ready oxidation to their corresponding acids in living organisms (Thommen, 1961).

On the basis of the observed activity of the enzyme towards various carotenoid substrates, some generalizations about the enzyme can be made. First of all, the enzyme is seemingly specific for the 15,15′ double bond of the carotenoid substrate. In all cases, retinal was detected as the sole major product of the cleavage reaction. Second, the enzyme is relatively nonspecific with respect to the length of the carotenoid chain or even of substituents on the β-ionone ring. Of all the compounds tested, including the hydroxylated derivative zeaxanthin, only the epoxides were not cleaved by the enzyme. Third, the enzyme is most active with relatively short β-apocarotenols. As noted, the activity of β-apo-10′-carotenol, the most active substrate, was about 20 times greater than that of β-carotene. Of the C40 carotenoids, however, β-carotene proved to be the best substrate.

Clearly, additional carotenoids must be tested before any broad generalization can be made about the enzymatic conversion of carotenoids into vitamin A in mammals, and the enzyme should be purified to a much greater degree. At the moment, however, it seems probable that a single enzyme specific for the 15,15′ double bond, rather than several enzymes, cleaves a wide variety of carotenoids into retinal. Furthermore, a reason-

TABLE 14.6. *Cleavage of β-apocarotenals by carotenoid 15,15′-dioxygenase of rabbit intestine*

Compound	Growth-promoting activity	Relative rate of retinal formation
β-apo-12′-carotenal	125	235
β-apo-10′-carotenal	> 100	535
β-apo-8′-carotenal	40, 72	510
β-apo-4′-carotenal	ca. 100	125
β-carotene	100	100

able correlation exists between the relative enzymatic rate of retinal formation and the biological activity of a given carotenoid, at least in the few cases tested. Thus the actual enzymatic cleavage rate may be one of the major factors determining the growth-stimulating activity of a given provitamin.

Since many carotenals and other partially degraded forms of carotenoids have been identified in plants (Thommen, 1967), it is apparent that other cleavage enzymes exist in nature which oxidize carotenoids at positions in the conjugated chain other than the 15,15′ double bond (Olson, 1968). None of these other carotene cleavage enzymes has yet been studied, however.

TISSUE LOCALIZATION OF THE CLEAVAGE ENZYME

Our second query, concerning where the conversion of β-carotene and other carotenoids into vitamin A takes place, has been the subject of considerable controversy during the past fifty years (Moore, 1957). It is quite clear now that the two major organs responsible for the conversion are the intestine and the liver. The carotene cleavage enzyme has been identified in both tissues, and, as we have noted, purified considerably from the intestinal mucosa. To varying degrees in different species, intact carotenoids can cross the intestinal barrier, enter the plasma, and be transported mainly to the liver and to adipose tissue. Carotenoids not transformed in the intestinal mucosa are probably cleaved mainly in the liver. The kidney may also cleave carotenoids to some degree, and possibly some other organs may be active as well.

MECHANISM OF CLEAVAGE

Our third query, regarding the mechanism of the enzymatic cleavage reaction, has also been largely resolved. The enzyme appears to be a typical dioxygenase (Goodman and Huang, 1965; Olson and Hayaishi, 1965). Molecular oxygen is required for the reaction, and the enzyme is inhibited by ferrous chelating agents such as α,α′-dipyridyl and *o*-phenanthroline, but not by cyanide. Unlike monooxygenases, no other redox cofactor is needed. During the oxidative cleavage of β-carotene into retinal, the two hydrogen atoms on the 15 and 15′ carbon atoms are not released (Goodman et al., 1966). In all likelihood the central double bond is attacked by oxygen to form transitorily a peroxy-β-carotene, which quickly rearranges into two molecules of retinal (Olson and Hayaishi, 1965). The enzyme has a *p*H optimum in a slightly alkaline region, and is half saturated with β-carotene at a concentration of 1–3 μM.

The enzyme has been partially characterized from four sources: rat intestine (Goodman and Huang, 1965), rat liver (Olson and Hayaishi, 1965), hog intestine (Goodman, 1969), and rabbit intestine. The properties of the enzyme from all sources are very similar. However, the rabbit intestinal enzyme seems to be more resistant to a group of sulfhydryl binding reagents, while the hog mucosal enzyme is somewhat less so.

The nature of the β-carotene dispersion markedly affects the enzyme's activity (Goodman et al., 1967). Maximal enzymatic activity is obtained by an appropriate combination of a detergent and a polar lipid. This requirement is not specific, inasmuch as both bile salts and synthetic detergents are effective when combined with various kinds of phospholipids. The synthetic detergent sodium dodecyl sulfate, however, is able to replace the mixture of bile salts and lipid. Furthermore, when β-carotene is suspended in a water-clear ethanolic clathrate complex in the absence of any detergents, a slow but appreciable conversion of β-carotene into retinal takes place (J. L. Pope, unpublished observations). Under physiologic conditions, it is uncertain what micellar form of β-carotene is presented to the intestinal enzyme. Whether or not bile salt micelles transitorily enter the mucosal cells of the upper gut, where the cleavage enzyme is most active, has not been clearly defined.

Metabolism of retinal

We have paid considerable attention above to the oxidative cleavage of a single double bond, and thus far have not considered what happens in mammals to retinal, the major product of the cleavage reaction. Physiologically, the most important reaction of retinal is its interaction with an ε-lysine group of opsins in the eye to form a Schiff base or possibly a complex with both amino and sulfhydryl groups. Retinal is isomerized enzymatically to its 11-*cis* isomer in the eye, and retinol is isomerized as well in several tissues. Retinal may also be irreversibly oxidized to retinoic acid or it may be reduced by a group of alcohol dehydrogenases present in most, if not all, tissues. The major storage form of vitamin A is retinyl palmitate, which is probably formed by a transfer reaction involving phospholipids of the endoplasmic reticulum. Retinol and retinoic acid are excreted in the bile mainly in the form of glucuronides, which are formed in the intestinal mucosa and liver by typical glucuronyl transferases of the endoplasmic reticulum in the presence of uridine diphosphoglucuronic acid. The terminal carbon atoms of retinoic acid may also be oxidized by a peroxidase present in the endoplasmic reticulum of the kidney and liver (Roberts and DeLuca, 1967; DeLuca, 1969). A somewhat physiological depiction of the metabolism of carotenoids and vitamin A is shown in Figure 14.2. These various enzymatic processes, which have been considered in detail in recent reviews (Olson, 1967, 1968, 1969*a*, 1969*b*), shall not be treated further here.

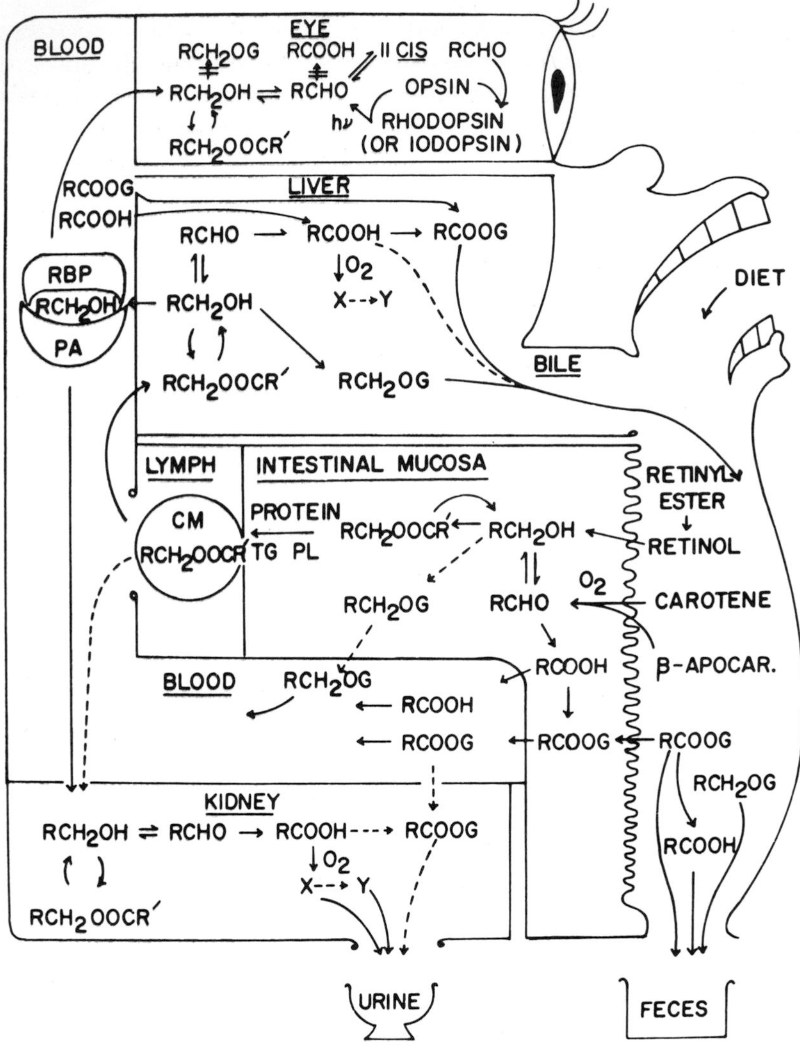

Fig. 14.2. Major metabolic reactions of carotenoids and vitamin A in the mammal. (Olson, 1969*b*. Reproduced by permission of the Federation of American Societies for Experimental Biology.)

Conclusions

We might summarize our thoughts in the following way. Steenbock's brilliant deduction that carotenoids might be converted to biologically active *leuko* forms was followed by the elucidation of the structure of retinol and by the realization that essentially all biologically active carotenoids contain either an unsubstituted retinyl or a 3-dehydroretinyl moiety. Most recently the catalytic transformation of carotenoids has been examined by use of a partially purified enzyme of the intestinal mucosa. The enzyme, termed carotenoid 15,15′-dioxygenase, specifically oxidizes the 15,15′ double bond of a large number of carotenoids into aldehydic products in the presence of molecular oxygen. The rate of enzymatic cleavage into retinal also correlates roughly with the biological activity of a given carotenoid. It is probable, although not proven, that a single enzyme mainly localized in the cytoplasm of the intestinal mucosa and of the liver is responsible in mammals for the conversion of provitamins into retinal and that the growth-stimulating activity of a given carotenoid significantly depends on its relative rate of enzymatic cleavage.

References

DeLuca, H. F. 1969. Pathways of retinoic acid and retinol metabolism. *Amer. J. Clin. Nutr. 22*:945.

Futterman, S., and L. D. Saslaw. 1961. The estimation of vitamin A aldehyde with thiobarbituric acid. *J. Biol. Chem. 236*:1652.

Glover, J. 1960. The conversion of β-carotene into vitamin A. *Vitamins Hormones 18*:371.

Glover, J., and E. R. Redfearn. 1954. The mechanism of the transformation of β-carotene into vitamin A in vivo. *Biochem. J. 58*:15P.

Goodman, D. S. 1969. The biosynthesis of vitamin A from β-carotene. *Amer. J. Clin. Nutr. 22*:963.

Goodman, D. S., and H. S. Huang. 1965. Biosynthesis of vitamin A with rat intestinal enzymes. *Science 149*:879.

Goodman, D. S., H. S. Huang, and T. Shiratori. 1966. Mechanism of the biosynthesis of vitamin A from β-carotene. *J. Biol. Chem. 241*:1929.

Goodman, D. S., H. S. Huang, M. Kanai, and T. Shiratori. 1967. The enzymatic conversion of all-*trans* β-carotene into retinol. *J. Biol. Chem. 242*:3543.

Goodwin, T. W. 1963. *The Biosynthesis of Vitamins and Related Compounds*, pp. 300, 302. Academic Press, New York.

Grangaud, R., M. Nicol, J. Le Gall, and A. Soussy. 1964. Chemical constitution and vitamin A activity [in French]. *Arch. Sci. Physiol. 18*:235.

Gross, J., and P. Budowski. 1966. Conversion of carotenoids into vitamins A_1 and A_2 in two species of freshwater fish. *Biochem. J. 101*:747.

Karrer, P., R. Morf, and K. Schopp. 1931. Vitamin A from fish oil II [in German]. *Helv. Chim. Acta 14*:1431.

Lakshmanan, M. R., J. L. Pope, and J. A. Olson. 1968. The specificity of a partially purified carotenoid cleavage enzyme of rabbit intestine. *Biochem. Biophys. Res. Commun. 33*:347.

Lakshmanan, M. R., J. A. Olson, and J. L. Pope. 1969. Specificity of the β-carotene cleavage enzyme. *Fed. Proc. 28*:490.

McCollum, E. V., and M. Davis. 1913. Necessity of certain lipins in the diet during growth. *J. Biol. Chem. 15*:167.

McCollum, E. V., and M. Davis. 1915. The nature of the dietary deficiencies of rice. *J. Biol. Chem. 23*:181.

Moore, T. 1930. Vitamin A and carotene. VI. The conversion of carotene to vitamin A *in vivo*. *Biochem. J. 24*:692.

Moore, T. 1957. *Vitamin A*, pp. 70–71. Elsevier, Amsterdam.

Olson, J. A. 1967. The metabolism of vitamin A. *Pharmacol. Rev. 19*:559.

Olson, J. A. 1968. Some aspects of vitamin A metabolism. *Vitamins Hormones 26*:1.

Olson, J. A. 1969*a*. The alpha and the omega of vitamin A metabolism. *Amer. J. Clin. Nutr.* 22:953.

Olson, J. A. 1969*b*. Metabolism and function of vitamin A. *Fed. Proc. 28*:1670.

Olson, J. A., and O. Hayaishi. 1965. The enzymatic cleavage of β-carotene into vitamin A by soluble enzymes of rat liver and intestine. *Proc. Nat. Acad. Sci. U.S.A. 54*:1364.

Roberts, A. B., and H. F. DeLuca. 1967. Pathways of retinol and retinoic acid metabolism in the rat. *Biochem. J. 102*:600.

Steenbock, H. 1919. White corn vs. yellow corn and a probable relationship between the fat soluble vitamins and yellow plant pigments. *Science 50*:352.

Steenbock, H., and P. W. Boutwell. 1920. Fat-soluble vitamine. III. The comparative nutritive value of white and yellow maizes. *J. Biol. Chem. 41*:81.

Steenbock, H., and E. G. Gross. 1920. Fat-soluble vitamine. IV. The fat-soluble vitamine content of green plant tissues together with some observations on their water-soluble vitamine content. *J. Biol. Chem. 41*:149.

Subbarayan, C., M. R. Lakshmanan, and H. R. Cama. 1966. Metabolism and biological potency of 5,6-monoepoxy-β-carotene. *Biochem. J. 99*:308.

Takahashi, K. 1922. Nutritive values of lipoids. IV. Separation and identification of active principle (vitamin A) of cod-liver oil. *J. Chem. Soc. (Japan) 43*:826.

Thommen, H. 1961. Research on the metabolism of β-apo-8′-carotenal [in French]. *Chimia 15*:433.

Thommen, H. 1967. Detection and identification of naturally occurring ketocarotenoids and carotenals [in German]. *Int. Z. Vitaminforsch. 37*:175.

15

METABOLISM OF RETINOL AND RETINOIC ACID

A. B. Roberts and H. F. DeLuca

Introduction

In recent years we have come to understand well the basic metabolic processes that are involved in the absorption, transport, and storage of vitamin A. We also understand the reactions of the vitamin in the visual cycle, as well as the oxidation-reduction reactions involved in the interconversion of the three principal forms of the vitamin—retinol, retinal, and retinoic acid. Despite the wealth of literature on these subjects, which has been recently reviewed by Olson (1968), the functions of vitamin A in growth and in reproduction remain unclear. Furthermore, it is not known whether the vitamin functions directly to produce certain responses or whether it must first be converted to an active species.

Since retinoic acid can support the growth of vitamin A–deficient rats (Arens and von Dorp, 1946) yet cannot be converted to either retinol or retinal (Sharman, 1949; Dowling and Wald, 1960; Futterman, 1962), it has been tempting to suppose that there might exist an "active" metabolite common to both retinol and retinoic acid. Such a compound would necessarily be formed by oxidative metabolism of retinol. There have been many and long searches for such a compound (Wolf and Johnson, 1960; Rogers et al., 1963; Yagishita et al., 1964; Zile and DeLuca, 1965; Sundaresan, 1966), but these have been hampered by two problems. First, under physiological conditions the utilization of retinol is tightly regulated and the amount of any circulating "active form" is probably minute (Roberts and DeLuca, 1967; Emerick et al., 1967). On the other hand, retinoic acid is metabolized so rapidly (Roberts and DeLuca, 1967; Zachman et al., 1966) that it is difficult to decide on an "active form" among its metabolic products. Secondly, attempts to isolate such a metabolite are further complicated by the ease of oxidation and other chemical alterations which occur during purification. To date, two metabolites of retinoic acid have been positively identified. Zile and co-workers (1967) have characterized 13-*cis* retinoic acid or its ester as a product of retinoic acid metabolism in the rat; and Olson and co-workers (Dunagin et al., 1965, 1966) have identified retinoyl-β-glucuronide as a major component of the bile metabolites of retinoic acid. It is unlikely that either of these, though both are biologically active (Zile and DeLuca, 1968), is the sought-after metabolite.

In vivo metabolism of retinol and retinoic acid

We have taken a more general approach and have investigated the over-all degradative metabolism of both retinol and retinoic acid in the rat (Roberts and DeLuca, 1967). It was thought that any similarities in their metabolism would be indirect evidence for their participation in common enzymatic pathways. The study was made possible by a generous gift from Hoffman-LaRoche Laboratories of both retinol and retinoic acid labeled in either the 15-^{14}C or 6,7-^{14}C positions and by the acquisition of 14-^{14}C retinoic acid from Tracerlab, Inc. By intravenously injecting physiological amounts (15 μg) of these radioactive compounds and measuring the radioactivity that subsequently appeared in the urine, feces, and expired carbon dioxide, we were able to make rough deductions about the over-all metabolism of retinol and retinoic acid and to compare them. The data from such experiments with retinoic acid are shown in Table 15.1. The important conclusions are that the degradation of the isoprenoid side chain to CO_2 is most extensive at the terminal 15-C, less at the 14-C, and stops before reaching the 6,7-C position on the β-ionone ring. On the other

TABLE 15.1. *Recovery of ^{14}C from rats given radioactive retinoic acid*

	Recovery of ^{14}C (% of dose)			
Retinoic acid	CO_2	Urine	Feces	Total
6,7-^{14}C	0.8 ± 0.4 (2)	38.0 ± 4.4 (4)	64.5 ± 1.3 (4)	103.3
14-^{14}C	18.9 ± 3.4 (3)	18.3 ± 0.3 (3)	61[a] (3)	98.2
15-^{14}C	35.0 ± 4.5 (2)	19.9 ± 1.7 (5)	43.7 ± 3.0 (4)	98.6

Notes: Male stock rats (250–300 g) received an intrajugular injection of 14.5 μg radioactive retinoic acid and were immediately placed in a glass metabolism cage for collection of urine, CO_2, and feces. Urine and CO_2 were collected for 48 hr, feces for 4 days.

Values are given as mean ± SD. Numbers in parentheses are the number of rats.

[a] The values obtained were all low, owing to bacterial decomposition of the radioactive products in the feces. Nevertheless, a plot of the three values obtained as a function of the time lapse (from the completion of the experiment to the time of combustion of the samples) was linear and extrapolated to a value of 61% recovery of the dose at zero time.

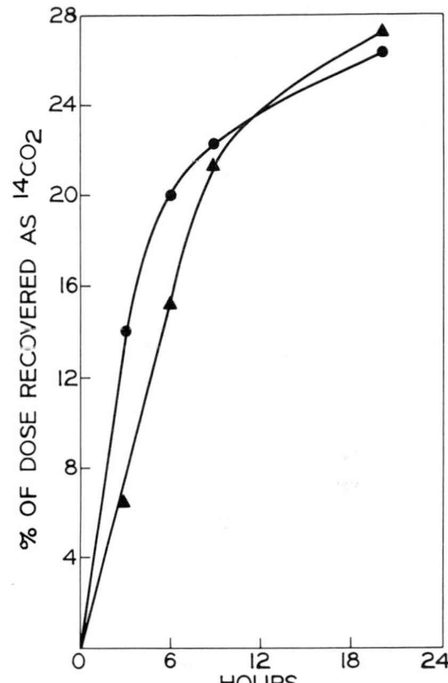

Fig. 15.1. Rate of $^{14}CO_2$ evolution from rats receiving either 15 μg (●) or 1.5 mg (▲) of 15-^{14}C retinoic acid. Doses were injected into the jugular vein and contained approximately the same amount of radioactivity.

hand, a larger proportion of the β-ionone ring (6,7-C) than of the side chain (14-C and 15-C) is excreted into the urine. The recovery of the radioactivity from ^{14}C retinoic acid was nearly complete 48 hr after injection of the dose, supporting the evidence that the acid cannot be stored in the rat.

To eliminate the possibility that side-chain oxidation resulted from non-enzymatic destruction of the small amount of retinoic acid, larger doses (1.5 mg) were injected (Fig. 15.1). Apart from a change in rate, there was no significant difference in the percentage of the dose metabolized to $^{14}CO_2$. This result is similar to that of Zachman et al. (1966), in which the percentage of the retinoic acid excreted as bile metabolites was unchanged over a 100-fold dose range. We were further able to show that the side-chain oxidation was unlikely to occur in the intestine, as oral administration of 15-^{14}C retinoic acid resulted in an excretion pattern not unlike that of an intravenous dose (Table 15.2). Finally, it could be shown that the decarboxylation of retinoic acid is distinct from its conjugation as bile metabolites, since the production of $^{14}CO_2$ from 15-^{14}C retinoic acid is not significantly different in either normal or bile-duct-cannulated rats (Fig. 15.2).

Table 15.2. *Distribution of radioactivity according to method of administration of the dose*

Method of dose administration	Recovery of ^{14}C (% of dose)			
	CO_2	Urine	Feces	Total
Oral	26.1 (1)	9.9 (1)	64.4 (1)	100.4
Intravenous	29.9 ± 1.4 (3)	12.2 ± 0.7 (6)	58.1 ± 4.0 (3)	100.2

Notes: Male stock rats (250–300 g) received 10–14 μg of 15-^{14}C retinoic acid in a 0.9% saline, 0.2% Tween 80 (polyoxyethylene sorbitan monooleate), 10% ethanol solution, either orally or injected into the jugular vein. Urine and CO_2 were collected for 48 hours, feces for 4 days.

Values are given as mean ± SD. Numbers in parentheses are the number of rats.

Interestingly, it could be shown that radioactive retinyl acetate is metabolized and excreted much the same as retinoic acid (Table 15.3) . Again, the side chain is oxidized to carbon dioxide, while the β-ionone ring portion of the molecule is excreted entirely through the urine and feces. In striking contrast to the metabolism of retinoic acid is that of retinyl acetate — a slow, controlled metabolism which continued at a nearly constant rate for 6–7 days (Roberts and DeLuca, 1967). Injection of smaller

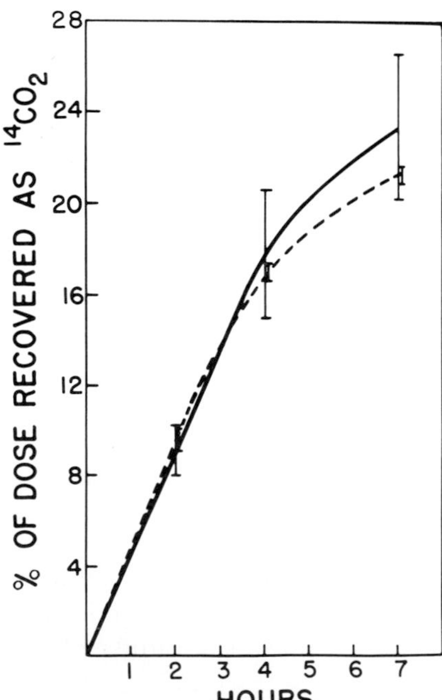

Fig. 15.2. Rate of $^{14}CO_2$ evolution in 4 bile-duct-cannulated rats (solid line) after the intrajugular injection of 10–15 μg of 15-^{14}C retinoic acid, as compared with that in 8 control rats (dashed line). The standard error of the mean is indicated for each point.

TABLE 15.3. *Recovery of ^{14}C from rats given radioactive retinyl acetate*

Retinyl acetate compound and dose	Recovery of ^{14}C			
	CO_2	Urine	Feces	Total
6,7-^{14}C (2.0 μg)				
% of dose	2.5 (2)	26.8 ± 2.8 (4)	26.3 ± 5.0 (4)	55.6
% of ^{14}C recovered[a]	4.5	48.2	47.3	100
15-^{14}C (2.0 μg)				
% of dose	15 (2)	15.0 ± 2.0 (2)	18.9 ± 2.6 (2)	48.9
% of ^{14}C recovered[a]	30.6	30.6	38.6	100
15-^{14}C (1.5 μg)				
% of dose	8.8 (2)	8.3 ± 0.8 (2)	10.3 ± 2.5 (2)	27.4
% of ^{14}C recovered[a]	32.1	30.3	37.6	100

Note: The values for urine and carbon dioxide represent the radioactivity recovered after 4 days. The values for the feces are based on collection after 5 days to allow for the time lag in elimination.

Values are given as mean ± SD. Numbers in parentheses are the number of rats.

[a] Recalculated as the percentage of the total amount of radioactivity recovered in 4 days.

doses of retinyl acetate resulted in a smaller percentage metabolized per day, thus indicating a rigorous conservation mechanism in the deficient rat. In order to facilitate comparison of the data for retinyl acetate with that for retinoic acid, we calculated the partitioning of only that portion of ^{14}C recovered after 4 days and thus eliminated any contribution from the stored vitamin.

Complete analysis of the data obtained for both retinoic acid and retinyl acetate suggests that at least three major pathways of metabolism can be described (Fig. 15.3). The basic assumption involved in arriving at this scheme is that the radioactivity that appears in the feces or urine from 15-^{14}C retinoic acid is part of an intact vitamin A skeleton. This is reasonable, since it has been demonstrated that the bile metabolites of retinoic acid and retinol—which account largely for the fecal and urinary excretion in an intact rat—contain a glucuronic acid conjugate of the intact

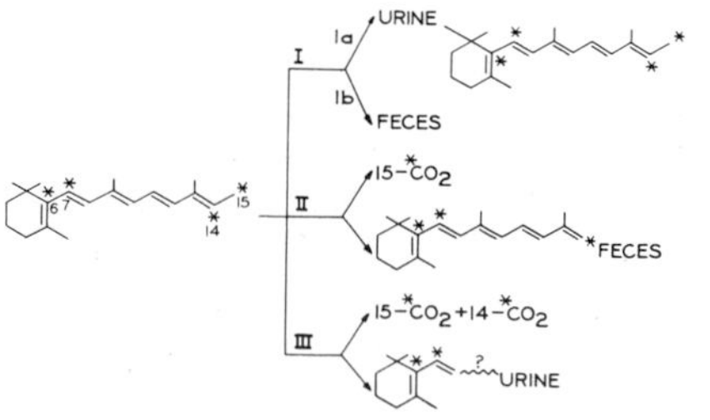

Fig. 15.3. Proposed pathways for the metabolism of retinoic acid or retinyl acetate in the rat. (Roberts and DeLuca, 1967. Reproduced by permission of the *Biochemical Journal.*)

molecule (Lippel and Olson, 1968). Pathways II and III are oxidative, and later evidence will indicate that they probably operate sequentially, with the 15-C being removed prior to oxidation of the 14-C.

The approximate partitioning of retinoic acid and retinyl acetate into these three pathways is shown in Table 15.4. That retinyl acetate metabolism contains contributions from the oxidative pathways II and III suggests that the terminal hydroxyl group might be oxidized and then decarboxylated, and therefore that retinoic acid or a similar compound could be an intermediate in retinol metabolism. Supporting this, Emerick and Zile (1967) in our laboratory have identified small amounts of retinoic acid formed by administration of physiological doses of retinol. Since the greater portion of the bile metabolites of retinol (pathway I) are distinct from those of retinoic acid, it would appear that not all of the retinol metabolized (and therefore excreted) has first been oxidized, but possibly only that portion described by pathways II and III. This leads to the suggestion that retinol is the storage form of the vitamin and that its release, which is under tight metabolic control, results in the formation of minute amounts of a more oxidized, rapidly metabolized form of the vitamin.

TABLE 15.4. *Postulated pathways for metabolism of low doses of retinoic acid and retinyl acetate*

Pathway	Retinoic acid (% of dose)	Retinyl acetate (% of dose)
I	62–65	67–69
Ia [a]	18–20	30–32
Ib [a]	43–45	36–38
II	18–20	9–12
III	18–20	17–19

[a] Pathways Ia and Ib are subdivisions of pathway I and represent the distribution of the proposed intact side chain into the urinary and fecal products, respectively.

Oxidative decarboxylation of ${}^{14}C$ and ${}^{15}C$ of retinoic acid in vitro

KIDNEY AND LIVER SLICES

Since evidence indicates the functioning of oxidative pathways in vivo, it was of obvious interest to determine whether these reactions could be studied in vitro. The progress of such reactions could easily be measured by the trapping and counting of ${}^{14}CO_2$ released from either 15-${}^{14}C$ retinoic acid or 14-${}^{14}C$ retinoic acid during the incubation. The oxidations were first studied in tissue slices of rat liver and kidney (Roberts and DeLuca, 1968*a*). As was found to be the case for the in vivo metabolism, no difference was observed whether the tissues were taken from vitamin A–deficient rats, stock rats, or deficient rats that had been fed retinoic acid. Liver and kidney were the most convenient tissues for study, and decarboxylation of retinoic acid was found to occur at a linear rate for 1–2 hr when a solution of Krebs-Ringer bicarbonate buffer, *p*H 7.4, with a 95% O_2, 5% CO_2 atmosphere was used. The rate of decarboxylation is proportional both to the amount of tissue and to the retinoic acid concentration. Oxidation of the 14-C to CO_2 can also be carried out in this system, though it occurs to a much smaller extent. As indicated in Table 15.5, the response to

TABLE 15.5. *Effect of inhibitors on the production of* CO_2 *from retinoic acid by tissue slices*

	Percentage of ^{14}C recovered as $^{14}CO_2$			
Retinoic acid	No inhibitor	Malonate (2×10^{-2} M)	Fluoroacetate (1×10^{-3} M)	DPPD (2×10^{-7} M)
14-^{14}C				
Kidney	4.1	1.0	0.8	0.3
Liver	1.6	0.6	1.1	0
15-^{14}C				
Kidney	20.9	27.6	20.5	0.5
Liver	17.9	20.1	19.2	0.8

Note: Each flask contained Krebs-Ringer bicarbonate buffer, 0.1 ml of either inhibitor solution or saline, and 100 mg of tissue slices from a stock rat. The incubation was carried out for 2 hr at 30 C in a 95% O_2, 5% CO_2 atmosphere. The concentration of retinoic acid was 3 μM.

inhibitors is very different between the decarboxylation of retinoic acid and the oxidation of the 14-C. Inhibitors of the Krebs cycle, malonate and fluoroacetate, are without effect on the decarboxylation but strongly inhibit the production of CO_2 from the 14-C. On the other hand, DPPD (*N,N′*-diphenyl-*p*-phenylene diamine), an inhibitor of free-radical reactions, completely blocks both reactions even though it has no influence on the metabolism of succinate under identical reaction conditions. This suggests that the decarboxylation might be initiated by a free-radical mechanism prior to oxidation of the 14-C through the Krebs cycle. Support for this idea was obtained by a study of the two reactions; it was found that the rate of decarboxylation is initially very rapid, whereas the oxidation of 14-C to CO_2 does not achieve its maximum rate until one hour after the start of the incubation (Fig. 15.4). This is more evident when the rate of CO_2 production in each 20-min period is plotted against incubation time (Fig. 15.5).

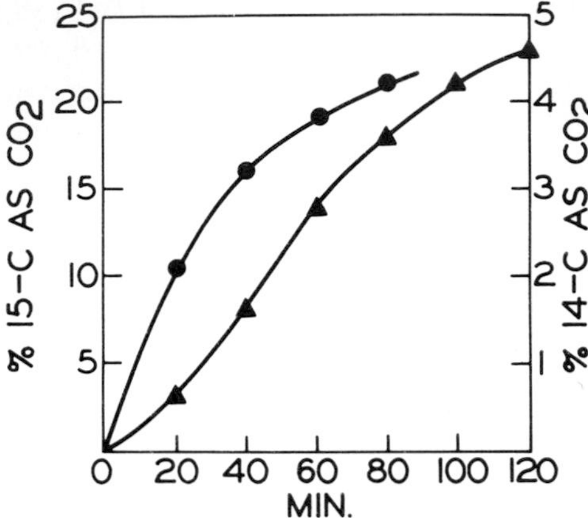

Fig. 15.4. Rate of $^{14}CO_2$ production in kidney slices from 15-^{14}C retinoic acid (●) and 14-^{14}C retinoic acid (▲).

All this evidence is summarized in a possible reaction scheme in Figure 15.6. Decarboxylation could occur by some free-radical mechanism resulting in oxidation of the 14-C. Some of the decarboxylation might result in the formation of a product which can undergo no further reaction, but possibly another product could then form an acyl-CoA derivative. By the mechanism of mitochondrial β-oxidation of branched methyl compounds (Pattison and Buchanan, 1964), this could lead to the production of a molecule of propionyl-CoA, which upon carboxylation and rearrangement to succinyl-CoA could then be catabolized by the Krebs cycle, in agreement with the experimental observations.

Although all these experiments were carried out with liver and kidney slices, decarboxylation also takes place in tissue slices of brain, skin, bone, and spleen, but not in tissue slices of intestine, lung, heart, diaphragm, or adrenals (Table 15.6) (Roberts and DeLuca, 1969). The re-

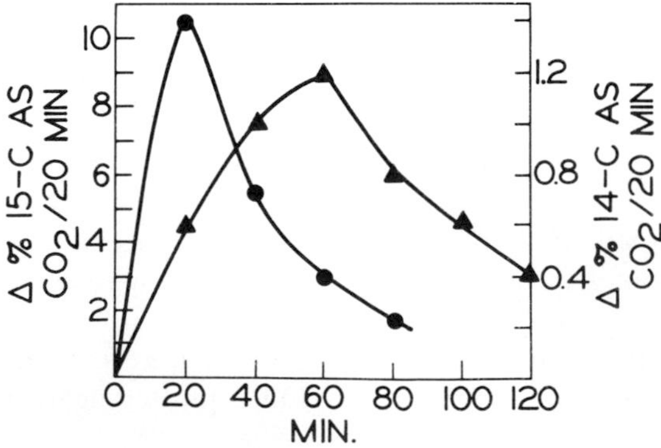

Fig. 15.5. Rate of production of $^{14}CO_2$ in a 20-min period as a function of incubation time. 15-^{14}C retinoic acid (●) and 14-^{14}C retinoic acid (▲) were used.

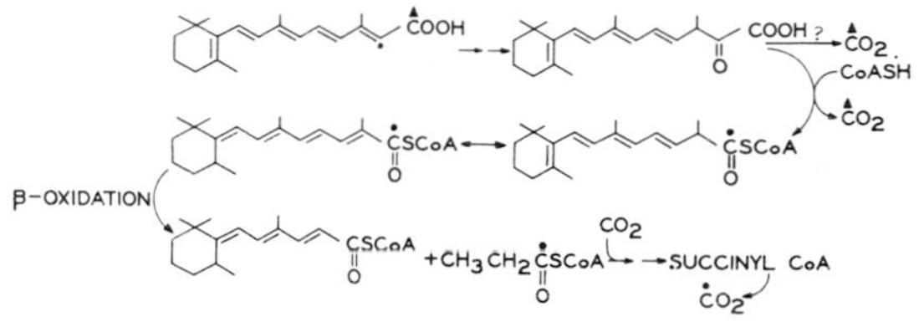

Fig. 15.6. Suggested pathway for the production in tissue slices of 15-CO_2 and 14-CO_2 from retinoic acid.

actions in each of these tissues could be inhibited with DPPD, indicating a mechanistic similarity.

LIVER AND KIDNEY MICROSOMES

The decarboxylation of retinoic acid was next studied in a microsomal enzyme system from rat kidney or rat liver (Roberts and DeLuca, 1968*b*). It is seen in Table 15.7 that the system requires Fe^{2+}, NADPH, a pyrophospate group, and O_2 for decarboxylation to occur to the maximum extent. For the requirement for pyrophosphate, PP_i is most active, but more complex pyrophosphates such as thiamine pyrophosphate or ATP can be substituted. Under no conditions does this system release any $^{14}CO_2$ from 14-^{14}C retinoic acid or 6,7-^{14}C retinoic acid. The microsomal reaction,

TABLE 15.6. *Decarboxylation activity of various tissues in vitro and the effect of DPPD*

Tissue	Decarboxylation activity[a]	+ DPPD[b] (% of control)
Liver	++	4.7
Kidney	++	2.3
Brain	+++	3.1
Bone	+	0
Skin	+	2.3
Spleen	+	—
Intestine	+—	n.a.
Heart	+—	n.a.
Adrenals	+—	n.a.
Lung	+—	n.a.
Diaphragm	+—	n.a.

Note: The preparation and incubation of the tissue slices was as described by Roberts and DeLuca (1969).

[a] Activity was judged in comparison with values for approximately equal amounts of liver or kidney (++: 26% decarboxylation in 2 hr). Greater activity than that of the liver or kidney (on a weight basis) has been designated +++, lesser activity as +. No significant decarboxylation was catalyzed by tissues designated +—.

[b] DPPD was added to the flask in 5 μl ethanol to a final concentration of 2×10^{-7} M.

TABLE 15.7. *Components essential for the decarboxylation of retinoic acid in liver microsomes*

Medium	Percentage of control initial velocity
All components	100
Less Fe^{2+}	50
Less NADPH	10
Less PP_i	55
Less Fe^{2+}, PP_i	27
Less NADPH, Fe^{2+}, PP_i	10
Less microsomes	10
Less O_2[a]	37

Note: Reaction mixture contained 50 mM KCL, 5 mM $MgCl_2$, 5 mM phosphate buffer (*p*H 7.3), 88 μM NADP, glucose-6-phosphate dehydrogenase, 1mM glucose-6-phosphate, 0.3 mM pyrophosphate (PP_i), 10 μM $FeSO_4$, and liver microsomes. The concentration of 15-^{14}C retinoic acid was 3.3 μM. Results were based on a 2-min incubation at 30 C.

[a] The reaction was carried out in nitrogen atmosphere.

under the conditions employed, reaches completion in about 4 min, at which time approximately 50% of the added retinoic acid has been decarboxylated (Fig. 15.7). Other oxidative reactions not resulting in decarboxylation are undoubtedly occurring in this system, as less than 10% of the original radioactivity can be recovered as retinoic acid after the incubation. The reaction rate is proportional to retinoic acid concentration as well as to microsome concentration. From the use of inhibitors it was possible to make deductions as to the nature of this reaction. Table 15.8 illustrates the response to the key inhibitors. Electron acceptors $K_3Fe(CN)_6$ and phenazine methosulfate are able to block the decarboxylation completely, as is EDTA. Competition for NADPH can be observed with aminopyrine, a drug metabolized by the microsomal hydroxylase enzymes. Most important, however, is the lack of inhibition in the presence of carbon monoxide – a condition under which hydroxylase activity is severely reduced. Equally important is the complete inhibition provided by very low concentrations of DPPD, which, we were able to demonstrate, had no effect on the demethylation of aminopyrine in an identical incubation. Thus, both in its requirements and in its inhibition pattern, the behavior of the decarboxylation is similar to a microsomal peroxidase system (Hochstein et al., 1964) rather than to the drug hydroxylating system (Ernster and Orrenius, 1965). This finding is enforced by the inhibitory

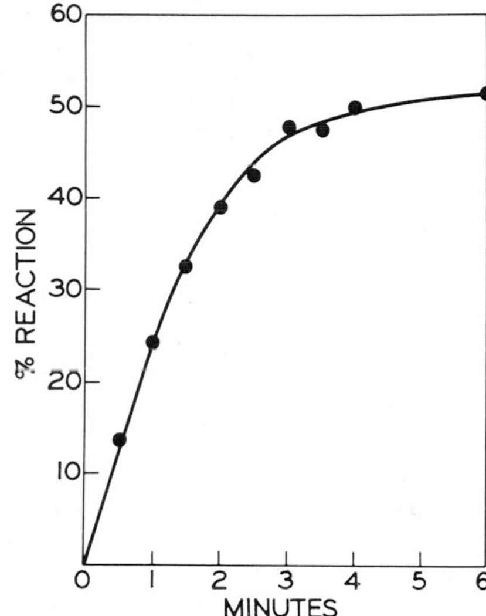

Fig. 15.7. Rate of decarboxylation of 15-^{14}C retinoic acid by a liver microsomal system. (Roberts and DeLuca, 1968*b*. Reproduced by permission of the *Journal of Lipid Research*.)

action of α-tocopherol, Mn^{2+}, and α,α-dipyridyl, all established peroxidase inhibitors.

Although some work regarding the identity of the product of this microsomal decarboxylation has been published (Roberts and DeLuca, 1968*b*), its relation to the actual in vivo metabolites of retinoic acid must be questioned. The most obvious objections are, first, that the possibilities for over-oxidation in such a rapidly peroxidizing system are enormous,

TABLE 15.8. *Inhibitors of microsomal decarboxylation of retinoic acid*

Inhibitor	Concentration (mM)	Percentage of control initial velocity
$K_3Fe(CN)_6$	0.2	0
Phenazine methosulfate	0.02	0
EDTA	0.2	0
Aminopyrine	10	39
Aminopyrine	1	63
CO and O_2 mixture[a]	—	100
DPPD	1.3×10^{-4}	0
α-tocopherol[b]	—	10
Mn^{2+}	1	0
α,α-dipyridyl	1	2

Note: The reaction conditions are described in Table 15.7.

[a] The ratio of CO to O_2 was 2:1.

[b] The α-tocopherol was homogenized (10 mg per 10 ml suspension) with the re-suspended microsomal pellet.

and second, that under no conditions of combined cell fractions and additional cofactors is any $^{14}CO_2$ released from 14-^{14}C retinoic acid when the microsomal system is operative. Although the inhibition by DPPD of the tissue slice decarboxylation indicates that it, too, is initiated by a free-radical attack, the reaction as it occurs in the slice system must be more limited in extent, as it can produce a product capable of further reaction similar to the pattern observed in vivo.

Effect of DPPD on in vivo oxidative decarboxylation of retinoic acid

Having characterized the in vitro decarboxylation, it was desirable to see whether feeding DPPD to a rat could result in a decrease of the in vivo decarboxylation (Roberts and DeLuca, 1969). DPPD is commonly used as a vitamin E substitute and can be administered to a rat with no adverse effects. The DPPD treatment causes a significant but small reduction of the in vivo decarboxylation, as seen in Figure 15.8. In vitro preparations of either tissue slices or microsomes from such a DPPD-treated rat have no decarboxylation activity, indicating that the level of DPPD in the various tissues is sufficient (Table 15.9).

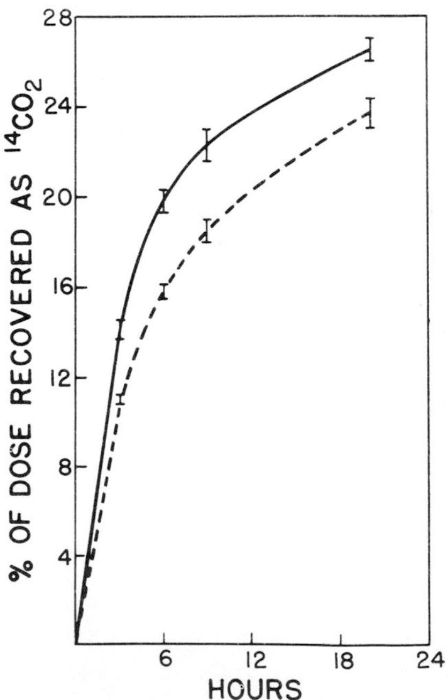

Fig. 15.8. Effect of DPPD on the in vivo decarboxylation of retinoic acid for 5–10 control rats (solid line) and for 5 rats maintained on a 0.01%–0.05% DPPD diet and given an oral dose of 2 mg DPPD in oil 3 hr before the intravenous injection of 10–14 μg of 15-^{14}C retinoic acid (dashed line). The standard error of the mean is indicated for each point.

TABLE 15.9. *Effect of DPPD on the in vitro decarboxylation of retinoic acid*

System	Percentage of control decarboxylation	
	DPPD in vitro[a]	DPPD in vivo[b]
Kidney slices	2.3	4.5
Liver slices	4.7	0
Kidney homogenate[c]	14.8	12.1
Liver microsomes	0	0

Note: Reaction conditions for the tissue slice and microsomal systems have been described in Tables 15.5 and 15.7, respectively. The tissue homogenates were incubated in a medium identical to that for the microsomes, less the NADPH-generating system, Fe^{2+}, and PP_i. All reactions were carried out at 30 C, but the microsomal reactions were stopped after 2–3 min, the homogenate reactions after 15–20 min, and the tissue slice reactions after 1.5–2 hr.

[a] DPPD was added to the flask in 5 μl ethanol to a final concentration of 2×10^{-7} M.

[b] DPPD (1 mg) was injected into the jugular vein of the rat 1–2 hr before it was killed (Roberts and DeLuca, 1969).

[c] The concentration of the homogenate in the reaction flask was 3.5%. Total inhibition could be provided by 1×10^{-5} M of DPPD.

Thus, although unknown factors could be masking a greater effect of DPPD in vivo, we are left to conclude that the in vitro oxidative pathways of retinoic acid metabolism as derived from tissue slice and microsomal systems can account only in part for the mechanism in vivo. It is hoped that the products of these reactions may soon be isolated and identified so that their role in the growth-supporting function of retinoic acid may be assessed. With the identification of these products will also come certainty as to whether the oxidative pathways for retinol and retinoic acid are identical or only similar, as is the case for the bile metabolites. This will also answer the question of whether free retinoic acid is a real intermediate in retinol metabolism or merely a very excellent substitute.

References

Arens, J. F., and D. A. van Dorp. 1946. Synthesis of some compounds possessing vitamin A activity. *Nature 157*:190.

Dowling, J. E., and G. Wald. 1960. The biological function of vitamin A acid. *Proc. Nat. Acad. Sci. U.S.A. 46*:587.

Dunagin, P. E., Jr., E. H. Meadows, Jr., and J. A. Olson. 1965. Retinoyl-beta-glucuronic acid: A major metabolite of vitamin A in rat bile. *Science 148*:86.

Dunagin, P. E., Jr., R. D. Zachman, and J. A. Olson. 1966. The identification of metabolites of retinol and retinoic acid in rat bile. *Biochim. Biophys. Acta 124*:71.

Emerick, R. J., Maija Zile, and H. F. DeLuca. 1967. Formation of retinoic acid from retinol in the rat. *Biochem. J. 102*:606.

Ernster, L., and S. Orrenius. 1965. Substrate-induced synthesis of the hydroxylating enzyme system of liver microsomes. *Fed. Proc. 24*:1190.

Futterman, S. 1962. Enzymatic oxidation of vitamin A aldehyde to vitamin A acid. *J. Biol. Chem. 237*:677.

Hochstein, P., K. Nordenbrand, and L. Ernster. 1964. Evidence for the involvement of iron in the ADP-activated peroxidation of lipids in microsomes and mitochondria. *Biochem. Biophys. Res. Commun. 14*:323.

Lippel, K., and J. A. Olson. 1968. Biosynthesis of beta-glucuronides of retinol and of retinoic acid *in vivo* and *in vitro*. *J. Lipid Res. 9*:168.

Olson, James A. 1968. Some aspects of vitamin A metabolism. *Vitamins Hormones 26*:1.

Pattison, F. L. M., and R. L. Buchanan. 1964. Toxic fluorine compounds: The use of the ω-fluorine atom in the study of the metabolism of branched-chain fatty acids. *Biochem. J. 92*:100.

Roberts, A. B., and H. F. DeLuca. 1967. Pathways of retinol and retinoic acid metabolism in the rat. *Biochem. J. 102*:600.

Roberts, A. B., and H. F. DeLuca. 1968*a*. Decarboxylation of retinoic acid in tissue slices from rat kidney and liver. *Arch. Biochem. Biophys. 123*:279.

Roberts, A. B., and H. F. DeLuca. 1968*b*. Oxidative decarboxylation of retinoic acid in microsomes of rat liver and kidney. *J. Lipid Res. 9*:501.

Roberts, A. B., and H. F. DeLuca. 1969. Effect of DPPD on the decarboxylation of retinoic acid *in vitro* and *in vivo*. *Arch. Biochem. Biophys. 129*:290.

Rogers, W. E., M. C. Chang, and B. C. Johnson. 1963. A biologically active metabolite of vitamin A. *Fed. Proc. 22*:433.

Sharman, I. M. 1949. The biological activity and metabolism of vitamin A acid. *Brit. J. Nutr. 3*:viii.

Sundaresan, P. R. 1966. Vitamin A and the sulphate-activating enzymes. *Biochim. Biophys. Acta 113*:95.

Wolf, G., and B. C. Johnson. 1960. Metabolic transformation of vitamin A. *Vitamins Hormones 18*:403.

Yagishita, K., P. R. Sundaresan, and G. Wolf. 1964. A biologically active metabolite of vitamin A and vitamin A acid. *Nature 203*:410.

Zachman, R. D., P. E. Dunagin, and J. A. Olson. 1966. Formation and enterohepatic circulation of metabolites of retinol and retinoic acid in bile duct-cannulated rats. *J. Lipid Res. 7*:3.

Zile, Maija, and H. F. DeLuca. 1965. A biologically active metabolite of retinoic acid from rat liver. *Biochem. J. 97*:180.

Zile, Maija, and H. F. DeLuca. 1968. Retinoic acid: Some aspects of growth-promoting activity in the albino rat. *J. Nutr. 94*:302.

Zile, Maija, R. J. Emerick, and H. F. DeLuca. 1967. Identification of 13-cis retinoic acid in tissue extracts and its biological activity in rats. *Biochim Biophys. Acta 141*:639.

16

VITAMIN A DEFICIENCY IN THE GERM-FREE STATE

W. E. Rogers, Jr., J. G. Bieri, and E. G. McDaniel

Introduction

The tide of research on the role of vitamin A in nonvisual processes has flowed and ebbed and now seems to be flowing once again. The first wave, peaking in the early sixties, was characterized by experiments designed to test the premise that vitamin A, like the B vitamins, may act as a coenzyme (Johnson and Wolf, 1960). This approach was based on the theory that in the absence of a coenzyme, metabolic paths in vivo will be blocked at specific sites, and that certain enzymes in vitro will be found to be either less active or in decreased amounts in the subcellular fractions where they are normally found. These theories were tested and led to the identification of certain enzymes whose activity seemed related to the amount of vitamin A present in the animal. Some of these enzymes are involved in sulfate activation, steroid synthesis, cholesterol and ubiquinone formation, ascorbic acid synthesis, and drug detoxification. The efforts of several investigators provided data that seemed to corroborate the predictions that this vitamin functioned as a coenzyme, but subsequently a sequence of observations was made that began to weaken this hypothesis.

Scientists, in repeating certain of these experiments, found that they could not obtain distinct differences in enzyme activity that could be clearly attributed to the level of vitamin A in the organism. From many of these experiments, there developed an increased appreciation of several complications inherent in work on vitamin A–deficient animals. There is evidence that vitamin A has membrane-active properties which may be responsible for many of its effects on animals, and these must be considered when designing experiments and interpreting results. Also, there is a potential problem in that rates of reaction may not be linear when the specific activity of enzyme fractions are compared in normal and vitamin A–deficient tissue. A final major concern is the preparation of control animals which will adequately compensate for the profound differences in the physiological state of vitamin A–deficient animals. A distinction must be made between those effects which are the secondary, rather than the primary, results of deficiency.

After depressed enzyme activity was first observed, attempts were made to isolate a coenzyme form of vitamin A, but progress has been slow. Furthermore, the correlation of vitamin A activity to enzyme activity during purification has not been completely suggestive of a classical coenzyme function. Thus, as the first tide of research expressing the coenzyme concept has ebbed, scientists have turned to examine alternative hypotheses of vitamin A action that might provide a more profitable basis for further experiments.

Now the tide of vitamin A research seems to be welling again. Regardless of whether one's enthusiasm is directed toward exploring new coenzyme functions, the role of vitamin A as an inducer, or its effect on membranes, or other mechanisms, a requirement for clear results will be an experimental animal in which vitamin A deficiency can be studied without concomitant inanition and infection. For several years we have compensated for inanition through the use of various types of tube-fed and pair-fed controls. In the last year and a half, however, we have become increasingly interested in the use of germ-free animals for investigations on the primary lesion in vitamin A deficiency. Our work is pointed toward development of an animal suitable for detection of phenomena induced by vitamin A, and this report describes our progress toward that goal.

Vitamin A deficiency in germ-free rats

ADULT RATS

Beaver (1961) first reported on the pathology and survival of vitamin A–deficient rats in the germ-free state. Though much valuable data was presented, there were several key bits of information, such as growth curves, that were missing. This omission, together with observations such as the relatively constant food consumption in germ-free vitamin A–deficient rats, stimulated our initial investigations (Bieri et al., 1969).

Germ-free rats at weaning were fed an autoclaved vitamin A–deficient diet R–9 (st.) (Table 16.1). Some rats served as conventionalized controls and were transferred from the isolator to cages in the regular animal room where they were fed the same autoclaved diet. In both the germ-free and conventionalized groups, some animals were given this diet supplemented with stabilized vitamin A (6 mg/kg diet). This level was used in all experiments.

In the first experiment, the rats were of two litters from dams fed deficient diet after parturition. The 3 male conventionalized rats on the

TABLE 16.1. *Vitamin A–deficient rat diet for autoclave sterilization (R–9 (st.))*

Ingredient	Percentage
Casein, vitamin free	22.0
Vitamin mixture [a]	6.0
Fox and Briggs salt mixture	6.0
Corn oil plus antioxidant [b]	4.0
Corn starch	58.0
Cellulose	4.0

[a] At three times customary level.
[b] *dl* α tocopherol acetate.

deficient diet stopped growing in five weeks, lost weight rather quickly, and died by the seventh week post-weaning (Fig. 16.1). These animals exhibited the usual signs of vitamin A deficiency such as periorbital encrustation with porphyrin pigment, xerophthalmia, and diarrhea, but not ataxia or incoordination. In contrast, the 4 male germ-free rats on a deficient diet did not stop growing until the ninth or tenth week, at which time they exhibited a mild head wobble, weakness in their hind legs, and

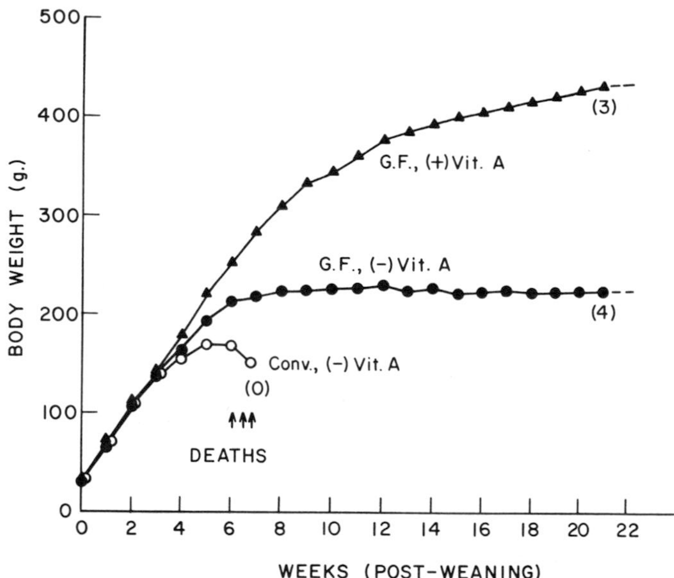

Fig. 16.1. Growth and survival of 4 germ-free vitamin A–deficient male rats. Controls were 3 conventionalized vitamin A–deficient male rats (bottom curve) and 3 germ-free vitamin A–supplemented male rats (top curve). The basic diet for all rats was R–9 (st.). Numbers in parentheses indicate the surviving rats.

difficulty in coordination, most evident when they attempted to right themselves after being placed on their backs. The deficient rats maintained a relatively constant body weight for long periods, in contrast to the vitamin A–supplemented controls, which grew at a normal rate, with the 3 males reaching about 440 g in 22 weeks. Though manifestations of the nerve disorder did not intensify, depilitation around the eyes and depigmentation of the incisor teeth increased. Feces became somewhat fluid. Alopecia did not develop but the hair coat was thin, silky, and loose. Testes were extremely atrophic, and the death of deficient rats was preceded by sharp weight loss. Autopsy revealed that approximately half of the deaths seemed to have been caused by urinary bladder stones or strangulation of the intestines caused by twisting of the cecum; in the other cases the cause of death was not apparent. The histological examination of tissues from these animals is still incomplete but results so far generally confirm those of Beaver (1961).

After the rats had been on the deficient diet for 22 weeks (including about 15 weeks during which the weight levels were stabilized), several trials were carried out to establish whether growth potential was intact. When retinoic acid (6 mg/kg) was added to the diet of two rats, one rat did not gain significantly (Fig. 16.2), but subsequently gained about 50 g in four weeks when retinyl palmitate was introduced. The second rat displayed a marked growth response to retinoic acid. In three separate tests with this rat, growth commenced within three days of the addition of retinoic acid to the diet and ceased promptly upon its removal.

Since the control vitamin A–supplemented rats and the deficient rats were housed in the same isolator, it was possible that the prolonged maintenance of life in the deficient animals might be explained by their consumption of traces of the control diet somehow transferred within the isolator. In order to test this possible explanation, a new experiment was conducted with the deficient rats and the normal controls housed in separate isolators. In this arrangement, the deficient rats still maintained their body weight for as long as seven months, and their physical condition was not different from that of the deficient rats in the first experiment.

SURVIVAL OF RATS ON AMINO ACID DIETS

The next experiments were designed to eliminate the possibility that there might be hidden sources of vitamin A in the R–9 (st.) diet. All three major components of this diet (protein, carbohydrate, and lipid) conceivably could carry traces of vitamin A, but attention was given first to casein. Initial experiments were carried out with a mixture of 4% casein and 18% L-amino acids substituted for the 22% casein of R–9 (st.). This diet autoclaved successfully. It was fed to germ-free rats that had been on

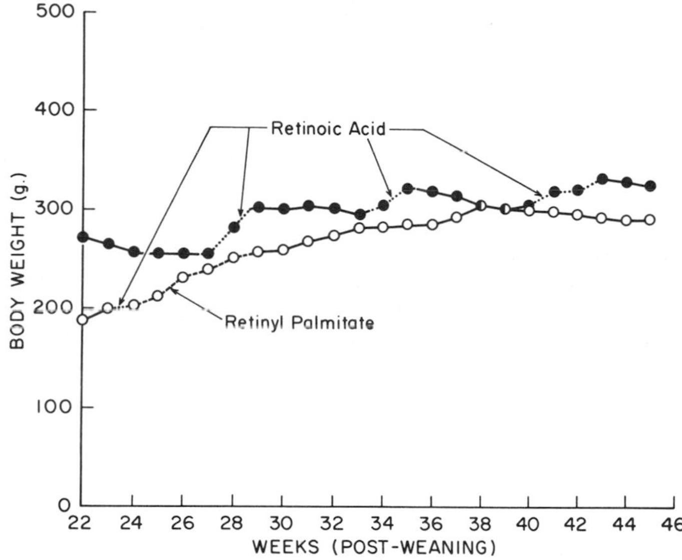

Fig. 16.2. Growth response of 2 germ-free male rats after 22 weeks on a vitamin A–deficient diet (see Fig. 16.1), upon re-alimentation with vitamin A (either retinoic acid or retinyl palmitate).

R–9 (st.) for a long period to eliminate stored vitamin A. Some of the rats maintained body weight for several weeks on the substituted diet, but others did not. It was thought that the latter result might be due to poor adaptation to the new diet because of the weakened condition of these rats after 17 weeks on a deficient diet.

To examine more thoroughly the possibility of trace amounts of vitamin A in diet R–9 (st.), life maintenance was investigated with a more purified diet, R–16, to which rats were transferred at an earlier age. In diet R–16 (Table 16.2), casein is replaced by a mixture of L-amino acids, corn starch is replaced by sucrose, and corn oil is replaced by a mixture of coconut oil and stripped corn oil. This diet, with or without vitamin A, was sealed in polyethylene bags, sterilized by γ-irradiation, and introduced into the isolator with peracetic acid. Weanling rats of two litters from dams that had been on the R–9 (st.) diet since conception were conventionalized or kept germ-free and maintained on R–9 (st.) for two and a half weeks, which allowed them to deplete the small stores of vitamin A they had accumulated from the dam. At the end of this period, all of the conventionalized and half of the germ-free rats were transferred to the amino acid diet.

By the eighth week after weaning, all of the conventionalized rats had

TABLE 16.2. *Vitamin A–deficient rat diet for sterilization by irradiation (R–16)*

Ingredient	Percentage
L-amino acid mixture	19.1
L-asparagine	0.6
L-arginine•HCl	1.3
Vitamin mixture [a]	6.0
Fox and Briggs salt mixture	4.0
Hydrogenated coconut oil	6.0
Stripped corn oil plus antioxidants [b]	4.0
Sodium acetate	1.3
Cellulose	4.0
Sucrose	53.7

[a] At three times customary level.

[b] *dl*-α-tocopherol, *dl*-α-tocopheryl acetate, and ethoxyquin.

died (Fig. 16.3). Conversely, each of the four rats on R–16 had grown to approximately 190 g in five weeks. Three of these gradually lost an average of 45 g over the next ten weeks (12½ weeks on R–16), at which point the experiment was stopped. The fourth rat died after 6½ weeks. A male germ-free control receiving this diet with stabilized retinyl acetate, but in a separate isolator, gained 3–4 g daily and appeared normal in all respects. Deficient rats fed the casein-starch diet (R–9 (st.)) grew for a significantly longer period than did the rats fed the amino acid diet (R–16).

YOUNG RATS

It was of interest to establish whether growth would stop in juvenile rats if vitamin A deficiency could be invoked very early in life. In order to prepare young rats with extremely low body reserves of retinyl esters, advantage was taken of the observations by Thompson and associates (1963–64) that female rats depleted of retinyl esters and maintained on retinoic acid conceive normally. Pregnancy continues normally and live young are born if the dam is provided with traces of retinyl ester, in addition to the supplement of retinoic acid, during the last half of pregnancy. We have found that young rats prepared in this way survive if they are given vitamin A (Rogers, 1967). This indicates that the vitamin A stores of the newborn are small and that the retinoic acid in the milk of the dams is inadequate, at least in a conventional environment, for rats treated in this way. If the nurselings are not supplied with vitamin A, they usually die during the first week of life with few pathologic signs other than a swollen abdomen; however, if they survive into the second week they frequently develop an unusual crippling of the forelimbs before dying (Rogers and Bieri, 1969).

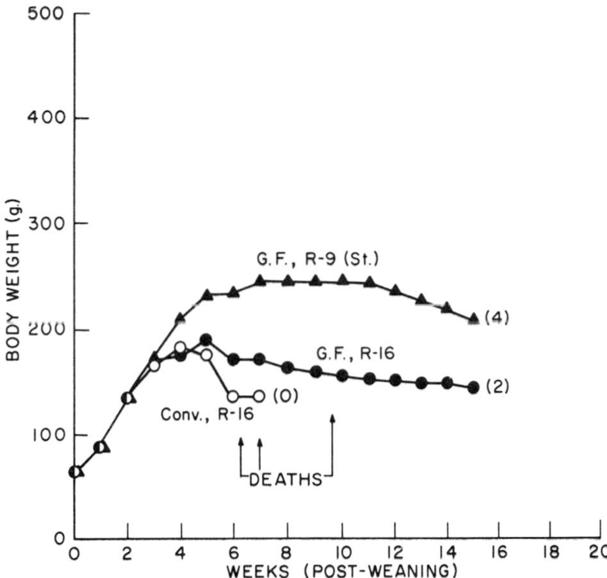

Fig. 16.3. Growth and survival of 3 germ-free vitamin A–deficient male rats on diet R–16. Controls were 2 conventionalized vitamin A–deficient male rats on R–16 (bottom curve) and 4 germ-free vitamin A–deficient male rats on R–9 (st.) (top curve). For the first 2½ weeks, all rats were on the R–9 (st.) diet. Numbers in parentheses indicate the surviving rats.

In order to see if growth in juvenile rats would be blocked by vitamin A deficiency, we prepared young rats by the procedures above, but under germ-free conditions. Germ-free female rats were fed the casein–cornstarch–corn oil diet until a vitamin A deficiency was established (as evidenced by cessation of growth), and then transferred to this diet supplemented with retinoic acid. They were bred with normal males and, from the ninth to the twentieth day of pregnancy, were given 1 μg retinyl acetate per day in addition to the retinoic acid in the diet. Commencing on the sixth day of life the baby rats were given either (a) 5 μg retinoic acid each day throughout the experiment, (b) 5 μg retinoic acid each day until weaned, or (c) the vehicle (corn oil) alone. From the twelfth day after parturition the dam was given her daily supplement of retinoic acid *per os* in order to prevent the young rats from obtaining retinoic acid from her diet.

In these experiments litters of rats were not removed from the isolator to serve as conventionalized controls, since the number of litters was lim-

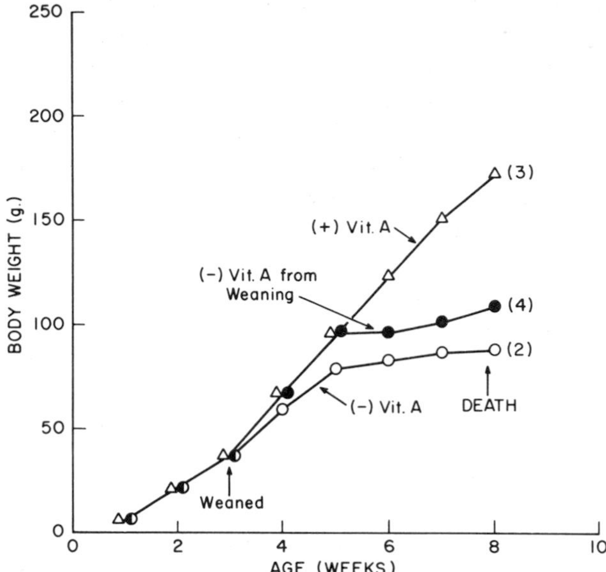

Fig. 16.4. Growth and survival of germ-free vitamin A–deficient rats from one litter from a dam that was depleted of vitamin A stores prior to breeding and then maintained with retinoic acid. From the sixth day of life, 4 of the offspring were given retinoic acid daily only until weaning and then the vehicle (middle curve); and 3 were given the vehicle only (bottom curve). Controls were 3 rats of the same litter given retinoic acid daily (top curve). Numbers in parentheses indicate the surviving animals. Results for the other three litters in the experiment were closely similar.

ited and similar experiments had been done previously with young rats from conventional dams (Rogers and Bieri, 1969). As shown in Figure 16.4, the rats supplemented with retinoic acid until weaning gained very little more than those given only the vehicle. Average weights of rats in these groups were 40 g and 37 g, respectively, in three litters, and 37 g and 36 g in the fourth litter. However, after weaning the difference in growth became marked.

Prior to weaning there was one instance of transient, mild wrist flexure among 14 vitamin A–deficient rats. However, weakness in the front legs appeared universally about the thirty-first day of life in the groups never given retinoic acid, and about two days later in the groups given retinoic acid until they were weaned. For about a week in the former groups and more slowly in the latter groups, forelimb weakness increased until the rats were hardly able to use these legs for support. The front legs occasionally dragged backwards from the shoulder, but more frequently were extended forwards with elbows and wrists on the cage floor (Fig. 16.5). Difficulty in climbing at this time required that food and water cups be placed on the floor of the cages. Outside of the specific crippling of the forelegs, the physical condition of these young rats resembled that of older deficient rats. On the fifty-sixth day of life the average weights of the rats were as follows: in groups given retinoic acid continuously, 170–200 g; in groups given the supplement until weaning, 99–125 g; and in unsupplemented groups, 85–90 g. At the time of writing, some of these rats have been without vitamin A supplementation for over 12 weeks.

Response of vitamin A deficient rats to hormones

A simple explanation for the diminished growth caused by vitamin A deficiency is that an endocrine gland is not producing sufficient hormone or, conversely, that production of hormones is intact, but a target tissue has become unresponsive. Through the administration of suspected hor-

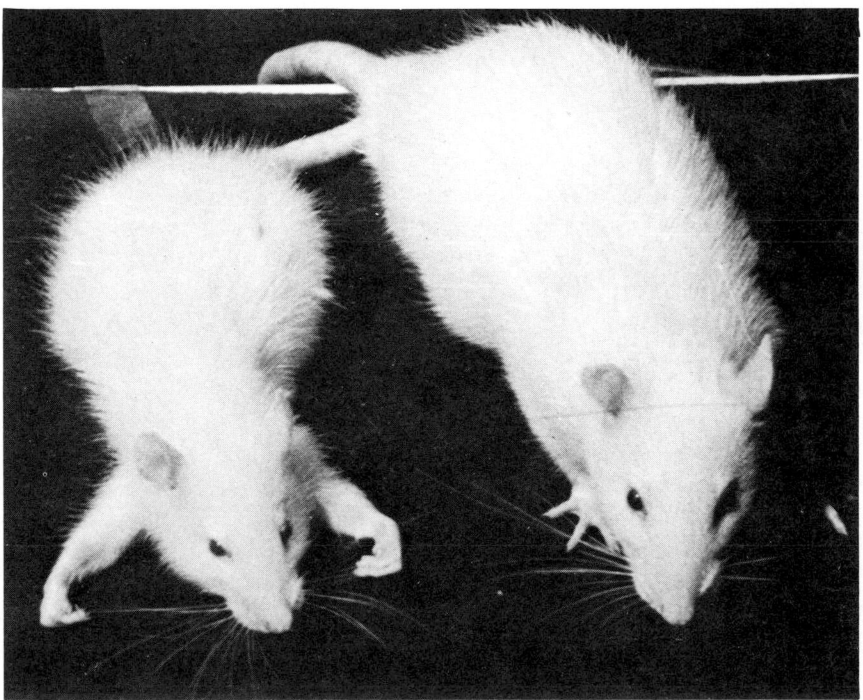

Fig. 16.5. Rats of litter represented in Figure 16.4 at fifty-sixth day of life. The crippled animal (left) was given no vitamin A after birth.

mones and the analysis of plasma hormone levels these possible explanations can be tested.

In a preliminary experiment, bovine growth hormone* was given to vitamin A–deficient germ-free rats after the weight level had stabilized for 11–12 weeks. For ten days an amount was given that customarily supports growth in a hypophysectomized rat, but no change in body weight resulted. Because of the possibility that these animals were too old to respond significantly to the hormone, the experiment was repeated in male rats that had been on the deficient diet for nine weeks and whose weight level had just stabilized. For nine days, pairs of these rats were given either L-thyroxine, testosterone propionate, or dexamethasone at supporting levels, or growth hormone in tenfold excess. None of these treatments promoted growth, and dexamethasone and thyroxine caused marked weight loss. In addition, protamine zinc insulin appeared to be poorly tolerated by these animals.

Vitamin A deficiency in germ-free chicks

In a conventional environment, chicks on a vitamin A–deficient diet become ataxic between the second and third week of life (Krishnamurthy et al., 1963; Havivi and Wolf, 1967; Howell and Thompson, 1967*b*). The uncoordinated chicks' difficulty in obtaining food contributes to their weight loss and early death. It has been reported that, in a germ-free environment, vitamin A–deficient chicks developed ataxia in about the same length of time as conventional chicks, and half of the birds died shortly (Reyniers et al., 1960). Despite their weakness, however, the surviving birds were reported to have had a satisfactory appearance and were still growing at 39 days of age when the experiment was stopped. Since to our knowledge these interesting observations have not been confirmed, we undertook a re-examination of the response of germ-free chicks to vitamin A deficiency.

Eggs fertile for 17 days were washed in peracetic acid and activated iodine solutions (Wescodyne), and either passed into a germ-free metal isolator or kept in a conventional environment. The composition of the soy protein–cottonseed oil–corn starch diet used in this experiment is shown in Table 16.3. One week after hatching, the germ-free chicks were transferred to a large, plastic-film isolator, and the conventional chicks were placed in a similar, unsterilized isolator. Equal illumination, temperature, and humidity were provided. At this time, supplementation of some chicks with retinyl acetate commenced.

* All hormones were supplied through the courtesy of the Endocrinology Study Section of the National Institutes of Health.

TABLE 16.3. *Vitamin A–deficient chick diet for autoclave sterilization (C–22)*

Ingredient	Percentage
Soy protein	30.0
L-cystine	0.3
DL-methionine	0.2
Vitamin mixture	2.0
Choline chloride	0.1
Fox and Briggs salt mixture	6.0
Cottonseed oil plus antioxidants[a]	4.0
Corn starch	57.4

[a] *dl*-α-tocopheryl acetate and ethoxyquin.

In both the germ-free and the conventional isolators, the chicks given vitamin A grew well and were vigorous (Fig. 16.6). Among the four vitamin A–deficient conventional chicks, ataxia appeared on the fourteenth day, and the birds soon had difficulty walking and squatted much of the time. All were dead by the twenty-eighth day. In contrast, three of four deficient birds in the germ-free isolator were relatively free of ataxia and grew as

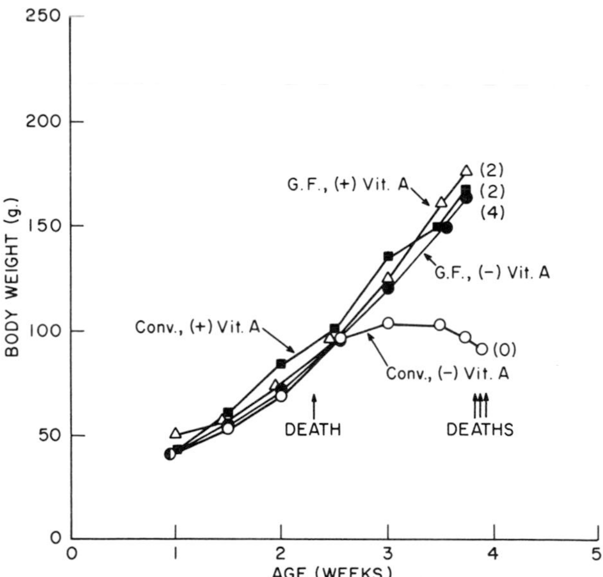

Fig. 16.6. Growth and survival of chicks hatched on the same day under germ-free or conventional conditions and raised on diet C–66 with or without vitamin A. Numbers in parentheses indicate the surviving animals; the 4 deaths were all in the conventional vitamin A–deficient group.

well as supplemented controls for almost four weeks. Ataxia, however, appeared in this group just before the twenty-eighth day, when a sudden weight loss occurred among all the germ-free chicks. An assay for sterility then revealed contamination of the isolator by an anaerobe, and the experiment was terminated.

Discussion

One of the intriguing relationships observed in these experiments is the appearance of mild nerve involvement at the time when appetite decreases and growth stops. Crippling and growth failure have been recognized for many years as aspects of the vitamin A deficiency syndrome, but the relationship between these phenomena is still unclear. It has been suggested that vitamin A deficiency affects nerves directly, and evidence for this conclusion still exists (Takeshita and Ko, 1965; Clausen, 1969). On the other hand, impressive evidence has accumulated that supports the concept that vitamin A deficiency causes a disproportionate growth of the central nervous system and of the skull and vertebral system that encases it, and that this overcrowding results in damage to the nerves. The mechanism suggested by Wolbach (1947) involves failure of endochondral bone growth and decreased remodeling of bone chambers while appositional growth of bone of periosteal origin continues in the normal pattern as long as food consumption remains adequate. In confirmation of this hypothesis, it was demonstrated that animals do not become crippled if the level of intake of the vitamin A–deficient diet is restricted in order to prevent the growth of soft tissue (Wolbach and Bessey, 1941; Wolbach and Hegsted, 1952).

Mellanby (1944) suggested that vitamin A deficiency is accompanied by the failure of osteoclastic enlargement of bone chambers, whereas Howell and Thompson (1967*a*) suggested that there is an abnormal development of cancellous bone from the periosteal lining of these cavities. In the latter report, vitamin A deficiency was rapidly induced in mature nongrowing chickens. In this situation, lack of endochondral bone growth cannot be the explanation for crippling, whereas the development in two weeks of sheets or spicules of cancellous bone from the periosteal lining of the vertebral canal does provide a plausible basis for the symptoms.

In the experiments on germ-free rats reported here, incoordination in adult (but not fully grown) animals, and crippling of front legs in young animals was observed uniformly. The incoordination in older animals did not develop into crippling during prolonged exposure to a vitamin A–deficient diet, and it was corrected rapidly by supplementation with vitamin A. The lack of exacerbation of crippling and the rapidity of its cure suggests that abnormal periosteal bone growth is not an invariable result of vitamin A deficiency. Furthermore, the moderately severe and somewhat progressive crippling observed in the young animals during their period of most intense growth suggests that levels of food intake and relative growth of soft tissues and the skeleton are significant factors in the etiology of crippling as postulated by Wolbach.

It is possible that the animals in our germ-free experiments were not completely vitamin A–deficient. In the casein–cornstarch–corn oil diet there are several possible sources of trace amounts of vitamin A. Under germ-free conditions these traces might be sufficient for maintenance of vital functions even though many nonvital systems deteriorate. In the germ-free state, rats show a decreased metabolic rate (Wostmann et al., 1968). This may be pertinent, since Johnson and Baumann (1948) reported that feeding desiccated thyroid or thiouracil seemed to hasten or delay, respectively, the utilization of liver stores of vitamin A. Furthermore, these investigators demonstrated a very clear effect between growth restriction and decreased utilization of liver stores of the vitamin. Cold-temperature stress seems to increase the rate of depletion of liver vitamin A when initial stores of the vitamin are normal (Sundaresan et al., 1967), but not when the stores are low (Phillips, 1962). Other factors such as dietary antioxidants (Davies and Moore, 1941) also have been observed to modify the rate at which vitamin A stores are consumed. A combination of decreased metabolic rate and stress, lack of growth and infection, and a high dietary level of α-tocopherol might allow the germ-free animal to survive for long periods on traces of vitamin A that would be quite ineffective for animals in a conventional environment.

Though some recent evidence (Clausen, 1969) suggests that vitamin A stores are conserved, a prevailing opinion is that under normal conditions, liver stores of vitamin A in weanling rats are consumed at a constant rate. Dowling and Wald (1958) reported that when stock weanling rats were placed on a vitamin A–deficient diet, their liver stores of the vitamin decreased linearly to zero in about 3½ weeks. At this time the blood level of the vitamin fell precipitously to zero and rhodopsin commenced a linear decrease, reaching 16% of normal at about the eighth week, when all the classic signs of deficiency were manifested. In the Dowling and Wald experiment, the liver depletion rate was 2–2.5 μg of vitamin A per day. A lower value has been cited as the minimum requirement for restoration of growth in a young rat (Moore, 1957). This value is given as 1–2 IU per day, though liver stores are not detected unless the supplement is 20–30 IU per day. Finally, data are available on the transfer of vitamin A to rats during gestation. Henry and associates (1949) found a total liver store of approximately 1 IU in newborn rats from dams given levels of vitamin A sufficient for growth but not storage. In our germ-free studies of rats born in the isolator, it is probable that maternal liver stores of retinyl esters were extremely low prior to breeding and that the young rats commenced life with a maximum of 1 μg of the ester. The only source of vitamin A for continued growth observed in these animals seems to be small amounts of retinoic acid in the milk or excreta of the dam or, subsequent to weaning, traces of vitamin A in the casein–cornstarch–corn oil diet. For conventional vitamin A–deficient young rats, these possible traces of the vitamin were always inadequate.

In conclusion, it seems possible that the pattern of slow growth in the young rats and the prolonged survival of the older rats might be due to a combination of traces of vitamin A in the casein–cornstarch–corn oil diet and greatly decreased requirements for the vitamin under germ-free conditions. In evaluating this possibility, the long survival of rats on the amino acid–sucrose–stripped fat diet should be kept in mind. Furthermore, in these experiments all the classic signs of full-blown vitamin A deficiency were exhibited except weight loss, early death, and the lesions associated with bacterial infection. These interesting observations make it apparent that many concepts regarding vitamin A requirements will have to be re-investigated in the germ-free state. One of the most intriguing observations is that of prompt growth response to vitamin A. This seems to indicate that time-consuming repair processes are not required before recovery of growth, provided that the central nervous system has not grown appreciably during the interim when skeletal growth has been blocked. Under these conditions it appears that the germ-free animal will be an extremely useful experimental model with which to study phenomena induced by, or otherwise responsive to, vitamin A.

References

Beaver, D. L. 1961. Vitamin A deficiency in the germ-free rat. *Amer. J. Pathol.* *38*:335.

Bieri, J. G., E. G. McDaniel, and W. E. Rogers, Jr. 1969. Survival of germfree rats without vitamin A. *Science 163*:574.

Clausen, J. 1969. The effect of vitamin A deficiency on myelination in the central nervous system of the rat. *European J. Biochem.* 7:575.

Davies, A. W., and T. Moore. 1941. Interaction of vitamins A and E. *Nature* *147*:794.

Dowling, J. E., and G. Wald. 1958. Vitamin A deficiency and night blindness. *Proc. Nat. Acad. Sci. U.S.A. 44*:648.

Havivi, E., and G. Wolf. 1967. Vitamin A, sulfation and bone growth in the chick. *J. Nutr. 92*:467.

Henry, K. M., S. K. Kon, E. H. Mawson, J. E. Stanier, and S. Y. Thompson. 1949. The passage of vitamin A from mother to young in the rat. *Brit. J. Nutr. 3*:301.

Howell, J. McC., and J. N. Thompson. 1967*a*. Observations on the lesions in vitamin A deficient adult fowls with particular reference to changes in bone and central nervous system. *Brit. J. Exp. Pathol. 45*:450.

Howell, J. McC. and J. N. Thompson. 1967*b*. Lesions associated with the development of ataxia in vitamin A–deficient chicks. *Brit. J. Nutr. 21*:741.

Johnson, B. C., and G. Wolf. 1960. The function of vitamin A in carbohydrate metabolism; its role in adrenocorticoid production. *Vitamins Hormones 18*:457.

Johnson, R. M., and C. A. Bauman. 1948. Relative significance of growth and metabolic rate upon the utilization of vitamin A by the rat. *J. Nutr. 35*:703.

Krishnamurthy, S., J. G. Bieri, and E. L. Andrews. 1963. Metabolism and biological activity of vitamin A acid in the chick. *J. Nutr. 79*:503.

Mellanby, E. 1944. Nutrition in relation to bone growth and the nervous system. *Proc. Roy. Soc.* [*Biol.*] *132*:28.

Moore, T. 1957. *Vitamin A*, p. 227. Elsevier, Amsterdam.

Phillips, W. E. J. 1962. Low-temperature environmental stress and the metabolism of vitamin A in the rat. *Can. J. Biochem. Physiol. 40*:491.

Reyniers, J. A., M. Wagner, T. D. Luckey, and H. A. Gordon. 1960. Survey of germfree animals: the White Wyandotte Bantam and White Leghorn chicken. *LOBUND Reports 3*:140.

Rogers, W. E., Jr. 1967. Accelerated vitamin A deficiency in rats. *Fed. Proc. 26*:636.

Rogers, W. E., Jr., and J. G. Bieri. 1969. Vitamin A deficiency in the rat prior to weaning. *Proc. Soc. Exp. Biol. Med. 132*:622.

Sundaresan, P. R., V. G. Winters, and D. G. Therriault. 1967. Effect of low environmental temperature on the metabolism of vitamin A (retinol) in the rat. *J. Nutr. 92*:474.

Takeshita, T., and J. Ko. 1965. On the lesion of peripheral nervous tissues of vitamin A deficiency, using rats. *Bitamin 31*:50.

Thompson, J. N., J. McC. Howell, and G. A. J. Pitt. 1963–64. Vitamin A and reproduction in rats. *Proc. Roy. Soc.* [*Biol.*] *159*:510.

Wolbach, S. B. 1947. Vitamin A deficiency and excess in relation to skeletal growth. *J. Bone Joint Surg. 29*:171.

Wolbach, S. B., and O. A. Bessey. 1941. Vitamin A deficiency and the nervous system. *Arch. Pathol. 32*:689.

Wolbach, S. B., and J. M. Hegsted. 1952. Vitamin A deficiency in the chick. *Arch. Pathol. 54*:13.

Wostmann, B. S., E. Bruckner-Kardoss, and P. L. Knight, Jr. 1968. Cecal enlargement, cardiac output and O_2 consumption in germfree rats. *Proc. Soc. Exp. Biol. Med. 128*:137.

17

RECENT STUDIES ON SOME METABOLIC FUNCTIONS OF VITAMIN A

G. Wolf and L. De Luca

Introduction

Many of us in vitamin research are connected with the science of nutrition. As nutritionists we are frequently beset by what psychologists call an identity crisis: Are we physiologists or biochemists or physiological chemists or none of these or a combination?

Professor Steenbock wrote a succinct and convincing answer to this problem (Steenbock and Gross, 1920):

> It is true that much of immediate practical importance in vitamin relations may be gained by a study of the dietary properties of various foodstuffs fed singly and in combinations, but it is not to be questioned that ultimately a true conception of problems in nutrition is dependent on the determination of the occurrence of various substances in foods and a development of an appreciation of their physiological role. We refer here to the effect of various substances on secretion, motor activity, irritability, conductivity, permeability, and cell proliferation, all of which are concerned in such a gross physiological process as growth.

This prophetic remark about secretion and cell proliferation in connection with vitamin A, made in 1920, is a true mark of Steenbock's scientific genius.

There is now, we believe, general agreement that vitamin A is to be regarded as a hormone rather than a vitamin in the classical sense of a coenzyme. By "hormone" we mean a substance secreted into the bloodstream which influences tissues and organs so as to differentiate and elaborate new cell types and new enzymes. There is no a priori reason why a hormone should have to be made by the animal itself. It is quite conceivable that a hormone can be taken in the diet, stored in the liver, and secreted into the bloodstream when needed. The liver then acts as the endocrine organ.

Vitamin A—or perhaps "hormone A"—has four distinct physiological functions. Again, we have a precedent: cortisone, for instance, has a variety of functions, such as regulation of gluconeogenesis and amino acid metabolism. These functions of vitamin A are (1) maintenance of proper vision; (2) maintenance of spermatogenesis in the male and prevention of resorption of the fetus in the female; (3) maintenance of bone growth, in particular the activity of the osteoblasts (Hayes et al., 1968) and, therefore, prevention of deficiency-caused nerve disorders due to pressure of overgrown bone on nerve cells; and (4) maintenance of the mucus-secreting cells of epithelia and prevention of keratinization (as so well explored by Fell and her collaborators).

When we consider the response of epithelial tissues to the vitamin, it seems as if basal cells of epithelia had two pathways of cytodifferentiation open to them: without the vitamin they keratinize, and with the vitamin they form columnar, mucus-secreting cells. A most persuasive series of experiments supporting this view was recently reported by Saffiotti and associates (1968). They found that, in the course of inducing lung tumors in hamsters, carcinogenic hydrocarbons first cause squamous metaplasia of the columnar, mucus-secreting epithelia of the lung. By feeding the hamsters excess vitamin A, however, metaplasia and the subsequent tumor induction can be inhibited, presumably by supplying enough of the vitamin to the affected cells to stimulate them to form mucus and maintain their columnar differentiation. This reasoning leads to the idea, first proposed by Parnell and Sherman (1962), that different tissues have different thresholds for vitamin A. The tissue with the lowest threshold is the epithelial lining of the gastrointestinal tract; in the presence of normal levels of vitamin A, its basal cells produce mucus-secreting (goblet) cells. A higher threshold is found in the columnar epithelium of the trachea, which changes to stratified, squamous epithelium under vitamin A deficiency (Parnell and Sherman, 1962). Next higher in threshold is the corneal epithelium, normally consisting of stratified, squamous epithelium, but producing keratin under vitamin A deficiency. Finally, the epidermis has the highest threshold. This tissue produces keratin even under normal vitamin A–sufficient conditions; production increases under vitamin A deficiency. Fell (1957) showed that even epidermis from chick embryo in organ culture, exposed to massive doses of the vitamin, can be made to produce columnar, mucus-secreting cells.

Protein synthesis by intestinal mucosa

In our experiments, the behavior of intestinal mucosa towards vitamin A deficiency was in some ways similar to that of chick embryo skin explants transferred from a vitamin A–rich to a vitamin A–free medium: the mucus-secreting cells degenerate and are shed. Histologically, we found only about one-half the number of goblet cells in the intestinal wall of deficient rats (De Luca et al., 1969), although there is no evidence of subsequent keratinization.

We regard the intestinal mucosa as a model for mucous membranes and are investigating the response to vitamin A deficiency. Since glycoprotein is the principal constituent of the mucus produced by intestinal cells, we attempted to determine the hypothetical action of vitamin A on glycoprotein synthesis. Attention focused initially on the protein core. We studied in vitro protein synthesis in subcellular fractions from the small intestine of pair-fed normal and vitamin A–deficient rats.

In summary, the intestines of vitamin A–deficient rats whose common bile ducts had been ligated yielded normal polyribosomes and synthesized protein normally. Isolated rough endoplasmic reticulum (RER), on the other hand, showed a very depressed rate of protein synthesis in deficiency. This is reasonable, since the recognized locus of synthesis of the glycoproteins is the vesicles formed by the RER. By combining RER from normal animals with the *p*H 5 fraction from the supernatant solu-

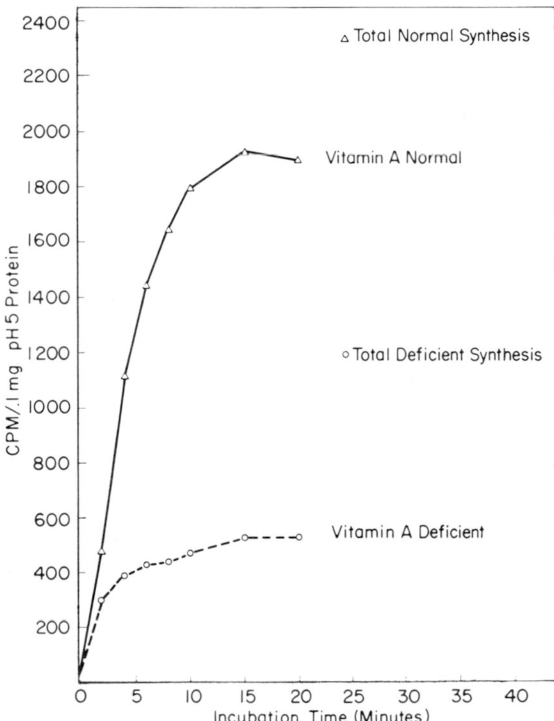

Fig. 17.1. The incorporation of radioactive leucine into leucyl-tRNA, using tRNA from mucosa of the small intestine of normal and vitamin A–deficient rats.

tion of deficient mucosa, and vice versa, we located the lesion due to the deficiency in the *pH* 5 fraction. This fraction principally contains transfer ribonucleic acid (tRNA) and the enzymes which activate amino acids and esterify them to tRNA (aminoacyl-tRNA synthetases).

The cell fractions were prepared and incubated with radioactive leucine as previously described by De Luca and associates (1969) except that guanosine triphosphate and RER were omitted. The *pH* 5 fraction used had a protein concentration of 1 mg/ml. Aliquots of 0.05 ml were removed at different times, diluted with nonradioactive leucine, and precipitated with ice-cold trichloroacetic acid. The precipitates were counted on Millipore filters. In parallel, the total level of protein synthesis was determined by incubating RER (0.25 mg protein) with 0.5 mg *p*H 5 fraction protein as described by De Luca and associates (1969), followed by trichloroacetic acid, plating, and counting. Figure 17.1 shows that the activity of the *p*H 5 fraction in forming aminoacyl-tRNA's is depressed in vitamin A deficiency.

To test whether this effect is due to the tRNA or the synthetases, we fractionated normal intestinal tRNA on DEAE-cellulose (Fig. 17.2). Ten

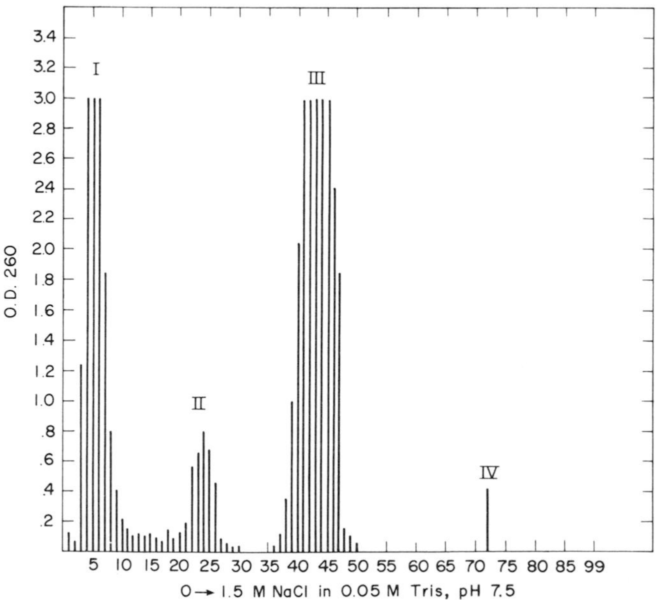

Fig. 17.2. Fractionation of normal rat intestinal tRNA on DEAE-cellulose. Only peak III was active in accepting radioactive leucine with the intestinal *p*H 5 fraction.

male rats, each 60 g, were prepared by having their common bile ducts ligated 24 hr before they were killed. The extraction method for the tRNA was that of Strehler and associates (1967), and involved phenol extraction of the intestinal mucosal homogenate, alcohol precipitation, re-extraction in 1 N NaCl, and re-precipitation. The final precipitate was chromatographed on a DEAE-cellulose (Cl^-) column (1 × 20) equilibrated with 0.01 M tris chloride at *p*H 7.5. The tRNA was eluted with a linear NaCl gradient (0–1.5 M), 5 ml fractions were collected, and the OD was read at 260 mμ and 280 mμ. The ratio of the OD at 260 mμ to that at 280 mμ was about 2.3. The four major peaks were pooled separately and precipitated in the presence of ethanol. We obtained one RNA peak, No. III, which has high activity for accepting ^{14}C leucine with the *p*H 5 enzymes.

With this normal tRNA, it was possible to titrate the activity of the synthetase from deficient and normal intestine. The cell fractions were prepared and incubated as described earlier. The concentration of the *p*H 5 fraction protein was 200 μg per incubation. Figure 17.3 shows that, with a large excess of normal intestinal tRNA, the difference between deficient and normal charging of tRNA by amino acids is reduced from 57% to 28%. At earlier stages of deficiency, the difference in charging

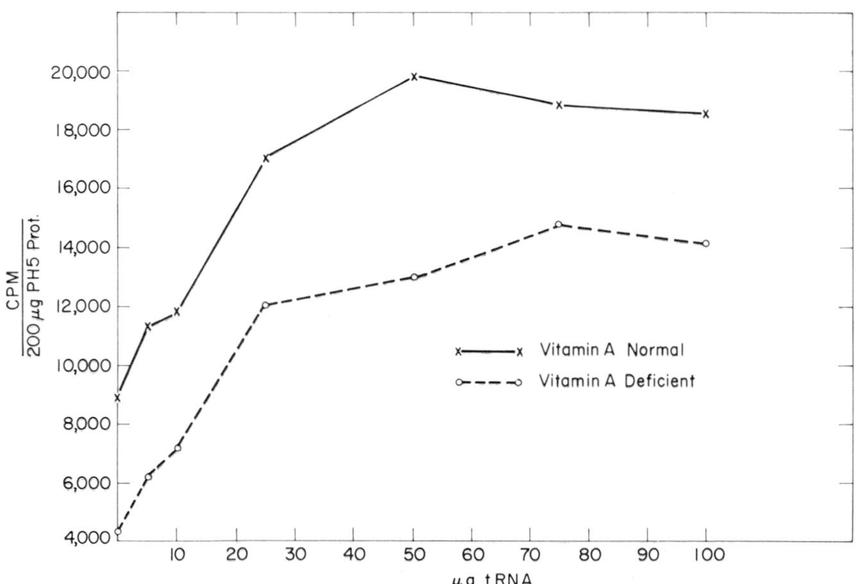

Fig. 17.3. The effect of increasing concentrations of normal intestinal tRNA (peak III) on the formation of ^{14}C leucyl-tRNA with normal and vitamin A–deficient intestinal *p*H 5 fractions.

was initially 25% and could be totally removed with increasing amounts of normal tRNA.

As more is learned about the regulation of protein synthesis, one important difference is becoming apparent between bacterial and animal systems: messenger RNA (mRNA) in bacteria is short-lived, and protein synthesis is regulated through control of the rate of synthesis of new mRNA (transcription). The mRNA of animal cells appears to have a much longer life. Regulation of protein synthesis by hormones, for instance, can frequently occur through control of the rate of protein synthesis on existing mRNA. Thus, Turkington (1969) found that modification of tRNA controlled mammary gland differentiation in organ culture; and O'Malley and co-workers (1968) showed that the chick oviduct differentiates through estrogen-dependent changes in tRNA.

As a result of code degeneracy, each amino acid can have more than one tRNA and a corresponding multiplicity of synthetases. We are at present testing the hypothesis that in vitamin A deficiency one type of charged tRNA in intestinal mucosa disappears. Therefore, any mRNA requiring that specific aminoacyl-tRNA cannot be translated. It is conceivable that another tRNA (for the same amino acid) can then be charged, leading to translation of another type of mRNA and hence to a new protein and ultimately to a new cell type.

Glycopeptide biosynthesis in rat intestine

Characteristic glycopeptides secreted by the cells of the small intestine have not yet been investigated. Vitamin A–deficient and normal, pair-fed control rats were injected intraperitoneally with 25 μc per 200 g body weight of ^{14}C-glucosamine-HCl (30 mc per nmole) 2 hr before being killed. Glycopeptides were prepared as shown in Table 17.1, and about the same

TABLE 17.1. *Preparation of glycopeptides from rat intestinal mucosa*

1. Scrape mucosa; dilute 1:10 with 80% ethanol; homogenize (virtis); heat to 100 C for 15 min.
2. Centrifuge; discard supernatant.
3. Re-extract precipitate with 80%, 100% ethanol, and ether.
4. Suspend in water; digest with trypsin 5 hr at 30 C; add $CaCl_2$ to get final concentration of 0.01 M at *p*H 8; digest with pronase 42 hr at 37 C; dilute to 7% strength with trichloroacetic acid.
5. Centrifuge; discard precipitate.
6. Cool supernatant; add 2 volumes of ethanol.
7. Glycopeptides will precipitate.

Note: Method is adapted from the one described by Inoue and Yosizawa (1966).

amount (10 mg per rat) was obtained from the two types of animal. Purification yielded a mixture of glycopeptides with about 2% protein content. The glycopeptides were then chromatographed on a DEAE-Sephadex A–50 (Cl^-) column, prepared as described by Inoue and Yosizawa (1966), and stepwise elution with increasing concentrations of LiCl was carried out. Fractions of 15 ml each were collected. Maximum labeling of the intestinal glycopeptides occurred 2 hr after the rats were injected with the labeled glucosamine. When the purified glycopeptides were chromatographed after such a 2-hour ^{14}C-glucosamine pulse, five major peaks of radioactivity were isolated (Fig. 17.4). In the deficient intestine, peak III eluted with 0.4 N LiCl was much lower, while peak V eluted with 1 N LiCl had increased in size. The ratio III/V in deficiency is about 1:10, whereas it is 1:2 in normal conditions. Analysis showed that peak III is rich in uronic acid, glucosamine, and hexose but is poor in sialic acid and has almost no sulfate. Peak V is similar except for being poor in hexose as well. The only sulfate-rich peak is IV. We are presently attempting to get

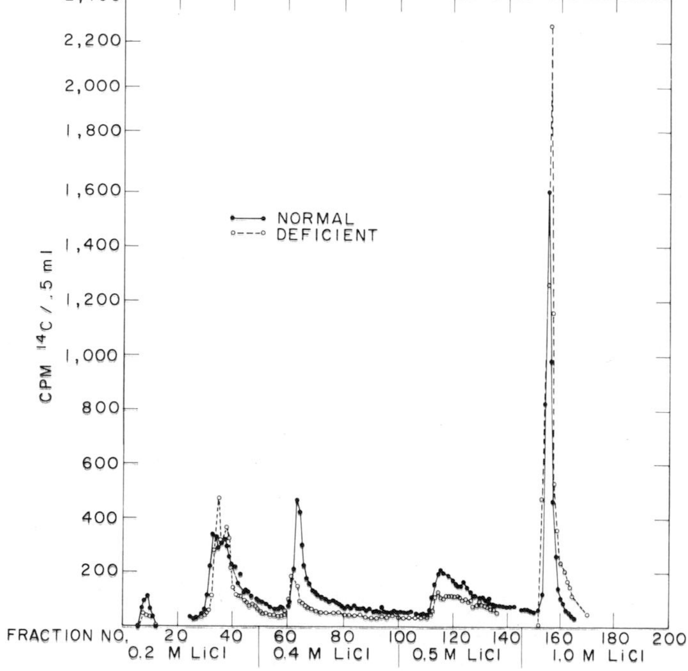

Fig. 17.4. Fractionation of glycopeptide from normal and deficient rat intestinal mucosa.

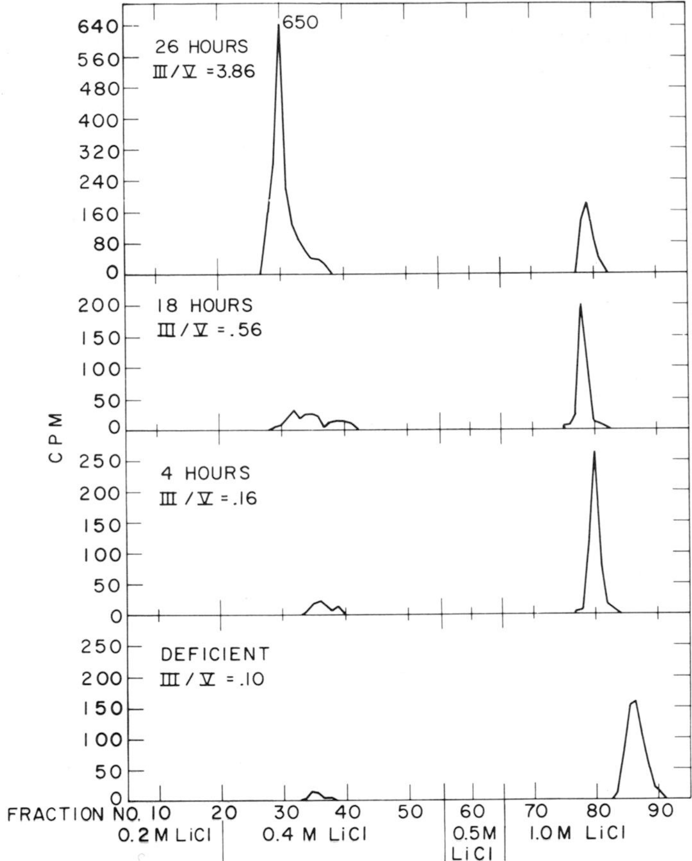

Fig. 17.5. Incorporation of ^{14}C-glucosamine into glycopeptide in vitamin A–deficient rat intestinal mucosa, various times after injection of vitamin A.

exact molar ratios of these constituents and to determine their turnover in vitamin A–deficient and normal intestine.

Vitamin A–deficient rats were intraperitoneally injected with 500 μg retinol dissolved in Tween 80–ethnol saline. The preparation of the glycopeptides was as for the previous experiment. The first indication of recovery in peak III was observed after 18 hr (Fig. 17.5). Considering the short half-life of intestinal mucosal cells, this time is certainly long enough for the appearance of a new cell-type rather than a new constituent of existing cells in response to the vitamin.

We can do no better than to close with a remark from Steenbock about his own work (Steenbock and Black, 1924): "The suggestions carried by the data presented in this paper are obvious. As we realize that we have already indulged extensively in unorthodox speculations we shall withhold further statement of probabilities. . . ."

References

De Luca, L., E. P. Little, and G. Wolf. 1969. Vitamin A and protein synthesis by rat intestinal mucosa. *J. Biol. Chem. 244*:701.

Fell, H. B. 1957. The effect of excess vitamin A on cultures of embryonic chicken skin explanted at different stages of differentiation. *Proc. Roy. Soc.* [*Biol.*] *146*:242.

Hayes, K. C., S. W. Nielsen, and H. D. Eaton. 1968. Pathogenesis of the optic nerve lesion in vitamin A–deficient calves. *Arch. Ophthalmol. 80*:777.

Inoue, S., and Z. Yosizawa. 1966. Purification and properties of sulfated sialopoly saccharides isolated from pig colonic mucosa. *Arch. Biochem. Biophys. 117*:257.

O'Malley, B. W., A. Aronow, A. C. Peacock, and C. W. Dingman. 1968. Estrogen-dependent increase in t-RNA during differentiation of the chick oviduct. *Science 162*:567.

Parnell, J. P., and B. S. Sherman. 1962. Effect of vitamin A on keratinization in the A–deficient rat, p.113. *In* E. O. Butcher and R. F. Sognnaes (ed.), *Fundamentals of Keratinization*. Publication No. 70. Amer. Ass. for the Advance. of Science, Washington, D.C.

Saffiotti, U., R. Montesano, A. R. Sellakumar, and S. A. Borg. 1967. Experimental cancer of the lung. *Cancer 20*:857.

Steenbock, H., and A. Black. 1924. Fat-soluble vitamine. XVII. The induction of growth-promoting and calcifying properties in a ration by exposure to ultraviolet light. *J. Biol. Chem. 61*:405.

Steenbock, H., and E. G. Gross. 1920. Fat-soluble vitamine. IV. The fat-soluble content of green plant tissues together with some observations on their water-soluble vitamine content. *J. Biol. Chem. 41*:149.

Strehler, B. L., D. D. Hendley, and G. P. Hirsch. 1967. Evidence of a codon restriction hypothesis of cellular differentiation: multiplicity of mammalian leucyl-sRNA-specific deficiency in an alanyl-sRNA synthetase. *Proc. Nat. Acad. Sci. U.S.A. 57*:1751.

Turkington, R. W. 1969. Methylation of t-RNA during hormone-dependent differentiation of mammary gland *in vitro. Fed. Proc. 28*:724.

18

THE ROLE OF VITAMIN A IN REPRODUCTION

J. N. Thompson

Introduction

Nutritionists usually associate reproduction with vitamin E rather than with vitamin A. Nevertheless, in many species vitamin A plays important roles both in the formation of spermatozoa and in the maintenance of pregnancy. It is needed also in avian eggs for normal development of the embryos. In the past, research workers and reviewers have justifiably emphasized the vitamin's other interesting and dramatic roles, such as controlling bone growth, maintaining epithelial tissues, and forming visual pigments. The action of vitamin A in reproduction has received less attention. One reason is that many abnormalities of reproduction in vitamin A–deficient animals result from deficiency lesions that are not specific to the reproductive system, and it has not been possible to recognize the direct effects of avitaminosis on reproduction or sometimes even to be aware of their existence.

A new approach to the study of the effects of vitamin A deficiency on reproduction emerged during tests of the biological activity of retinoic acid. Retinoic acid can substitute for the true vitamin (retinol) in many, but not all, of its functions. Thus retinoic acid maintains growth and general health (Arens and van Dorp, 1946), but it does not maintain vision because animals are unable to reduce it to the aldehyde retinal, the prosthetic group of the visual pigments (Dowling and Wald, 1960), and in some species, it does not maintain reproduction (Thompson et al., 1964). Animals given vitamin A–free diets containing retinoic acid or methyl retinoate are normal in growth, overt appearance, and longevity, but

The experiments reported in this chapter were devised and conducted in collaboration with Dr. W. A. Coward, Dr. J. McC. Howell, and Dr. G. A. J. Pitt of the University of Liverpool, England, and were supported in part by the Agricultural Research Council, United States Public Health Service Grant AM–05632, the British Egg Marketing Board, and F. Hoffmann-La Roche and Company.

visual pigment formation and some aspects of reproduction are affected as in the absence of vitamin A. These animals are thus very suitable for the demonstration and investigation of certain specific effects of vitamin A deficiency on reproduction and vision.

Several reviews, notably those by Mason (1939), Rubin and Bird (1942), and Moore (1957), describe the reproductive disorders in conventional vitamin A–deficient animals. The following reappraisal of the roles of vitamin A in reproduction has been made in the light of recent studies with animals maintained on retinoic acid or its methyl ester. Table 18.1

TABLE 18.1. *Comparison of the biological properties of retinoic acid, methyl retinoate, and vitamin A*

Property	Vitamin A (retinol, retinyl acetate, retinal, etc.)	Retinoic acid	Methyl retinoate
Maintains body growth and prevents infection, epithelial metaplasia, overgrowth of bone, loss of appetite, etc.	+	+	+
Forms visual pigment	+	—	—
Maintains testes in rats, guinea pigs, and hamsters	+	—	—
Maintains testes in roosters	+	+	+
Maintains pregnancy in rats and guinea pigs	+	—	—
Maintains seminal vesicle size in rats	+	—	—
Is transferred by birds to their eggs	+	—	—
Stimulates development of avian embryos	+	+	+
Has high toxicity to avian embryos	—	+	—

Note: The signs indicate the presence (+) or absence (—) of the property.

compares the biological properties of retinoic acid with those of retinol and methyl retinoate.

Reproduction in males

In the rat, and probably in many other species, vitamin A deficiency results in three major abnormalities in the male reproductive system: metaplasia of epithelia and infection, atrophy of the accessory sexual organs, and degeneration of the germinal epithelium of the testes. These changes are important in that they can impair fertility, but they are brought about by different mechanisms, not all of which arise because of truly specific roles of vitamin A in reproduction.

THE ACCESSORY SEXUAL ORGANS

Infection in the reproductive tract is probably a secondary effect of keratinizing metaplasia, an abnormality occurring in many epithelial tissues of vitamin A–deficient animals. Its prevention does not represent a specific role of vitamin A in reproduction.

The accessory sexual organs in deficient animals, such as the seminal vesicles, are sometimes smaller than normal. This abnormality is not related to either the degree of infection in the glands or the severity of the lesions in the testes. Mason (1939) suggested that it results from inanition and general debility in the deficient animal. When he administered vitamin A to deficient animals, the restoration of the seminal vesicles to their normal size was considerably impeded when the food supply was restricted. In contrast, the germinal epithelium of the testes was repaired even during starvation. Endocrine abnormalities are probably involved in the reduction in size of the accessory sexual organs because injections of extracts of urine from pregnant women or daily implants of pituitary tissue into deficient rats produced marked hypertrophy of the interstitial tissue of the testes and enlargement of the atrophied prostate and seminal vesicles (Mason, 1939). A similar response to sources of gonadotropin was reported by van Os (1934) and by Mayer and Goddard (1951) . The accessory sexual organs in deficient rats also increase in size when testosterone is administered (Mayer and Truant, 1949). These experiments suggest that vitamin A deficiency lowers the level of circulating hypophyseal gonadotropins, and thus depresses androgen production in the interstitial cells of the testes.

The mechanisms involved in the reduction of gonadotropin levels have not been adequately explained. There are histological abnormalities in the hypophyses of deficient animals (Sutton and Brief, 1939; Hodgson et al., 1946; Erb et al., 1947) but the gonadotropin activity of the gland in vitamin A–deficient rats is apparently abnormally high (Mason and Wolfe, 1930).

Although inanition may be responsible for some of these changes (Leatham, 1961), other factors must be involved in rats given vitamin A–deficient diets containing retinoic acid. They are well nourished and yet they have smaller seminal vesicles than controls given retinol (Thompson et al., 1965*a*). This effect is illustrated by the seminal vesicle weights listed in Table 18.2. In rats given methyl retinoate the reduction in size of the accessory sexual organs could be a secondary effect of damage to the germinal epithelium, or perhaps loss of vision (Coward et al., 1966), but these are tentative explanations which may or may not be relevant to the changes in completely deficient animals.

When all the findings are considered together, one is left with the impression that vitamin A deficiency has inconsistent effects on the accessory sexual organs because of complicated interactions of major and minor disturbances in the endocrine system. This view is substantiated by a recent report that cockerels marginally deficient in vitamin A have enlarged combs and testes (Nockels and Kienholz, 1967), and that changes in the activity of the adrenal gland were thought to be responsible (Nockels and Herrick, 1969).

THE TESTES

In vitamin A deficiency the testes become edematous, and the germinal epithelium is lost. Although this lesion has been observed in various species, the most detailed investigations have been made with rats. Mason (1933) found that as the deficiency disease advanced, spermatogenesis was slowed, and the more mature sperm-forming cells fell away from the germinal epithelium so that eventually only a few primitive forms, spermatogonia and spermatocytes, remained in the tubules. These losses were readily repaired after the rats were fed vitamin A, and this served to distinguish these losses from the lesions in the testes due to vitamin E deficiency which, even in their early stages, cannot be cured.

The special nature of the role of vitamin A in the testes became apparent when it was discovered that retinoic acid was unable to replace retinol in maintaining the germinal epithelium (Thompson et al., 1964), although it does maintain other epithelial tissues affected during vitamin A deficiency. Male rats given vitamin A–deficient diets containing retinoic acid or its ester were found to be sterile.

Degeneration of the germinal epithelium occurred in these animals when tissue stores of retinol and its esters were exhausted, and the lesions in their early stages were histologically similar to the changes occurring in the testes during complete deficiency (Howell et al., 1963). Rats given retinoic acid (either as a sodium salt or as a methyl ester) remained in good general health, and they had a normal life span. Thus it was possible to allow the degeneration of the testes to continue for a much longer time than was possible in orthodox deficient animals, which died soon after the onset of deficiency disease. Eventually, in the rats given retinoic acid, most of the sperm-forming cells disappeared and the lumen of the testes tubules was obliterated by a syncytium of Sertoli cells; this advanced lesion must be assumed to be irreversible.

When rats given the vitamin A–deficient diet containing retinoic acid were also provided with retinol (as retinyl acetate) they had normal testes. Therefore the degeneration of the testes in the animals given retinoic acid was not due to a toxic effect of the acid. This conclusion was confirmed by the absence of testicular lesions in rats given normal diets containing large amounts of retinoic acid.

On the basis of experiments with retinoic acid and methyl retinoate, vitamin A was believed to have a special role in the germinal epithelium of the testes. This role was fundamentally different from the prevention of keratinizing metaplasia, in which retinoic acid is almost as effective as retinol. Similar abnormalities were found in the testes of guinea pigs (Howell et al., 1967), boars (Palludan, 1966), and hamsters given vitamin A–deficient diets containing retinoic acid. Thus vitamin A may have a special role in the testes in most higher animals. Roosters, however, were found to have essentially normal testes when they were maintained with retinoic acid or methyl retinoate instead of retinol (Thompson et al., 1969).

The fundamental biochemistry of the effect of vitamin A on the testes has yet to be explored in detail. A primary effect on the endocrine system seems to have been eliminated (Coward et al., 1966): neither testosterone nor FSH had beneficial effects on the histological appearance of the testes tubules in rats maintained with methyl retinoate, although testosterone did increase the size of the seminal vesicles (Table 18.2). The evidence available at the present time favors the hypothesis that retinol or one of its metabolites may act directly on the germinal epithelium. This has been dramatically confirmed in recent experiments with vitamin A–deficient boars given retinoic acid. Palludan (1966) injected either retinol or retinal into the testicles and after several months the germinal epithelium, at the site of the injections but not elsewhere, was found to have been repaired.

TABLE 18.2. *Effects of hormones and retinyl acetate on the testes and seminal vesicles of rats maintained with methyl retinoate*

Treatment	Number of rats with: Essentially normal testes	Partly degenerate testes	Degenerate testes	Average weight of testes (g)	Average weight of seminal vesicles (g)
Experiment 1					
Untreated	0	1	9	1.61	0.83
TP	1	1	8	1.13	2.38
Retinyl acetate	9	1	0	2.49	1.03
Retinyl acetate + TP	7	3	0	1.83	2.07
Experiment 2					
Untreated	0	0	10	1.43	0.75
FSH	0	1	9	1.72	1.42
Retinyl acetate	8	2	0	2.43	1.33
Retinyl acetate + FSH	9	0	0	2.79	1.30

Source: Coward et al. (1966).

Notes: The rats, from weaning, were on a vitamin A–deficient diet containing methyl retinoate. They were given the treatments daily (5 μg retinyl acetate, 1 mg TP, and 1 mg FSH) when 39–67 days old in experiment 1 and 45–75 days old in experiment 2. TP = testosterone propionate; FSH = follicle-stimulating hormone.

The testes of most species do not contain high concentrations of vitamin A, but this is not an argument against a direct action; indeed it is difficult to detect vitamin A in many other tissues, such as the epithelia, in which it is needed. Rats given small but nutritionally effective quantities of radioactively labeled retinyl acetate have been shown to incorporate significant amounts of retinol into the testes (Coward and Thompson, 1967).

Reproduction in the female

PREGNANCY

Vitamin A deficiency has been shown to have dire effects on pregnancy. The outcome depends on the severity of the deficiency, and the defects described range from delivery of living, congenitally malformed young to total resorption of all fetuses. Vitamin A deficiency has been produced in several species during pregnancy but, as in the study of reproduction in the male, the most comprehensive investigations have been done with rats. In vitamin A–deficient female rats the vaginal epithelium becomes permanently keratinized, and the changes which are normally associated with the estrus cycle are obliterated. The estrus cycle, nevertheless, continues uninterrupted until the terminal stages of deficiency, and often deficient female rats will mate with normal males and conceive. Mason (1935) found that these animals frequently resorb their fetuses during the second week of pregnancy.

Fetal resorption and other abnormalities of pregnancy could, until recently, be reasonably attributed to the combined effects of inanition, debility, epithelial keratinization, infection, and endocrine disturbances, all of which are known to occur in the vitamin A–deficient animals. Rats given vitamin A–deficient diets and retinoic acid, however, do not suffer from these general deficiency signs but they also resorb their fetuses (Thompson et al., 1964). Fetal resorption is therefore not merely a secondary consequence of the general effects of deficiency disease, but occurs because of the direct role played by vitamin A in pregnancy. In animals maintained with retinoic acid, fetal resorption is unlikely to be due to a toxic effect of the acid, even though large amounts of retinoic acid have been shown to have deleterious effects on normal pregnant animals (Kochhar, 1967), because supplements of the small amounts of retinol will prevent resorption.

Injections of estrone and progesterone, alone and in combination, did not prevent resorption in rats given vitamin A–deficient diets containing retinoic acid or methyl retinoate (Coward et al., 1966; Calaustro and Lichtan, 1968). In contrast, Hays and Kendall (1956) found that progesterone maintained pregnancy in vitamin A–deficient rabbits, and Juneja and associates (1969) found that pregnenolone, 17β-estradiol, transplants of pituitary homografts and, in some experiments, progesterone prevented resorption in rats maintained with retinoic acid. The positive effect of progesterone in the experiments with rabbits may have been due to nonspecific improvement in metabolism and to mobilization of trace reserves of vitamin A. Similar mechanisms may explain some of the responses obtained in rats given retinoic acid, but the beneficial effects of pregnenolone were clear-cut. Vitamin A as retinol or retinal probably has a direct effect in maintaining pregnancy. However, little is known about its mode of action other than that the earliest changes in its absence are found in the placenta (Howell et al., 1964; Calaustro and Lichtan, 1968), and that it may involve the biosynthesis of steroid hormones.

The chick embryo

Poultry nutritionists have long been aware that vitamin A deficiency in birds leads to a marked drop in egg production. The mechanisms involved have not been investigated in any detail, but cessation of egg production could be reasonably accounted for as a secondary effect of reduced feed intake, endocrine disturbances, or other vitamin A deficiency lesions not specifically concerned with reproduction.

The failure of vitamin A–deficient hens to produce eggs has prevented investigation of the effects of avitaminosis on chick embryos. Indeed, it could perhaps be justifiably concluded that vitamin A deficiency does not directly affect hatchability before it prevents egg production (Rubin and Bird, 1942).

When the biological activity of retinoic acid was investigated, it was discovered that in poultry, as in other animals, the acid maintained growth and general health and prevented the occurrence of overt vitamin A deficiency lesions other than blindness (Thompson et al., 1969). Furthermore, hens given vitamin A–deficient diets containing retinoic acid or methyl retinoate produced eggs at a normal rate and had high fertility after artificial insemination. These eggs, which for convenience may be called "retinoic acid eggs," invariably failed to hatch. Development was normal during the first 48 hr of incubation, but then was suddenly arrested (Thompson, 1969; Thompson et al., 1969). Normally, at this stage, large blood vessels make their appearance in the membrane surrounding the embryo, the *area vasculosa,* and they remain as conspicuous features in eggs incubated beyond this stage. These vessels never appeared in the retinoic acid eggs: the *area vasculosa* contained blood in islands and at the periphery, but in spite of continued expansion it did not appear to have an active circulatory system. The embryo grew markedly abnormal in appearance and eventually it died.

The embryos in the eggs of quail maintained with methyl retinoate die at exactly the same stage (Figs. 18.1, 18.2, 18.3; cf. Thompson, 1969). In order to insure complete absence of retinol and its derivatives from the eggs, it is essential that the hens themselves be reared, from the time they are hatched, on vitamin A–free diets containing retinoic acid or methyl retinoate. This takes 6 months in the domestic hen but only 6 weeks in quail. Thus, quail is a more convenient species than the domestic hen for the production of retinoic acid eggs. A diet containing methyl retinoate which is suitable for quail is shown in Table 18.3.

The abnormal development of the embryos in the retinoic acid eggs was shown to be due to a deficiency of vitamin A, which occurred because birds do not transfer retinoic acid to their eggs. When the hens were given supplements of retinol (as retinyl acetate), their eggs hatched normally. Thus the original abnormalities of embryonic development could not have been due to a toxic effect of the acid.

TABLE 18.3. *Composition of vitamin A–deficient diet containing methyl retinoate for quail*

Ingredients	Percentage
Soybean meal	45.00
Glucose	31.71
Soybean oil	8.00
DL-methionine	0.50
Mineral mixture [a]	6.04
Vitamin mixture [b]	0.50
$CaCO_3$ [c]	6.15
$CaHPO_4 \cdot 2H_2O$ [c]	1.60
Choline chloride	0.50

[a] Contains (per 100 g diet): $CaHPO_4 \cdot 2H_2O$, 2.722 g; $CaCO_3$, 1.355 g; KH_2PO_4, 0.868 g; NaCl, 0.713 g; $KHCO_3$, 0.21 g; MgO, 0.085 g; $MnCl_2 \cdot 4H_2O$, 46.6 mg; ferric citrate, 26.7 mg; ZnO, 6.9 mg; copper acetate, 3.4 mg; KI, 0.26 mg.

[b] A mixture in glucose containing (per 100 g diet): inositol, 25 mg; nicotinic acid, 5 mg; calcium pantothenate, 3 mg; thiamine•HCl, 1 mg; riboflavin, 1 mg; pyridoxine•MCl, 1 mg; folic acid, 0.4 mg; menadione, 0.12 mg; biotin, 0.011 mg; cholecalciferol 0.002 mg; vitamin B_{12}, 0.0014 mg; *dl*-α-tocopheryl acetate, 1 mg; ethoxyquin, 10 mg; and methyl retinoate, 1 mg.

[c] $CaCO_3$ and $CaHPO_4 \cdot 2H_2O$ should be replaced by glucose until egg production.

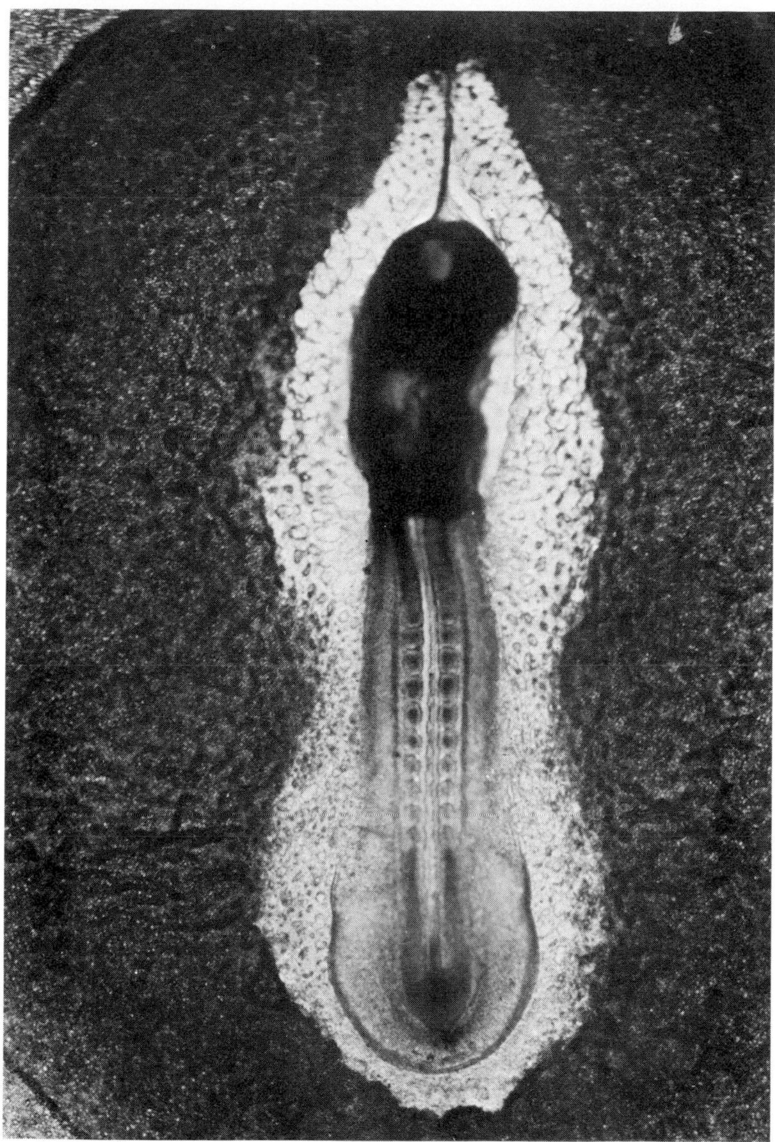

Fig. 18.1. Embryo after 2 days' incubation in egg from a quail given a vitamin A–deficient diet containing methyl retinoate. The embryo has reached the stage at which development ceases to be normal. A conspicuous feature is the absence of major blood vessels in the *area vasculosa*.

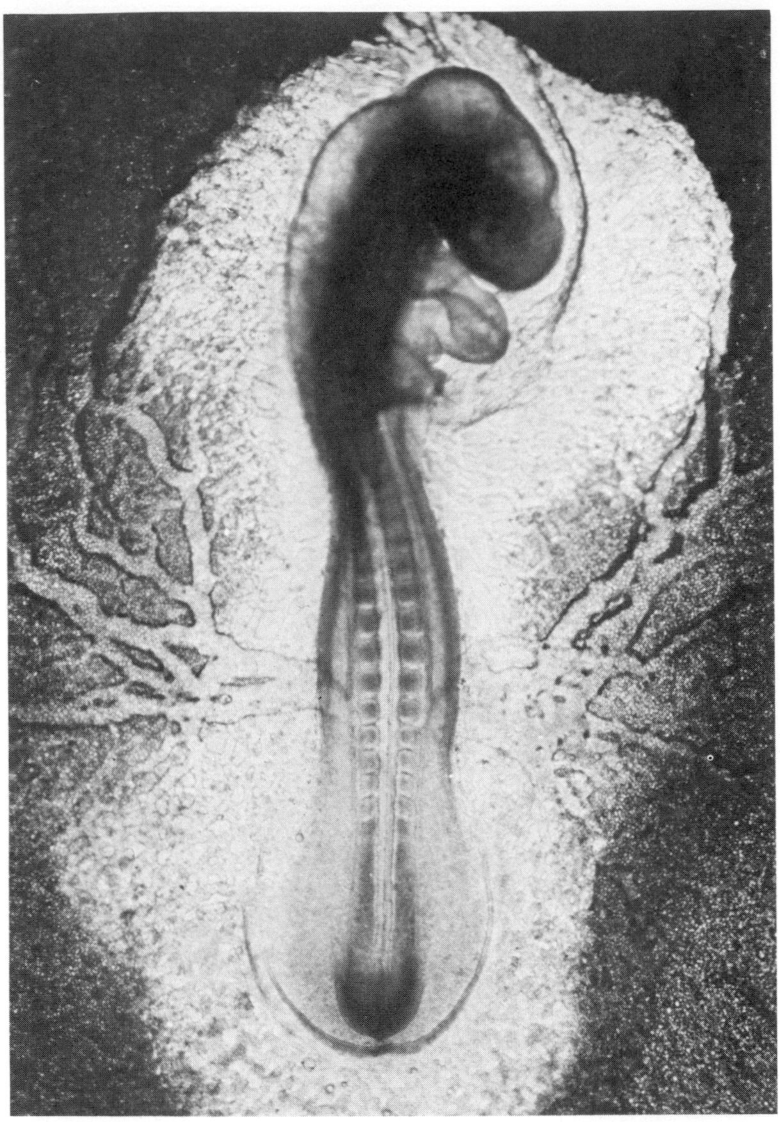

Fig. 18.2. Embryo after 3 days' incubation in egg from a quail given a vitamin A–deficient diet containing retinyl acetate, showing normal extra-embryonic circulatory system.

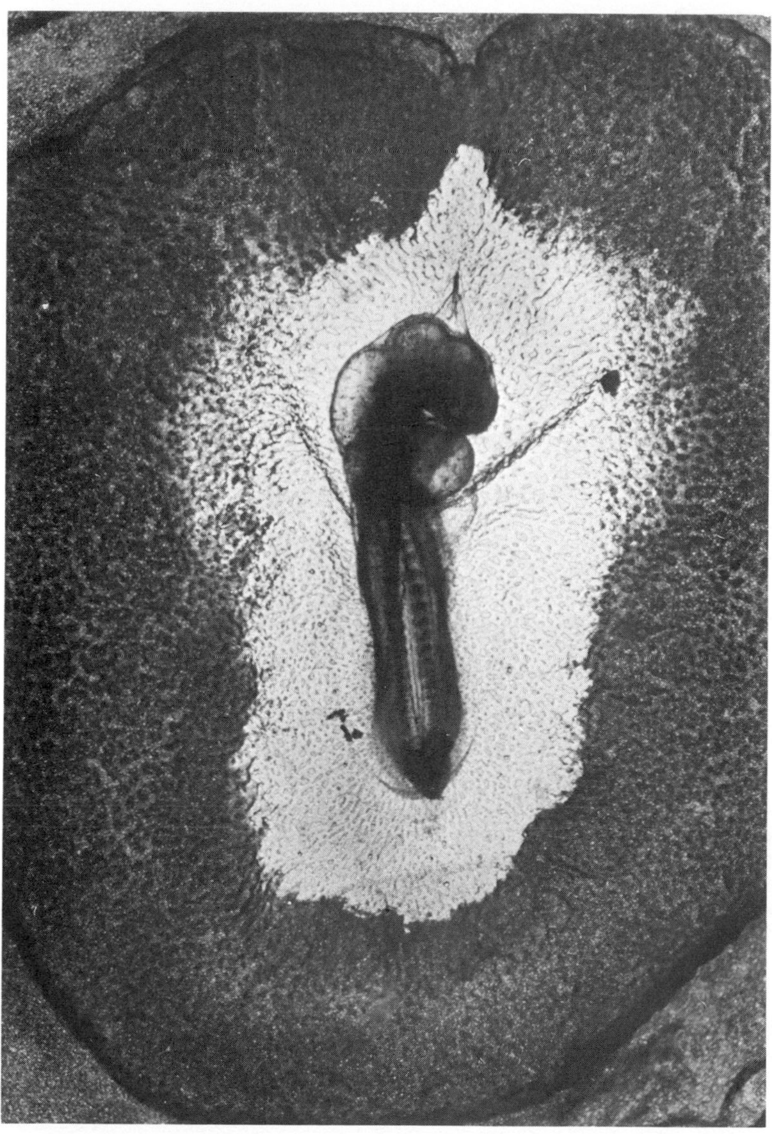

Fig. 18.3. Embryo after $2\frac{1}{2}$ days' incubation in egg from a quail given a vitamin A–deficient diet containing methyl retinoate. The embryo is malformed, and the *area vasculosa* still lacks major blood vessels.

The development of embryos in retinoic acid eggs could also be prolonged, although not always to hatching, by injecting vitamin A–active substances into the eggs before incubation. In tests of this kind it was demonstrated that retinol, retinal, retinyl acetate, and other sources of vitamin A would stimulate development, whereas substances lacking vitamin A activity had no beneficial effects (Table 18.4). Retinoic acid was slightly effective when small amounts were injected. Larger quantities of retinoic acid, since they are extremely toxic to normal-developing embryos, could not be meaningfully tested for activity in the retinoic acid eggs. An unexpected finding was that the ester of retinoic acid, methyl retinoate, was relatively innocuous in normal-developing eggs and was very effective in stimulating development of the embryos in retinoic acid eggs. Hitherto

TABLE 18.4. *Effect of vitamin A derivatives and other substances on embryonic development in retinoic acid eggs*

Substance administered [a]	Quantity (μg/egg)	Number of fertile eggs injected	Embryos stimulated (%)[b]
Untreated	—	470	0
Saline solution alone	—	120	0
Miscellaneous [c]	100 or 1000[c]	146	0
Retinol	20	35	34
	2	135	74
	0.5	30	40
	0.15	25	8
Retinyl acetate	20	36	25
Retinal	100	111	32
	50	27	56
	4	22	45
	2	28	43
β-carotene	100	112	12
Retinoic acid	2	60	2
	1	73	3
	0.5	42	2
	0.2	46	2
Methyl retinoate	100	196	20
	50	85	39
	10	68	31
	4	9	33
	2	40	45

Source: Thompson et al. (1969).

[a] Injected in 0.1 ml saline before incubation.

[b] Percentage of fertile embryos developing normally beyond 48 hr incubation.

[c] Eggs were injected with lutein (0.1 mg), folic acid (1 mg), vitamin B_{12} (0.1 mg), or biotin (0.1 mg).

methyl retinoate has been considered to be merely a stable source of retinoic acid when added to animal diets. Clearly, however, the free acid and the ester do not always have identical biological effects.

Conclusion

Primary functions of vitamin A in maintaining epithelial tissues, regulating bone growth, and forming visual pigment were recognized early in nutrition research. There is no doubt, however, that vitamin A has other roles in reproduction. The inability of retinoic acid to act in reproduction while being fully effective in other systemic roles of the vitamin implies that independent mechanisms are involved.

The inactivity of the acid in reproduction is in itself an interesting phenomenon. The inability of the acid to maintain the testes and the placenta suggests that they, like the retina, require retinol or retinal specifically. Alternatively, it is possible that in these tissues the acid merely fails to reach the active sites. This is almost certainly the explanation of the production of vitamin A–deficient embryos in the eggs of hens maintained with retinoic acid. The acid, especially when esterified, is able to satisfy at least some of the needs of the embryo when it is injected into the eggs. It must be concluded that the hen given retinoic acid in the diet is unable to deposit a useful quantity in her eggs.

Does the hen transfer a small amount of retinoic acid, or is the deficiency in the egg absolute? This is an important question in that the total absence of vitamin A derivatives from the retinoic acid eggs would imply that normal development of the embryos during the first two days of incubation does not require vitamin A.

The fundamental nature of the vitamin A requirement in embryos at and beyond two days of incubation and the relationship of this requirement to the need for vitamin A in growing and adult animals remain unexplained. These topics, together with the remarkable differences in biological activity between retinoic acid and its methyl ester, are suggested as starting points for new theory and experiment.

References

Arens, J. F., and D. A. van Dorp. 1946. Activity of vitamin A acid in the rat. *Nature 158*:622.

Calaustro, E. Q., and I. J. Lichten. 1968. Effects of retinoic acid and progesterone on reproductive performance in retinol-deficient female rat. *J. Nutr. 95*:517.

Coward, W. A., J. McC. Howell, G. A. J. Pitt, and J. N. Thompson. 1966. Effects of hormones on reproduction in rats fed a diet deficient in retinol (vitamin A alcohol) but containing methyl retinoate (vitamin A acid methyl ester). *J. Reprod. Fert. 12*:309.

Coward, W. A., and J. N. Thompson. 1967. Retinol and retinyl esters in rats fed small amounts of retinyl acetate. *Biochem. J. 103*:35P.

Dowling, J. E., and G. Wald. 1960. The biological function of vitamin A acid. *Proc. Nat. Acad. Sci. U.S.A. 46*:587.

Erb, R. E., F. N. Andrews, S. M. Hauge, and W. A. King. 1947. Observations on vitamin A deficiency in young dairy bulls. *J. Dairy Sci. 30*:687.

Hays, R. L., and K. A. Kendall. 1956. Beneficial effect of progesterone on pregnancy in the vitamin A deficient rabbit. *J. Nutr. 59*:337.

Hodgson, R. E., S. R. Hall., W. J. Sweetman, H. G. Wiseman, and H. T. Converse. 1946. The effect of vitamin A deficiency on reproduction in dairy bulls. *J. Dairy Sci. 29*:669.

Howell, J. McC., J. N. Thompson, and G. A. J. Pitt. 1963. Histology of the lesions produced in the reproductive tract of animals fed a diet deficient in vitamin A alcohol but containing vitamin A acid. I. The male rat. *J. Reprod. Fert. 5*:159.

Howell, J. McC., J. N. Thompson, and G. A. J. Pitt. 1964. Histology of the lesions produced in the reproductive tract of animals fed a diet deficient in vitamin A alcohol but containing vitamin A acid. II. The female rat. *J. Reprod. Fert. 7*:251.

Howell, J. McC., J. N. Thompson, and G. A. J. Pitt. 1967. Changes in the tissues of guinea-pigs fed on a diet free from vitamin A but containing methyl retinoate. *Brit. J. Nutr. 21*:37.

Juneja, H. S., N. R. Moudgal, and J. Ganguly. 1969. Studies on metabolism of vitamin A: The effect of hormones on gestation in retinoate-fed female rats. *Biochem. J. 111*:97.

Kochhar, D. M. 1967. Teratogenic activity of retinoic acid. *Acta Pathol. Microbiol. Scand. 70*:398.

Leathem, J. H. 1961. Nutritional affects on endocrine secretions, p. 666. *In* W. C. Young (ed.), *Sex and Internal Secretions*, 3rd ed. Vol. 1. Williams and Wilkins, Baltimore.

Mason, K. E. 1933. Differences in testis injury and repair after vitamin A–deficiency, vitamin E–deficiency, and inanition. *Amer. J. Anat. 52*:153.

Mason, K. E. 1935. Foetal death, prolonged gestation, and difficult parturition in the rat as a result of vitamin A–deficiency. *Amer. J. Anat. 57*:303.

Mason, K. E. 1939. Relation of the vitamins to the sex glands, p. 1149. *In* E. Allen (ed.), *Sex and Internal Secretions*, 2nd ed. Williams and Wilkins, Baltimore.

Mason, K. E., and J. N. Wolfe. 1930. The physiological activity of the hypophyses of rats under various experimental conditions. *Anat. Rec. 45*:232.

Mayer, J., and J. W. Goddard. 1951. Effects of administration of gonadotrophic hormone on vitamin A–deficient rats. *Proc. Soc. Exp. Biol. Med. 76*:149.

Mayer, J., and A. P. Truant. 1949. Effects of administration of testosterone on vitamin A–deficient rats. *Proc. Soc. Exp. Biol. Med. 72*:436.

Moore, T. 1957. *Vitamin A*. Elsevier, Amsterdam.

Nockels, C. F., and R. B. Herrick. 1969. Increased adrenal Δ^5-3β-hydroxysteroid dehydrogenase in vitamin A–deficient cockerels. *Proc. Soc. Exp. Biol. Med. 130*:410.

Nockels, C. F., and E. W. Kienholz. 1967. Influence of vitamin A deficiency on testes, bursa fabricius, adrenal and hematocrit in cockerels. *J. Nutr. 92*:384.

van Os, P. M. 1934. The influence of the gonadotrophic hormone from the urine on the testis with degenerated seminal tubules. *Acta Brev. Neerl. Physiol. 6*:151.

Palludan, B. 1966. Direct effect of vitamin A in boar testis. *Nature 211*:639.

Rubin, M., and H. R. Bird. 1942. Relation of vitamin A to egg production and hatchability. *Univ. Md. Agr. Exp. Sta. Bull. A12*:339.

Sutton, T. S., and B. J. Brief. 1939. Physiologic changes in the anterior hypophysis of vitamin A–deficient rats. *Endocrinology 25*:302.

Thompson, J. N. 1969. Vitamin A in development of embryo. *Amer. J. Clin. Nutr. 22*:1063.

Thompson, J. N., J. McC. Howell, and G. A. J. Pitt. 1964. Vitamin A and reproduction in rats. *Proc. Roy. Soc.* [*Biol.*] *159*:510.

Thompson, J. N., J. McC. Howell, and G. A. J. Pitt. 1965. Nutritional factors affecting fertility: Vitamin A, p. 34. *In* C. R. Austin and J. S. Perry (eds.), *Biological Council Symposium on Agents Affecting Fertility*. J. & A. Churchill, London.

Thompson, J. N., J. McC. Howell, G. A. J. Pitt, and C. I. McLaughlin. 1969. The biological activity of retinoic acid in the domestic fowl and the effects of vitamin A deficiency on the chick embryo. *Brit. J. Nutr. 23*:471.

C

VITAMIN A DEFICIENCY IN GERM-FREE RATS

N. Raica, Jr., M. A. Stedham, Y. F. Herman, and H. E. Sauberlich

Studies on the characteristics of vitamin A–deficient, germ-free rats have been reported by Beaver (1961) and by Bieri and co-workers (1969). There were two significant differences noted in germ-free rats as compared with conventional rats. The most interesting finding was that of Bieri and co-workers, who reported that although both types of rats stopped growing after a comparable period of time, the germ-free rats were able to survive for many weeks with a vitamin A deficiency. Beaver did not find any differences in longevity. Although the lesions which developed as a result of vitamin A deficiency were comparable in germ-free and conventional rats, they were more extensive in the germ-free rat. In neither study with germ-free rats were data presented on tooth or bone development.

The study being reported in this note was undertaken to determine whether germ-free rats utilize β-carotene as effectively as do conventional rats. Data are also presented to support the finding of increased longevity in the vitamin A–deficient germ-free rats. Pathological data, particularly on tooth development, is included as well.

Preparation of germ-free animals

Mature germ-free female and male rats of the Fisher strain were purchased from Charles River Breeding Laboratories and bred in a sterile environment. During lactation the mothers were fed the steam-sterilized vitamin A–deficient diet described in Table C.1. The young were weaned at about

The assistance of Capt. R. R. Maronpot in initiating the pathological investigations and of Sp5 D. Rath in working with the germ-free animals is very much appreciated.

The principles of laboratory animal care as promulgated by the National Society for Medical Research were observed.

TABLE C.1. *Vitamin A–deficient diet for germ-free rats*

Ingredient	Percentage
Casein, vitamin free	22.0
Starch	61.8
Cottonseed oil	5.0
Salt mix (U.S.P. IV)	4.0
Cellulose	3.0
DL-methionine	0.2
Starch-vitamin mix[a]	4.0

Note: the diet was steam sterilized at 252 F for 30 min. This is the standard diet for germ-free rats except that the standard diet includes 0.50 mg of retinyl palmitate per 100 g of diet.

[a] The vitamin content per 100 g of diet was as follows: vitamin D_3, 2.5 μg; α-tocopherol, 50 mg; menadione, 10 mg; thiamine HCl, 6 mg; riboflavin, 3 mg; nicotinamide, 5 mg; nicotinic acid, 5 mg; calcium pantothenate, 30 mg; inositol, 100 mg; choline chloride, 200 mg; pyridoxine HCl, 2.0 mg; pyridoxamine HCl, 0.4 mg; biotin, 0.1 mg; folic acid, 1.0 mg; PABA, 5 mg; cyanocobalamine, 2.5 μg.

21 days and were maintained in groups of 2–4 rats in sterile, wire-bottomed, metal cages. After the rats had been maintained on the vitamin A–deficient diet for a period of 80 days, growth of the animals leveled off. They were continued on the vitamin A–free diet for a total of 148 days, at which time they were divided into two equal groups and provided a daily oral supplement of either 15 μg of retinol as retinyl acetate or 28 μg of β-carotene in cottonseed oil. The oil solutions were sterilized by filtration. After 19 days of supplementation, the animals were not fed for 24 hr and were then killed. Tissues were removed for pathological examination and measurement of liver retinol stores. Livers were saponified and extracted with ether, and the retinol was determined by the trifluoroacetic acid procedure of Neeld and Pearson (1963).

Liver stores of vitamin A in the germ-free state

After 140 days on the vitamin A–deficient diet, two males showed symptoms of cecal volvulus (lethargy, extended abdomen, no fecal droppings, reduced food consumption, and porphyrin accumulation around the eyes). These rats were killed and their livers analyzed for total content of vitamin A, which was found to be less than 0.5 μg per liver. A similar value was observed for a germ-free female rat that was maintained on the vitamin

TABLE C.2. *Liver vitamin A stores in the depleted germ-free rat*

Rats studied	Period of depletion	Weight (g)	Retinol per liver (μg)
Males (2)	140 days	182[a]	< 0.5
Females (1)	168 days[b]	188	< 0.5

[a] Average body weight of two rats.
[b] Study terminated.

A–deficient diet until termination of the study (168 days). Data are presented in Table C.2.

Table C.3 shows body weights at selected intervals during the depletion period. The body weights of the four remaining males declined after first leveling off. Early in the supplementation period all four males showed symptoms of volvulus complication. These complications may have been related to the weight loss noted during the final phase of the depletion period.

TABLE C.3. *Body weights of germ-free rats during vitamin A depletion*

	Weight of rats (g)	
Time on deficient diet	Males (4)	Females (6)
10 days	77 ± 22	76 ± 14
80 days	236 ± 9	158 ± 4
110 days	225 ± 14	169 ± 6
148 days[a]	203 ± 22	170 ± 8

Note: Values are given as mean ± SD.
[a] End of depletion period.

Of the two males that died, only one had a volvulus. The two surviving males receiving retinol were killed and were found to have volvulus. Their total liver retinol content after 6 and 13 days of supplementation were 9.6 μg and 16.2 μg, respectively.

Weight gains and liver retinol stored after supplementation are shown in Table C.4. Although the weight gains in the two groups are essentially

TABLE C.4. *Effect of vitamin A repletion in germ-free rats*

Supplement	Starting weight (g)	Ending weight (g)	Total retinol per liver (μg)
Carotene	174 ± 4	195 ± 3	70.8 ± 1.4
Retinol	166 ± 9	185 ± 14	85.3 ± 11.3

Notes: Six female germ-free rats were fed a vitamin A–deficient diet (Table C.1) for 148 days and then a supplemented diet for 19 days. The daily individual supplement was 28 μg of β-carotene for half the rats and 15 μg of retinol for the other half.

Values are given as mean ± SD.

equal, total liver retinol stores were slightly less in the carotene-supplemented group. These data are consistent with the conclusions of the Expert Committee on Biological Standardization (1950) that retinol, when fed to rats at relatively low levels, was twice as effective biologically as β-carotene, i.e., 1 IU of vitamin A is equal to 0.6 μg of β-carotene or 0.3 μg of retinol.

Pathology of vitamin A deficiency in the germ-free state

Necropsy showed an absence of gross lesions in the females, except for worn, chalky, white teeth. In the two males, in addition to the abnormal teeth, there were enlarged accessory sex glands and flaky proteinaceous material in the urinary bladder. Eye lesions were absent in the animals examined both grossly and microscopically. Other lesions caused by vitamin A deficiency were seen in each of the nine rats examined microscopically.

Odontopathy of the incisor teeth was consistently present. The changes consisted of an excess labial dentin and a reduced amount of lingual dentin, as shown in sagittal section (Fig. C.1). The hyperplastic labial dentin was knobby and irregularly stained at its anterior surface. On the pulp side of the labial dentin, various odontoblast configurations deviating from the normally palisaded arrangement of the cells were observed.

Salivary glands were examined in four rats, and in each case squamous metaplasia of ductular epithelium was seen. In one rat mucous glands of the soft palate had squamous metaplasia and cornification of the glandular acini, or small ducts. In two rats in which adequate pancreatic tissue was submitted, squamous metaplasia of interlobular pancreatic ducts was present.

In all females, kidneys contained numerous lamellate mineral crystals primarily at the cortico-medullary junction. These crystals were positive on both Von Kossa and alizarin red stained sections, indicating the presence of calcium salts. One of the two males had a very small number of crystals. Lesions were not seen in the two urinary bladders submitted.

Uterine or vaginal lesions were absent in the four female animals examined. Sperm production was not evident in either male. In one male rat, atrophy and contraction of the seminiferous tubules were indicated by a pronounced separation between the basement membranes and interstitium. Dilation and accumulation of proteinaceous materials were seen in the bulbo-urethral glands of both rats. Other male accessory sex organs had degrees of epithelial hyperplasia and metaplasia with cornification.

The liver of one female had undergone severe fatty changes and ballooning degeneration of a few subscapular hepatocytes, but no inflammation seen. The liver of another female contained multiple accumulations of

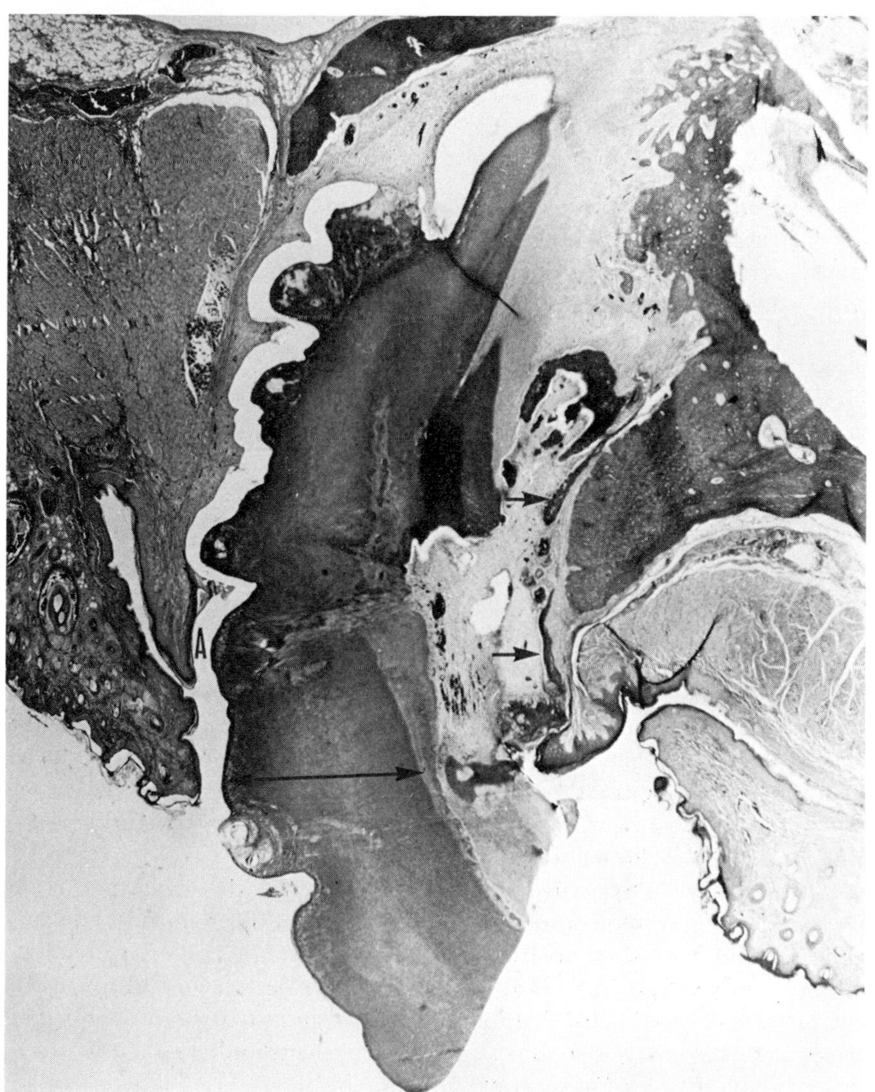

Fig. C.1. Incisor tooth of vitamin A–deficient germ-free rat, sagittal section (18×). The greatly thickened labial dentin (double-pointed arrow) has an irregular, knobby surface. The knobs are irregularly stained and some contain cells of the enamel organ. The enamel space, A (vacated by routine tissue processing), is also irregular. The lingual dentin (arrows) is thinner than normal and is discontinuous. The lesions of the pulp cavity (odontoblast proliferation and hemorrhage) are not seen in detail at this magnification.

mononuclear inflammatory cells but no cellular degeneration. All livers contained some degree of hemosiderosis.

Discussion

Prior to the initiation of this study, eight germ-free rats were maintained on a vitamin A–deficient diet for several months. Growth ceased about 40 days after weaning and remained constant until the study was terminated by vitamin A supplementation. The only overt symptoms of vitamin A deficiency were transient diarrhea, slight paralysis of the hind quarters, loss of hair around the eyes, worn, chalky, white teeth, and growth arrest. In the present study growth did not stop until 80 days after weaning.

Although adequate controls were not utilized, the data support the conclusion that vitamin A deficiency was established and also confirm the findings of Bieri and co-workers in regard to the longevity of vitamin A–deficient germ-free rats. Other studies in this laboratory with the same strain of germ-free rat on an identical diet (supplemented with vitamin A) resulted in normal growth, tooth development, and tooth pigmentation.

In our studies, the eye lesions (xerophthalmia) described by Beaver (1961) and Bieri and co-workers (1969) did not occur; this cannot be explained. A transient porphyrin accumulation around the eyes was observed in some of our rats; however, this accumulation was also found to occur in vitamin A–sufficient germ-free rats that developed a volvulus. Moore (1957) has stated that eye lesions may not always occur in rats because death may occur before the lesions can develop. Therefore, the rate of onset of severe vitamin A deficiency and its attendant complications may influence the development of xerophthalmia.

In his review Moore cited data which suggested that vitamin A may be required for detoxification. If this is a function of vitamin A, the conventional rat may then succumb not only to infection, as suggested by various studies (e.g., Bieri et al., 1969), but also to toxicants of microbial origin. The reduced detoxification load in the germ-free rat probably contributes to longevity, but also suggests that the germ-free rat may have reduced vitamin A requirements.

The lesions seen in these vitamin A–deficient rats are similar to those described by Beaver (1961), but enough differences are present to be noteworthy. In Beaver's study the most remarkable changes were in the liver, where hyalin droplet degeneration to frank liver necrosis was seen. In our rats, only one had degenerative hepatocytes. The reneal calcification seen in all females and one of the males in our study may or may not have been due to vitamin A deficiency. Nephritis, nephrosis, and mineral deposition are commonly seen in rats, although usually in older rats. Beaver reported rather extensive tubular calcification in three out of ten vitamin A–deficient germ-free rats, the oldest of which were about four months; our rats were killed at about seven months. Incisor teeth lesions, a characteristic of vitamin A–deficient rats previously described by Schour and Massler (1942), occurred most frequently.

Conclusions

Germ-free vitamin A–deficient rats utilize β-carotene and retinol as effectively as do conventional rats, as measured by growth and liver retinol stores. The presence of vitamin A deficiency was established by very low liver stores of retinol, growth arrest, mild hindquarter paralysis, transient diarrhea, response to oral supplementation with retinol or β-carotene, and pathological data. Xerophthalmia was not found in this study when rats were examined either grossly or microscopically. Longevity of the vitamin A–deficient germ-free rat has been confirmed.

References

Beaver, D. L. 1961. Vitamin A deficiency in the germ-free rat. *Amer. J. Pathol. 38*:335–357.

Bieri, J. G., E. G. McDaniel, and W. E. Rogers, Jr. 1969. Survival of germfree rats without vitamin A. *Science 163*:574–575.

Expert Committee on Biological Standardization. 1950. World Health Organ. Tech. Rep. Series No. 3.

Moore, T. 1957. *Vitamin A*. Elsevier, Amsterdam.

Neeld, J. B., and W. N. Pearson. 1963. Macro- and micromethods for the determination of serum vitamin A using trifluoroacetic acid. *J. Nutr. 79*:454–462.

Schour, I., and M. Massler. 1942. The teeth, chap. 6. *In* J. Q. Griffith and E. J. Farris (ed.), *The Rat in Laboratory Investigation*. J. B. Lippincott, Philadelphia.

VITAMIN E

19

VITAMIN E AND THE BIOLOGICAL ANTIOXIDANT THEORY

J. Green

The problem of the biological role of vitamin E in animals is still unsolved, and it is well known that two schools of thought exist. Some workers consider that, although the pathological effects of deficiency are diverse, the vitamin's action may well involve a specific biochemical mechanism (or perhaps several such mechanisms) yet to be discovered. Other workers, on the basis of arguments to be discussed below, consider that vitamin E functions in vivo solely as a physiological lipid antioxidant (Tappel, 1962). According to this hypothesis, random, free radical–catalyzed lipid peroxidation is a continual biological process, which damages cellular and intracellular structures and destroys certain enzymes and other labile intracellular components. It is suggested that vitamin E inhibits this process and that, in its absence, the various pathological signs of disease occur. Many workers consider that both theories of vitamin E action are viable and that they may not be either inconsistent or mutually exclusive.

Basis of the antioxidant theory

There are five types of evidence that provide the theoretical and practical basis for the theory. They are as follows:

1. The fact that α-tocopherol is a lipid antioxidant, albeit not a very powerful one, in vitro.

2. The well substantiated nutritional relationship between dietary unsaturated fat and the onset and incidence of vitamin E deficiency disease in numerous species. This relationship, which has been quantified by Harris and Embree (1963), is, in fact, a complex one, involving factors such as the peroxidative effects of unsaturated fat on vitamin E in the diet, the continuation and enhancement of these effects in the intestinal tract, and probably more than one facet of a physiological interdependence.

3. The demonstration that the tissues of vitamin E–deficient animals are more peroxidizable than those of supplemented animals and the apparent demonstration that the former tissues contain more lipid peroxides than do the latter.

4. Suggestions that labile substances – such as vitamin A, SH–containing enzymes, ascorbic acid, and ATP – are protected by vitamin E from peroxidative destruction in the tissues.

5. The fact that certain other substances, which show antioxidant properties in vitro, can fulfill part of the function of vitamin E in some species.

Although a wealth of largely circumstantial detail has been gathered in support of the above ideas, examination reveals many anomalies that are difficult to explain. There is, in fact, little direct evidence that lipid peroxidation is a continuing process in all tissues or that vitamin E prevents it or that the proposed process is damaging. Nor have there been many attempts to test the validity of the theory's postulates and predictions by direct experiment. A critical examination of the theory now follows.

The peroxidation process

Direct tests for peroxidation in tissues have been singularly uninformative. Dam and Granados (1945) first attempted direct measurement of true lipid peroxides in the adipose tissue of vitamin E–deficient rats and chicks given diets containing cod-liver oil, and they found up to 190 μ-equiv per g. Emmel and LaCelle (1961) reported much larger values in the adipose tissue of rats given large amounts of unsaturated fats. Bunyan and coworkers (1967*b*) found very much lower peroxide values in adipose tissue even when the diet contained large amounts of polyunsaturated fatty acids, and they showed that extreme care was necessary to prevent peroxidation of tissue lipids after death and during the subsequent analytical procedure. They found that rat liver, kidneys, testes, and leg muscle normally contained peroxides in the range of 10–40 μ-equiv per g lipid and the values were not altered by substantial changes in the unsaturation of the dietary lipid or by vitamin E or synthetic antioxidants. They found no increase in the peroxide value of tissues in nutritional liver necrosis or testicular degeneration in the rat nor in chicks with exudative diathesis or encephalomalacia. The adipose tissue of rats given oleic acid as the only dietary lipid was almost peroxide-free, and even large quantities of dietary polyunsaturated fatty acids only raised the peroxide value to a maximum of 40 μ-equiv per g lipid. In contrast to the absence of effect in other tissues, vitamin E readily reduced the peroxide value of adipose tissue.

Bunyan and co-workers (1968) gave multiple doses of cod-liver-oil esters or corn-oil esters to vitamin E–deficient rats for 4 weeks, under conditions in which the lipids did not mix with other food. They found that, even when the esters were peroxidized before use, lipid peroxides did not accumulate in the adipose tissue. They suggested that the peroxides normally accumulating in the adipose tissue of vitamin E–deficient animals may be largely exogenous.

Effects on polyunsaturated fatty acid (PUFA) metabolism

If vitamin E is a generalized tissue antioxidant, vitamin E deficiency in animals might perhaps lead to a generalized loss of PUFA from the tissues, especially those of target organs. Certain specific effects of vitamin E deficiency on the PUFA composition of tissues have been demonstrated. Hove and Hove (1953) found lowered linoleate in rabbit and rat brains. Bieri and Andrews (1964) found lowered docosopentaenoate levels and raised linoleate, arachidonate, and docosatetraenoate levels in rat testis, but little change in other organs. Witting and Horwitt (1964) found less total PUFA in the muscle of vitamin E–deficient rats given unsaturated lipids than in the muscle of vitamin E–supplemented controls. There is no evidence, however, of a generalized loss of PUFA in vitamin E deficiency. Bernhard (1958) found no change in rat brain, liver, lungs, spleen, or depot fat, and this was confirmed by Bunyan and co-workers (1967*a*). Recently, Lee and Barnes (1969) have studied rats for 14 months, and they also found little consistent change in the PUFA composition of vitamin E–deficient animals during this period.

Metabolism of α-tocopherol

If lipid peroxidation in vivo is mechanistically and kinetically identical with the process in vitro, it follows that in vitamin E–deficient tissues its rate must be enhanced (Witting, 1965). Factors that exacerbate vitamin E deficiency could be regarded as "prooxidant" and would thus be expected to increase the peroxidative destruction of vitamin E in the tissues (Dam and Granados, 1945; Hove, 1955; Weber et al., 1962).

There is, in fact, little evidence that this is the case, except in experiments in which admixture of unsaturated fat into the diet could be expected to lead to destruction of vitamin E before feeding or in the gastrointestinal tract. Thus, Markson and co-workers (1957) found no difference in vitamin E levels in the livers of chicks with and without encephalomalacia, and Fisher and Kaunitz (1965) reported similar findings in chicks with exudative diathesis. Blaxter and co-workers (1953) produced muscular dystrophy in calves with dietary cod-liver oil and found, in fact, more tocopherol in the muscles of affected animals than in those of controls. Harris and Mason (1956) state that kidney autolysis in rats, produced by feeding them large amounts of highly unsaturated fatty acids for long periods, is not associated with low tocopherol concentrations in the kidney. Fitch and Dinning (1963) found that the rate of depletion of serum tocopherol in vitamin E–deficient monkeys over 400 days was unaffected by the presence of unsaturated fat in their diet.

It has now been shown that a number of disease-inducing stresses in the vitamin E–deficient animal do not, in fact, increase the rate of metabolism of previously administered small doses of radioactive α-tocopherol. This has been shown for dietary polyunsaturated fatty acids in the rat (Green et al., 1967*a*) and in the chick (Diplock et al., 1967*a*). Selenium deficiency, likewise, does not increase tocopherol metabolism in the chick (Diplock et al., 1967*a*) or in the rat (Green et al., 1967*b*).

Metabolism of secondary antioxidants and hydrogen donors

As seen above, the direct evidence does not appear to support the concept that dietary-fat stress is associated with an increase in tocopherol metabolism, as is required by the antioxidant theory. Tappel (1962) suggested that α-tocopherol might be potentiated in vivo by hydrogen donors such as ascorbic acid or sulfhydryl compounds, which might act as secondary antioxidants for the inhibitory reactions. However, there is no evidence that there is either increased metabolism or lowered levels of these compounds in the vitamin E–deficient animals. Lindan and Work (1953) found no relation between the incidence of liver necrosis and hepatic ascorbic acid or glutathione levels in the rat. Although Budowski and Mokadi (1961) found lowered hydrazyl-reactive compounds in the cerebella of chicks with encephalomalacia, Glavind and Søndergaard (1964*a*, 1964*b*) found no relationship between lipid-soluble antioxidant levels in chick brain and the incidence of encephalomalacia, nor between antioxidant levels in rat liver and the onset of liver necrosis. Calvert and Scott (1962) found glutathione levels to be increased in the skeletal muscle of vitamin E–deficient chicks with muscular dystrophy. Green and co-workers (1967*a*) showed that an increase in dietary PUFA did not affect ascorbic acid or sulfhydryl group levels in the rat.

Anti–vitamin E stress factors

A number of dietary and environmental stress factors have been shown to lead to clinical signs of disease and death in animals deprived of vitamin E. Others have since been demonstrated, and selenium is now known also to counteract, at least in part, such vitamin E "antagonists."

Hove (1955) suggested that anti–vitamin E stress factors might act as prooxidants, preventing lipid peroxidation in tissues. However, there has been no experimental demonstration that this occurs in vivo. Diplock and co-workers (1967*c*) were able to produce a high incidence of liver necrosis and death in weanling rats given a low-casein diet and silver acetate (0.15% in the drinking water or 130 ppm in the diet). Vitamin E and selenium prevented the disease. Nevertheless, it was found that the silver treatment did not increase the metabolism of small doses of radioactive α-tocopherol administered previously; in fact, the silver-treated animals contained more hepatic α-tocopherol than did the controls. Diplock and co-workers (1967*b*) made a similar study of iron toxicity in the vitamin E–deficient rat. Golberg and Smith (1958), who studied the toxic effects of iron given by injection, showed that it could be counteracted by vitamin E and suggested that the toxicity was caused by a prooxidant effect on lipid peroxidation. However, Diplock and co-workers (1967*b*) showed that iron overloading did not cause an increase in tocopherol metabolism, nor was there any increased destruction of tocopherol when the rats were given dietary cod-liver oil as well as the iron injections. In fact, as was observed with silver, the tissues of the iron-treated animals contained significantly more tocopherol than did those of the controls.

Synthetic antioxidants and vitamin E function

Of the five classes of evidence that can be considered to provide a basis for the biological antioxidant theory, four have now been examined and appear to fail to support the theory adequately. The problem of the vitamin E–like action of certain synthetic antioxidants remains. It is still difficult to decide whether these substances function in place of vitamin E, whether they merely spare vitamin E, or, indeed, whether, these substances have some other functions. Detailed examination of the problem yields a number of anomalies. If synthetic antioxidants are active simply because they spare vitamin E, that is likely to take place, in my opinion, before absorption rather than in the tissues. The distinction is important, since the evidence already examined above does not support the idea that α-tocopherol or any other substance can be shown to be protected from peroxidation in the tissues. In a review of the activity of antioxidants in vitamin E–deficiency diseases, Dam (1957) showed that many of their effects could certainly be attributed to the protection of traces of vitamin E in the diet and, possibly, in the gastrointestinal tract.

The two most active antioxidants, which might be considered to have true physiological activity, are DPPD (*N,N′*-diphenylphenylenediamine) and ethoxyquin (6-ethoxy-1,2-dihydro-2,2,4-trimethylquinoline). The former substance has been shown to have vitamin E–like activity in many deficiency diseases in different species, and, according to Draper and coworkers (1964), it prevents gestation-resorption in the rat even on highly purified amino acid diets, without fat and rigorously purified from traces of vitamin E. However, the remarkable synergistic effects discovered to exist between vitamin E, selenium, and antioxidants (Bieri, 1964; Thompson and Scott, 1969) must still impose a note of caution, and it is desirable that the interesting experiment of Draper and co-workers (1964) be repeated in the presence of vitamin E–free dietary fat. Questions still remain, however, even concerning the roles of DPPD and ethoxyquin. DPPD, for example, is apparently only poorly active against exudative diathesis in the chick, whereas much more poorly active antioxidants, such as Antabus (tetraethylthiuram disulfide) and NDGA (nordihydroguaiaretic acid) are effective against this disease. DPPD, moreover, is virtually inactive against muscular dystrophy in the chick or the rabbit. Ethoxyquin, similarly, is highly active against diseases like encephalomalacia in the chick but is inactive against many other deficiency diseases. Green and Bunyan (1969) have recently reviewed the whole field of antioxidant activity and have drawn attention to many such problems, to which the generalized antioxidant theory is unable to give adequate answers.

Carbon tetrachloride toxicity, vitamin E function, and synthetic antioxidants

For the purpose of further examining the possible roles of vitamin E and synthetic antioxidants, we studied CCl_4 toxicity in the rat. This substance, in small doses, is a liver poison, producing a centrilobular necrotic lesion and extensive hepatic fat accumulation. Larger doses produce death in coma, usually in about 24 hr. Hove (1948) showed that survival in CCl_4-treated rats could be increased by pretreatment for several weeks with dietary vitamin E, and Hove (1955) suggested that CCl_4 might be toxic because it increased tissue lipid peroxidation. Gallagher (1961) found that large doses of vitamin E given intraperitoneally to rats 40 hr before CCl_4 was administered significantly increased survival, and he found that DPPD was also highly active, even when given later than the vitamin E. Recknagel (1967) and Slater (1966) have recently revived the lipid peroxidation theory of CCl_4 toxicity.

Green and co-workers (1969) studied the relationship between CCl_4 toxicity and peroxidation. They showed that malondialdehyde production by microsomal fractions of rat liver during incubation with CCl_4 could not be related to the hepatotoxic action of CCl_4 in vivo, nor could evidence be found of increased lipid peroxides in the livers of CCl_4-treated rats.

Furthermore, toxic doses of CCl_4 did not increase the catabolism of previously administered ^{14}C-α-tocopherol, and, in fact, significantly more α-tocopherol was found in the liver of CCl_4-treated animals than in that of untreated controls. (Cf. the results with silver and iron.)

Critical examination of the literature on the relationship between CCl_4 toxicity and vitamin E reveals many contradictory reports.

1. It seems that, although long-term treatment with dietary vitamin E may increase survival, very large doses given prophylactically may also have some effect, provided the dose is given about 40 hr before CCl_4 is administered.

2. Most reports suggested that vitamin E is ineffective against the hepatic fat accumulation, and the evidence concerning the effect of vitamin E on the liver necrosis is conflicting.

Cawthorne and co-workers (1970) have made a detailed study of the problem and the following tables summarize much of our work. Young adult rats of both sexes were used, and CCl_4 was given orally, as were the pretreatments. Two levels of CCl_4 were used: 2.0 ml/kg to produce sub-acute toxicity with hepatic lesions and larger doses to produce acute toxicity and death. The LD_{80} was about 4.0 ml/kg in males and about 8.5 ml/kg in females. Survival was measured after 72 hr, and necrotic de-

TABLE 19.1. *Effect of oral doses of vitamin E on the acute toxicity of CCl_4 in male and female rats*

		Vitamin E given		Survival [a]	
Test	Sex	Dose (mg/kg)	Time before CCl_4 (hr)	Controls	Vitamin E–treated rats
1	Male	450	72, 48, 24	13/35	24/24[b]
2	Male	450	72	12/20	8/10
3	Male	450	48	12/20	10/10
4	Male	450	24	12/20	9/10
5	Female	450	72, 48, 24	8/34	21/30[b]
6	Female	450	72, 48, 24	5/14	3/9
7	Female	450	96, 72, 48, 24	3/20	0/9
8	Female	450	72	11/31	6/20
9	Female	450	48	11/30	3/19
10	Female	2000	48	6/17	3/10
11	Female	450	24	16/44	6/29
12	Female	2000	24	11/31	3/19
13	Female	450	6	16/44	4/27[c]
14	Female	2000	6	6/17	2/8

Note: The rats, weight range 160–220 g, were given a stock diet. Males were given 3.5 ml/kg of CCl_4 and females 8.5 ml/kg orally, after preliminary doses of D-α-tocopheryl acetate, as described.

[a] No. alive 72 hr after CCl_4 / Total no. in group.

[b] Significantly greater than the survival of rats not given vitamin E, $P < 0.001$.

[c] Significantly less than the survival of rats not given vitamin E, $P < 0.05$.

generation was assessed (in the experiments on subacute toxicity) by histological examination, according to an arbitrary scale as follows: +++, severe; ++, moderate; +, slight. Neutral triglycerides in liver were measured by the usual methods.

Table 19.1 summarizes the effects of pretreatment with oral D-α-tocopheryl acetate on survival in rats. There is clearly a considerable difference in effect on males and on females; only the former are adequately protected. Table 19.2 summarizes the effects of vitamin E against subacute toxicity in female rats, when the vitamin E was given in single and multiple doses at various times before CCl_4 was administered. There was virtually no prevention of the necrosis and none of the fatty accumulation. Indeed, as the vitamin E dose was increased to very large levels, there was a significant increase in hepatic triglycerides. These findings confirm the large majority of literature reports (cf. McLean, 1967). The most important feature of the results was that the level of vitamin E in the liver appeared not to be related to the effect. Thus, a comparison of Tables 19.1 and 19.2

TABLE 19.2. *Liver necrosis and hepatic triglyceride (TG) levels in female rats treated with CCl_4 and with vitamin E*

Vitamin E given					
Dose (mg/kg)	Time before CCl_4 (hr)	Liver weight (%body weight)	Liver TG (mg/g)	Liver tocopherol [a] (μg/g)	Necrosis
		TEST 1			
—	[b]	3.7 ± 0.2[b]	22.4 ± 6.7[b]	—	—
—	—	4.2 ± 0.2	82.6 ± 24.0	13 ± 1	+++
450	72, 48, 24	4.9 ± 0.6[c]	73.9 ± 34.9	313 ± 93	+++
450	72	3.8 ± 0.1	67.7 ± 19.2	5 ± 6	+++
450	24	4.3 ± 0.3	72.8 ± 18.6	117 ± 36	++
450	6	4.2 ± 0.4	97.0 ± 13.1	141 ± 60	+++
		TEST 2			
—	[b]	—	20.1 ± 5.7[b]	—	—
—	—	4.0 ± 0.2	49.7 ± 19.0	—	+++
2000	48	4.0 ± 0.4	53.9 ± 30.6	210 ± 168	+++
2000	24	4.2 ± 0.4	52.7 ± 21.7	499 ± 143	+++
2000	6	4.0 ± 0.2	105.3 ± 27.7[c]	105 ± 57	+++

Notes: The rats, six in each group, were given a stock diet and were dosed with 2.0 ml/kg of CCl_4. They were killed 24 hr later. D-α-tocopheryl acetate was given before CCl_4 at the times shown.

Values are given as mean ± SD.

[a] These analyses in parallel similar groups killed at the same time as CCl_4 was given to other groups in the table.

[b] No CCl_4 given.

[c] Significantly greater than controls, $P < 0.001$.

shows that, although the hepatic level of α-tocopherol is very low 72 hr after dosage with vitamin E, the treatment is highly effective in preventing mortality in male rats. In females the treatment is ineffective, even though higher hepatic levels can be attained.

A similar series of experiments was then carried out with ethoxyquin, and Tables 19.3 and 19.4 summarize the results with female rats. Parallel experiments showed that there was no difference in the response of males and females to this antioxidant. The effects on survival are completely clear-cut and they are paralleled by the effects on the necrotic and fatty lesions. Ethoxyquin pretreatment gave almost complete protection against both mortality and the liver lesions, provided that it was given at least 48 hr before CCl_4. Hepatic ethoxyquin levels were measured, and they clearly demonstrated that there was very little ethoxyquin in the liver at the time the CCl_4 was given. The liver increased significantly in weight after ethoxyquin treatment, and it is apparent that the substance is acting not as an antioxidant (for it is not present in the liver at the critical time) but by some indirect means.

A similar series of experiments was carried out with butylated hydroxytoluene (BHT) which, unlike ethoxyquin, has very little activity in vitamin

TABLE 19.3. *Effects of oral doses of ethoxyquin and BHT on the acute toxicity of CCl_4 in female rats*

Pretreatment		Survival [a]	
Dose (mg/kg)	Time before CCl_4 (hr)	Controls	Pretreated
ETHOXYQUIN			
300	72, 48, 24	6/27	19/20[b]
500	72	5/40	16/19[b]
500	48	3/20	9/9[b]
500	24	5/40	4/17
500	6	2/20	0/10
BHT			
400	72, 48, 24	4/34	10/16[b]
600	72	1/14	6/19[c]
600	48	1/14	7/8[b]
600	24	1/24	0/18
600	6	3/30	0/17

Note: The rats were given a stock diet and were dosed with 8.5 ml/kg of CCl_4 orally. Pretreatment with the antioxidants was before CCl_4 at the times shown.

[a] Number alive 72 hr after CCl_4 / Total number in group.

[b] Significantly greater than controls, $P < 0.001$.

[c] Significantly greater than controls, $P < 0.01$.

TABLE 19.4. *Liver necrosis and hepatic triglyceride (TG) levels in female rats treated with CCl_4, ethoxyquin, and BHT*

Pretreatment					
Dose (mg/kg)	Time before CCl_4 (hr)	Liver weight (% body weight)	Liver TG (mg/g)	Liver antioxidant[a] level (μg/g)	Necrosis
		ETHOXYQUIN (TEST 1)			
—	[b]	3.9 ± 0.5[b]	13.7 ± 3.8	—	0
—	—	4.4 ± 0.4	59.3 ± 17.8[c]	—	+++
300	72, 48, 24	6.8 ± 0.8[c]	25.3 ± 7.9[d]	< 5	+
500	72, 48, 24	8.3 ± 0.4[c]	38.9 ± 13.8[d]	< 5	+
500	72	5.5 ± 0.6[c]	32.8 ± 7.7[d]	< 5	+
500	48	5.5 ± 0.8[c]	33.8 ± 5.8[d]	< 5	+
500	24	5.6 ± 0.7[c]	59.1 ± 17.6	18 ± 7	+
500	6	4.9 ± 0.4[c]	54.6 ± 31.0	17 ± 7	++
		BHT (TEST 2)			
—	[b]	—	20.9 ± 3.2[b]	—	0
—	—	4.5 ± 0.4	90.4 ± 20.6[c]	—	+++
400	96	4.3 ± 0.1	64.7 ± 13.9[d]	< 1	+++
400	72	4.7 ± 0.5	59.4 ± 9.1[d]	< 1	+++
		BHT (TEST 3)			
—	[b]	4.5 ± 0.5[b]	12.3 ± 2.6[b]	—	0
—	—	4.8 ± 0.5	42.3 ± 8.4[c]	—	+++
400	48	5.2 ± 0.6	40.4 ± 14.9	< 1	++
400	24	5.6 ± 0.3[c]	85.1 ± 25.6[e]	< 1	++
400	6	5.1 ± 0.5	80.9 ± 21.7[e]	< 1	+++

Notes: The rats, six in a group, were given a stock diet and were dosed orally with 2.0 ml/kg of CCl_4. They were killed and analyzed 24 hr later. The antioxidant was given orally at the times stated before the CCl_4.

Values are given as mean ± SD.

[a] These analyses in parallel groups of animals killed at same time as CCl_4 was given to other groups in the table.

[b] No CCl_4 given.

[c] Significantly greater than controls, $P < 0.05–0.01$.

[d] Significantly less than CCl_4-treated controls, $P < 0.05–0.01$.

[e] Significantly greater than CCl_4-treated controls, $P < 0.05–0.01$.

E deficiency diseases. Tables 19.3 and 19.4 summarize the results with female rats (once again, the response of male rats was similar). This antioxidant had a significant effect on increasing survival, although the protection was rarely as complete as with ethoxyquin. As with ethoxyquin, BHT had to be administered no later than 48 hr before CCl_4. It also significantly inhibited the hepatic triglyceride rise, and, once again, there was a clear-cut time threshold of activity, 48–72 hr before CCl_4. There was virtually no effect of BHT on the liver necrosis, however. As with ethoxyquin, the liver weight increased after treatment with BHT. When the

BHT was administered only shortly before CCl_4, this produced a remarkable increase in hepatic triglycerides, which was significantly higher than the rise produced by CCl_4 itself. The liver in many of these experiments was analyzed for BHT, and less than 1 $\mu g/g$ was found during the critical period of activity. It is clear that this substance acts, not as an antioxidant, but by some indirect mechanism.

The above experiments demonstrate that synthetic antioxidants can prevent CCl_4 toxicity in the rat in different ways and in ways that may also be different from those of vitamin E. The analytical evidence discounts the idea that any of the three substances is active because it prevents lipid peroxidation in vivo. Their action is certainly indirect, probably involving induction of microsomal mixed-function oxidases. Carpenter (1966) drew attention to the role of vitamin E in increasing the hepatic concentration of these enzymes, and we have confirmed this for vitamin E, ethoxyquin, and other antioxidants (Cawthorne et al., 1970).

A role for vitamin E in specific protein synthesis is possible.

References

Bernard, K. 1958. Biochemistry of the polyunsaturated fatty acids. *Oléagineaux 13*:19.

Bieri, J. G. 1964. Synergistic effects between antioxidants and selenium or vitamin E. *Biochem. Pharmacol. 13*:1465.

Bieri, J. G., and E. L. Andrews. 1964. Fatty acids in rat testes as affected by vitamin E. *Biochem. Biophys. Res. Commun. 17*:115.

Blaxter, K. L., F. Brown, and A. M. Macdonald. 1953. The nutrition of the young Ayrshire calf. 13. The toxicity of the unsaturated acids of cod-liver oil. *Brit. J. Nutr.* 7:287.

Budowski, P., and S. Mokadi. 1961. Detection of free-radical damage in the vitamin E–deficient chick. *Biochim. Biophys. Acta 52*:609.

Bunyan, J., A. T. Diplock, and J. Green. 1967 [Bunyan et al., 1967*a*]. Effects of vitamin E deficiency on total polyunsaturated fatty acids in rats and chicks. *Brit. J. Nutr. 21*:217.

Bunyan, J., J. Green, A. Murrell, A. T. Diplock, and M. A. Cawthorne. 1968. On the postulated peroxidation of unsaturated lipids in the tissues of vitamin E–deficient rats. *Brit. J. Nutr.* 22:97.

Bunyan, J., E. A. Murrell, J. Green, and A. T. Diplock. 1967 [Bunyan et al., 1967*b*]. On the existence and significance of lipid peroxides in vitamin E–deficient animals. *Brit. J. Nutr. 21*:475.

Calvert, C. C., and M. L. Scott. 1962. Studies on glutathione in tissues of dystrophic chicks. *Poultry Sci. 41*:633.

Carpenter, M. P. 1966. Polyenoic fatty acids of rat testis, the effect of d-tocopherol. *Fed. Proc. 25*:764 (Abstr.)

Cawthorne, M. A., J. Bunyan, M. V. Sennitt, J. Green, and P. Grasso. 1970. *Brit. J. Nutr. 24*:352.

Dam, H. 1957. Influence of antioxidants and redox substances on signs of vitamin E deficiency. *Pharmacol. Rev. 9*:1.

Dam, H., and H. Granados. 1945. Peroxidation of body fat in vitamin E deficiency. *Acta Physiol. Scand. 10*:162.

Diplock, A. T., J. Bunyan, D. McHale, and J. Green, 1967. [Diplock et al., 1967*a*]. Vitamin E and stress. 2. The metabolism D-α-tocopherol and the effects of stress in vitamin E deficiency in the chick. *Brit. J. Nutr. 21*:103.

Diplock, A. T., J. Green, J. Bunyan, M. A. Cawthorne, and J. Dawson. 1967 [Diplock et al., 1967*b*]. Vitamin E and stress. 6. Iron overloading and the metabolism of D-α-tocopherol in the rat. *Brit. J. Nutr. 21*:725.

Diplock, A. T., J. Green, J. Bunyan, D. McHale, and I. R. Muthy. 1967 [Diplock et al., 1967*c*]. Vitamin E and stress. 3. The metabolism of D-α-tocopherol in the rat under dietary stress with silver. *Brit. J. Nutr. 21*:115.

Draper, H. H., J. G. Bergan, M. Chiu, A. S. Csallany, and A. V. Boaro. 1964. A further study of the specificity of the vitamin E requirement for reproduction. *J. Nutr. 84*:395.

Emmel, V. M., and P. L. LaCelle. 1961. Studies on the kidney in vitamin E deficiency. 2. Renal tocopherol content in relation to vitamin E deficiency changes in the kidney. *J. Nutr. 75*:335.

Fisher, H., and H. Kaunitz. 1965. Dietary saturated medium-chain triglycerides and vitamin E deficiency in chicks and rats. *Proc. Soc. Exp. Biol. Med. 120*:175.

Fitch, C. D. and J. S. Dinning. 1963. Vitamin E deficiency in the monkey. 5. Estimated requirements and the influence of fat deficiency and antioxidants on the syndrome. *J. Nutr. 79*:69.

Gallagher, C. H. 1961. Protection by antioxidants against lethal doses of carbon tetrachloride. *Nature 192*:881.

Glavind, J. and E. Søndergaard. 1964*a*. Effect of nutrition on antioxidant levels of the body. 1. Tissue oxidants in chicks on an encephalomalacia-producing diet. *Acta Chem. Scand. 18*:2173.

Glavind, J., and E. Søndergaard. 1964*b*. Effect of nutrition on antioxidant levels of the body. 2. Antioxidant levels in the livers of rats on a necrogenic diet. *Acta Chem. Scand. 18*:2179.

Golberg, L. and I. P. Smith. 1958. Changes associated with the accumulation of excessive amounts of iron in certain organs of the rat. *Brit. J. Exp. Pathol. 39*:59.

Green, J., and J. Bunyan. 1969. Vitamin E and the biological antioxidant theory. *Nutr. Abstr. Rev. 39*:321.

Green, J., J. Bunyan, M. A. Cawthorne, and A. T. Diplock. 1969. Vitamin E and hepatotoxic agents. 1. Carbon tetrachloride and lipid peroxidation in the rat. *Brit. J. Nutr. 23*:297.

Green, J., A. T. Diplock, J. Bunyan, D. McHale, and I. R. Muthy. 1967 [Green et al., 1967*a*]. Vitamin E and stress. 1. Dietary unsaturated fatty acid stress and the metabolism of α-tocopherol in the rat. *Brit. J. Nutr. 21*:69.

Green, J., A. T. Diplock, J. Bunyan, I. R. Muthy, and D. McHale, 1967 [Green et al, 1967*b*]. Vitamin E and stress. 4. The metabolism of D-α-tocopherol during nutritional hepatic necrosis in the rat and the effects of selenium, methionine and unsaturated fatty acids. *Brit. J. Nutr. 21*:497.

Harris, P. L., and N. D. Embree. 1963. Quantitative consideration of the effect of polyunsaturated fatty acid content of the diet upon the requirements for vitamin E. *Amer. J. Clin. Nutr. 13*:385.

Harris, P. L., and K. E. Mason. 1956. Vitamin E and metabolic processes, p. 1. *Vitamina E. Atti del terzo Congresso Internazionale Venezia. 1955*. Edizioni Valdoneza, Verona.

Hove, E. L. 1948. Interrelation between α-tocopherol and protein metabolism. 3. The protective effect of vitamin E and certain nitrogenous compounds against carbon tetrachloride poisoning in rats. *Arch. Biochem. Biophys. 17*:457.

Hove, E. L. 1955. Anti-vitamin E stress factors as related to lipid peroxides. *Amer. J. Clin. Nutr. 3*:328.

Hove, E. L., and Z. Hove. 1953. Effect of dietary protein level and tocopherol on unsaturated fatty acid content of rat tissues. *Fedn. Proc. 12*:417.

Lee, D. J. W., and M. McC. Barnes. 1969. The effects of vitamin E deficiency on the total fatty acids and the phospholipid fatty acids of rat tissues. *Brit. J. Nutr. 23*:289.

Lindan, O., and E. Work. 1953. Experimental liver necrosis in rats. 1. Changes in liver, blood and spleen glutathione and ascorbic acid levels in dietetic liver necrosis. *Biochem. J. 55*:554.

Markson, L. H., R. B. A. Carnaghan, and W. H. Parr. 1957. Studies on encephalomalacia in poultry. 2. The tocopherol status of normal and affected chicks. *Brit. Vet. J. 113*:303.

McLean, A. E. M. 1967. Effect of diet and vitamin E on liver injury due to carbon tetrachloride. *Brit. J. Exp. Pathol. 48*:632.

Recknagel, R. O. 1967. Carbon tetrachloride hepatotoxicity. *Pharmacol. Rev. 19*:145.

Slater, T. F. 1966. Necrogenic action of carbon tetrachloride in the rat: a speculative mechanism based on activation. *Nature 209*:36.

Tappel, A. L. 1962. Vitamin E as the biological lipid antioxidant. *Vitamins Hormones 20*:493.

Thompson, J. N., and M. L. Scott. 1969. Role of selenium in the nutrition of the chick. *J. Nutr. 97*:335.

Weber, F., U. Gloor, and A. Wiss. 1962. Vitamin E and essential fatty acids. *Fette Seifen Anstr-Mittel 64*:1149.

Witting, L. A. 1965. Biological availability of tocopherol and other antioxidants of the cellular level. *Fed. Proc. 24*:912.

Witting, L. A., and M. K. Horwitt. 1964. Effect of degree of fatty acid unsaturation in tocopherol deficiency–induced creatinuria. *J. Nutr. 82*:19.

20

BIOLOGICAL ACTIVITY AND METABOLISM OF *N*-SUBSTITUTED TOCOPHERAMINES: IMPLICATIONS ON VITAMIN E FUNCTION

J. G. Bieri

During the past thirty years, over a hundred modifications of the α-tocopherol molecule have been synthesized. None of these compounds (with one exception, to be mentioned later) has exhibited biological activity approaching that of α-tocopherol. Among the tocopherols themselves, the considerably greater biological activity of α-tocopherol compared with its β, γ, and δ homologs has led over the years to the concept that the α-structure, with three methyl groups on the chroman ring, represents the ultimate in molecular specificity for vitamin E activity.

In the tocotrienol series, greatest biological activity is found with the trimethyl homolog, α-tocotrienol, but the activity is less than half that of α-tocopherol, indicating the importance of the saturated side chain. A few compounds with structures not related to tocopherol have been shown to possess limited vitamin E activity, for example, the commercial antioxidants ethoxyquin and *N,N′*-diphenylphenylenediamine, but compared with α-tocopherol their potencies are erratic in different species.

It has been known that the utilization of the tocopherols, i.e., their deposition in the liver when the tocopherols are included in the diet, was roughly proportional to their biological activities (Bolliger and Bolliger-Quaife, 1955; Griffiths, 1959). This has suggested that the rates of intestinal absorption and deposition in the tissues may be more important factors in determining activity than any structural specificity necessary to perform their biochemical function. Wiss and co-workers (1962) and Gloor and co-workers (1966) have shown, however, that another factor must be considered in evaluating utilization, namely, the retention or turnover of the compounds in the tissues. Their studies indicated that absorption and deposition of the various tocopherols may not be very different but that α-tocopherol is retained longer by the tissues than are the less active tocopherols.

From these considerations, the relationship between structure and biological activity appears to have two components. First, there are certain aspects of molecular structure which facilitate absorption, transport to the tissues, and binding to essential cellular components, and, second, there must be a functional group necessary for biochemical reactivity. In the case of the tocopherols, it is apparent that, for optimal utilization and retention, the saturated side chain and three methyl groups on the ring (as in α-tocopherol) are essential, while for a functional group, the hydroxyl is critical.

An exception to the essentiality of the hydroxyl group was provided in 1942 when Smith and co-workers (1942) synthesized α-tocopheramine and found it to be approximately as active as α-tocopherol This compound, however, received little attention. In 1966, Schwieter and co-workers (1966) prepared the amine derivatives of the four tocopherols, and also substituted one or two methyl or ethyl groups on the amino group. The structures of these derivatives of γ-tocopherol are shown in Figure 20.1.

Biological activity of the tocopheramines

In testing these derivatives in the erythrocyte hemolysis test, Schwieter and co-workers (1966) found α-, β-, γ-, and δ-tocopheramines to have biological activities similar to their hydroxy analogs, the tocopherols. Among

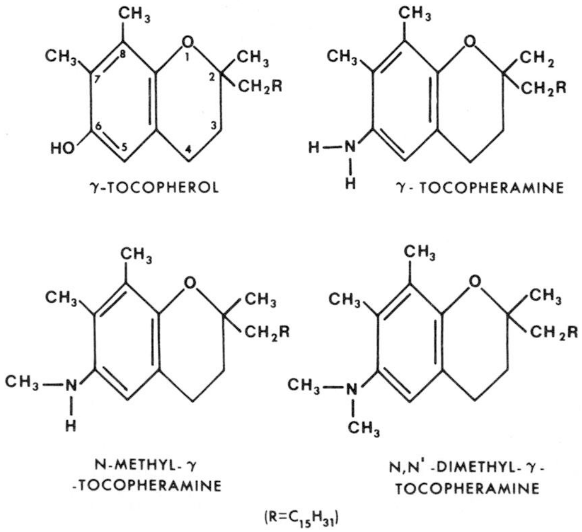

γ-TOCOPHEROL

γ-TOCOPHERAMINE

N-METHYL-γ-TOCOPHERAMINE

N,N'-DIMETHYL-γ-TOCOPHERAMINE

$(R=C_{15}H_{31})$

Fig. 20.1. Structural formulas for the tocopheramine, *N*-methyl-tocopheramine, and *N,N'*-dimethyl-tocopheramine derivatives of γ-tocopherol.

the *N*-alkyl-substituted tocopheramines, only two had significant activity: *N*-methyl-β-tocopheramine and *N*-methyl-γ-tocopheramine. These compounds had 125%–130% of the activity of α-tocopherol.

The hemolysis test has been shown to correlate well with other vitamin E biological assays; we felt it was important, however, to explore the activity of these compounds further in several whole-animal assays. This was done in both the chick and the rat. Two different vitamin E–deficiency syndromes were studied with the chick (Bieri and Prival, 1967). In the prevention of exudative diathesis, three amine derivatives – α-tocopheramine, *N*-methyl-β-tocopheramine and *N*-methyl-γ-tocopheramine – had activity essentially the same as that of α-tocopherol (Table 20.1). β- and γ-tocopheramines were considerably less active. In the prevention of encephalomalacia (Table 20.2), α-tocopheramine and *N*-methyl-β-tocopheramine were again as active as α-tocopherol, while β-tocopheramine was much less active.

TABLE 20.1. *Relative vitamin E activities of tocopheramines in preventing chick exudative diathesis*

Compound	Relative activity			
	Exp. 1	Exp. 2	Exp. 3	Average
dl-α-tocopherol	100	100	100	100
dl-α-tocopheramine	112	109	—	110.5
dl-β-tocopheramine	—	—	50	50
dl-γ-tocopheramine	—	—	38	38
dl-*N*-methyl-β-tocopheramine	86	116	—	101
dl-*N*-methyl-γ-tocopheramine	90	87	—	88.5

Source: Bieri and Prival (1967).

Since some investigators are reluctant to accept any estimate of vitamin E biological activity other than that obtained by the classic rat-fertility test, we compared *N*-methyl-β-tocopheramine and α-tocopherol in this assay (Bieri and Mason, 1968). As seen in Table 20.3, this methyl-substituted

TABLE 20.2. *Relative vitamin E activities of tocopheramines in preventing chick encephalomalacia*

Compound	Relative activity
dl-α-tocopherol	100
dl-α-tocopheramine	98
dl-β-tocopheramine	20
dl-*N*-methyl-β-tocopheramine	110

Source: Bieri and Prival (1967).

TABLE 20.3. *Relative vitamin E activity of N-methyl-β-tocopheramine in the rat reproduction assay*

Dose (mg)	Number of rats	Number of positive responses	Fertility (%)	Relative potency
		dl-α-TOCOPHEROL		
0.24	5	0	0	100.0
0.36	6	2	33.3	
0.53	8	6	75.0	
0.80	6	6	100.0	
		dl-N-METHYL-β-TOCOPHERAMINE		
0.24	5	0	0	88.7 ± 7.4[a]
0.36	8	1	12.5	
0.53	7	5	71.4	
0.80	6	6	100.0	

Source: Bieri and Mason (1968).
[a] Confidence limits = 77%–107% ($P = 0.05$).

amine derivative of β-tocopherol was essentially just as active as α-tocopherol.

We thus confirmed the full biological activities of α-tocopheramine, *N*-methyl-β-tocopheramine, and *N*-methyl-γ-tocopheramine found by Schwieter and co-workers (1966). This equivalency of activity in four different vitamin E assays leaves little doubt that the *N*-methyl-β- and *N*-methyl-γ-tocopheramines would be effective substitutes for α-tocopherol in all physiological requirements for the vitamin. Our results did not show the activity of the two *N*-methyl compounds to be greater than that of α-tocopherol. This may be due to the somewhat more limited aspects of the whole-animal assays, with regard to numbers of animals, compared with the hemolysis assays.

Metabolism of the tocopheramines

The question next arose, are these active amines converted to their corresponding tocopherols in the body? The thin-layer chromatographic separation of these compounds is very effective (as shown in Figure 20.2 for the various derivatives of γ-tocopheramine), so that their determinations are quite uncomplicated. Furthermore, all of these compounds can be separated and quantified by gas chromatography (Bieri and Prival, 1967), so that the combination of thin-layer and gas chromatography gives a sensitive procedure for identification of submicrogram amounts. When rats depleted of α-tocopherol were fed α-tocopheramine or *N*-methyl-β-tocopheramine and their livers were analyzed by this procedure, no evidence for α- or β-tocopherols was found. Similarly, Gloor and co-workers

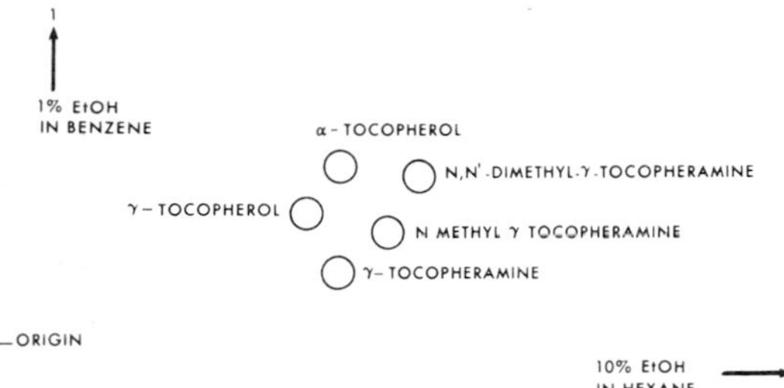

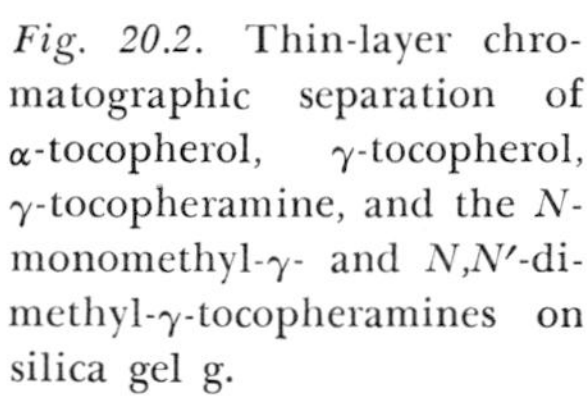
Fig. 20.2. Thin-layer chromatographic separation of α-tocopherol, γ-tocopherol, γ-tocopheramine, and the *N*-monomethyl-γ- and *N,N'*-dimethyl-γ-tocopheramines on silica gel g.

(1966), using ^{14}C-labeled compounds, also were unable to demonstrate that either the tocopheramines or the *N*-methyl-tocopheramines were converted to tocopherols.

In the thin-layer analysis of liver from rats fed *N*-methyl-β-tocopheramine, a second, unidentified, spot was always noted in addition to the spot of the compound that was fed. Isolation of this material permitted its identification, from the ultraviolet absorption curve and gas chromatographic retention time, as β-tocopheramine. Thus, the *N*-methyl compound was demethylated in vivo and stored in the liver (Table 20.4). We have consistently found that 15%–25% of these *N*-methyl-tocopheramines are deposited in the liver as the demethylated tocopheramines.

TABLE 20.4. *Evidence for in vivo demethylation of N-methyl-β-tocopheramine*

	Liver concentration (μg/g)	
Compound fed	*N*-Me-β-NH_2[a]	β-NH_2[b]
dl-N-methyl-β-tocopheramine	62.3	15.2[c]
dl-β-tocopheramine	0	12.1

Note: Rats depleted of vitamin E for 3 weeks were fed 2.33 μmole of the compounds for 4 days.

[a] *N*-methyl-β-tocopheramine.

[b] β-tocopheramine.

[c] This material when isolated had an absorption maximum and a gas chromatographic retention time identical to those of authentic β-tocopheramine.

Analyses of both chick and rat livers indicated that *N*-methyl-β- and *N*-methyl-γ-tocopheramines are stored more efficiently than is α-tocopherol (Table 20.5). There was no difference in the intracellular distribution of these compounds. Further information on utilization was provided in an experiment in which α-tocopherol and *N*-methyl-β-tocopheramine were fed to lactating rats one day after delivering their litters. Each litter was reduced in size to six, and the young rats and their mothers were sacrificed after sixteen days of feeding the compound in the maternal diet. Care was taken to prevent the baby rats from obtaining the mother's diet, so that

TABLE 20.5. *Storage of tocopherol and tocopheramines in liver of rats and chicks*

Compound fed	Liver concentration (μg/g)
CHICKS	
dl-α-tocopherol	23.0 ± 1.3
dl-α-tocopheramine	31.5 ± 4.3
dl-*N*-methyl-β-tocopheramine	53.5 ± 6.8
RATS	
dl-α-tocopherol	23.0 ± 1.3
dl-α-tocopheramine	28.0 ± 4.5
dl-β-tocopheramine	17.2 ± 4.5
dl-γ-tocopheramine	14.9 ± 2.8
dl-*N*-methyl-β-tocopheramine	55.5 ± 7.2
dl-*N*-methyl-γ-tocopheramine	40.9 ± 1.8

Source: Bieri and Prival (1967).

Notes: Compounds were fed for 4 days to α-tocopherol–depleted chicks (100 mg/kg diet) or rats (1 mg (2.33 μmole)/day).

Values are given as mean ± SE.

the liver analyses represent compounds obtained only through the milk. Since the mothers were depleted of α-tocopherol for only four days before the birth of their young, all of the baby rats had some α-tocopherol stores at birth.

As seen in Table 20.6, the amount of *N*-methyl-β-tocopheramine deposited in the maternal livers was more than five times the amount of

TABLE 20.6. *α-Tocopherol and β-tocopheramines in liver and plasma of lactating rats*

Compound fed[a]	Liver (μg/g)			Plasma (μg/100 ml)		
	α-T[b]	β-NH_2[c]	*N*-Me-β-NH_2[d]	α-T[b]	β-NH_2[c]	*N*-Me-β-NH_2[d]
dl-α-tocopherol						
Rat A	24[e]	—	—	252[e]	—	—
Rat B	16[e]	—	—	161[e]	—	—
dl-*N*-methyl-β-tocopheramine						
Rat C	6	6	38	107	57	84
Rat D	10	14	79	132	31	117

[a] Normal pregnant rats were depleted of vitamin E for 4 days before birth of the young. 1 mg (2.33 μmole) of each compound was fed daily during days 1–16 of lactation.

[b] α-tocopherol.

[c] β-tocopheramine.

[d] *N*-methyl-β-tocopheramine.

[e] These values should be corrected for the amounts of α-tocopherol found in the tissues of rats fed *N*-methyl-β-tocopheramine.

α-tocopherol. Since these rats were fasted 24 hr before sacrificing, it would appear that the methyl derivative is not eliminated very rapidly from the liver. Again, a significant amount of demethylated tocopheramine was found in the liver.

The proportion of β-tocopheramine was even greater in the plasma. When the plasma and liver α-tocopherol values of the mothers fed α-tocopherol are corrected for the amounts present in the tissues of the mothers fed the methyl tocopheramine, the superior utilization of *N*-methyl-β-tocopheramine is even more apparent.

Analyses of livers from the baby rats (Table 20.7) again confirmed the more efficient retention of *N*-methyl-β-tocopheramine. Littermates of these rats had an average of 5 μg of α-tocopherol per liver at birth. When this value is subtracted from the values found after 16 days, it can be seen that only 1–6 μg of additional α-tocopherol was stored, compared with 7–11 μg of *N*-methyl-β-tocopheramine.

In their initial screening of the tocopheramines in the hemolysis test, Schwieter and co-workers (1966) found all of the dimethyl tocopheramines to be much less active than the monomethyl tocopheramines. Subsequently, Søndergaard and Dam (personal communication) reported that *N,N′*-dimethyl-γ-tocopheramine had 65% of the activity of α-tocopherol in preventing muscle dystrophy in chicks. Since it is known that vitamin E activity is dependent on a reactive hydrogen atom (vitamin E ethers, for example, are inactive), either attached to oxygen as in the tocopherols or to nitrogen as in the tocopheramines, one would expect that the dimethyl tocopheramine should be demethylated in order to be biologically active.

TABLE 20.7. *α-Tocopherol and β-tocopheramines in livers of nursing rats*

	μg/total liver			
Compound fed [a]	α-T [b]	*N*-Me-β-NH_2 [c]	β-NH_2 [d]	Total NH_2
α-tocopherol				
Litter A	10.8 [e]	—	—	—
Litter B	5.8 [e]	—	—	—
N-methyl-β-tocopheramine				
Litter C	4.6	5.6	1.5	7.1
Litter D	4.1	8.4	2.3	10.7

[a] Compounds were fed to mothers for 16 days after birth of young. Values are averages of 4 rats from litters of 6.

[b] α-tocopherol.

[c] *N*-methyl-β-tocopheramine.

[d] β-tocopheramine.

[e] These values should be corrected for the average 4.3 μg of α-tocopherol found in livers of the rats fed *N*-methyl-β-tocopheramine.

To test this hypothesis, *N,N′*-dimethyl-γ-tocopheramine and also *N*-methyl-γ-tocopheramine were fed to vitamin E–depleted rats and the livers were analyzed. As seen in Table 20.8, the dimethyl compound was demethylated, as was also the monomethyl tocopheramine. There was no γ-tocopheramine detected in the livers from the rats fed the dimethyl compound. These results, as well as other observations on liver and plasma levels, suggest that the monomethyl tocopheramine is the most active form of these compounds and that total demethylation is not essential in order to exert biochemical activity. It should be noted that the dimethyl compound was stored to the same extent as was the monomethyl derivative.

TABLE *20.8. Evidence for in vivo demethylation of N,N′dimethyl-γ-tocopheramine*

		Liver (μg/g)		
Compound fed [a]	Serum (μg/100 ml)	*N,N′*-Di-Me-γ-NH_2 [b]	*N*-Me-γ-NH_2 [c]	γ-NH_2 [d]
dl-N,N′-dimethyl-γ-tocopheramine	295 ± 11	21.5 ± 0.6	3.3 ± 0.2	0
dl-N-methyl-γ tocopheramine	238 ± 19	n.a.	18.7 ± 0.7	2.2 ± 1.4

[a] Rats depleted of vitamin E for 7 weeks were fed 2.33 μmoles of each compound daily for 4 days. Values are means ± SE for 3 or 4 rats.
[b] *N,N′*-dimethyl-γ-tocopheramine.
[c] *N*-methyl-γ-tocopheramine.
[d] γ-tocopheramine.

With regard to the further metabolism of *N*-methyl β- or *N*-methyl-γ-tocopheramines, Gloor and co-workers (1966) showed by the isotope-dilution procedure that these compounds were oxidized to their corresponding quinones, which in turn were converted to tocopheronolactones. A proposed scheme for the formation of the quinones via the oxime is shown in Figure 20.3.

The high biological activity of *N*-methyl-β- and *N*-methyl-γ-tocopheramines indicates that the α-tocopherol structure does not have as high a degree of specificity for vitamin E activity as has been thought. It appears, however, that three methyl groups are critical, either all on the chroman ring, as in α-tocopherol, or two on the ring and one on the amino group, as in *N*-methyl-β- and *N*-methyl-γ-tocopheramines. These three alkyl groups probably are responsible for the greater cellular affinity of such compounds, when compared with β- and γ-tocopherols or with tocopheramines which have only two methyl groups.

The relatively high storage of *N,N′*-dimethyl-γ-tocopheramine observed in these studies indicates that four methyl groups are just as favorable

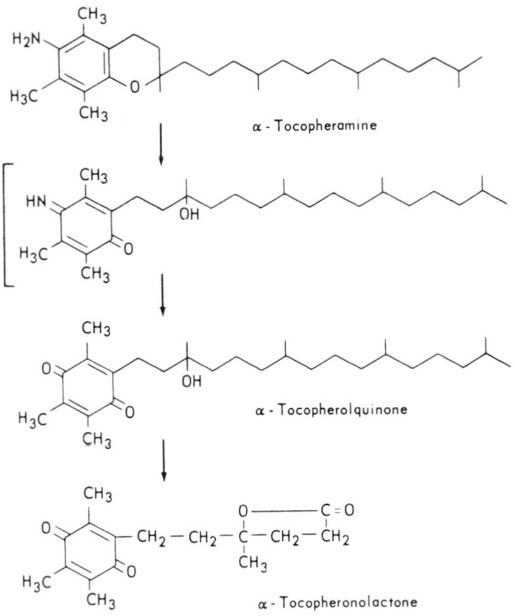

Fig. 20.3. Proposed scheme for the formation of tocopherolquinone and tocopheronolactone from tocopheramine.

for utilization and retention as are three methyls, but—probably because of the slow rate of demethylation to yield the monomethyl tocopheramine—the dimethyl compound has reduced biological activity.

Structure and function of vitamin E–active compounds

What are the implications of these observations with regard to the chemistry of vitamin E at the cellular level? In view of the high biological activities of these amine derivatives of β- and γ-tocopherol, we can conclude that reactions such as oxidation and dimerization, involving the methyl groups in positions 5 and 7 of α-tocopherol, are not essential to the functional activity of the vitamin. The fact that the hydroxyl group in the 6-position may be replaced by an amino group or an *N*-methyl amino group indicates that a reactive hydrogen is the functional atom of the molecule.

Inasmuch as the two methyl groups on the ring of *N*-methyl-β-tocopheramine and N-methyl-γ-tocopheramine can be in either the 5,8 or the 7,8 position without diminishing biochemical reactivity, there is not a high degree of structural specificity in the sense usually associated with protein-coenzyme interaction. On the other hand, the increased cellular retention bestowed by three, and perhaps four, methyl groups indicates that compounds with these configurations have a much greater affinity for certain subcellular structures than do other lipid-soluble antioxidants. This latter type of specificity should not be minimized in considerations of vitamin E function. Also, the fact that the tocopherols and the methyl-substituted tocopheramines are effective lipid antioxidants (Bieri and Prival, 1967) must not obscure the possibility that nonlipid oxidants or free radicals in tissues may also react with the active hydrogen of these compounds. Such a mechanism would effectively maintain a variety of essential compounds in the reduced state.

One further consideration from these studies should be mentioned. Since *N*-methyl-β-tocopheramine (and also the γ-isomer) are deposited and retained by the liver at least twice as effectively as is α-tocopherol, it would seem that, if the activity of these derivatives at the molecular level is equal to that of α-tocopherol, then they should be considerably more efficient in total biological activity as assayed in the whole animal. The fact that their activities by bioassay are only equal to, or perhaps slightly greater than, that of α-tocopherol suggests that the amine derivatives do not function as efficiently as α-tocopherol in the cell.

References

Bieri, J. G., and K. E. Mason. 1968. Vitamin E activity of *N*-methyl-β-tocopheramine in the rat reproduction assay. *J. Nutr. 96*:192.

Bieri, J. G., and E. L. Prival. 1967. Vitamin E activity and metabolism of *N*-methyl-tocopheramines. *Biochemistry 6*:2153.

Bolliger, H. R., and M. L. Bolliger-Quaife. 1955. Vitamin E. *Atti del terzo congresso internazionale. Venezia 1955*:30.

Gloor, U., J. Wursch, U. Schwieter, and O. Wiss. 1966. Resorption, retention, verteilung und stoffwechsel das *d*,l-α-tocopheramins, *d*,l-*N*-methyl-γ-tocopheramins und des γ-tocopherols im vergleich zum *d*,l-α-tocopherol bei der ratte. *Helv. Chim. Acta 49*:2303.

Griffiths, T. W. 1959. Relative rates of liver storage of pure α-, β-, γ-, and δ-tocopherols in the growing chick. *Nature 183*:1061.

Schwieter, U., R. Tamm, H. Weiser, and O. Wiss. 1966. Zur synthese und vitamin-E-wirksamkeit von tocopheraminen und ihren *N*-alkyl-derviaten. *Helv. Chim. Acta 49*:2297.

Smith, L. I., W. B. Renfrow, and J. W. Opie. 1942. The chemistry of vitamin E. XXXVIII. α-Tocopheramine, a new vitamin E factor. *J. Amer. Chem. Soc. 64*:1082.

Wiss, O., R. H. Bunnell, and U. Gloor. 1962. *Vitamins Hormones 20*:440.

21

KINETIC STUDIES ON MITOCHONDRIAL ENZYMES DURING RESPIRATORY DECLINE RELATING TO THE MODE OF ACTION OF TOCOPHEROL

Klaus Schwarz and Werner Baumgartner

The work reported here had its beginnings in 1939 when dietary liver necrosis was discovered by one of us (see Schwarz, 1944*a*) as a new deficiency disease and an investigation of the nutritional factors which protected against it was begun. Wheat-germ oil was found to be highly effective; by fractionation of the protective agent from this source, using the prevention of death from liver necrosis as an assay, tocopherol was reisolated between 1940 and 1943 (Schwarz, 1944*a*, 1944*b*). Other investigators showed that the sulfur amino acids exerted protective effects against the same disease (Daft et al., 1942; see Daft, 1954). Our early studies, leading to the identification of vitamin E as a liver-protecting agent, were followed by fractionation studies on factor 3, a distinctly different natural principle which independently prevented the same deficiency disease (Schwarz, 1951). These efforts culminated in 1957 in the discovery of selenium as an important dietary agent (Schwarz and Foltz, 1957). The existence of an interdependence between vitamin E and selenium was thus first established in dietary liver necrosis. Soon thereafter, the effectiveness of selenium was demonstrated in several other diseases previously attributed solely to lack of vitamin E. The most notable examples are exudative diathesis in chicks and other fowl, white muscle disease in sheep and cattle, and "hepatosis dietetica" in swine. The latter deficiency com-

These studies were supported in part by United States Public Health Service Grant AM–08669.

We acknowledge the excellent technical assistance of Mrs. Virginia Hill and Mrs. Martha Duckworth. We also thank Miss Maureen Conley and Mr. Moses Jordan for their capable management of diets and laboratory animals.

bines the syndromes of liver necrosis and muscular dystrophy with those of exudative diathesis.

The mode of action of vitamin E in the prevention of the severe tissue changes seen in all such deficiency diseases has been the subject of investigation in the senior author's laboratory since 1943. It is obvious that a full understanding of its mode of action on the molecular level within the organism has not yet been achieved, in spite of the huge amount of "data" on vitamin E published in the literature. The dichotomy of opinion about its functions is well documented by the papers on the subject presented in this book. Similar confrontations have taken place elsewhere (Schwarz, 1961, 1962*a*, 1962*b*, 1965, 1969). Some believe that vitamin E functions merely as a lipid-soluble antioxidant. We have maintained for years, on the other hand, that vitamin E may function as a catalytic agent in intermediary metabolism, at a specific metabolic site which is of fundamental importance for energy metabolism.

There are many findings which mitigate against the assumption that, in the prevention of dietary liver necrosis and related disturbances, tocopherol is effective simply because of its antioxidant properties. Much time has been spent in our laboratory in the search for valid evidence of random peroxidation in vivo and of an in vivo antioxidant function of tocopherol—with negative results. For instance, we have never been able to demonstrate the presence of peroxides or their breakdown products such as malondialdehyde in liver tissue of animals dying of liver necrosis induced by vitamin E (and selenium) deficiency. Only some of these studies have been published (Corwin, 1962; Schwarz, 1962*a*).

Our attempts to define the function of vitamin E centered on the study of livers from animals during the latent phase of necrotic-liver degeneration. The main participants in these studies (carried out until 1963 at the former Section of Experimental Liver Diseases, NIAMD, at the National Institutes of Health, and since then at the Laboratory of Experimental Metabolic Diseases, VA Hospital, Long Beach, California) have been S. Chernick, W. Mertz, L. Corwin, and C. Lee. The experiments have progressed step by step from the whole animal, through tissue slices, homogenates, subcellular fractions, and membrane structures (primarily of mitochondria), to well defined enzyme systems, whereby we hope to arrive eventually at the site of action of tocopherol on the molecular level. The main aspects of the earlier phases of this work have been summarized elsewhere (Schwarz, 1962*a*, 1965).

Respiratory decline

The investigations have been confined largely to studies on respiratory decline, a phenomenon characteristic of the latent phase of dietary necrotic liver degeneration. During this phase, seven to ten days preceding the onset of gross, acute necrosis and sudden death, changes of mitochondria and microsomal structures are detectable by electron microscopy, and liver tissue shows a peculiar inability to maintain normal oxygen consumption in vitro (Fig. 21.1).

A working hypothesis has evolved which permits the interpretation of a great many—at first seemingly unrelated—observations. The phenomenon of respiratory decline is observed with liver slices and also with homogenates, but not so readily with isolated mitochondria from the livers of animals during the latent phase of the disease. Under the conditions of experimentation, respiratory decline is not related to the rate of peroxide formation in the homogenate (Corwin, 1962; Schwarz, 1962*a*). Combination experiments disclosed that microsomes exert a deleterious effect on the respiring vitamin E–deficient mitochondria. This effect is prevented by complexing agents such as EDTA, diethyldithiocarbamate, and *o*-phenanthroline. It was concluded that respiratory decline is related to a disturbance of trace-element balance (Schwarz, 1962*a*). Very small amounts of

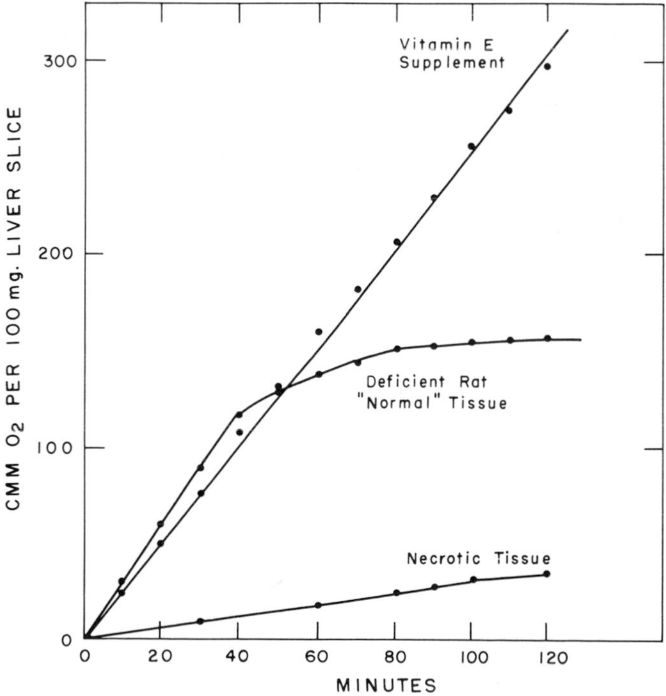

Fig. 21.1. Respiratory decline of rat liver slices in the Warburg respirometer. Substrate: 0.01 M glucose.

certain elements of the transition-metal series, for example, Cd^{++} and Hg^{++}, and also of AsO_2^-, produce respiratory decline artificially in isolated mitochondria. A loss of titrable sulfhydryl groups is related to the breakdown of respiratory activity. Reduced glutathione and dimercaptopropanol prevent respiratory failure.

As a working hypothesis, it was assumed that the immediate cause of respiratory failure was a block of sulfhydryl sites or of other highly sensitive loci on certain enzymes indispensable to respiration. Vitamin E, either supplemented in the diet or added to in vitro systems (liver homogenate, combinations of mitochondria with microsomes, or trace elements), protects against respiratory decline under the conditions of these earlier experiments. A comparison of the potencies of various tocol derivatives, dimethylbenzoquinones and trimethylbenzoquinones with isoprenoid side chains, K vitamins, ubiquinones, and related compounds has been carried out. In the in vitro system using liver homogenate and α-ketoglutarate as substrate, the various tocopherols showed an order of potency identical to that in the dietary resorption-sterility assay. A synthetic α-tocopherol analog (α_3-tocopherol) with an unsaturated side chain was more potent than α-tocopherol itself. Two mechanisms for the mode of action of the tocopherols and other naturally occurring quinonoid substances were taken into consideration, namely, oxidation-reduction and formation of addition products of sulfhydryl groups with quinones which are well known (for example, 1,4 addition reactions).

Through these investigations, it has been established that vitamin E has a direct and immediate effect on intermediary metabolism of mitochondria. This effect is not mediated through, or related to, the mechanics of genetic transcription. Studies relating to the role of vitamin E (and selenium) in oxidative metabolism of liver tissue, especially with β-hydroxybutyrate as a substrate, have also been carried out by Johnson and his collaborators (Grove et al., 1965, 1966; Grove and Johnson, 1967). The effect of selenium and vitamin E on the oxidation of tricarboxylic acid cycle intermediates, with emphasis on pyruvate and succinate, has been studied by Bull and Oldfield (1967).

The present review contains a reassessment of mitochondrial enzyme levels, studies on respiratory decline of liver homogenates (minus the nuclear fraction) with various substrates, results obtained with respiratory failure in mitochondria, and data on a vitamin E activator found in cytoplasmic supernatant. The influence of microsomes, heavy metals, and complexing agents is not treated in detail. The primary emphasis is on reaction kinetics and the application of kinetic criteria in identifying the primary metabolic lesion and the site and mode of action of vitamin E.

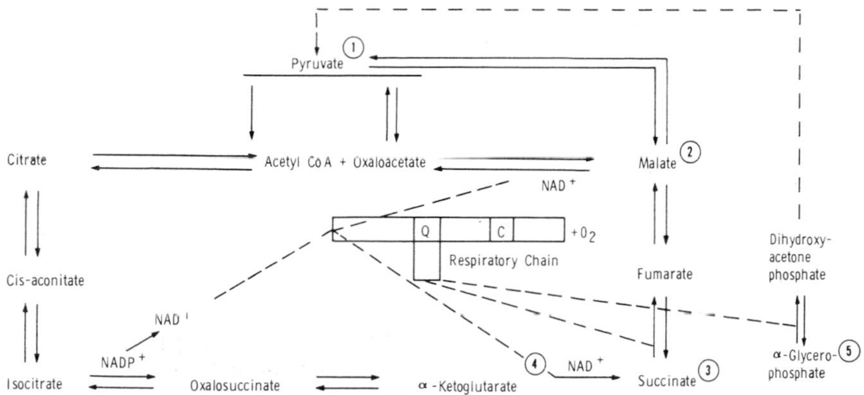

Fig. 21.2. Reactions investigated in the study of respiratory decline. 1: pyruvic oxidase, lipoyl dehydrogenase; 2: malic oxidase, malic dehydrogenase; 3: succinic oxidase, succinic dehydrogenase; 4: α-ketoglutarate oxidase, lipoyl dehydrogenase; 5: α-glycerophosphate oxidase. (After West et al., 1966.)

The main areas of intermediary metabolism investigated in this study are shown in Figure 21.2.

Enzyme activities and permeability of mitochondria during the latent phase of liver necrosis

The possibility that key enzymes change in activity during the latent phase of liver necrosis was reexamined by experiments wherein dehydrogenase and oxidase activities per unit mitochrondria were determined during the interval from the fourteenth to the twenty-first day of deficiency period. A method for the quantification of mitochondria, based on light-scattering properties, was developed. Existing techniques for measuring mitochondrial concentration, such as the biuret method or succinic dehydrogenase activity, were also employed.

The state of the mitochondrial membrane during the latent phase described above was monitored by measuring so-called latency effects (Greville, 1966). The term "membrane control ratio" (MC ratio) is suggested in its place; it is defined by R/I, where R is the enzyme activity with ruptured mitochondria and I the reaction rate with intact mitochondria. The magnitude of this ratio depends, of course, on the chosen substrate concentration. Also, considerable care has to be taken to assure that the enzyme is not deactivated by the methods used for the removal of the permeability barrier. Sonification, treatment with $CaCl_2$, or repeated freezing with dry ice–acetone and thawing were used to rupture mitochondria, as indicated.

SPECIFIC ACTIVITIES OF SUCCINIC, LIPOYL, MALIC, AND NADH DEHYDROGENASES AND OF NADH OXIDASE

Succinic oxidase is an enzyme system which exhibits respiratory decline under conditions of the Warburg assay (Corwin and Schwarz, 1958). The possibility that succinic dehydrogenase and/or the membrane deteriorate during the latent phase was investigated by the experiments listed in Table 21.1. Different electron acceptors (dichlorophenol indophenol (DCPIP) or phenazine methosulfate) and different substrate concentrations were used to monitor different rate-determining steps, as well as to safeguard against possible reagent-induced modifications of the membrane or enzyme. Liver mitochondria were obtained from animals maintained on deficient diets or on diets supplemented with vitamin E and selenium.

The results in Table 21.1 indicate that no significant differences in succinic dehydrogenase activities or MC ratios exist between the various diets at different stages of the latent phase. The accuracy with which MC ratios were measured was generally not as high as the accuracy of reaction rates determined under ruptured conditions. This is partly due to the difficulty

TABLE 21.1. *Reaction rates of dehydrogenase and oxidase systems in deficient and in vitamin E and selenium supplemented liver mitochondria*

		MC ratio		Reaction rate	
Enzyme	Assay system	No dietary supplement	Vitamin E + Se supplement	No dietary supplement	Vitamin E + Se supplement
Succinic dehydrogenase	DCPIP	2.30	2.30	4.1	4.1
	Phenazine methosulfate	1.95	2.00	23.2	24.4
Malic dehydrogenase	OAA + NADH	—	—	2.0	1.9
Lipoyl dehydrogenase	Lipoamide + NADH	15.3	15.0	4.1	4.7
NADH dehydrogenase	$K_3[Fe(CN)_6]$	—	—	13.6	14.0
	DCPIP (diaphorase)	—	—	18.4	18.6
NADH oxidase system	NADH	—	—	29.0	30.1

Note: Determinations were made after 5 days of supplementation following 12 days of predepletion.

of measuring initial reaction rates under the conditions of the nonlinear kinetics produced by the low substrate concentrations used in MC ratio determination and partly due to the difficulty of making adequate corrections for light-scattering effects. In the present case, MC ratios were also adversely affected by the relatively high permeability of the mitochondrial membrane to the reagents.

Table 21.1 also contains rates and MC ratios of lipoyl dehydrogenase assays. This enzyme was investigated because of its previous implication as a key enzyme in the respiratory decline of the α-ketoglutarate oxidase system (Schwarz et al., 1962). The large MC ratios observed with lipoyl dehydrogenase are attributed to the low permeability of the mitochondrial membrane to NADH. Lipoamide was used as substrate. Once again, no significant differences were observed in enzyme activities or MC ratios between diets at different stages of the latent phase. This result is in agreement with the previous observations which showed normal levels of lipoyl dehydrogenase activity at the beginning of the Warburg experiments (Schwarz et al., 1962).

NADH dehydrogenase activity was investigated with two different electron acceptors, $K_3[Fe(CN)_6]$ and DCPIP, while oxygen served as acceptor in the NADH oxidase assay. The use of $K_3[Fe(CN)_6]$ increased the permeability of the membrane to such an extent that no MC ratios could be measured. A potentially good system for the study of membrane parameters is afforded by the NADH oxidase system, since the natural substrate and electron acceptor are used. In practice, however, the reaction with unsonified mitochondria proved to be too slow in relation to mitochondrial scatter changes, and accurate MC ratios could not be determined. Once again, no significant differences in enyzme activities were observed with the various diets.

The enzyme system responsible for malate oxidation in the Warburg respirometer also shows in vitro respiratory decline during the latent phase. No difference in malic dehydrogenase activity between deficient and supplemented animals could be detected in the present study (Table 21.1). Malic dehydrogenase activity was measured from the thermodynamically more favorable side, i.e., by use of oxaloacetate and NADH. It was found that 98% of the measured activity is due to the cytoplasmic counterpart of this mitochondrial enzyme. In view of the high activity in the cytoplasm, malic dehydrogenase can play an important role in the shuttle mechanisms linking cytoplasmic pyridine nucleotide to the respiratory chain, as demonstrated in Figure 21.3 (Greville, 1966). Subsequent analysis of respiratory-decline kinetics shows that the shuttle reaction is presently the only mechanism capable of explaining the decline observed with the malate substrate in the homogenate system (see below).

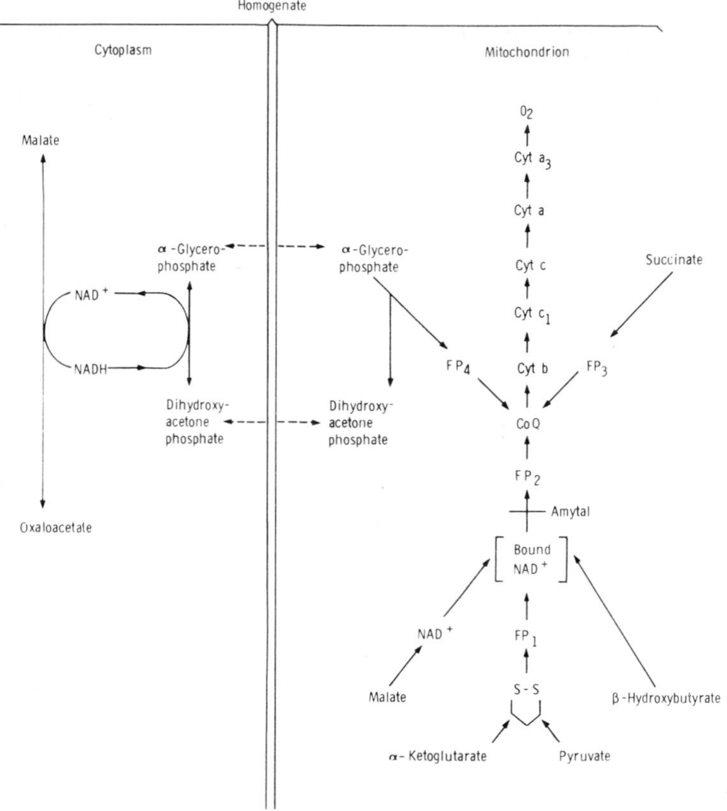

Fig. 21.3. Pathways involved in mitochondrial respiratory decline, including the α-glycerophosphate shuttle. (After Lehninger, 1965.)

Enzyme activities and MC ratios in partially necrotic livers

Failure to demonstrate differences in dehydrogenase and oxidase activities per unit mitochondria, and in permeability during the latent phase of liver necrosis, prompted the study of these parameters during the brief necrotic phase. Experiments were performed with mitochondria prepared from livers containing approximately 1/8 to 1/4 necrotic tissue. The results of these studies are listed in Tables 21.2 and 21.3. It is evident from these data that the activities of succinic dehydrogenase or oxidase are not greatly affected by necrosis. The MC ratios are altered, however. They reach approximately unity with succinic acid, which is indicative of a drastic alteration of the mitochondrial membrane during the terminal phase. Similar results were obtained when MC ratios were studied in the

TABLE 21.2. *Succinic oxidase and dehydrogenase activities and MC ratios of necrotic and normal liver mitochondria*

	Liver normal [a]			Liver partially necrotic [b]		
	Reaction rate			Reaction rate		
	Mito-chondria intact	Mito-chondria ruptured [c]	MC ratio	Mito-chondria intact	Mito-chondria ruptured [c]	MC ratio
EXPERIMENT 1						
DCPIP	1.5	5.0	3.3	3.8	4.5	1.2
Warburg	17.0	—	—	15.6	—	—
EXPERIMENT 2						
DCPIP	—	7.0	—	—	5.9	—
Phenazine methosulfate	16.8	23.7	1.4	16.5	18.5	1.1
Warburg	8.7	—	—	8.5	—	—
EXPERIMENT 3						
DCPIP	1.9	3.3	1.7	2.4	2.6	1.1
Phenazine methosulfate	13.5	22.1	1.6	17.0	16.8	1.0

[a] Livers from animals on a supplemented Torula yeast diet containing, per 100 g of diet, 10 mg of synthetic α-tocopheryl acetate and 15 μg selenium as sodium selenite.

[b] Livers from animals on the unsupplemented, basal Torula yeast diet taken at start of the terminal phase of necrotic-liver degeneration. Animals outwardly still normal, but with livers containing distinct areas of massive necrosis.

[c] Mitochondria in Experiment 1 were ruptured by freezing (dry ice/acetone) and thawing. Mitochondria in Experiments 2 and 3 were ruptured by $CaCl_2$ treatment.

lipoyl dehydrogenase system. Values varying between 1 and 4 were observed (Table 21.3) instead of the usual ratio of 15 (Table 21.1). The decrease of activity in necrotic livers is more pronounced for lipoyl dehydrogenase (−43%, −63%) than for succinic dehydrogenase (−24%, −38%). It is possible to interpret this result in terms of the different locations of these enzymes on the mitochondrial membrane, succinic dehydro-

TABLE 21.3. *Differences in enzyme activities and MC ratios in mitochondria of normal-appearing and partially necrotic rat livers*

	Reaction rate [a]		MC ratio	
Enzyme	Experiment 1	Experiment 2	Normal	Partially necrotic
Succinic dehydrogenase	−24	−38	1.7	1.0
Lipoyl dehydrogenase	−43	−63	14–17	1–4
Ratio of reaction rates [b]	*1.8*	*1.7*	—	—

[a] Percentage difference between normal and partially necrotic liver.

[b] Percentage difference lipoyl dehydrogenase/percentage difference succinic dehydrogenase.

genase being situated on the inner membrane and lipoyl dehydrogenase on the more fragile outer membrane (Allmann and Bachmann, 1967).

Our investigations of the necrotic and prenecrotic state indicate that abrupt changes appear to be characteristic of necrosis-related phenomena. Necrosis, changes in membrane permeability, and several kinetic features to be discussed below all occur abruptly. All these changes suggest the involvement of zero-order reactions with respect to essential intermediates or protective agents. It is evident that such a mechanism affords considerable advantages to an organism, since it enables essential reactions to be maintained at a constant rate in spite of widely fluctuating substrate concentrations. However, zero-order dependence makes it difficult to analyze the exact nature of the changes in terms of the cause-effect interactions prior to the sudden change to the higher-order kinetics which prevail during the short time-interval prior to the termination of the reaction.

Kinetic study of respiratory decline and dehydrogenase deactivation in liver homogenates

ZERO-ORDER RESPIRATORY DECLINE

A kinetic study of respiratory decline in liver homogenates was made prior to investigating the underlying mechanism. Initially, kinetic interpretations were complicated by large endogenous reactions; the problem could be controlled through the proper choice of medium. In preceding studies of respiratory decline, phosphate buffers were used. Tris (hydroxymethyl) amino methane in place of phosphate buffer and a reduction of the NAD^+ concentration decreases the endogenous reaction considerably. The medium used for respiratory-decline studies presented here — with 100 mg of liver homogenate in a total volume of 3 ml — consisted of 10 mM sodium phosphate, 1 mM NAD^+, 5mM Mg^{++}, 1 mM ATP, 66 mM Tris (*p*H 7.6), and sufficient substrate to saturate the enzyme. Homogenates (minus nuclei) were prepared by means of a constant-torque Eberbach motor and a Potter-Elvehjem homogenizer from minced liver and sufficient 0.25 M sucrose to give a 10% suspension. Blood cells, unbroken liver cells, and membranous and nuclear material were removed by centrifugation at 3000 rpm in a Servall SS–1 centrifuge at 700 × *g* for 10 min.

The endogenous oxygen consumption was subtracted from the main reaction. Results treated in this way reveal that respiratory decline occurs abruptly, in the characteristic fashion of a zero-order reaction. Figure 21.4 shows typical data for succinic and α-ketoglutarate oxidase reactions with vitamin E–deficient and in vitro–supplemented homogenates. Identical zero-order kinetics were also observed for the pyruvate and malate oxidase systems. Zero-order decline can be prevented by both dietary and in vitro

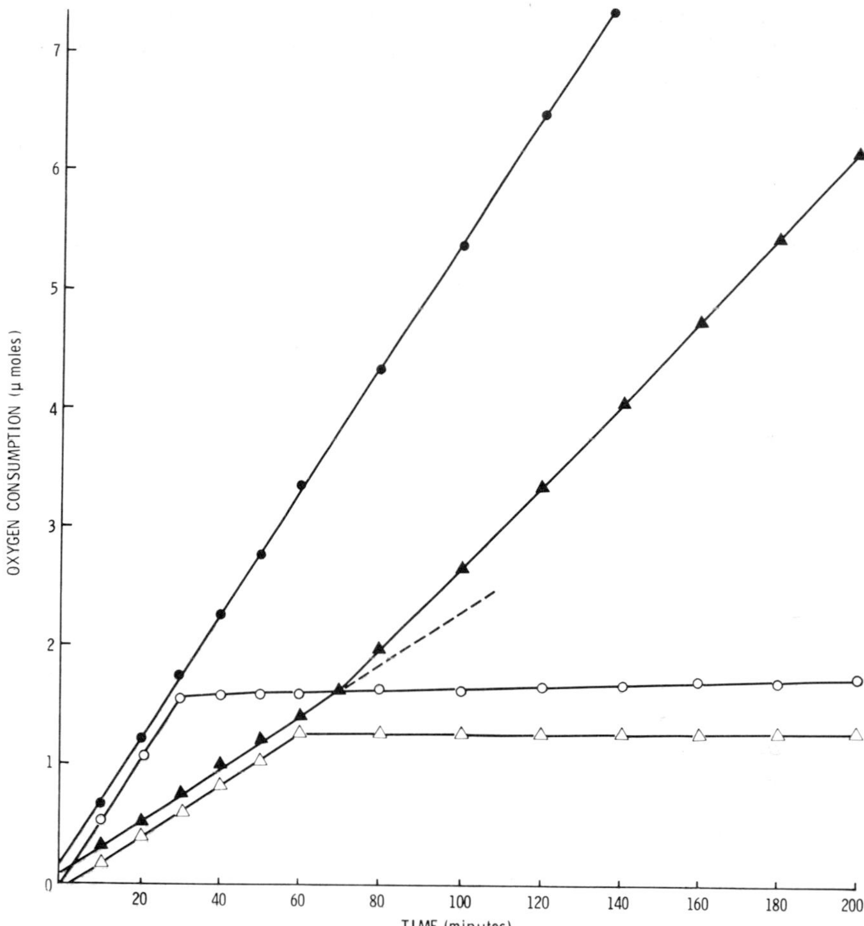

Fig. 21.4. Respiratory decline of succinic oxidase and α-ketoglutarate oxidase reactions in vitamin E–deficient rat liver homogenates, and its prevention by the addition of α-tocopherol (50 μg *DL*-α-tocopherol per vessel with 3 ml of reactions mixture). ○, succinic oxidase; ●, succinic oxidase + tocopherol; △, α-ketoglutarate oxidase; ▲, α-ketoglutarate oxidase + tocopherol. For medium composition, see text.

supplementation of α-tocopherol, provided that the mitochondrial membrane is left intact. Respiratory decline cannot be prevented by vitamin E when the mitochondrial membrane is ruptured by sonification of the homogenate. Under these conditions in the majority of cases, the reaction usually commences at the reduced rate characteristic of respiratory decline. In some cases, however, respiration occurs at normal rates for approximately the first 10 min.

REQUIREMENT FOR NAD+ AND PHOSPHATE IN RESPIRATORY DECLINE

Further studies of respiratory decline were made with the succinic oxidase system, where the kinetic situation is relatively simple in view of the absence of shuttle mechanisms between cytoplasmic and mitochondrial enzymes (as shown in Fig. 21.3). Previous studies had shown that respiratory decline is accentuated by the inclusion of NAD+ (Corwin and Schwarz, 1959). The possibility exists, therefore, that respiratory decline in succinic oxidase is due to an oxaloacetic acid feedback mechanism (Chance and Hagihara, 1962; Corwin, 1965). This possibility was investigated by removing oxaloacetic acid by transamination with exogenous transaminase and glutamic acid. Fig. 21.5 shows that preventing feedback inhibition

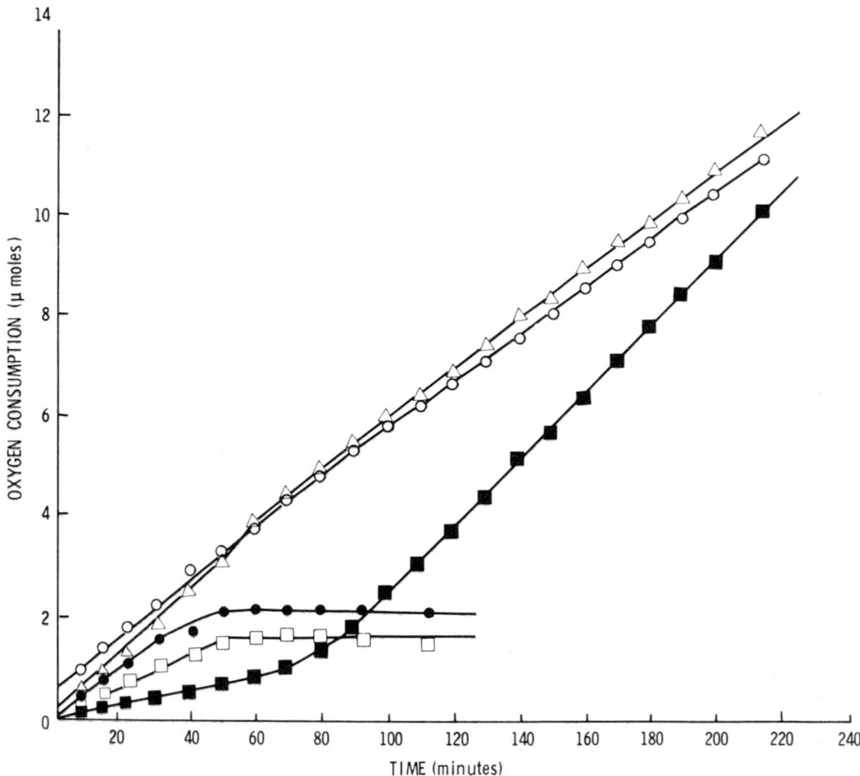

Fig. 21.5. The effect of oxaloacetic acid (OAA) removal by transamination on respiratory decline of succinic oxidase reactions in vitamin E–deficient rat-liver homogenates. ●, declining medium; □, declining medium + transamination; ■, non-declining medium + OAA; △, non-declining medium; O, non-declining medium + OAA + transamination.

has no effect on respiratory decline. The efficiency of oxaloacetic acid removal was tested in nondeclining reactions by adding of sufficient oxaloacetic acid to inhibit the succinate reaction and removing this inhibition by transamination. To guard against the permeability and compartmentalization effects, the experiments were also performed with sonified homogenates.

In order to further clarify the influence of NAD^+ on the respiratory decline of vitamin E–deficient liver homogenates, succinic oxidase reactions were performed in the Warburg respirometer with liver homogenates obtained from animals maintained on both the deficient and the α-tocopherol and selenium supplemented diets. Reactions were performed in different media, starting with the simplest containing only Tris and succinate, and successively adding the other cofactors until the full complement of Tris, Mg^{++}, ATP, ADP, and phosphate was reached. From these investigations, it became clear that respiratory decline does not occur in the absence of phosphate and NAD^+. In the absence of phosphate and NAD^+, but in the presence of Tris, Mg^{++}, and ATP, both deficient and supplemented homogenates gave identical, nondeclining respiration rates (Fig. 21.6). An interesting feature of these reactions is the initially slow, but linear, reaction rate, which increases abruptly after approximately 30–40 min. In the presence of 10 mM phosphate, the reaction starts immediately at its maximum rate. Increasing the concentration of phosphate to 30 mM produces no further increase in the initial reaction rate. The slight decline observed after 70 min with 10 mM phosphate became more accentuated at the higher concentration. This could be attributed to a potentiating effect of phosphate on the decline, producing endogenous NAD^+. Finally, with 1 mM NAD^+, the usual, drastic, zero-order decline following 30 min of normal oxygen consumption is observed. On the basis of these and earlier experiments, respiratory decline appears intimately connected with the presence of exogenous NAD^+.

NICOTINAMIDE ADENINE DINUCLEOTIDASE ACTIVITY

The possibility that destruction of NAD^+ by nicotinamide adenine dinucleotidase is related to respiratory decline has been investigated before, with negative results (Chernick et al., 1955). By assaying for NAD^+ with the alcohol dehydrogenase method, we established in the present series of experiments that α-tocopherol, Mn^{++}, and EDTA have no effect on the rate of NAD^+ losses. In addition, tests with nicotinamide supplements inhibitory to nicotinamide adenine dinucleotidase activity had no effect on the respiratory breakdown, nor was nicotinamide adenine dinucleotidase activity detectable in a mitochondrial system showing respiratory decline (see below). Grove and Johnson (1967), on the other hand, using

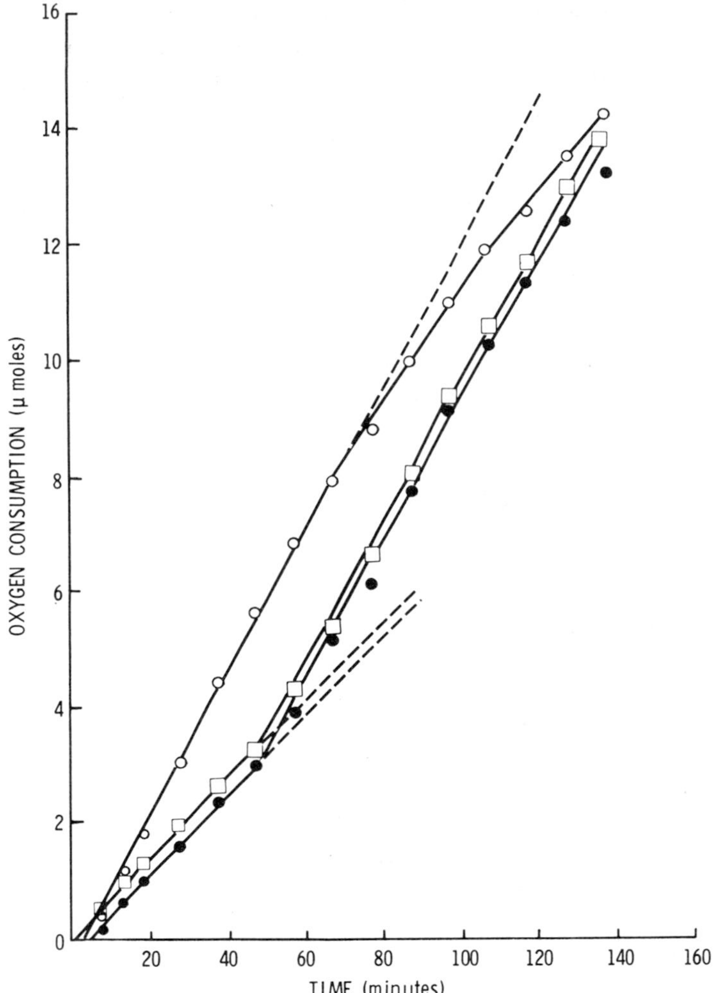

Fig. 21.6. Succinic oxidase reactions with liver homogenates obtained from rats maintained on a vitamin E–deficient or a vitamin E–supplemented diet. Reaction medium: tris buffer (*p*H 7.6), 5 mM Mg^{++}. □, vitamin E–deficient; ●, vitamin E–supplemented; O, vitamin E–deficient + 10 mM of sodium phosphate.

β-hydroxybutyrate as substrate, related the enhancement of respiratory decline by microsomes to nicotinamide adenine dinucleotidase effects. The β-hydroxybutyrate oxidase system requires NAD^+. It appears that different oxidase systems could vary in sensitivity to nicotinamide adenine dinucleotidase activity.

INDEPENDENCE OF RESPIRATORY DECLINE FROM EFFECTS OF 2,4-DINITROPHENOL

The above-mentioned abrupt increase in reaction rate (Fig. 21.6) at the point where decline usually takes place was further investigated. It was found that this increase could not be prevented by the in vitro addition of α-tocopherol. The reaction started immediately at its maximum rate, however, when the homogenate was sonified or when 0.05 mM 2,4-dinitrophenol was included. The graphs obtained from these experiments were identical to those in Fig. 21.6 with 10 mM of phosphate. It appears, therefore, that the above-mentioned increase in rate, without 2,4-dinitrophenol, could be due to an uncoupling of the mitochondria under Warburg conditions rather than to a sudden increase in permeability of the mitochondrial membrane. The latter possibility cannot be excluded, however, in view of the chemiosmotic theory of oxidative phosphorylation in which uncoupling is attributed to specific permeability changes (Lehninger, 1965). It is evident, then, that respiratory decline induced by the Warburg conditions and uncoupling occur at approximately the same time, i.e., after 30 to 40 min of respiration. It has yet to be established, however, whether these effects are causally interrelated or are only coincidentally parallel to each other.

In older experiments with liver slices (Chernick and Schwarz, 1956), it was shown that respiratory decline is not affected by 2,4-dinitrophenol. Both the stimulatory and inhibitory effects of the drug were masked by the failure of oxygen uptake. It was inferred that the site of the metabolic lesion in respiratory decline is separate and distinct from that of 2,4-dinitrophenol action. A reexamination of the question of the link between uncoupling and respiratory decline was carried out, under present experimental conditions, using liver homogenates and concentrations of 2,4-dinitrophenol which uncouple but are not inhibitory to oxygen consumption. In agreement with the previous results, respiratory decline occurred as usual after 30 to 40 min, in spite of uncoupling by 2,4-dinitrophenol. These results seem to exclude the direct participation of uncoupling in the respiratory-decline mechanism.

The finding by Azzone, Ernster, and Klingenberg (1960) that 2,4-dinitrophenol uncouples mitochondrial respiration from oxidative phosphorylation but does not inhibit energy-dependent reverse electron flow may be important in the interpretation of these results. It will be shown below that, under certain conditions, reverse electron flow is implicated in the initiation of respiratory decline. While only uncoupling occurs with 2,4-dinitrophenol, uncoupling caused by Warburg assay conditions could be associated with a breakdown in reverse electron flow. The occurrence of an increase in oxygen consumption (failure of respiratory control) at the 30 to 40 min mark on one hand and of a decrease in oxygen consumption in the presence of NAD+ and phosphate (respiratory decline) on the other could thus be understood.

TIME ELEMENT IN RESPIRATORY DECLINE

The dependence of respiratory decline on the NAD+ concentration (Fig. 21.7) is of considerable interest. Consistent with the above observation that decline appears related to the detrimental conditions of the Warburg assay, only the severity of decline and not the time of its occurrence is determined by the concentration of NAD+. The severity of decline is an abruptly changing function of the NAD+ concentration, not a continuous one. It appears to occur in at least two phases, suggesting critical threshhold effects at different NAD+ levels.

THE ROLE OF MICROSOMES

Under the standard conditions of the earlier experiments, isolated mitochondria from prenecrotic livers (in contrast to intact liver slices and liver homogenates) performed normally, i.e., they demonstrated a behavior which in almost all respects was indistinguishable from that of normal mitochondria (Corwin and Schwarz, 1959). A consistent loss of respiration was seen, however, when malate or succinate were used as substrate in the presence of NAD+. Since oxaloacetic acid is a potent inhibitor of succinate and malate, and since ATP, acetyl CoA, Mn^{++}, and Mg^{++} – which aid in the removal of oxaloacetate – prevented this phenomenon, it was postulated that one of the pathways of the enzymatic utilization of oxaloacetate was impaired by the absence of tocopherol.

Combination experiments with mitochondria and various subfractions such as microsomes and microsomal supernatants showed that the supernatant fraction by itself had only a small effect, but that the addition of the microsomes to the system produced respiratory decline which was preventable by tocopherol at near-physiological dose levels (Corwin, 1961; Schwarz, 1962*a*). These studies were carried out with oxaloacetic acid or α-ketoglutarate as substrate.

Under the present experimental conditions with succinate as substrate, we have not been able to demonstrate a deleterious effect of sonified or unsonified microsomes on the respiratory behavior of mitochondria. Carefully washed mitochondria with or without dietary vitamin E show a vitamin E–responsive respiratory breakdown (see below). While the differences between the previous results with microsome fractions and the more recent studies have not been fully explained, it is apparent that one of the components of the medium or some other experimental parameter is etiologically involved. Since different substrates have been used, it is also possible that different oxidase systems are not equally responsive to the addition of the microsomal fraction. This latter possibility is borne out by results

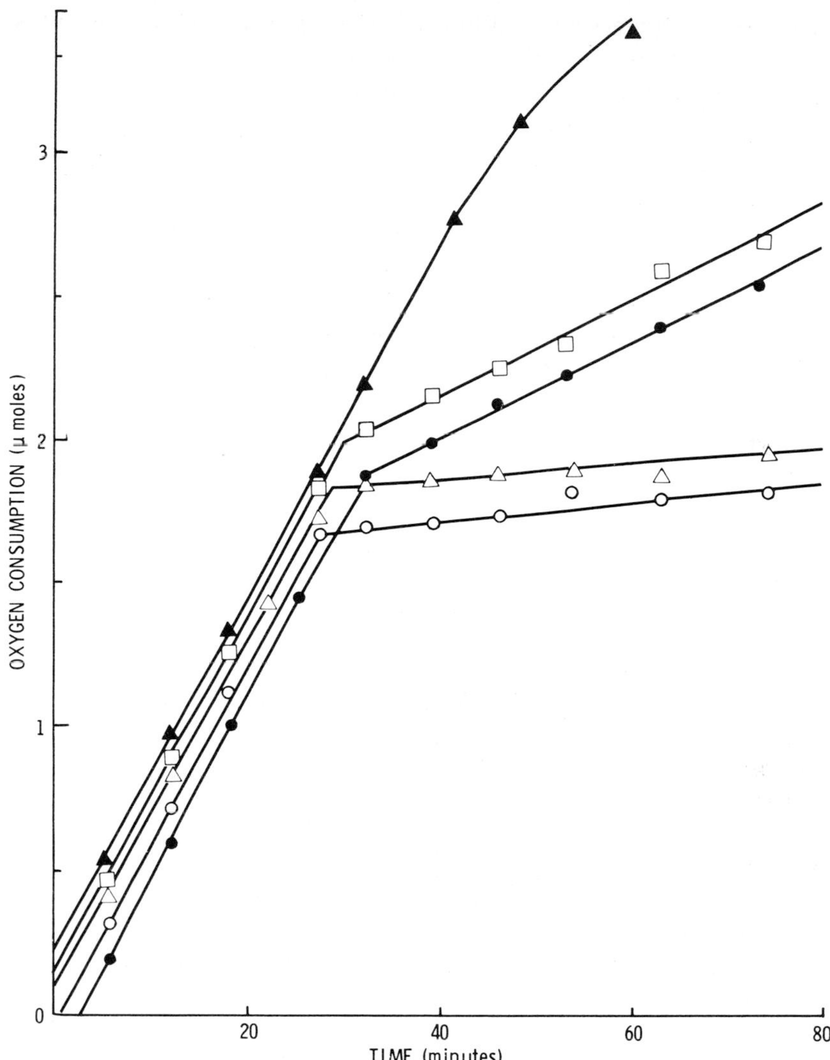

Fig. 21.7. Respiratory decline of the succinic oxidase reaction with vitamin E–deficient rat-liver homogenates at different NAD^+ concentrations. NAD^+ concentrations (mM): ▲, zero; ●, 0.17; □, 0.34; O, 0.68; △, 1.02.

of Grove and co-workers, who found that the addition of microsomes to mitochondria in reactions with succinate, α-ketoglutarate, or malate resulted in increased oxygen consumption but in no additional respiratory decline in the case of α-ketoglutarate and succinate. With β-hydroxybutyrate as substrate, on the other hand, no increase in respiration was seen, but addition of microsomes resulted in respiratory failure (Grove et al., 1966). In a subsequent paper, respiratory decline with β-hydroxybutyrate as substrate was related to NAD-ase activity associated with the microsomal fraction (Grove and Johnson, 1967).

THE EFFECT OF COMPLEXING AGENTS

The possibility that NAD^+ produces respiratory decline via ionic impurities was examined, particularly since the phenomenon can be prevented by EDTA, diethyldithiocarbamate, α,α'-dipyridyl, or *o*-phenanthroline (McLean, 1960; Schwarz, 1962*a*). Experiments were performed with NAD^+ from three different sources and grades of purities. Identical respiratory-decline patterns were obtained with all three samples. It is possible that the effect of EDTA is related to its well-documented effect on the state of the mitochondrial membrane (Hunter et al., 1969) or to its influence on the binding of NAD^+ to the latter (MacLennan and Tzagoloff, 1966). The significance of this binding will be discussed below.

DECLINE OF SUCCINIC DEHYDROGENASE VS. SUCCINIC OXIDASE

The activities of several key dehydrogenases were compared to the activity of their respective oxidases in the Warburg assay. Experiments were performed under declining and nondeclining conditions in the presence and absence of vitamin E. Samples of homogenate were removed during the Warburg assay for spectroscopic measurements of dehydrogenase activities with artificial electron acceptors. Several difficulties were encountered, caused by partial precipitation of the homogenate and changes in the mitochondrial membrane which take place during the Warburg assay. Techniques for sampling and membrane rupture were used which prevented scatter artifacts. Succinic dehydrogenase activity, measured with phenazine methosulfate as electron acceptor, did not decrease significantly within the 30–40 min interval in which respiratory decline regularly manifests itself in the succinic oxidase system (see Fig. 21.4). Therefore, a loss of succinic dehydrogenase activity is not directly linked to respiratory decline.

On extending the exposure of the homogenate to the respiratory-decline-producing Warburg medium for 180 min, however, the dehydrogenase activity decreased by 50%. This late decline in succinic dehydrogenase activity occurs only in the presence of the NAD^+ supplement, in analogy to respiratory decline per se under our experimental conditions. It also is prevented by in vivo or in vitro supplementation of tocopherol. The phenomenon is not observed when the Warburg vessels are not shaken. Whether respiratory decline occurs in the absence of shaking could not be established, since oxygen diffusion becomes rate limiting. There are numerous conditions, however, under which respiratory decline of vitamin E–deficient homogenates does not occur, in spite of vigorous shaking.

DECLINE OF LIPOYL DEHYDROGENASE VS. α-KETOGLUTARATE OXIDASE

It had been shown previously that lipoyl dehydrogenase activity decreases along with the respiratory decline of the α-ketoglutarate oxidase system (Schwarz et al., 1962). The kinetics of these declines were reinvestigated under the present, somewhat different, conditions.

The present determinations of lipoyl dehydrogenase were carried out after sonification of the samples taken from the Warburg medium, in contrast to the previous studies in which digitonin treatment was used to make the enzyme accessible to the participants in the assay reaction. A comparison of these two methods showed that sonification produced activities which were severalfold bigger than those obtained with the digitonin treatment. Using sonification, we found that lipoyl dehydrogenase differed in several important respects from other enzyme systems exhibiting decline under Warburg conditions (succinic dehydrogenase, NADH oxidase). With vitamin E–deficient homogenates, the enzyme declines slowly from the start of the Warburg assay, reaching approximately 50% of its original activity after 160 min of Warburg exposure. An almost identical loss of activity was observed in the absence of NAD^+ (−58%), i.e., under conditions where respiratory decline does not occur. Identical decreases in activity were obtained when the vessels were kept at rest. Dietary supplementation of α-tocopherol has only a slight protecting effect against the loss in enzyme activity (−42% of initial activity in 160 min with dietary vitamin E and −58% without it). This situation could not be improved by the in vitro addition of tocopherol.

It is obvious that the continuously declining lipoyl dehydrogenase activity observed in the present study with sonified samples does not parallel the zero-order kinetics of respiratory decline. While digitonin treatment in the earlier experiments produced results showing a close relationship between lipoyl dehydrogenase activity and respiratory decline, the present experiments indicate that there is no parallel between the total lipoyl dehydrogenase activity in the mitochondria and respiratory breakdown during the Warburg experiment. With α-ketoglutarate, the decrease in total lipoyl dehydrogenase activity is not low enough to be consistent with an explanation based on a changeover in the rate-determining step. This follows from the fact that the rate-determining-step approximation requires at least a tenfold difference in rates between the slowest and the second slowest steps in a reaction sequence before it can be applied with any kind of validity. Only if the overall activity of lipoyl dehydrogenase accurately reflects the lipoyl dehydrogenase activity within the α-ketoglutarate oxidase compartment would a consecutive kinetic mechanism without a rate-determining step be similarly excluded.

DECLINE OF NADH OXIDASE VS. α-KETOGLUTARATE OXIDASE

Enzyme systems such as α-ketoglutarate oxidase, which involve NAD+ as a cofactor, proceed via the NADH oxidase system (Fig. 21.3). In view of the known instability of NADH oxidase under in vitro conditions (Singer, 1966), one has to consider the possibility that respiratory decline with NADH-linked substrates is caused by the deterioration of the NADH oxidase system. Experiments showed that in vitamin E–deficient homogenates the deactivation observed in the NADH oxidase system (Fig. 21.8) is more closely related to the respiratory decline of α-ketoglutarate than to the previously noted deactivation of the overall activity of lipoyl dehydrogenase. In the present case, the NADH oxidase activity decreased rapidly to approximately 25% of its original activity within the first half hour, i.e., before the onset of respiratory decline. In the absence of exogenous NAD+, decline in NADH oxidase also occurred, but only at approximately half the rate. The biphasic curve describing the decline in enzyme activity reaches the 25% level after about 125 min. Addition of α-tocopherol to the diet or the medium prevents the rapid loss of NADH oxidase ac-

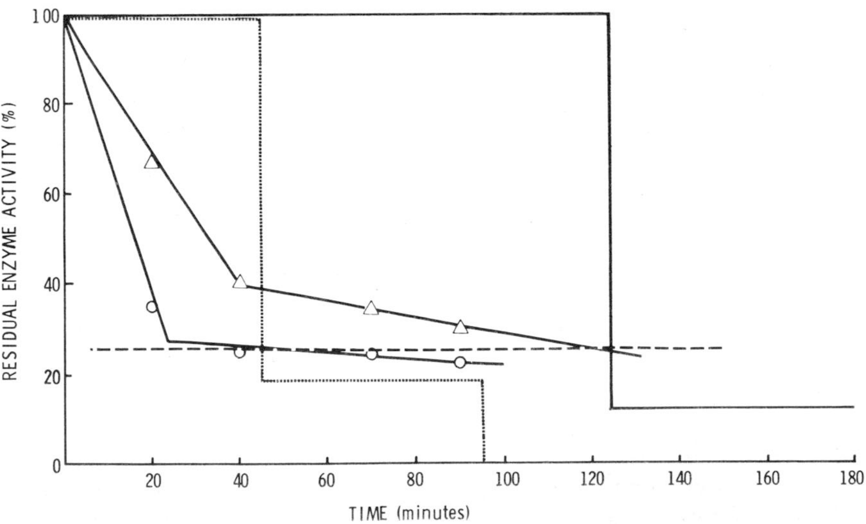

Fig. 21.8. NADH oxidase activity at different stages of α-ketoglutarate oxidation by vitamin E-deficient liver homogenates in the Warburg respirometer. Warburg assay: α-ketoglutarate without NAD^+, solid line, α-ketoglutarate + 1 mM NAD^+, dotted line. NADH oxidase assay: without NAD^+, △; with NAD^+, O.

tivity (not shown on graph). After 180 min of exposure to the Warburg medium with shaking, 60% of the initial activity is still present. No decrease in NADH oxidase activity was observed when the homogenate was incubated without shaking for 180 min in the Warburg respirometer. When NADH dehydrogenase activity was measured using $K_3[Fe(CN)_6]$ as an acceptor, no decrease in activity was observed under any of the above-described conditions.

From a kinetic point of view, the results show that NADH oxidase is not rate limiting in the respiration with α-ketoglutarate as substrate, since the decrease in α-ketoglutarate oxidase activity does not follow NADH oxidase deactivation. The decrease in NADH oxidase activity would, however, be sufficiently severe and fast to have resulted in a changeover in the rate-determining step prior to the incidence of respiratory decline. This means that, although NADH oxidase activity is not normally rate controlling, it may have approached this situation after 25 min in the presence of NAD^+, when the activity has decreased to 25% of its original value. However, since this level is now almost constant at 25%, it is not possible to explain the abrupt decrease in α-ketoglutarate activity in simple kinetic terms. This view is further supported by the observation that 80% of bound NAD^+ can be lost without influencing the respiration rate of NADH-linked enzymes (MacLennan and Tzagoloff, 1966).

Although the data in Figure 21.8 exclude the explanation of respiratory decline in terms of a changeover in rate-determining step, as well as in terms of a consecutive mechanism (no rate-determining step), they point to yet another conceivable mechanism. A mitochondrial-control mechanism may exist which operates on respiration according to a binary (off-on) control mechanism. The data suggest the existence of a threshhold value of minimum NADH oxidase activity. When this point is reached, at approximately 25% of its original activity, a sudden shutdown in electron transport takes place. This could be related to conformational changes in enzymes or to local critical changes of membrane potential with resultant alterations in membrane and enzyme structure (and function). In the presence of NAD^+ this occurs after 45 min, and in the absence of NAD^+, after 125 min.

ZERO-ORDER VS. NON-ZERO-ORDER DECLINE

From the data presented so far, it is clear that one should distinguish between zero-order-respiratory-decline and continuous-decline mechanisms. Certain important differences, as well as parallels, exist between these two phenomena. Zero-order decline shows abrupt and well-defined responses toward NAD^+ and α-tocopherol, suggestive of a physiologically important control mechanism of respiration. Continuous decline, on the other hand, shows less dramatic responses to vitamin E or NAD+. It appears that in continuous decline vitamin E could protect specific active sites against unspecific inactivating mechanisms, such as protein denaturation at the air-liquid interface during shaking.

Respiratory decline in isolated mitochondria

RESPIRATORY DECLINE

To more readily relate results obtained with isolated mitochondria to those of the homogenate system, it was decided to use an exclusively mitochondrial enzyme, such as succinic oxidase, in the attempt to demonstrate decline in mitochondria. Except for the use of 1mM ADP, an identical medium of Tris buffer, ATP, Mg++, sodium phosphate, and NAD+ was used in initial studies of respiratory decline. The differences between reactions in which NAD+ had been excluded (nondeclining medium) and those containing NAD+ (declining medium) were slight. For these experiments, mitochondria corresponding to 100 mg of liver tissue were used per 3 ml of medium. Mitochondria were prepared from the above-described liver homogenates by further centrifugation in a Servall SS–1 centrifuge at 9,000 rpm for a period of 15 min. The pellet was washed twice with 0.25 M sucrose which equaled the volume of removed supernatant prior to final resuspension. In view of the high MC ratio of isolated mitochondria for NAD+ (see above), the NAD+ concentration was doubled and that of phosphate trebled over that used in the initial experiments with isolated mitochondria. Under these conditions a significant zero-order decline was obtained (Fig. 21.9). Respiratory decline occurred not only in mitochondria from animals on diets deficient in α-tocopherol, however, but also in those from animals on diets supplemented with vitamin E or maintained on normal stock diets. Furthermore, decline could not be prevented in the isolated mitochondria by addition of α-tocopherol alone.

VITAMIN E–ACTIVATOR EFFECT

The cause for the absence of a vitamin E effect was investigated by reconstitution experiments. Mitochondria isolated from deficient and supplemented animals were recombined with their respective mitochondrial supernatants. The reconstituted sample was therefore identical to the homogenate (minus nucleus and cell debris), except for centrifugation and two washings of the isolated mitochondria with 0.25 M sucrose. Experiments performed with these "reconstituted homogenates" from vitamin E–deficient and from vitamin E–supplemented animals gave identical respiratory-decline patterns. These results indicate that diet differences in respiratory decline disappear as a consequence of either centrifugation, resuspension, or washing procedures. On investigating these possibilities

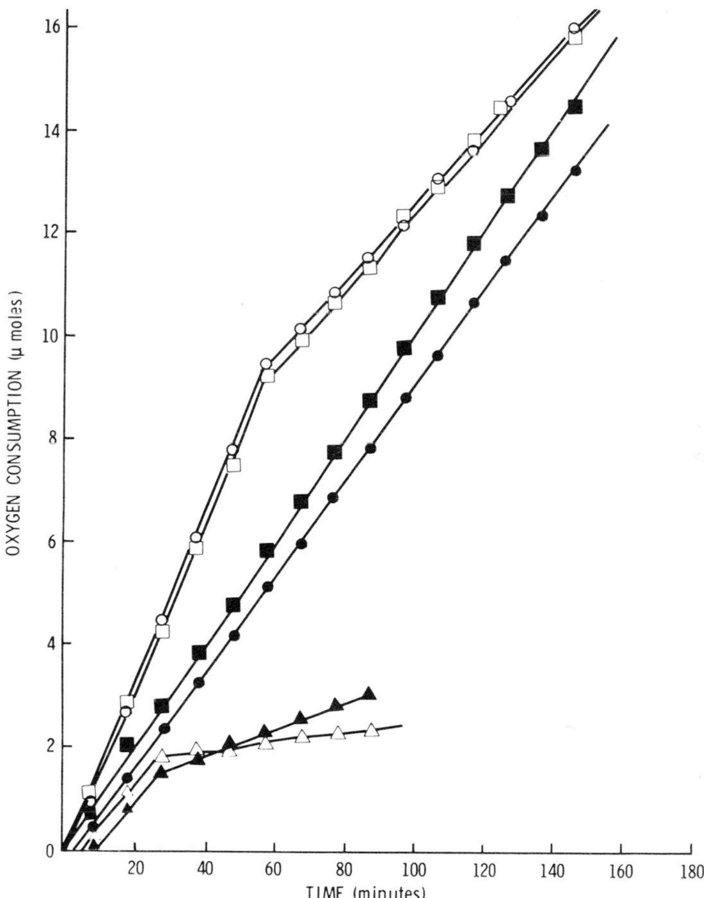

Fig. 21.9. The effect of different amounts of alcohol-precipitate in combination with 50 μg of α-tocopherol on respiratory decline of isolated mitochondria with succinate as substrate. Reaction medium: tris buffer (*p*H 7.6); 20 mM sodium phosphate; 3 mM Mg^{++}; 1 mM ATP; 1 mM ADP; and 2 mM NAD^+, as indicated. The amount of precipitate is expressed as the percentage of the amount present in the equivalent mass of liver tissue. Reactions were performed with NAD^+ and indicated percentage of precipitate: △, zero; ▲, 12%; ■, 25%; □, 50%; O, 100%. Reactions performed without NAD^+: ●, zero precipitate.

further, it was found that washing of the isolated mitochondria caused the disappearance of diet differences. It removes a loosely adhering layer of protein, as shown by biuret assays. This material could possibly contain vitamin E or a derivative of vitamin E. It has not been possible, to date, to reestablish normal functions by recombining mitochondria with the removed fraction. Addition of α-tocopherol to these reconstituted homogenates prevents respiratory decline.

The problem was further studied by partial reconstitution experiments, in which washed mitochondria were recombined with only one of the following constituent components: microsomes, microsomal supernatant, precipitate derived from the microsomal supernatant with treatment by either alcohol or heat, and the filtrate of the last-mentioned fraction. From the results of the above-described reconstitution experiments and the data shown in Figure 21.9, it is apparent that vitamin E requires the presence of an activating component before it can protect against respiratory decline. This activator is present in the microsomal supernatant. Dialysis experiments have shown that the vitamin E activator is tightly associated with the alcohol- or heat-precipitable material of the microsomal supernatant fraction. Furthermore, the activator appears not to be an enzyme, since boiling up to one hour does not destroy its effect.

The effects of varying activator concentrations on the protective effect of 50 μg of α-tocopherol are shown in Figure 21.9. It is seen that 100%, 50%, or 25% of the normal activator concentration produce almost identical results as far as vitamin E protection against respiratory decline is concerned. At a concentration of 12%, no vitamin E activation was observed. Experiments with activator concentrations in the 12%–24% interval (not shown) indicate an abrupt termination of the effect within a 3% concentration range. The cutoff point in effective vitamin E–activator concentration varies somewhat from one preparation to another. No significant difference in efficiency could be detected in vitamin E–activator preparations from deficient and from vitamin E–supplemented rats. It is also evident from Figure 21.9 that the kinetics of respiration change with increasing vitamin E–activator concentration. At a concentration of 50% or more, an increase of respiration for a period of 57 min occurs in addition to the vitamin E–activation effect. Respiration then returns abruptly to a normal rate. Increasing the concentration to 100% does not influence the duration of the period of increased respiration. The abrupt return to normal respiration rates at the 57 min mark occurs both in the presence and in the absence of NAD^+, and may therefore be unrelated to respiratory decline.

To guard against effects of microsomal or other types of contamination, experiments were performed with three different fractions of mitochondria. Heavy, medium, and light mitochondria were prepared by centrifugation in 0.25 M sucrose at 3,000, 7,000, and 10,000 rpm, respectively, for sufficient time to give approximately three equal fractions. Identical patterns of respiratory decline were obtained with all three mitochondrial fractions.

Since it was essential to perform these experiments with the same mitochondria/NAD+ ratio, mitochondria were quantified according to their succinic dehydrogenase activity rather than by their light-scattering properties or their protein content.

NADH OXIDASE VS. SUCCINIC OXIDASE AND SUCCINIC DEHYDROGENASE

In order to further narrow down the area in which respiratory decline originates, experiments were performed with the NADH oxidase system (as measured in the Warburg respirometer with isolated mitochondria) in the absence of other substrates. The decline-producing medium with high NAD+ and phosphate levels was used. Low shaking rates of 80 cycle/min were used, since deactivation through coagulation was observed at higher speeds. It was also necessary to employ sufficiently high NADH concentrations (15 μmoles) to avoid control of the reaction rate by diffusion processes.

Under these conditions, constant NADH oxidase activity was obtained for 50 min of incubation. No respiratory decline was observed. This is noteworthy since, with succinate as a substrate, the same mitochondria exhibited respiratory decline in the succinic oxidase assay but maintained a constant succinic dehydrogenase activity. The latter enzyme was determined with phenazine methosulfate as an electron acceptor. The enzyme systems involved are shown in Figure 21.3. Phenazine methosulfate draws electrons from the flavoprotein designated as FP_3. The latter, succinic dehydrogenase, is a complex enzyme containing not only flavin adenine dinucleotide but also Mo^{++} and labile, nonheme iron as participants in the electron-transfer operation. Since (a) respiratory decline does not occur with NADH as a substrate and (b) the succinate dehydrogenase reaction (with phenazine methosulfate) is intact in declining mitochondria when succinate is a substrate, two possibilities apparently exist for the location of the primary metabolic lesion:

1. It is possible that the mechanism linking succinic dehydrogenase and coenzyme Q (CoQ reductase system) breaks down and is the site of action of α-tocopherol.

2. It is also possible that changes in membrane-bound NAD+ control the mitochondrial respiration of succinate.

At present, it is not possible to indicate which of these two alternatives for locating the primary metabolic lesion and the site of action of vitamin E is really involved. Both concepts are consistent with most of the experimental findings and with the working hypothesis developed at a much earlier phase of these studies, which indicated that the active site of tocopherol in the respiratory-decline system is located neither in the main parts of the citric acid cycle nor in the electron-transfer chain, but rather in the mechanisms which connect these two systems to each other (Schwarz,

1962*a*). The first alternative (see also Corwin, 1965), i.e., the involvement of the succinic dehydrogenase/CoQ reductase, will not be discussed further here.

MEMBRANE-BOUND NAD+

Respiratory decline could be the result of an increase in membrane-bound NAD+ through adsorption from the Warburg medium. A shift of the NAD+/NADH equilibrium towards the reduced form via reverse electron flow could also be involved in these interrelationships. Electron microscopic observations from the laboratories of Green (Green et al., 1968) and of Hackenbrock (1968) recently indicated that vast changes in the configuration of the inner mitochondrial membrane occur, depending on, and connected with, changes in respiration rates. It is conceivable that the changes in membrane configuration are the consequence of shifts in the NAD+/NADH equilibrium. Membrane-bound, oxidized NAD+ contains a strong positive charge which could be the cause of alterations in the inner mitochondrial membrane.

NAD+/NADH EQUILIBRIUM

Several findings would support the concept that bound NAD+ is of importance in triggering the stoppage of oxygen consumption when respiratory decline occurs. For instance NADH itself, as well as substrates which shift the NAD+/NADH equilibrium from the oxidized toward the reduced form (such as β-hydroxybutyrate), will not show respiratory decline. In the presence of Amytal, with succinate as a substrate, the inclusion of small amounts (6 μmoles) of NADH or of β-hydroxybutyrate will prevent respiratory decline in the absence of vitamin E. This effect can even be produced in sonified mitochondria. Further, Amytal has a potentiating effect on the tocopherol activator, making it possible to prevent decline with 50μg of α-tocopherol in vitro in the presence of only 2.5 of the activator concentration normally present. Since under these conditions there is no endogenous respiration, this effect is not due to reduction of NAD+ by the endogenous substrate.

RESPIRATORY-CONTROL MECHANISMS

The exact mechanism whereby bound NAD+ exercises respiratory control is not quite clear. Chance and co-workers (Chance and Hollunger, 1960; Chance and Hagihara, 1962) have suggested that NAD+ controls succinate respiration via the oxaloacetic acid feedback inhibition. In this case, the degree of NAD+ reoxidation is controlled by reverse electron flow. Azzone and co-workers (1960) object to this mechanism on the basis of results with uncoupled mitochondria and transamination experiments. Our transamination experiments with homogenates as well as with isolated mitochondria also seem to exclude this explanation for zero-order respiratory decline. Furthermore, respiratory decline occurs also in enzyme systems which are not subject to oxaloacetic acid feedback inhibition, such as α-ketoglutarate oxidase and α-glycerophosphate oxidase. The latter was found to be particularly sensitive, since it shows respiratory decline even in the absence of NAD^+. Phosphate ions, however, still potentiate the respiratory breakdown. The α-glycerophosphate shunt is the main shuttle between cytoplasmic and intramitochondrial NAD^+/NADH, and thus between cytoplasmic substrates and the respiratory chain (see Fig. 21.3), and could contribute significantly to the decline observed with NADH-linked enzyme systems in homogenates. Whether or not uncoupling may be a phenomenon parallel to respiratory decline, or whether it is causally related to the latter, has been discussed above.

Summary and Conclusions

No differences in various dehydrogenase and oxidase activities were found between normal mitochondria and those from vitamin E–deficient livers during the latent phase of dietary necrotic liver degeneration, i.e., shortly before the onset of necrosis and death from acute liver injury. MC ratios were also unaltered. However, in animals at the beginning of the acute terminal phase which show partial necrosis of the liver, a distinct breakdown of the membrane control of enzyme activities was observed.

In liver homogenates of animals during the prenecrotic phase of liver necrosis, respiratory decline – i.e., breakdown of oxidation after initially normal periods of respiration – follows typical zero-order kinetics. In the medium used (Tris buffer with low phosphate) and with succinate as substrate, respiratory decline is observed only in the presence of added NAD^+. During respiratory decline in the Warburg respirometer with succinate as a substrate, succinic dehydrogenase activity remained unchanged. When α-ketoglutarate served as substrate, a direct parallel between respiratory decline and the activities of total lipoyl dehydrogenase or NADH oxidase was not found. However, NADH oxidase showed a steep decline preceding the respiratory breakdown. With the exception of the latter system, none of the enzyme systems measured showed a loss of activity commensurate with a changeover in the rate-determining step or with the rate of oxygen consumption, which is initially kept at a high level and drops very suddenly to approximately one-fifth of the initial rate. The results do not exclude the possibility that a crucial enzyme declines and reaches a critically low level which leads through some secondary triggering mechanism to the acute breakdown of respiration.

A new system for the production of respiratory decline in isolated mitochondria has been found. In contrast to previous methods based on application of arsenite or Cd^{++}, the present system uses the medium applied for homogenate studies, which contains high NAD^+ and sodium phosphate levels. Not only vitamin E– and selenium-deficient liver mitochondria, but also those from normal animals supplied with vitamin E, undergo respiratory failure. Vitamin E alone has no effect on this system but is fully protective against this respiratory impairment when combined with the cytoplasmic supernatant. The component indispensable for vitamin E activity on the isolated mitochondria (vitamin E activator) is precipitated from the supernatant, after removal of the microsomes, by means of ethanol or by heat treatment at 100 C. The activator is fully effective at approximately one-fifth of the amounts normally present. There is no significant difference in vitamin E–activator levels in livers from vitamin E– and selenium-deficient animals and from normal animals.

In this mitochondrial system, respiratory decline is observed with succinic acid as a substrate while succinic dehydrogenase levels remain steady. NADH oxidase, on the other hand, does not show respiratory failure. Respiratory decline also does not occur with succinate as a substrate in the presence of Amytal and small amounts of α-hydroxybutyrate or NADH.

These results would favor one of two modes of action of vitamin E in the prevention of respiratory decline.

It is possible that vitamin E is an active participant, a cofactor, in electron-transfer catalysis. Under the conditions of the present experiments, the area of the primary metabolic lesion in respiratory decline could be located between succinic dehydrogenase and coenzyme Q (CoQ reductase), if succinic acid is the substrate.

The alternate explanation based on changes in membrane-bound NAD^+ which could control mitochondrial utilization of succinate via configurational changes of enzymes or membrane structures.

At present, it is not possible to decide which of these two alternatives for locating the primary metabolic lesion and the site of action of vitamin E is really involved. Both are consistent with most of the experimental findings and with the working hypothesis, developed at a much earlier phase of these studies, which indicated that the active site of tocopherol in the respiratory-decline system is located neither in the main parts of the citric acid cycle, nor in the electron-transfer chain, but rather in the mechanisms which connect these two systems to each other.

References

Allman, D. W., and E. Bachmann. 1967. Isolation of a mitochondrial membrane fraction containing the citric acid cycle and ancillary enzymes, p. 443. *In* R. W. Estabrook and M. E. Pullman (eds.), *Methods in Enzymology*, Vol. X. Academic Press, New York.

Azzone, G. F., L. Ernster, and M. Klingenberg. 1960. Energetic aspects of the mitochondrial oxidation of succinate. *Nature 188*:552.

Bull, R. C., and J. E. Oldfield. 1967. Selenium involvement in the oxidation by rat liver tissue of certain tricarboxylic cycle intermediates. *J. Nutr. 91*:237.

Chance, B., and B. Hagihara. 1962. Activation and inhibition of succinate oxidation following adenosine disphosphate supplements to pigeon heart mitochondria. *J. Biol. Chem. 237*:3540.

Chance, B., and G. Hollunger. 1960. Energy-linked reduction of mitochondrial pyridine nucleotide. *Nature 185*:666.

Chernick, S. S., J. G. Moe, G. P. Rodnan, and K. Schwarz. 1955. A metabolic lesion in dietary necrotic liver degeneration. *J. Biol. Chem 217*:829.

Chernick, S. S., and K. Schwarz. 1956. Dinitrophenol and the site of the respiratory lesion in dietary necrotic liver degeneration. *Fed. Proc. 15*:754.

Corwin, L. M. 1961. Role of microsomes in decline of oxidation in vitamin E–deficient rat liver homogenates. *Fed. Proc. 20*:145.

Corwin, L. M. 1962. Studies on peroxidation in vitamin E–deficient rat liver homogenates. *Arch. Biochem. Biophys. 97*:51.

Corwin, L. M. 1965. Further studies on the regulation of succinate oxidation by vitamin E. *J. Biol. Chem. 240*:34.

Corwin, L. M., and K. Schwarz. 1958. Vitamin E, Factor 3 and succinate oxidation. *Fed. Proc. 17*:206.

Corwin, L. M., and K. Schwarz. 1959. An effect of vitamin E on the regulation of succinate oxidation in rat liver mitochondria. *J. Biol. Chem. 234*:191.

Daft, F. S. 1954. Experimental differentiation between liver necrosis and liver cirrhosis and some dietary factors affecting their development. *Ann. N.Y. Acad. Sci. 57*:623.

Daft, F. S., W. H. Sebrell, and R. D. Lillie. 1942. Prevention by cystine or methionine of hemorrhage and necrosis of the liver in rats. *Proc. Soc. Exp. Biol. Med. 50*:1.

Green, D. E., J. Asai, R. A. Harris, and J. T. Pennison. 1968. Conformational basis of energy transformations in membrane systems. *Arch. Biochem. Biophys. 125*:684.

Greville, G. D. 1966. Factors affecting the utilization of substrates by mitochondria, p. 88. *In* J. M. Tager, S. Papa, E. Quagliariello, and E. C. Slater (eds.), *Regulation of Metabolic Processes in Mitochondria*. American Elsevier, New York.

Grove, J. A., and R. M. Johnson. 1967. Vitamin E deficiency in the rat. III. The relationship of nicotinamide adenine dinucleotide to respiratory decline. *J. Biol. Chem. 242*:1623.

Grove, J. A., R. M. Johnson, and J. H. Cline. 1965. Vitamin E deficiency in the rat. I. Effect of substrate concentration on respiratory decline in liver homogenates from rats fed a vitamin E–deficient diet. *Arch. Biochem. Biophys. 110*:357.

Grove, J. A., R. M. Johnson, and J. H. Cline. 1966. Vitamin E deficiency in the rat. II. The effect of rat liver microsomes and cytoplasmic supernatant on respiratory decline. *J. Biol. Chem. 241*:5564.

Hackenbrock, C. R. 1968. Ultrastructural bases for metabolically linked mechanical activity in mitochondria. II. Electron transport-linked ultrastructural transformations in mitochondria. *J. Cell Biol. 37*:345.

Hunter, F. E., J. F. Levy, J. Fink, B. Schutz, F. Guerra, and A. Hurwitz. 1959. Studies on the mechanism by which anaerobiosis prevents swelling of mitochondria *in vitro*: Effects of electron transport chain inhibitors. *J. Biol. Chem. 234*:2176.

Lehninger, A. L. 1965. *The Mitochondrion: Molecular Basis of Structure and Function*, 2nd ed., p. 128. W. A. Benjamin, New York.

McLean, A. E. M. 1960. Phenergan and versene in dietary liver necrosis. *Nature 185*:191.

MacLennan, D. H., and A. Tzagoloff. 1966. Studies on the electron transfer system. LXVI. Effect of diphosphopyridine nucleotide deficiency on respiration, respiratory control, and phosphorylation in mitochondria. *J. Biol. Chem. 241*:1933.

Schwarz, K. 1944*a*. Über einen ernährungsbedingten, tödlichen Leberschaden und seine Verhütung durch Leberschutzstoffe. Hoppe-Seyler's *Physiol. Chem. 281*:101.

Schwarz, K. 1944*b*. Tocopherol als Leberschutzstoff. Hoppe-Seyler's *Physiol. Chem. 281*:109.

Schwarz, K. 1951. A hitherto unrecognized factor against dietary necrotic liver degeneration in American yeast (Factor 3). *Proc. Soc. Exp. Biol. Med. 78*:852.

Schwarz, K. 1961. A possible site of action for vitamin E in intermediary metabolism. Conference on "The Metabolism and Function of the Fat-Soluble Vitamins A, E, and K." *Am. J. Clin. Nutr. 9*:71.

Schwarz, K. 1962*a*. Vitamin E, trace elements and sulfhydryl groups in respiratory decline (An approach to the mode of action of tocopherol and related compounds). *In* "Symposium on Vitamin E and Metabolism." *Vitamins Hormones 20*:463.

Schwarz, K. 1962*b*. Lipids and antioxidants in dietary necrotic liver degeneration, p. 387. *In* H. W. Schultz (ed.), *Symposium on Foods: Lipids and Their Oxidation*. Avi, Westport, Conn.

Schwarz, K. 1965.The role of vitamin E, selenium and related factors in experimental nutritional liver diseases. *Fed. Proc. 24*:58.

Schwarz, K. 1969. Biochemistry and intermediary metabolism of vitamin E, pp. 28–43. *In* Symposium Proceedings. The Biochemistry, Assay and Nutritional Value of Vitamin E. Association of Vitamin Chemists. Chicago, Ill.

Schwarz, K., and C. M. Foltz. 1957. Selenium as an integral part of α-Factor 3 against dietary necrotic liver degeneration. *J. Amer. Chem. Soc. 79*:3292.

Schwarz, K., C. E. Lee, and J. P. Stesney. 1962. Lipoyl dehydrogenase as a site of enzymatic breakdown in respiratory decline. *Z. Naturforsch 17b*:788.

Singer, T. P. 1966. Flavoprotein dehydrogenases of the respiratory chain, p. 132. *In* M. Florkin and E. H. Stotz (eds.), *Comprehensive Biochemistry: Biological Oxidations*, Vol. *14*. American Elsevier, New York.

West, E. S., W. R. Todd, H. S. Mason, and J. T. Van Bruggen. 1966. *Textbook of Biochemistry*, p. 959. Macmillan, New York.

22

METABOLISM OF VITAMIN E

H. H. Draper and A. Saari Csallany

Introduction

It is a familiar paradox that, whereas the fat-soluble vitamins were the first to be discovered, their functions are destined to be the last to be elucidated. It is only in the last decade that substantial progress has been made in this field, and, in large part, advances have been made possible by the availability of new experimental tools: radiochemical forms of the vitamins for detection of metabolites in the tissues; new chromatographic methods for their isolation; nuclear magnetic resonance and mass spectroscopy for their characterization. These techniques have been of great value in identifying the metabolites formed in various tissues. On the other hand, the state of knowledge concerning the functional mechanisms of the fat-soluble vitamins is still in marked contrast to that concerning their water-soluble counterparts.

This situation is well illustrated by the present status of research on vitamin E. While several metabolites have been isolated and identified, they all appear to be biologically inactive metabolic end products rather than active forms. Not only has the search for an enzymatically active metabolite been unsuccessful, but there has been an increasing skepticism regarding its existence. The present paper contains a review of current knowledge of the metabolism of this vitamin and an evaluation of the significance of this information for the function of vitamin E in animals.

Metabolites of vitamin E

NATURAL FORMS

Following the studies of Pennock and co-workers (1964), there appear to be eight naturally occurring forms of vitamin E (Fig. 22.1). Nearly all information on the metabolism of the vitamin pertains to the α-isomer, but it is likely that the metabolic reactions of the other isomers are generally analogous. The superiority of the biological activity of α-tocopherol over that of the other forms evidently is due largely to differences in efficiencies

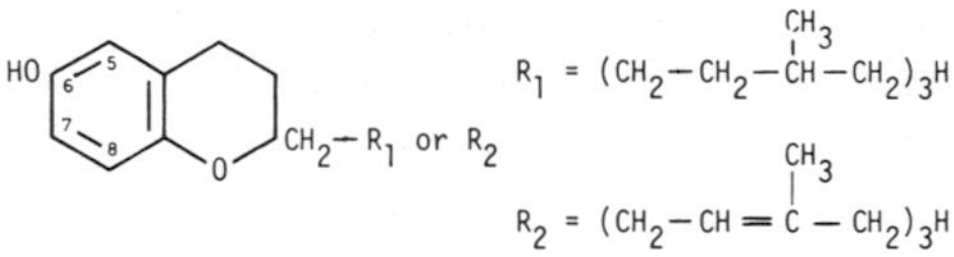

HO (ring positions 5, 6, 7, 8) chroman–CH_2–R_1 or R_2

$R_1 = (CH_2{-}CH_2{-}CH(CH_3){-}CH_2)_3H$

$R_2 = (CH_2{-}CH{=}C(CH_3){-}CH_2)_3H$

Tocols (R_1)	Tocotrienols (R_2)	CH_3 Substitution
α -T	α - T - 3	5, 7, 8
β -T	β - T - 3	5, 8
γ -T	γ - T - 3	7, 8
δ -T	δ - T - 3	8

Fig. 22.1. Naturally occurring forms of vitamin E. (After Pennock et al., 1964.)

of intestinal absorption and in rates of elimination from the tissues. The potencies of the various tocopherols in vitro, as reflected in the erythrocyte hemolysis assay or in the stabilization of unsaturated oils, are much more uniform. In evaluating nutritional status with respect to vitamin E, it is therefore probably more accurate to consider the total circulating plasma titer rather than only that of α-tocopherol.

α-TOCOPHEROL QUINONE AND α-TOCOPHERONIC ACID

Although the presence of α-tocopherol-*p*-quinone in lipid extracts of animal tissues is reported in a number of older publications, its formation as an isolation artifact on various chromatographic adsorbents left its natural occurrence in animal tissues in doubt for many years. Persuasive evidence for its formation in rat liver and in adipose tissue has been obtained, however, using ^{14}C-α-tocopherol (Csallany et al., 1962; Weber and Wiss, 1963). This compound is the major product of chemical oxidation with such agents as $FeCl_3$, $AuCl_3$, and $AgNO_3$ (Figure 22.2). It is readily reduced to the hydroquinone form, both chemically and biologically, and there is evidence that it may participate in electron transport in chloroplasts, where it is present in substantial concentrations (Dilley and Crane, 1963). In animal systems, on the other hand, it is a minor metabolite of α-tocopherol and is essentially devoid of biological activity.

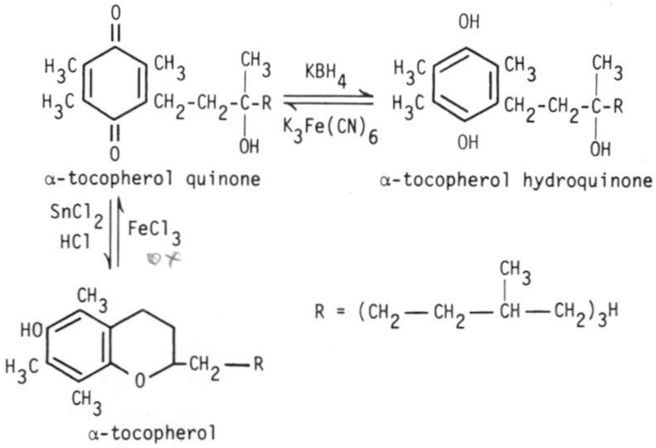

α-tocopherol quinone ⇌ (KBH_4 forward; $K_3Fe(CN)_6$ reverse) α-tocopherol hydroquinone

α-tocopherol quinone ⇌ ($SnCl_2$, HCl; $FeCl_3$) α-tocopherol

$R = (CH_2{-}CH_2{-}CH(CH_3){-}CH_2)_3H$

Fig. 22.2. Interconversions of α-tocopherol, α-tocopherol quinone, and α-tocopherol hydroquinone.

Studies on the metabolism of ^{14}C-*d*-α-tocopherol quinone (Chow et al., 1967) showed that there is no conversion to α-tocopherol in rat liver. The compound was metabolized partially by reduction to the hydroquinone, conjugation with glucuronic acid, secretion in the bile, and elimination in the feces. Another portion was degraded, apparently in the kidney, to α-tocopheronic acid and was eliminated in the urine. This urinary metabolite (Fig. 22.3) was first isolated by Simon and co-workers (1956) after administration of massive doses of α-tocopherol to rabbits and humans. It is biologically inactive for animals and may be regarded as a product of α-tocopherol quinone catabolism. As the latter is itself only a minor metabolite of α-tocopherol and is eliminated partially through the feces, it follows that α-tocopheronic acid is ordinarily an extremely minor product of vitamin E metabolism. Its presence in the urine does serve, incidentally, as prima facie evidence for the natural occurrence of α-tocopherol quinone in the tissues.

The fate of α-tocopherol hydroquinone is of particular interest in view of the finding of Mackenzie and Mackenzie (1959, 1960) that this compound is active in the prevention of sterility and muscular dystrophy if administered in frequent doses. These authors concluded that the hydroquinone per se can serve as an antisterility and antidystrophic factor. Studies by Chow and co-workers (1967) on the metabolism of ^{14}C-*d*-α-tocopherol hydroquinone by rats showed that it was more rapidly eliminated from the liver than was the corresponding quinone. Conjugates of tocopheronic acid in the urine and of the hydroquinone in the feces were the main excretory forms. In contrast to the results obtained with ^{14}C-α-tocopherol quinone, little, if any, free compound was eliminated in the feces. Reduction of the quinone evidently was closely coupled with conjugation and apparently gave rise to no free hydroquinone in the tissues. This may account for the lack of biological activity of the oxidized form. When exogenous hydroquinone is administered in doses of sufficient size and frequency, however, it evidently persists in the free form long enough to exert a biological effect. Considering the slow rate of α-tocopherol quinone formation and the efficiency with which it is reduced and conjugated in the liver and kidneys, it is unlikely that the free hydroquinone exists, un-

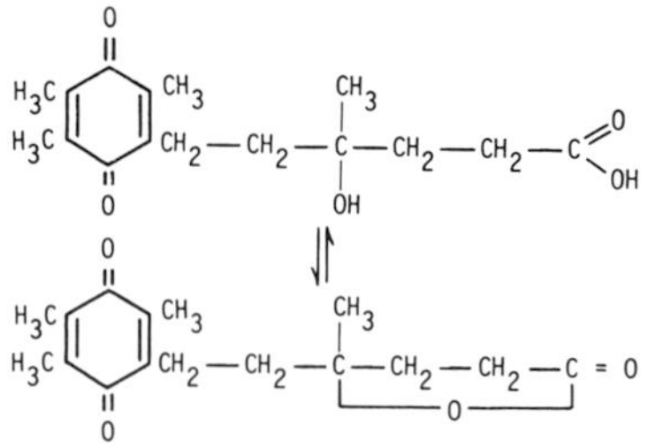

Fig. 22.3. α-Tocopheronic acid and its γ-lactone. (After Simon et al., 1956.)

der normal physiological conditions, in biologically active concentrations in animal tissues.

DIMER AND TRIMER

A metabolite of ^{14}C-*d*-α-tocopherol which was chromatographically distinguishable from α-tocopherol quinone and α-tocopheronic acid was detected in rat- and pig-liver extracts by Alaupovic and co-workers (1961). The presence of this material was confirmed by Csallany and Draper, who further observed that it could be obtained synthetically by oxidation of α-tocopherol with alkaline $K_3Fe(CN)_6$. Additional investigation indicated that this "metabolite" was a mixture of a dimer and trimer (Csallany and Draper, 1963; Draper et al., 1967). Neither compound possesses biological activity and both, like α-tocopherol quinone, appear to be end products of α-tocopherol oxidation in vivo.

The nature of the condensation between the two monomers (and consequently the structure of the trimer) has been a subject of much investigation. The proposed formation of a carbon-carbon bond between the two 5-methyl groups (Nelan and Robeson, 1962; Schudel et al., 1963) was confirmed by use of α-tocopherol-5-methyl-^{3}H (Csallany and Draper, unpublished), but recent evidence obtained by near-infrared spectroscopy, deuterium labeling, silylation, and mass spectroscopy indicates that the condensation mechanism is unusually complex.

Administration of synthetic ^{14}C-labeled dimer and dihydroxy dimer to rats has shown that the oxidized and reduced forms are interconvertible in the liver. The oxidized compound was the main form recovered from the tissues after ^{14}C-α-tocopherol administration, but traces of dihydroxy dimer also were consistently detected (Draper et al, 1967). The dimer is poorly absorbed from the intestine, indicating that its presence in the tissues cannot be accounted for by oxidation of α-tocopherol in the lumen of the gut. Following intraperitoneal administration of ^{14}C-labeled trimer, only the unchanged compound was recovered from the liver.

Oxidation of vitamin E by lipid free radicals

Although the stabilizing effect of vitamin E on unsaturated oils has been known for many years, little information has been forthcoming regarding the products generated from tocopherols as a result of their antioxidant action in autoxidizing lipids. The literature contains references to the presence of α-tocopherol-*p*-quinone and the red *o*-quinone in oxidized oils. The latter apparently arises in some natural oils from the oxidation of γ-tocopherol.

The observation that α-tocopherol oxidation in vivo and by mild oxidizing agents leads to dimer and trimer formation prompted a search for

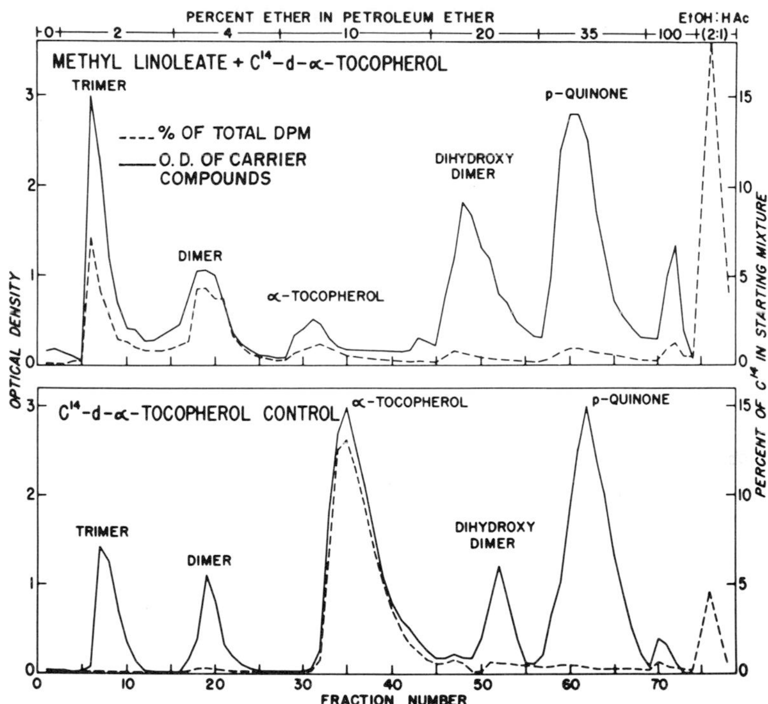

Fig. 22.4. ^{14}C elution pattern obtained by alumina column chromatography of a mixture of methyl linoleate and ^{14}C-α-tocopherol (2:1) after incubating at 60 C for 70 hr in an air oven. (From Draper, 1969, Metabolism and function of vitamin E. *Fed. Proc. 28*:1690.)

these compounds in autoxidizing lipids. Controlled oxidation of vitamin E was induced by incubating a 2:1 (w/w mixture of methyl linoleate and ^{14}C-α-tocopherol at 60 C for 70 hr. Fractionation of the oxidation products by alumina column chromatography revealed the presence of dimer, trimer, and highly polar oxidation products (Fig. 22.4). The unidentified polar compounds eluted with ethanol–acetic acid (2:1) may represent decomposition products of ^{14}C-α-tocopherol quinone. Under similar conditions of incubation, ^{14}C-α-tocopherol and pure methyl linoleate hydroperoxide yielded the dimer and the trimer as the main products of oxidation (Fig. 22.5). There was a strong correlation between the rate of decrease in peroxide value and the rate of oxidation of α-tocopherol.

Implications for the function of vitamin E in animals

These results show that there is an analogy between the oxidation products of vitamin E formed in vivo and those formed in the presence of autoxidizing fatty acids or their peroxides. This finding implies that the

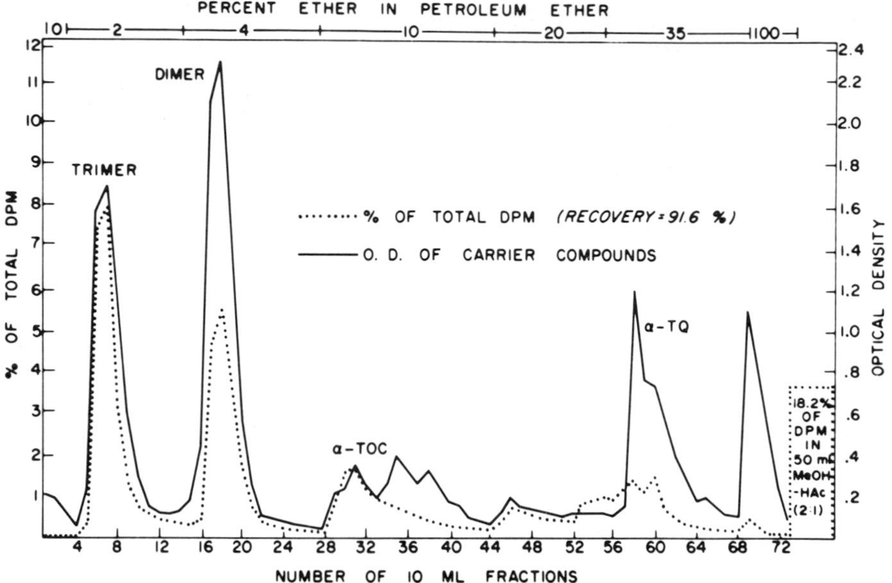

Fig. 22.5. [14]C elution pattern obtained by alumina column chromatography of a mixture of methyl linoleate hydroperoxide and ^{14}C-α-tocopherol (2:1) after incubating at 60 C for 70 hr in an air oven. (From Draper, 1969, Metabolism and function of vitamin E. *Fed. Proc. 28*:1690.)

products formed in vivo arise from reactions between α-tocopherol and lipid free radicals or peroxides, and it is in harmony with the results of nutritional studies which indicate that, at least in some experimental animals, vitamin E can be replaced with certain synthetic antioxidants. Both lines of investigation point to the conclusion that the function of the vitamin in animals is associated with its antioxidant properties. There is little information, however, concerning the precise mechanism of its action. The acyl reactant may be a fatty-acid free radical, a preformed peroxide, or a peroxy free radical. In any event, it appears that many cell constituents are susceptible to denaturation by lipid peroxides and that the suppression of these moieties is an essential biochemical requirement. The diverse symptoms of vitamin E deficiency seen in animals share a common incipient histopathological feature: the degeneration of cellular and subcellular membranes which are known to be rich in polyunsaturated fatty acids.

References

Alaupovic, P., B. C. Johnson, Q. Crider, H. N. Bhagavan, and B. J. Johnson. 1961. Metabolism of alpha-tocopherol and the isolation of a nontocopherol-reducing substance from animal tissues. *Amer. J. Clin. Nutr. 9*:76.

Chow, C. K., H. H. Draper, A. Saari Csallany, and Mei Chiu. 1967. The metabolism of C^{14}-α-tocopheryl quinone and C^{14}-α-tocopheryl hydroquinone. *Lipids* 2:390.

Csallany, A. Saari, and H. H. Draper. 1963. Dimerization of α-tocopherol *in vivo*. *Arch. Biochem. Biophys. 100*:335.

Csallany, A. Saari, H. H. Draper, and S. N. Shah. 1962. Conversion of *d*-α-tocopherol-C^{14} to tocopheryl-*p*-quinone *in vivo*. *Arch. Biochem. Biophys. 98*:142.

Dilley, R. A., and F. L. Crane. 1963. Light-induced changes of α-tocopherylquinone in spinach chloroplasts. *Biochim Biophys. Acta 75*:142.

Draper, H. H., A. Saari Csallany, and Mei Chiu. 1967. Isolation of a trimer of α-tocopherol from mammalian liver. *Lipids* 2:47.

Mackenzie, J. B., and C. G. Mackenzie. 1959. The effect of α-tocopherol, α-tocopherylhydroquinone and their esters on experimental muscular dystrophy in the rat. *J. Nutr. 67*:223.

Mackenzie, J. B., and C. G. Mackenzie. 1960. The antisterility activity of alphatocohydroquinone in the female rat. *J. Nutr. 72*:322.

Nelan, D. R., and C. D. Robeson. 1962. The oxidation product from α-tocopherol and potassium ferricyanide and its reaction with ascorbic and hydrochloric acids. *J. Amer. Chem. Soc. 84*:2963.

Pennock, J. F., F. W. Hemming, and J. D. Kerr. 1964. A reassessment of tocopherol chemistry. *Biochem. Biophys. Res. Commun. 17*:542.

Schudel, P., H. Mayer, J. Metzger, R. Rüegg, and O. Isler. 1963. Die Struktur des Kaliumferricyanid-Oxydationsphoduktes von α-Tocopherol. *Helv. Chim. Acta 46*:636.

Simon, E. J., A. Eisengart, L. Sundheim, and A. T. Milhorat. 1956.The metabolism of vitamin E. II. Purification and characterization of urinary metabolites of α-tocopherol. *J. Biol. Chem. 221*:807.

Weber, F., and O. Wiss. 1963. Über den Stoffwechsel des Vitamins E in der Ratte. *Helv. Physiol. Acta 21*:131.

23

STUDIES ON VITAMIN E AND RELATED FACTORS IN NUTRITION AND METABOLISM

M. L. Scott

Vitamin E is involved in maintaining the health of the brain, the vascular system, the erythrocytes, the skeletal muscles, the liver, the heart, the gonads, and the incisor teeth of rats, and in preventing yellow fat and ceroid in adipose and other tissues. It appears to function in at least two different metabolic roles: (a) as a fat-soluble antioxidant, and (b) in a more specific role interrelated with the metabolism of selenium and sulfur amino acids.

In a thorough review of the evidence for and against a "biological antioxidant theory" as a possible explanation of all functions of vitamin E, Green and Bunyan (1969) concluded that the antioxidant theory cannot possibly explain all functions of the vitamin. They pointed out that only circumstantial evidence supports its role as a biological antioxidant even in certain specific functions. I believe, however, that the evidence that α-tocopherol acts as a biological antioxidant in such functions as prevention of encephalomalacia is sufficiently strong to permit its use in a working hypothesis to explain *certain* functions of the vitamin. Although the second function of vitamin E may be related to its capacity to control oxidation-reduction potentials in one or more metabolic systems, the nature of these systems is unknown, and the vitamin is functioning in a much more specific role than that of a simple antioxidant.

Factors affecting vitamin E requirements

In its role as an antioxidant, the amount of vitamin E required in the diet depends to a large extent upon two factors: (a) the amount of dietary polyunsaturated fatty acid (PUFA), especially linoleic acid, and (b) the presence of other natural or synthetic fat-soluble antioxidants in the diet and in the animal body. The quantitative dietary requirement for vitamin E to perform its functions thus depends upon the status of other factors in the diet. As the PUFA content of the diet increases, the vitamin E requirement increases; as the amounts of natural or synthetic fat-soluble antioxidants are increased in the diet, the requirement for vitamin E decreases. Harris and Embree (1963) suggested that each gram of dietary PUFA increases the *d*-α-tocopherol requirement by about 0.6 mg. Effective synthetic antioxidants appear to eliminate the need for vitamin E as an antioxidant.

In its more specific role, as in prevention of nutritional muscular dystrophy in rabbits, guinea pigs, monkeys, and chicks, the amount of vitamin E required is not influenced by the level of polyunsaturated fatty acids unless these are actively peroxidizing and thereby destroying the dietary vitamin E. The vitamin E requirement for these specific functions also is not altered by dietary synthetic antioxidants, except insofar as these protect the vitamin from oxidation destruction.

Recently it has been shown in our laboratory that the dietary requirement for vitamin E also depends to a very great extent upon the state of the animal's selenium nutrition. When synthetic amino acid diets fed to chicks and Japanese quail are extremely low in selenium, very high dietary levels of vitamin E are completely ineffective in prevention of vitamin E–deficiency disease, because of failure to absorb the vitamin. This report summarizes the influences of PUFA, antioxidants, selenium and the sulfur amino acids on vitamin E nutrition in the chick and in other animals and discusses in detail recent studies on the effects of selenium upon vitamin E nutrition and metabolism in the chick.

Vitamin E–deficiency diseases

Most vitamin E–deficiency diseases are now quite well delineated. Information also is available concerning the influences of PUFA, selenium, antioxidants, and sulfur amino acids upon these various diseases. A summary of this information is presented in Table 23.1. As indicated in the table, some deficiency diseases respond to vitamin E and other suitable antioxidants; others require vitamin E in a more specific function; some require selenium as the primary factor; and certain diseases may require both vitamin E and selenium for complete prevention.

ANTIOXIDANT-RESPONSIVE DISEASES

Encephalomalacia. The degenerative changes of the cerebellum in the chick termed encephalomalacia respond to dietary vitamin E or to suitable

TABLE 23.1. *The vitamin E–deficiency diseases*

Disease	Experimental animal	Tissue affected	Severity dependent upon dietary PUFA	Prevented by: Vitamin E	Selenium	Synthetic antioxidants	Sulfur amino acids
		REPRODUCTIVE FAILURE					
Embryonic degeneration							
Type A	Female rat, hen, turkey	Vascular system of embryo	Yes	Yes	No	Yes	No
Type B	Cow, ewe	Vascular system of embryo	No	No[a]	Yes[b]	No	No
Sterility	Male rat, guinea pig, hamster, dog, cock	Male gonads	No	Yes	No	No	No
		LIVER, BLOOD, BRAIN, CAPILLARIES, ETC.					
Liver necrosis	Rat, pig	Liver	No	Yes	Yes	No	No
Erythrocyte hemolysis	Rat, chick man (premature infant)	Erythrocytes	Yes	Yes	No	Yes	No
Plasma protein loss	Chick, turkey	Serum albumen	No	Yes	Yes	No	No
Anemia	Monkey	Bone marrow	No	Yes	No	Yes	No
Encephalomalacia	Chick	Cerebellum	Yes	Yes	No	Yes	No
Exudative diathesis	Chick, turkey	Vascular system	No	Yes	Yes	No	No
Kidney degeneration	Rat, monkey, mink	Kidney tubular epithelium	Yes	Yes	Yes	No	No
Depigmentation	Rat	Incisors	Yes	Yes	No	Yes	No
Steatitis (yellow fat disease)	Mink, pig, chick	Adipose tissue	Yes	Yes	No	Yes	No
		NUTRITIONAL MYOPATHIES					
Nutritional muscular dystrophy							
Type A	Rabbit, guinea pig, monkey, duck, mouse, mink	Skeletal muscle	No	Yes	No	No?	No
Type B	White muscle disease of lamb, calf, kid	Skeletal and heart muscles	No	No[a]	Yes[b]	No	No
Type C	Turkey	Gizzard, heart	No	No[a]	Yes	No	No
Type D	Chicken	Skeletal muscle	No[c]	Yes	No	No	Yes

[a] Not effective in diets severely deficient in selenium.

[b] When added to diets containing low levels of vitamin E.

[c] A low level (0.5%) of linoleic acid is necessary to produce dystrophy; higher levels did not increase vitamin E required for prevention.

fat-soluble antioxidants but not to selenium or to sulfur amino acids in the diet. Encephalomalacia does not occur in chicks fed fat-free, vitamin E–deficient diets. The incidence and severity of this disease is markedly increased as the level of linoleic acid in the diet increases. In the prevention of encephalomalacia there is little doubt that vitamin E is functioning as an antioxidant and that the disease can be prevented by any antioxidant which can prevent peroxidation of linoleic acid. However, the primary metabolic defect which causes the cerebellar degeneration and hemorrhage is not known.

Kokatnur and associates (1960) and Nishida and co-workers (1960) obtained evidence indicating that a specific oxidation product of linoleic acid creates the symptoms of encephalomalacia through a toxic action on the cerebellar vascular system. However, this explanation is not consistent with the finding of Scott and Stoewsand (1961) that di-phenyl-para-phenylene diamine (DPPD) effectively prevented encephalomalacia even when given daily to chicks receiving a vitamin E–deficient purified diet high in PUFA and free of antioxidants. This diet developed complete oxidative rancidity during the course of the experiment, and without the addition of DPPD to the daily diet, 75% of the chicks died of encephalomalacia.

Erythrocyte hemolysis. The in vitro hemolysis of vitamin E–deficient erythrocytes in isotonic dialuric acid, hydrogen peroxide, or oxygen-containing saline solution is prevented by dietary α-tocopherol or by synthetic antioxidants.

Yellow fat, ceroid, and lipofuscins (steatitis). Peroxidation of fat and formation of yellow to brown pigments occurs in animals fed vitamin E–deficient diets containing cod-liver oil or other sources of PUFA. The color which develops in the adipose tissues has been found to be a mixture of two pigments; one is a fat-soluble yellow pigment showing yellow green fluorescence; the other is dark brown and is insoluble in both fat solvents and water. The latter pigment, termed ceroid, is apparently a polymerization of PUFA peroxides with lipoproteins. The lipofuscin age pigments may represent the presence of these ceroid pigments within the lysosomes of the cells where, because of their insolubility and indigestibility by the lysosomal enzymes, the ceroid pigments remain and accumulate throughout the life of the animal (Tappel, 1968). Gedigk (1959) found the lipid components of ceroid and lipofuscin to be identical, with some differences in their protein components. The extent to which antioxidants, particularly vitamin E, can slow the formation of lipofuscins and perhaps delay aging remains to be determined. Attempts to show the existence of peroxides in adipose tissues in vivo have failed. Much further work is needed to identify the primary sources and the sequence of formation of these pigments.

Resorption-gestation. The question of whether or not reproductive failure in vitamin E–deficient female rats represents a simple antioxidant deficiency is the subject of much controversy. Søndergaard concluded in his review (1967) that "Antioxidants cannot protect against fetal resorption. They can, however, improve the reproductive capacity by protecting suboptimal amounts of vitamin E present in the diet or in the various organs of the rat." Draper and associates (1964) have shown, however, that the antioxidant diphenyl-*p*-phenylenediamine was effective in preventing this deficiency disease in rats which had received diets very low in vitamin E over a period of three generations and in bringing about normal gestations when added to diets which had caused fetal death and resorption in the previous gestation period. The fact that ethoxyquin, which readily prevents encephalomalacia, is not effective in preventing resorption gestation, only adds to the difficulty in trying to determine the possible mode of action of vitamin E in prevention of this deficiency disease.

Although recent information from New Zealand (Andrews et al., 1968) indicates that there are forms of reproductive failure in sheep which respond primarily to dietary or injected selenium, the classical reproductive failure characterized by death and resorption of the fetus in rats fed vitamin E–deficient diets appears to be primarily a vitamin E–responsive deficiency disease. Selenium compounds have no effect upon the resorption-gestation syndrome in rats (Harris et al., 1958; Christensen et al., 1958).

The most widely used biological assay for vitamin E has been a determination of the amount of an unknown material required to prevent fetal death and resorption in rats as compared to the amount of vitamin E required when added to a specific basal diet. The vitamin E level required for prevention of fetal resorption under these conditions is so critical that this assay method has been used widely for assessing the relative biopotencies of various forms of vitamin E. It is necessary, however, in a determination of the vitamin E content of an unknown material, that the linoleic acid and antioxidant present in the test material be eliminated or that appropriate controls be used. The primary metabolic defect which causes death and subsequent resorption of the embryo is not known. There are degenerative changes in the uterus. However, the vascular system of the embryo also undergoes degeneration, and the embryo suffers from a severe anemia.

The cause of death in vitamin E–deficient chicken and turkey embryos has not been studied extensively. The vascular system appears to be degenerated, as in rat embryos.

Depigmentation of rat incisors. When vitamin E–deficient rat diets contain added cod-liver oil, an iron-containing pigment which imparts the normal yellow orange color to rat teeth is markedly diminished. This depigmentation, which often accompanies liver necrosis in vitamin E–deficient rats, is usually not affected by dietary selenium, which prevents the necrosis. Instead, either vitamin E or a suitable antioxidant is needed to restore normal pigmentation.

Mitochondrial swelling. In the prevention of mitochondrial swelling and in some of its functions which have been shown to aid the action of the cytochrome C reductase system, vitamin E also probably acts simply as a biological antioxidant. Evidence largely obtained with in vitro studies indicates that factors which favor peroxidation act to increase mitochondrial swelling and thereby to reduce the activity of the cytochrome system, while factors which prevent peroxidation also prevent these abnormalities.

VITAMIN E–RESPONSIVE DISEASES

Muscular dystrophy in rabbits, guinea pigs, monkeys, chicks, ducks, mice, and mink. Two types of nutritional muscular dystrophy appear to exist. One responds primarily to vitamin E, the other responds primarily to selenium. Nutritional muscular dystrophy in rabbits, guinea pigs, chicks, and monkeys appears to be a vitamin E–responsive disease. Muscular dystrophy in these animals does not respond to selenium. In cases where synthetic antioxidants have been effective, this may have been due to protection of traces of vitamin E. A very special peculiarity of the dystrophy in chicks is that it can be prevented in the absence of vitamin E by supplementing the diet with cystine. The chick appears to be unique in this respect, since cystine has not been reported to be of any benefit in the prevention of nutritional muscular dystrophy in any other animal, including the turkey poult. Although dystrophy in ducks, mice, and mink is prevented by vitamin E, and not by selenium, little is yet known about the exact nature of these diseases.

Vitamin E–responsive muscular dystrophy does not appear to be due to a simple need for an antioxidant. This disease, as studied in the chick, does not respond to dietary synthetic antioxidants at levels several times those needed to prevent encephalomalacia; yet the disease is invariably prevented or cured by supplementing the diet with normal levels of vitamin E.

Extensive studies of nutritional muscular dystrophy in chicks have been conducted in my laboratory at Cornell University over the past twelve years (Scott, 1962*a*, 1962*b*). Brief summaries of some of the results of these experiments are given below.

1. Studies on phosphorus metabolism in dystrophic chicks showed that phosphorus turnover is much greater, the inorganic phosphorus is higher, but the organic, high-energy phosphates such as creatine phosphate and ATP are lower in the muscles of dystrophic chicks than in the muscles of chicks receiving sufficient vitamin E and selenium to prevent muscular dystrophy. The activity of the enzyme, phosphorylase, also has been shown to be reduced in dystrophic chick muscles (Nesheim et al., 1959; Calvert et al., 1961).

2. Addition of either cystine or methionine to a vitamin E–deficient diet (already supplemented with low levels of ethoxyquin and selenium to prevent encephalomalacia and exudative diathesis, respectively) completely prevents muscular dystrophy even in the absence of vitamin E. Cystine is about twice as effective as methionine on an equal-sulfur basis, and the requirement for cystine is not antagonized by arginine, whereas added arginine increases the amount of methionine needed to prevent dystrophy (Scott and Calvert, 1962).

3. Studies have been conducted in an effort to determine the role of cystine and methionine in the prevention of this disorder. The effects of dietary cholic acid, sodium taurocholate, and taurine on the severity of the myopathy of vitamin E–deficient chicks were studied in conjunction with determinations of taurine excretion rate. Dietary cholic acid significantly increased the severity of the myopathy. Sodium taurocholate and taurine both reduced the severity of the muscle lesions. Dystrophic chicks fed the basal diet excreted greater quantities of urinary taurine than chicks fed a vitamin E–supplemented diet. Chicks fed the basal diet with added cystine were nondystrophic but had taurine excretion rates similar to those of dystrophic chicks. Taurine excretion rates were related to cystine and vitamin E content of the diet rather than to severity of myopathy. These results suggest that prevention of nutritional muscular dystrophy in the chicks depends on the metabolic availability of cysteine or cystine. The effects of the bile salts and the taurine upon the severity of the myopathy were probably due to changes in rates of conversion of cysteine to taurine (Hathcock and Scott, 1966*a*).

Studies were conducted which show that creatinuria is not necessarily related to severity of nutritional muscular dystrophy in chicks. When conversion of methionine to cysteine was encouraged by dietary supplementation with the methyl acceptor, guanidoacetic acid, dystrophy was prevented but creatine excretion was increased. Guanidopropionic acid, a possible inhibitor of the above pathway, caused an increase in muscular dystrophy and a marked decrease in creatine excretion. Therefore, creatinuria in the nutritionally dystrophic chick is not primarily caused by muscle degeneration, or vice versa (Hathcock and Scott, 1966*b*).

In studies with methionine labeled with ^{35}S, it has been impossible to show that vitamin E is involved in the conversion of methionine to cystine.

In an effort to determine if any of the sulfhydryl-containing enzymes were directly concerned in prevention of muscular dystrophy, the addition of copper sulfate to the vitamin E–deficient, dystrophy-producing diet greatly increased the severity of muscular dystrophy. This effect was completely prevented by supplementing the diet with vitamin E. The succinic dehydrogenase content of chick breast muscles was found to be altered by various treatments which also affected the incidence and the severity of the dystrophy; there was no consistent relationship, however, between the occurrence or the severity of dystrophy and the succinic dehydrogenase content of the muscles (Scott, Søndergaard, and Dam, 1962).

An experiment was conducted to determine if the activity of cystine in prevention of muscular dystrophy is through the transfer of a sulfhydryl group from cysteine to some other compound in the animal body. Accordingly, graded levels of cystine were fed with or without the presence in the diet of 0.04%, and 0.08% sodium thioglycolate, which is known to be an effective inhibitor of the enzyme, cysteine desulfhydrase. This experiment showed that equivalent amounts of cystine were required for prevention of dystrophy in the presence and in the absence of sodium thioglycolate, thereby indicating that transsulfhydration is not involved in the prevention of muscular dystrophy by dietary cystine. In other experiments, several sulfhydryl antagonists were fed to chicks in the presence of graded levels of dietary cystine. These antagonists did not interfere with the amount of cystine required to prevent muscular dystrophy in the chick.

4. In another approach to the study of these interrelationships, graded levels of linoleic acid were fed in the presence and in the absence of graded levels of vitamin E. It was shown that, even when the diet contained the antioxidant ethoxyquin, approximately 0.5% of dietary linoleic acid was necessary to produce muscular dystrophy. Levels above 0.5% linoleic acid did not increase the amount of vitamin E required for prevention of dystrophy (Calvert and Scott, 1964).

Muscle tissues of chicks with muscular dystrophy produced by feeding a diet deficient in vitamin E and sulfur amino acids and containing excess dietary linoleic acid showed significant increases in peroxidation, as evidenced by the TBA* index of the muscle tissues, and also showed increased activities of the lysosomal enzymes, acid phosphatase, β-glucuronidase, cathepsin, β-galactosidase, and ribonuclease. The degree of peroxidation and the increases in lysosomal enzymes were in direct proportion to the increase in severity of muscular dystrophy. Addition of DL-methionine

* A standard test for peroxidation using thiobarbituric acid, which is believed to react with a decomposition product of peroxidized linoleic acid, malonyl dialdehyde.

or *d*-α-tocopheryl acetate to the diet prevented the dystrophy, reduced the peroxidation, and reduced the lysosomal enzyme activities. These results support the hypothesis that nutritional muscular dystrophy in the chick is initiated by peroxidative tissue damage. A question still remains, however, concerning the biochemical mechanism responsible for the protection of the muscle tissues from this degeneration, especially in regard to the role of sulfur amino acids, which prevent dystrophy in the absence of vitamin E, and of selenium, which markedly spares the amount of vitamin E required (Desai et al., 1964; Desai and Scott, 1964).

5. In the course of these studies it was found that, when the basal diet is supplemented with methionine until the chicks are three weeks of age, dystrophy is prevented as long as the methionine is in the diet. Sudden removal of the supplemental methionine from the diet causes immediate precipitation (within 48 hr) of severe muscular dystrophy. This finding was utilized to conduct a time-sequence study to determine whether the increases in lysosomal enzymes precede the onset of muscular dystrophy or if they occur after muscular dystrophy is initiated in the tissues.

The results of this experiment showed that, upon removal of methionine from the vitamin E–deficient diet, symptoms of muscular dystrophy occurred concurrently with the appearance of peroxidation and lysosomal enzymes. Appreciable dystrophy was observed with relatively low tissue levels of lysosomal enzymes. Upon returning the supplemental methionine or vitamin E to the diet of dystrophic chicks, rapid recovery from muscular dystrophy was observed with both treatments. The rate of recovery was faster following supplementation with methionine than with vitamin E. Lysosomal enzyme concentration in the muscles continued to rise sharply after methionine supplementation and remained at a fairly high level even after most of the symptoms of muscular dystrophy in the chicks had disappeared. Peroxidizability of the tissues also remained high in the chicks receiving the vitamin E–deficient diet, even though muscular dystrophy was cured by the addition of methionine. These results indicate that the lysosomal enzymes are not involved in producing the degeneration of the tissues but apparently are increased in dystrophic muscles simply to help to remove the products of degeneration from the muscles undergoing dystrophy.

The finding that methionine is completely effective not only in preventing, but also in reversing, nutritional muscular dystrophy under conditions of high peroxidizability and high lysosomal enzyme content of the muscle tissues indicates that methionine-cystine metabolism is the key to the primary mechanism of prevention and cure of nutritional muscular dystrophy (Desai and Scott, 1964).

6. Studies comparing *d*- and *l*-α-tocopheryl acetates in the prevention of

muscular dystrophy in chicks showed that *l*-α-tocopheryl acetate (the unnatural form) is only approximately 25% as effective as *d*-α-tocopheryl acetate (the natural form) for prevention of this disease. Studies of the total tocopherol content of the blood plasma of chicks receiving various forms of tocopherol showed that, regardless of the form of tocopherol in the diet, dystrophy was prevented when a total blood tocopherol level of approximately 1000 μg per 100 ml of blood was attained. These results indicate, therefore, that natural *d*-α-tocopheryl acetate is the active form of the vitamin simply because it is either absorbed or retained more efficiently than the other forms (Scott and Desai, 1964). With thin-layer chromatographic techniques, it was shown that the substance in the blood was indeed tocopherol, and not some other compound such as a ubiquinone or a ubichromenol.

7. Studies with ubiquinones and ubichromenols indicated that these substances were not directly concerned in the prevention of muscular dystrophy, although ubichromenols will prevent encephalomalacia (Søndergaard et al., 1962).

Testicular degeneration in the vitamin E–deficient male rat. According to Mason (1967), the irreversible testicular degeneration in male rats occurs with vitamin E–deficient diets whether or not they are supplemented with PUFA. This disease is not responsive to antioxidant action.

Anemia in the monkey. Although anemia in vitamin E–deficient rhesus monkeys responds to DPPD and to the 6-chromanol of hexahydrocoenzyme Q_4 (Fitch, 1968), vitamin E is vastly superior to these compounds in bringing about remission, and Fitch believes that they only have a sparing effect upon a basic, specific need for vitamin E.

The antioxidant effect of vitamin E in protecting the red blood cells from hemolysis has been referred to previously. Fitch and co-workers have shown, however, that anemia in monkeys stems from a lack of hematopoiesis in the bone marrow rather than from excessive red blood cell destruction. The role of vitamin E in hematopoiesis is not known.

SELENIUM-RESPONSIVE DISEASES

Necrotic liver degeneration. Liver necrosis in rats is the deficiency disease used by Schwarz and Foltz (1957) in the studies which led to the discovery of the nutritional nature of selenium. While this disease is prevented by vitamin E, it is now quite apparent that the disease is also prevented by selenium alone, and thus it is quite likely that selenium is the primary factor needed for prevention.

Muscular dystrophy (myopathies) in lambs, calves, and turkeys. Nutritional muscular dystrophies of lambs, kids, and calves, often termed "white muscle disease," have been a problem for many years in certain areas throughout the world. Although this disease responded somewhat to vitamin E, control was not always satisfactory. A similar myopathy of the gizzard and heart occurs in young turkeys (Scott et al., 1967).

It has now been demonstrated in numerous studies that selenium deficiency is the primary cause of these diseases. Since selenium has not been administered in the complete absence of vitamin E, it is not yet possible to say whether these diseases can be prevented by selenium alone, or if they require both selenium and vitamin E.

Exudative diathesis in chicks. The severe edema termed "exudative diathesis" has been shown in our laboratory to be a selenium deficiency disease (Thompson and Scott, 1969).

A basal, crystalline amino acid, vitamin E–deficient diet was developed which contained all other generally recognized nutrients at more than adequate levels. Special care was taken to add sufficient methionine to prevent muscular dystrophy. Ethoxyquin also was added at a level which prevents encephalomalacia and also prevents any peroxidation of the PUFA present in the 5% soybean oil in the diet.

This diet, which contained less than 0.002 ppm of selenium, was fed alone and was supplemented with vitamin E alone, with selenium alone, and with combinations of vitamin E and selenium.

Addition to the diet of 0.1 ppm of selenium alone produced maximum growth and prevented all deficiency symptoms, while vitamin E in the absence of selenium did not prevent mortality, even at levels up to 1360 IU per kg. (This is approximately 100 times the vitamin E in natural diets.) A relationship was shown between the selenium requirement and the amount of vitamin E in the diet. Using diets containing 136 IU vitamin E per kg the amount of supplemental selenium needed ranged from 0.005 ppm to 0.01 ppm, whereas, with diets containing 13.6 IU vitamin E per kg, 0.02–0.05 ppm of added selenium (as sodium selenite) was needed.

Effects of selenium upon absorption and retention of vitamin E and of triglyceride

Tissue uptake of oral doses of *dl*-α-tocopherol 3,4-^{14}C, or of the corresponding acetate, was low in chicks receiving the amino acid basal diet. In chicks receiving the same diet with added selenite, the blood and tissue uptake of vitamin E was as much as 100 times greater than that of the basal chicks.

In the course of these studies, it was also noted that the plasma of most of the chicks receiving the basal diet without selenium was water-clear, while that of chicks receiving selenite showed the usual turbidity caused by the lipemia resulting from fat absorption.

Further studies using chromic oxide as a marker in the basal diet showed that the chicks receiving the basal, selenium-deficient diet almost completely lacked the ability to hydrolyze triglyceride. After about 14 days on the deficient diet, neutral fat begins to increase in the feces until, at about 20 days of age, most of the dietary fat can be recovered, unhydrolyzed.

Lipase activity of the pancreas in selenium-deficient chicks has been shown to be reduced in comparison with that in chicks receiving selenium, but studies on the specific cause of the marked decrease in fat hydrolysis have not yet been completed.

It appears quite likely that the decreased absorption and retention of vitamin E referred to above and reported earlier from our laboratory is a secondary phenomenon resulting from the failure of formation of lipid–bile salt micelles in the intestinal tract and possibly from a low production of the particular plasma lipoproteins concerned in vitamin E transport.

Addition of sodium taurocholate to the basal diet produced an increase in vitamin E absorption but did not improve fat digestion or prevent mortality.

Conclusion

This research demonstrates that selenium is an essential nutrient in its own right. It is required in metabolic processes which are not protected by vitamin E. Indeed, the evidence from these studies strongly indicates that one of the important functions of vitamin E is concerned with protection of traces of selenium in the animal body.

References

Andrews, E. D., W. J. Hartley, and A. B. Grant. 1968. Selenium-responsive diseases of animals in New Zealand. *New Zeal. Vet. J. 16*:3.

Calvert, C. C., R. A. Monroe, and M. L. Scott. 1961. Studies on phosphorus metabolism in dystrophic chicks. *J. Nutr. 73*:355.

Calvert, C. C., and M. L. Scott. 1964. Effect of linoleic acid on nutritional muscular dystrophy in the chick. *J. Nutr. 83*:307.

Christensen, F., R. Dam, I. Prange, and E. Søndergaard. 1958. The effect of selenium on vitamin E–deficient rats. *Acta Pharmacol. Toxicol. 15*:181.

Desai, I. D., C. C. Calvert, M. L. Scott, and A. L. Tappel. 1964. Peroxidation and lysosomes in nutritional muscular dystrophy of chicks. *Proc. Soc. Exp. Biol. Med. 115*:462.

Desai, I. D., and M. L. Scott. 1964. Comparative effectiveness of vitamin E and sulfur amino acids in recovery from muscular dystrophy. *Poultry Sci. 43*:1312.

Draper, H. H., J. G. Bergan, Mei Chiu, A. Saari Csallany, and A. V. Boaro. 1964. A further study of the specificity of vitamin E requirement for reproduction. *J. Nutr. 84*:395.

Fitch, C. D. 1968. Experimental anemia in primates due to vitamin E deficiency. *Vitamins Hormones 26*:501.

Gedigk, P. 1959. Lipogenous pigments. *Verhandl. Deut. Ges. Pathol. 42*:430.

Green, J., and J. Bunyan. 1969. Vitamin E and the biological antioxidant theory. *Nutr. Abstr. Rev. 39*:321.

Harris, P. L., and N. D. Embree. 1963. Quantitative consideration of the effect of polyunsaturated fatty acid content of the diet upon the requirements for vitamin E. *Amer. J. Clin. Nutr. 13*:385.

Harris, P. L., M. I. Ludwig, and K. Schwarz. 1958. Ineffectiveness of factor 3–active selenium compounds in resorption-gestation bioassay for vitamin E. *Proc. Soc. Exp. Biol. Med. 97*:686.

Hathcock, J. N., and M. L. Scott. 1966*a*. Alterations of methionine to cysteine conversion rates and nutritional muscular dystrophy in chicks. *Proc. Soc. Exp. Biol. Med. 121*:908.

Hathcock, J. N., and M. L. Scott. 1966*b*. Lack of correlation of creatinuria and nutritional muscular dystrophy. *Fed. Proc. 25*:242.

Kokatnur, M. G., S. Okui, F. A. Kummerow, and H. M. Scott. 1960. Effect of long chain keto acids on encephalomalacia in chicks. *Proc. Soc. Exp. Biol. Med. 104*:170.

Mason, K. E. 1967. In discussion of paper by E. Søndergaard, p. 376. *In* O. H. Muth (ed.), *Selenium in Biomedicine*. Avi, Westport, Conn.

Nesheim, M. C., S. L. Leonard, and M. L. Scott. 1959. Alterations in some biochemical constituents of skeletal muscle of vitamin E–deficient chicks. *J. Nutr. 68*:359.

Nishida, T., H. Tsuchiyama, M. Inoue, and F. A. Kummerow. 1960. Effect of intravenous injection of oxidized methyl ester of unsaturated fatty acids on chick encephalomalacia. *Proc. Soc. Exp. Biol. Med. 105*:308.

Schwarz, K., and C. M. Foltz. 1957. Selenium as an integral part of factor 3 against dietary necrotic liver degeneration. *J. Amer. Chem. Soc. 79*:3292.

Scott, M. L. 1962*a*. Antioxidants, selenium and sulphur amino acids in the vitamin E nutrition of chicks. *Nutr. Abstr. Rev. 32*:1.

———. 1962*b*. Vitamin E in health and disease of poultry. *Vitamins Hormones 20*:621.

Scott, M. L., and C. C. Calvert. 1962. Evidence of a specific effect of cystine in the prevention of a nutritional muscular dystrophy in vitamin E–deficient chicks. *J. Nutr. 77*:105.

Scott, M. L., and I. D. Desai. 1964. The relative anti-muscular dystrophy activity of the *d*- and *l*-epimers of α-tocopherol and of other tocopherols in the chick. *J. Nutr. 83*:39.

Scott, M. L., G. Olson, L. Krook, and W. R. Brown. 1967. Selenium-responsive myopathies of myocardium and smooth muscle in the young poult. *J. Nutr. 91*:573.

Scott, M. L., E. Søndergaard, and H. Dam. 1962. A lack of relationship between muscle succinic dehydrogenase and nutritional muscular dystrophy in chicks. *Fed. Proc. 21*:473.

Scott, M. L., and G. S. Stoewsand. 1961. A study of the ataxias of vitamin A and vitamin E deficiencies in the chick. *Poultry Sci. 40*:1517.

Søndergaard, E. 1967. Selenium and vitamin E interrelationships, p. 365. *In* O. H. Muth (ed.), *Selenium in Biomedicine.* Avi, Westport, Conn.

Søndergaard, E., M. L. Scott, and H. Dam. 1962. Effects of ubiquinones and phtyl-ubichromenol upon encephalomalacia and muscular dystrophy in the chick. *J. Nutr. 78*:15.

Tappel, A. L. 1968. Will antioxidant nutrients slow aging processes? *Geriatrics 23*:97.

Thompson, J. N., and M. L. Scott. 1969. Role of selenium in the nutrition of the chick. *J. Nutr. 97*:335.

24

REACTIONS OF VITAMIN E, UBIQUINOL, AND SELENOAMINO ACIDS, AND PROTECTION OF OXIDANT-LABILE ENZYMES

A. L. TAPPEL

Vitamin E is a focal point for two broad topics, namely, biological antioxidants and lipid-peroxidation damage. Vitamin E is related by its reactions to other biological antioxidants and reducing compounds. These compounds stabilize polyunsaturated lipids and minimize lipid-peroxidation damage. Relationships between biological antioxidants and lipid-peroxidation damage are very complex. Knowledge of similar, but non-biological, relationships between oxidant-labile olefinic compounds and antioxidant protection systems has developed to a sophisticated level, however (Scott, 1965; Lundberg, 1961; Schultz, 1962), and provides a valuable background for biological studies. In vivo lipid peroxidation has been identified as a basic deteriorative reaction in cellular mechanisms of aging processes (Packer et al., 1967; Tappel, 1968); in some phases of atherosclerosis (Hartroft, 1965; Perkins et al., 1965); in chlorinated hydrocarbon hepatotoxicity (Recknagel, 1967); in ethanol-induced liver injury (Di Luzio and Hartman, 1967); and in oxygen toxicity (Haugaard, 1968). Of these the greatest impact in human nutrition may come from increasing knowledge of lipid-peroxidation aging processes. These processes may be a universal disease of which the chemical deteriorative effects might be slowed by use of increased amounts of antioxidants (Harman, 1968; Tappel, 1968).

Vitamin E and lipid peroxidation

As a biochemical model of these deteriorative reactions, we have studied lipid-peroxidation damage to proteins and enzymes. Free radical intermediates of lipid peroxidation react with proteins and enzymes. As the extent of oxidation progresses, soluble polymeric products, incorporating low levels of lipid, give way to firmly cross-linked polymeric products containing moderate amounts of occluded and complexed lipid material. Automated Sephadex gel filtration and solubility studies of oxidized lipid-protein reaction products show that they are best characterized as protein-protein cross-linked polymers, and the polymerization mechanism is characterized as a free-radical chain-polymerization (Roubal and Tappel, 1966*a*). The pattern of damage to proteins induced by peroxidizing lipid is similar to that observed in radiation damage; proteins and enzymes lose solubility and constitutent amino acids are destroyed. Lipid-peroxidation damage is about one-tenth as effective as radiation damage. Amino acid destruction was measured in lipid-peroxidation damaged γ-globulin, catalase, serum albumin, hemoglobin, and ovalbumin. Among the most labile amino acids are methionine, histidine, cystine, and lysine (Roubal and Tappel, 1966*b*).

Further studies (Chio, 1968; Chio and Tappel, 1969*a*, 1969*b*) of quantitative enzyme inactivation by lipid peroxidation showed that sulfhydryl enzymes are most susceptible to inactivation. Oxidation products of polyunsaturated lipids also inactivate nonsulfhydryl enzymes; ribonuclease A was used as an experimental model. Concomitant with the loss of ribonuclease activity is the appearance of fluorescence in the enzyme-lipid reaction mixture. The inactivated ribonuclease shows fluorescent monomer, dimer, and higher molecular weight species in the Sephadex G–100 fractionation pattern. The fluorescence maximum is at 470 mμ when excited at 395 mμ. Ribonuclease, inactivated by malonaldehyde, has fluorescence and a gel-filtration pattern similar to that of the enzyme inactivated by polyunsaturated lipids. Malonaldehyde from peroxidizing lipids is probably the reactant for the intramolecular and intermolecular cross-linking of ribonuclease. The fluorescence produced by the cross-linking is attributed to the conjugated imine structure formed in protein between two ϵ-amino groups and malonaldehyde. In studies by Dr. K. S. Chio (1969*b*), the structure of the fluorescent chromophore was determined. Amino acids or their esters and *n*-hexylamine were reacted with malonaldehyde to yield conjugated Schiff bases. The Schiff bases possess characteristic absorption in the ultraviolet and visible regions. In solutions, Schiff bases derived from amino acids show spectral shifts on standing at room temperature, with an isosbestic point at 402 mμ. *Cis-trans* isomerization about the C=C bond or the C=N bond may account for the observed spectral shift. The electronic absorption in the 360 mμ region and fluorescence in the 470 mμ region have been attributed to the chromophoric system N–C=C–C=N, which contains six π-electrons. Infrared spectra contain a band in the 1650 cm^{-1} region, indicating the presence of a C=N bond. After the Schiff bases were reduced with sodium borohydride, mass spectral analyses were carried out to confirm that 1 mole of malonaldehyde reacts with 2 moles of amino acid ester or *n*-hexylamine to yield *N,N′*-disubstituted 1-amino-3-iminopropenes. The fluorescent chromophore, R—N=CH—CH=CH—NH—R, develops from the cross-linking reaction of malonaldehyde with many biologically important amines—including RNA, DNA, and phospholipids. Fluorescent products form in many biological systems—including mitochondria, microsomes, and lysosomes—when they undergo lipid peroxidation in vitro. This research allows qualitative identification of this fluorescent chromophore as a molecular lesion in lipofuscin age pigments which accumulate in tissues, especially in the brain and the heart of animals, as a function of age (Wolman, 1964). Age pigments have similar characteristic fluorescence spectra as those found in model systems, with a fluorescence maximum at 470 mμ when excited at 365 mμ.

Relationship between vitamin E and other antioxidants

Vitamin E, the major biological antioxidant, shows complex relationships with other antioxidants and reducing compounds (Tappel, 1962). These relationships are described in the classification of the following reactions. The major biological function of vitamin E in its inhibition of lipid peroxidation can be described as radical chain-breaking. As an ancillary function of ubiquinol, small amounts can react as a chain-breaking lipid antioxidant and can provide important homosynergism with vitamin E. Vitamin C can act as a synergist for vitamin E. Sulfhydryl compounds, mainly glutathione, sulfhydryl proteins, and cysteine, apparently react in small amounts as a free radical scavenger and as peroxide decomposers. Small amounts of methionine can also react as a peroxide decomposer and free radical scavenger. Selenoamino acids are powerful catalysts of sulhydryl-disulfide exchange, and they react as free radical scavengers and as peroxide decomposers, as well (Tappel and Caldwell, 1967).

To further explore the reactions of vitamin E with lipid hydroperoxyl radicals, free radical oxidations of several biological antioxidants were carried out with ferric iron–catalyzed dissociation of preformed lipid hydroperoxides (Gruger, 1968; Gruger and Tappel, 1970*a*, 1970*b*). In reactions of methyl linoleate hydroperoxides at 37 C, the relative rates of the following antioxidants were found: ubiquinol-6, 4.5; α-tocopherol hydroquinone, 2.9; ubichromenol-6, 1.1; ubichromenol-10, 1.0; and α-tocopherol, 1.0. Rates were measured for α-tocopherol oxidation by dissociating hydroperoxides of methyl linoleate, methyl linolenate, ethyl arachidonate, methyl eicosapentaenoate, and a highly unsaturated fraction of ethyl esters of fish-oil fatty acids. The degree of unsaturation of the lipid hydroperoxides had little effect on rates of α-tocopherol oxidation, except for the fish-oil fraction. Concentrations of ubiquinol, α-tocopherol, and polyunsaturated fatty acids present in the mitochondrial membrane are in the range for reasonable protective influence by biological antioxidants. In further studies by Dr. E. H. Gruger (Gruger and Tappel, 1970*a*, 1970*b*), free radical oxidations of α-tocopherol were carried out with ferric iron–catalyzed dissociations of preformed methyl linoleate hydroperoxides in various ethanolic solvent systems. Initial reaction rates, which were determined spectrophotometrically, were kinetically treated as first-order reaction dependent. Examinations of reaction parameters demonstrate a rate-inhibitory influence due to increased water levels in the reaction media. Also, increased acidity of reaction media causes increased rates of oxidation of antioxidants. At acid levels near *p*H 3, evidence suggests a transition from one predominant reaction mechanism to another, which may involve principally hydronium-ion catalysis at high acid levels.

Small amounts of ubiquinols may function as antioxidants in the mitochondrion. Ubiquinol-6 was more effective than ubiquinone-6 and almost as effective as α-tocopherol in reducing the stable free radical diphenyl-*p*-picrylhydrazyl. Antioxidant activity of ubiquinol-6, as measured at low oxygen concentrations with an oxygen electrode, was found to be as efficient as that of α-tocopherol as an inhibitor of the heme-catalyzed peroxidation of arachidonic acid emulsions (Mellors and Tappel, 1966). Ubiquinol-6 was oxidized to ubiquinone-6 by free radical products of the heme-catalyzed decomposition of cumene hydroperoxide α-Tocopherol did not inhibit this reaction. Light was used to catalyze the peroxidation of mitochondrial lipids at low concentrations of oxygen. This peroxidation was inhibited by the addition of ubiquinol-6 or of α-tocopherol to the mitochondria. Light-induced mitochondrial peroxidation was inhibited by ubiquinol-6 produced from exogenous ubiquinone-6 by the electron transport–linked oxidation of β-hydroxybutyrate. These reactions of ubiquinol as a chain-breaking antioxidant may explain why ubiquinones and related compounds have been found effective in the relief of certain vitamin E–deficiency syndromes in some species.

Vitamin E and selenoamino acids

In the function of vitamin E as a biological lipid antioxidant, its relationship with selenoamino acids is very important. A number of reactions of selenium compounds have been described (Tappel and Caldwell, 1967). Recent research (Dickson and Tappel, 1969*a*, 1969*b*) showed that in the presence of sulfhydryl compounds selenocystine increases the rate of activation and the time-integrated activity of the sulfhydryl enzymes papain and glyceraldehyde-3-phosphate dehydrogenase. Selenocystine also increases the rate and extent of inactivation of ribonuclease with cysteine. The effects on activation of papain by selenomethionine, by variation of the selenoamino acid concentration, and by the presence of N_2, O_2, and EDTA are consistent with a general mechanism of activation involving catalytic participation of selenocystine in sulfhydryl-disulfide exchange reactions. Papain activated in the presence of selenocystine and selenomethionine is partially protected against oxidative inactivation. The characteristics of the assay plots of substrate hydrolysis versus time, the effects of variation of assay parameters, and the dialysis of solutions containing protected papain indicate that the selenoamino acids bind reversibly to enzyme sulfhydryl groups to provide protection. Further, cysteine and glutathione reduce selenocystine to selenocysteine, with reaction equilibria attained rapidly. The extent of reduction is a function of the concentrations of the sulfhydryl compounds.

Maximum protection against oxidant and lipid-peroxidation damage is to be achieved by optimization of biological antioxidants, most of which are dietary components. Development of knowledge about these integrated qualitative and quantitative functions of the biological antioxidants is a major challenge of future research, and increased knowledge of vitamin E is the key to understanding this web of interactions.

References

Chio, K. S. 1968. Malonaldehyde reactions with amino acids and inactivation of ribonuclease and other enzymes by lipid peroxidation. Ph.D. thesis. University of California.

Chio, K. S., and A. L. Tappel. 1969*a*. Inactivation of ribonuclease and other enzymes by peroxidizing lipids and by malonaldehyde. *Biochemistry 8*:2827.

Chio, K. S., and A. L. Tappel. 1969*b*. Synthesis and characterization of the fluorescent products derived from malonaldehyde and amino acids. *Biochemistry 8*:2821.

Dickson, R. C., and A. L. Tappel. 1969*a*. Reduction of selenocystine by cysteine or glutathione. *Arch. Biochem. Biophys. 130*:547.

Dickson, R. C., and A. L. Tappel. 1969*b*. Effects of selenocystine and selenomethionine on activation of sulfhydryl enzymes. *Arch. Biochem. Biophys. 131*:100.

Di Luzio, N. R., and A. D. Hartman. 1967. Role of lipid peroxidation in the pathogenesis of the ethanol induced fatty liver. *Fed. Proc. 26*:1436.

Gruger, E. H., Jr. 1968. Reactions of biological antioxidants with aliphatic hydroperoxides. Ph.D thesis. University of California.

Gruger, E. H., Jr., and A. L. Tappel. 1970*a*. Reactions of biological antioxidants. I. Fe(III)-catalyzed reactions of lipid hydroperoxides with α-tocopherol. *Lipids 5*:326.

Gruger, E. H., Jr., and A. L. Tappel. 1970*b*. Reactions of biological antioxidants. II. Fe(III)-catalyzed reactions of methyl linoleate hydroperoxides with derivatives of coenzymes Q and vitamin E. *Lipids 5*:332.

Harman, D. 1968. Free radical theory of aging: Effect of free radical reaction inhibitors on the mortality rate of male LAF_1 mice. *J. Gerontol. 23*:476.

Hartroft, W. S. 1965. Atheroma begins at birth, p. 18. *In* F. A. Kummerow (ed.), *Metabolism of Lipids as Related to Atherosclerosis*. Charles C Thomas, Springfield, Ill.

Haugaard, N. 1968. Cellular mechanisms of oxygen toxicity. *Physiol. Rev. 48*:311.

Lundberg, W. O. (ed.). 1961. *Autoxidation and Antioxidants*. 2 vols. John Wiley (Interscience Publishers), New York.

Mellors, A., and A. L. Tappel. 1966. The inhibition of mitochondrial peroxidation by ubiquinone and ubiquinol. *J. Biol. Chem. 241*:4353.

Packer, L., D. W. Deamer, and R. L. Heath. 1967. Regulation and deterioration of structure in membranes. *Advances Gerontol. Res. 2*:77.

Perkins, E. G., T. H. Joh, and F. A. Kummerow. 1965. The composition of the extractable and bound lipids of the human aorta, p. 48. *In* F. A. Kummerow (ed.), *Metabolism of Lipids as Related to Atherosclerosis*. Charles C Thomas, Springfield, Ill.

Recknagel, R. O. 1967. Carbon tetrachloride hepatoxicity. *Pharmacol. Rev. 19*:145.

Roubal, W. T., and A. L. Tappel. 1966*a*. Polymerization of proteins induced by free-radical lipid peroxidation. *Arch. Biochem. Biophys. 113*:150.

Roubal, W. T., and A. L. Tappel. 1966*b*. Damage to proteins, enzymes, and amino acids by peroxidizing lipids. *Arch. Biochem. Biophys. 113*:5.

Schultz, H. W. (ed.). 1962. *Symposium on Foods: Lipids and Their Oxidation*. Avi, Westport, Connecticut.

Scott, G. 1965. *Atmospheric Oxidation and Antioxidants*. American Elsevier, New York.

Tappel, A. L. 1962. Vitamin E as the biological lipid antioxidant. *Vitamins Hormones 20*:493.

Tappel, A. L. 1968. Will antioxidant nutrients slow aging processes? *Geriatrics 23*:97.

Tappel, A. L., and K. A. Caldwell. 1967. Redox properties of selenium compounds related to biochemical function, p. 345. *In* O. H. Muth (ed.), *Selenium in Biomedicine*. Avi, Westport, Conn.

Wolman, M. 1964. The chromolipids, p. 96. *In* M. Wolman (ed.), *Handbuch der Histochemie*. Vol. V, Pt. 2 [in English]. Gustav Fischer Verlag, Stuttgart, Germany.

VITAMIN K

25

OCCURRENCE AND BIOPOTENCY OF VARIOUS FORMS OF VITAMIN K

John T. Matschiner

The story of vitamin K began in 1929, when Dam reported that chicks fed diets made deliberately low in fat for use in cholesterol-balance studies developed hemorrhages and gave samples of blood which were slow to coagulate (Dam, 1929, 1930). Work on this observation progressed leisurely for several years, but by 1935 it was clear that a fat-soluble vitamin designated K by Dam was responsible for preventing hemorrhages in normal, well fed animals (Dam, 1935*a*, 1935*b*; Almquist and Stokstad, 1935). Progress in this first phase of research on vitamin K reached its peak in 1939 and 1940, when the vitamin was isolated and characterized and when vigorous attempts were made to provide material for clinical use (Rosenberg, 1945). Associated studies had shown that vitamin K is valuable in the treatment of hemorrhages caused by bile-duct obstruction (Warner et al., 1938; Butt et al., 1938; Dam and Glavind, 1938*a*, 1938*b*) and in minimizing the hemorrhagic tendency of the newborn infant (Waddell et al., 1939). The important use of vitamin K in the control of anticoagulant therapy lay just ahead (Link, 1959; Meyer, 1959; Allen, 1959).

The structure of vitamin K_1 was proved by synthesis in 1939 (Almquist and Klose, 1939; Binkley et al., 1939; Fieser, 1939), but it was nearly twenty years before Isler and his collaborators reported the synthesis of vitamin K_2 (Isler et al., 1958). That vitamin, originally isolated in Doisy's laboratory from putrefied fish meal (McKee et al., 1939), was menaquinone-7. The classic synthetic work in Isler's laboratory led to the establishment of that structure and made available a series of vitamins ranging out to menaquinone-10, which has 50 carbons in the side chain and a molecular weight of 852 (Langemann and Isler, 1965). The menaquinones are bacterial vitamins and have been found to occur with side chains ranging from

Research in this report was supported in part by grants AM–09909 and AM–11311 from the National Institutes of Health.

20 carbons in menaquinone-4 to 65 carbons in menaquinone-13. Phylloquinone is the plant vitamin and has only been found as the phytyl (C_{20}) derivative.

Despite extensive clinical interest in vitamin K, nutritional and biochemical aspects remained undeveloped through the intervening decades. When Metta, Mameesh, and Johnson (1959) reported hemorrhages in young rats fed diets containing irradiated beef, a simple nutritional deficiency of vitamin K was not the accepted explanation. Rather, several laboratories painstakingly attempted to evaluate all factors in the expectation that development of the disease may have been due to a toxic principle (Johnson et al., 1960; Mellette and Leone, 1960; Doisy, 1961). Simple nutritional deficiency of vitamin K *was* the probable answer (Johnson et al., 1960; Mameesh et al., 1962; Matschiner and Doisy, 1966*a*), however, and the real, but elusive, requirement for vitamin K in mammalian species was affirmed. In those years, metabolic studies by Martius and co-workers (Martius, 1961*a*, 1961*b*) gave evidence that menaquinone-4 is the animal form of vitamin K. This compound is formed from menadione, and, more remarkably, from alkylated forms of vitamin K as well. Corroborating evidence has been presented for the conversion of menadione to menaquinone-4 in animal tissue (Griminger and Brubacher, 1966; Horth et al., 1966; Taggart and Matschiner, 1969), including the isolation and the physical and chemical identification of the metabolite by Dialameh and associates in 1968; but the relationship between the occurrence of menaquinone-4 and the function of vitamin K has not been clarified.

The only well established symptom of vitamin K deficiency in animals is defective blood coagulation – more specifically, a reduction in the activity of four plasma clotting factors presently designated II, VII, IX, and X (see Doisy and Matschiner, 1965). Measurement of any one of these factors may be used to estimate the action of vitamin K, so that an assay may be chosen because of its precision and because of the singular way in which it measures response to the vitamin.

Figure 25.1 shows the response in chicks fed dietary vitamin K in a typical bioassay (Matschiner and Doisy, 1966*b*). In this assay, prothrombin, or factor II, was measured in plasma by a one-stage procedure using Russell's viper venom as an extrinsic activator (Hjort et al., 1955). Day-old chicks were fed a deficient diet for 10 days, followed for 4 days by a diet supplemented with vitamin K. The curve shown here has been used for several years in our laboratory to estimate vitamin K in a variety of test substances. The assay is sensitive enough for plant and bacterial sources; in animal tissues, however, the amount of vitamin is often too small to be detected.

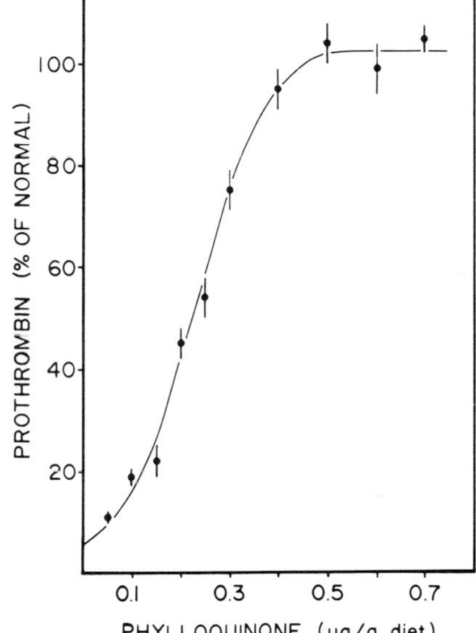

Fig. 25.1. Response of vitamin K–deficient chicks to diets containing controlled amounts of phylloquinone. Each point is accompanied by the standard error of the mean. (Matschiner and Doisy, 1966*b*. Reproduced by permission of the American Institute of Nutrition.)

Isolation of vitamin K from animal tissue

In 1967 we were able to isolate vitamin K from beef liver (Matschiner et al., 1967). From this source, the vitamin was obtained as a mixture of menaquinones with high molecular weights. On the basis of mass spectra and of other evidence, we proposed that most of the vitamin K present in beef liver is present as menaquinones-10, -11, and -12 (Matschiner and Amelotti, 1968). The origin of these vitamins appears to be in the rumen, since similar preparations of vitamin K were obtained from that source. Figure 25.2 shows portions of mass spectra containing the regions of the molecular ions from three samples of vitamin K purified from beef rumen. The values correspond in molecular weight to menaquinones-10, -11, -12, and -13.

From these data one can imagine that the vitamin K content of liver is determined by nutritional sources and is not dependent on metabolic events. If this is true, the liver of herbivores which are not ruminants should contain principally phylloquinone, the plant vitamin. Figure 25.3 shows a partition chromatogram (Matschiner and Taggart, 1967) of lipid from horse liver, along with a trace of radioactive phylloquinone. All of the biological activity recovered from this column was eluted in those fractions containing the radioactive phylloquinone. No biological activity was detected in the column wash, where lipophilic vitamins from beef

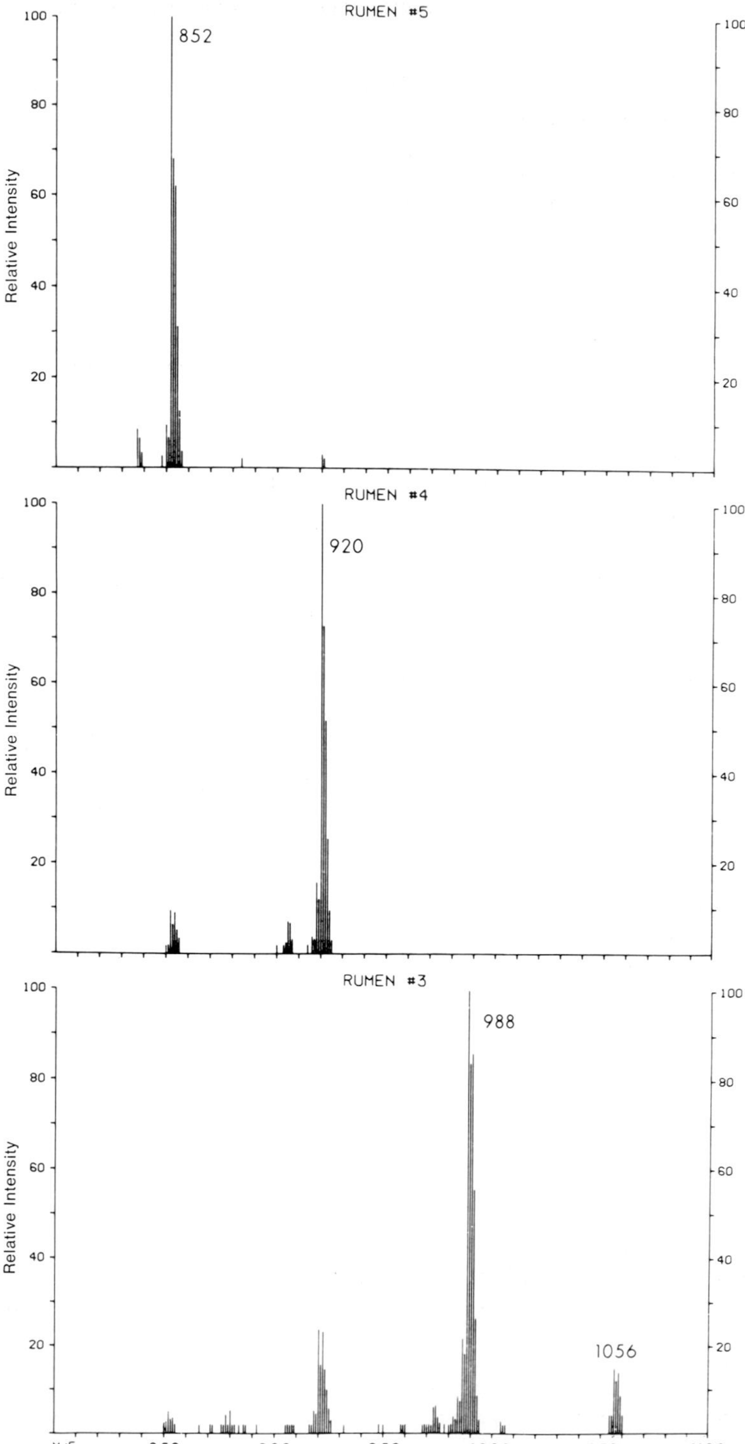
RUMEN #5
852
RUMEN #4
920
RUMEN #3
988
1056
Relative Intensity
100
80
60
40
20
M/E
850
900
950
1000
1050
1100

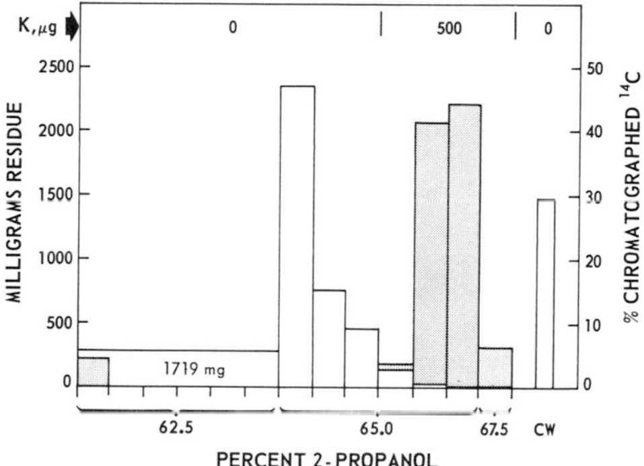

Fig. 25.3. Partition chromatography of vitamin K and associated lipids from horse liver. Recovery of radioactivity from added tracer ^{14}C phylloquinone is shown by the shaded bars; associated lipids, by the open bars. The amount of vitamin K determined by chick bioassay for groups of fractions and for the column wash (CW) is shown across the top.

liver would be found. More of these columns were run, and the vitamin from those fractions containing radioactivity and biological activity were combined and purified further. The mass spectrum of the final product, along with that of authentic phylloquinone, is shown in Figure 25.4.

These data support the identification of phylloquinone from horse liver. Along with the earlier results with beef liver, they support the view that liver contains mainly that vitamin K which is absorbed from the gut and does not, principally at least, contain biologically active forms of the vitamin which are metabolic in origin. As vitamin K is characterized from the liver of other species, however, this view may not be universally supported. Hamilton and Dallam (1968) reported that three species studied by them contained a naphthoquinone for which they proposed a dehydrophytyl structure. Since the compound they propose has not been identified elsewhere as a natural product, it would be suspected of having a metabolic origin. In any event, direct examination of liver has finally yielded some definitive information regarding the occurrence of vitamin K in animal tissue. These results follow by nearly thirty years the isolation of vitamin K from plant and bacterial sources.

Metabolic studies toward the occurrence and function of vitamin K

Although direct examination of liver has provided satisfying data regarding the occurrence of vitamin K, this approach is limited by the low concentration of the vitamin in animal tissue and by the dependence of each procedure on a biological assay to evaluate its success and to point the direction for the next experiment. Metabolic studies to estimate the occurrence of vitamin K in animal tissues have been reported from several

Fig. 25.2 (facing page). Molecular ions of menaquinones from beef rumen. Accelerating voltage, 3.0 kv; ion source, 70 ev, 310 C. (Reproduced by permission of the American Institute of Nutrition.)

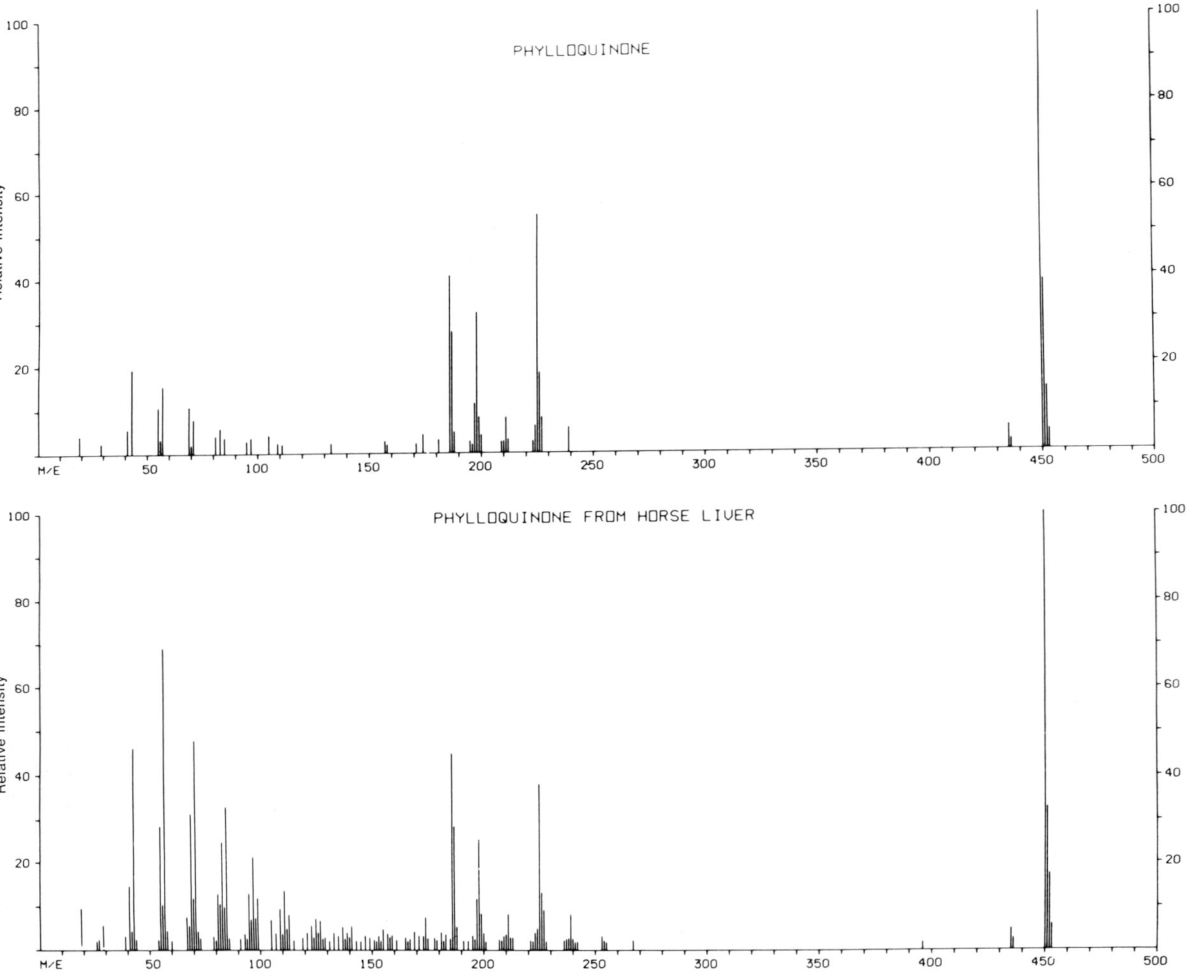
PHYLLOQUINONE
Relative Intensity
M/E
PHYLLOQUINONE FROM HORSE LIVER
Relative Intensity
M/E

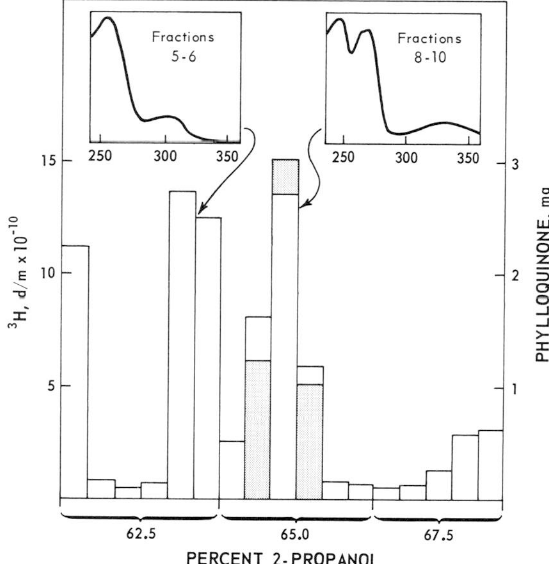

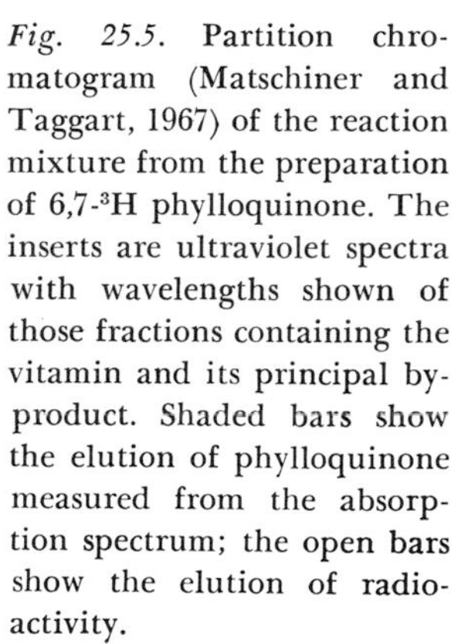
Fig. 25.5. Partition chromatogram (Matschiner and Taggart, 1967) of the reaction mixture from the preparation of 6,7-^{3}H phylloquinone. The inserts are ultraviolet spectra with wavelengths shown of those fractions containing the vitamin and its principal by-product. Shaded bars show the elution of phylloquinone measured from the absorption spectrum; the open bars show the elution of radioactivity.

laboratories, but the amount of vitamin K used in these experiments has generally been high. It seemed important to us to find a labeled form of vitamin K which could be used at concentrations really present in animal tissue. In a separate study in England (see Mitchell and Marrian, 1965), synkayvite, the diphosphate ester of menadiol, was prepared labeled with tritium with high specific activity. The most useful of these preparations, the 6,7-ditritio compound, has been available for several years from the Radiochemical Centre in Amersham. It can be used directly or can be hydrolyzed to yield menadione for metabolic studies. This substance also provides the starting material for a preparation of highly labeled phylloquinone.

PREPARATION OF RADIOACTIVE PHYLLOQUINONE

The reaction for the formation of phylloquinone had previously been carried out with as little as 30–40 mg of menadione, but in the preparation shown in Figure 25.5 we used only 6 mg of radioactive menadione with a specific activity of 10 Ci/mmole. Phylloquinone, with its characteristic absorption spectrum (in alcohol), was obtained in 31% yield. About an equal amount of a by-product (probably 2-methyl-2-phytyl-2,3-dihydro-1,4-naphthoquinone, Tishler et al., 1940*a*), shown with its absorption spectrum, was also obtained. In order to do double-label studies, the

Fig. 25.4 (facing page). Mass spectra of authentic phylloquinone (top) and phylloquinone isolated from horse liver (bottom). Accelerating voltage, 3.5 kv; ion source, 45 ev, 310 C.

same reaction was carried out with uniformly labeled phytol purified from algae grown in the presence of radioactive CO_2. From 13 mg of radioactive phytol, the vitamin was obtained in 27% yield. It had a specific activity of 70 mCi/mmole.

With these compounds available, particularly the tritiated form, it has been possible for the first time to follow vitamin K at steady-state concentrations and after curative doses through its turnover in liver and other tissues. One of the first experiments was reported by Taggart (1968).

RELATIONSHIP BETWEEN PROTHROMBIN LEVELS AND TISSUE VITAMIN CONCENTRATIONS

If vitamin K–deficient rats with prothrombin levels 30%–40% of normal are given just enough radioactive phylloquinone to correct the coagulation defect (Matschiner and Taggart, 1968), the presence of radioactive phylloquinone in liver assumes the curve shown in Figure 25.6. About 50% of the administered vitamin appears rapidly in liver and dies away along a curve which is not quite first order with respect to the concentration of the vitamin. The first half-life is about 2 hr, but subsequent half-lives are progressively longer. The appearance of prothrombin follows the curve described by the open circles. The initial rate of its appearance is more rapid than that predicted from the half-life of prothrombin in normal rats.* That calculated rate is shown by the dashed lines. A number of observations can be made from these data, but the connection between vitamin K in the liver and the appearance of prothrombin in plasma is not clear. It may be that the burst of vitamin K in liver which results from a single injected dose is responsible for a transient high rate of prothrombin synthesis, but we have not been able to obtain consistent evidence of a similar increase in prothrombin by giving excess vitamin K to normal rats. Figure 25.6 was purposely drawn with a base line corresponding to 200 picomoles of vitamin K because that is the amount of vitamin which we estimate may be present in the liver of a normal adult male rat.

Figure 25.7 shows a different response to vitamin K, which occurs in deficient rats given a single injection of menadione. In this case, plasma prothrombin does not rise immediately, but is delayed for 4 hr (Matschiner and Taggart, 1968). During this time, menaquinone-4 appears in the liver, but at concentrations much lower than those shown for phylloquinone in Figure 25.6. Finally, the rise in plasma prothrombin, when

* For use of the half-life of prothrombin to calculate the theoretical kinetics of induction of that protein see Pyorala (1966). The induction of other enzymes has been treated in a similar manner (Recheigl and Price, 1963; Schimke et al., 1964; Segal and Kim, 1965).

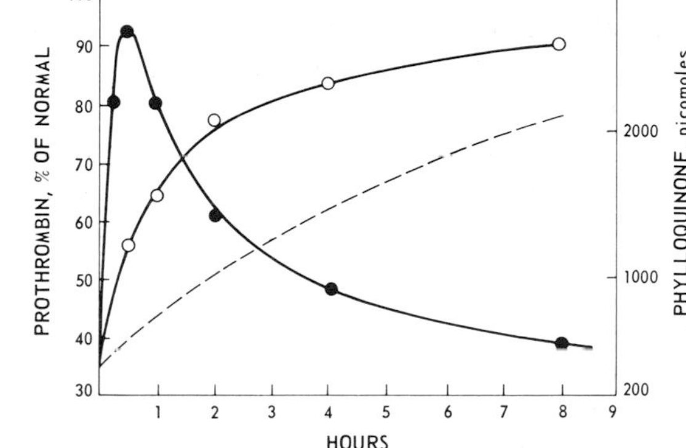

Fig. 25.6. Phylloquinone in liver (●) and prothrombin in plasma (O) of deficient rats after the injection of 3 μg of 6,7-^{3}H phylloquinone. The theoretical rate of appearance of prothrombin, based on its half-life in normal rats, is shown by the dashed line.

it does occur, is slower and closely resembles the theoretical rate. If menaquinone-4 is an active vitamin, as we believe, it is not clear why the lag in response occurs. Although the concentrations are low, the vitamin is present during the entire period. It may be that an infusion of phylloquinone in deficient rats at a level which would mimic the concentrations of menaquinone seen when menadione is administered would reveal a similar lag in prothrombin response. Certainly, deficient rats placed on a diet containing minimal amounts of vitamin K eventually achieve normal prothrombin concentrations without the opportunity for a large hepatic concentration of the vitamin. The kinetics of this type of feeding experiment have not been determined in detail, however.

All of these considerations have to do with the question: Is vitamin K, as we know that structure from classical studies, the active form of the vitamin? There has been no evidence that it is not; but these experiments with physiological levels of radioactive vitamin K constitute the first direct examination of that question. Figures 25.8 and 25.9 show the de-

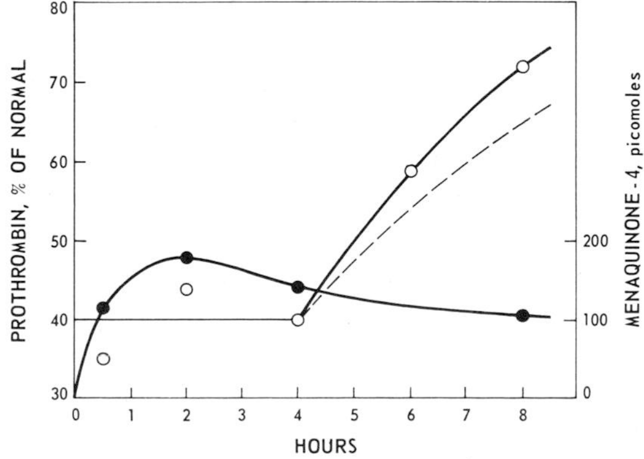

Fig. 25.7. Menaquinone-4 in liver (●) and prothrombin in plasma (O) of deficient rats after the injection of 10 μg of 6,7-^{3}H menadione. The theoretical rate of appearance of prothrombin, based on its half-life in normal rats, is shown by the dashed line. It is arbitrarily drawn to commence after the apparent lag period shown by the experimental values.

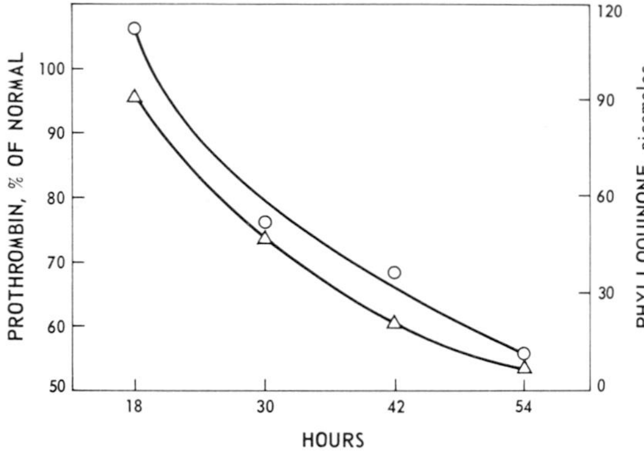

Fig. 25.8. Correlation of phylloquinone in liver (O) and prothrombin in plasma (△) during depletion of vitamin K after a single injection of 6,7-^{3}H phylloquinone in deficient rats.

cline of prothrombin and the decline of vitamin K in liver during the late phases of the experiments shown in Figures 25.6 and 25.7 and suggest that the known forms may be the active vitamins. In the experiment with phylloquinone (Fig. 25.8), the decline of that vitamin in the liver during the late period is approximately first order with respect to the concentration of the vitamin, with a half-life of about 13 hr. The decline of prothrombin is parallel to that of the vitamin, and, since the half-life of prothrombin itself is about 5 hr, these data support the view that the rate of synthesis of prothrombin in this phase of the experiment is declining in proportion to the concentration of phylloquinone in the liver. The data are circumstantial, but a direct correlation between vitamin K and the appearance, or in this case the disappearance, of prothrombin is evident.

In Fig. 25.9, the same correlation is shown for the late phase of the experiment with menadione. The half-life for menaquinone-4 from this figure is about 23 hr, and the curve is approximately paralleled by the drop in prothrombin concentration.

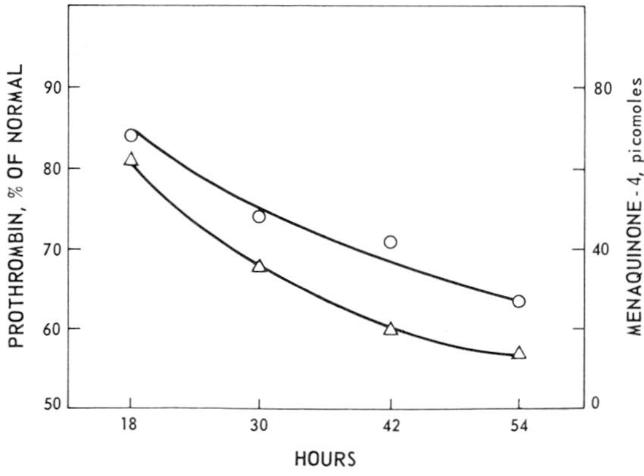

Fig. 25.9. Correlation of menaquinone-4 in liver (O) and prothrombin in plasma (△) during depletion of vitamin K after a single injection of 6,7-^{3}H menadione in deficient rats.

There are few metabolic forms of vitamin K known to occur in animal tissue. One is menaquinone-4; despite its metabolic origin, however, it bears no unique structural features to suggest a specific role in cellular processes. Given the formation of menaquinone-4, there is also the possibility of the natural occurrence of menadione, since it may be a metabolic intermediate. Finally, Gloor and associates (1966) recently identified a lactone which is formed from menaquinone or phylloquinone. This substance is apparently an excretory form of vitamin K and does not possess biological activity.*

IDENTIFICATION OF PHYLLOQUINONE OXIDE

The figures describing the time course of vitamin K in liver were prepared from data which excluded radioactivity not identified as phylloquinone or menaquinone-4. In fact, however, as much as 50% of the total radioactivity in liver may not be identified as vitamin K. Some radioactivity is not extracted from the liver, some has a different chromatographic mobility from that of the vitamin, and some radioactive vitamin decomposes during the experiment. Until recently, we had no evidence of the identity of other radioactive compounds. However, as a result of experiments with radioactive vitamin K which also involved the administration of warfarin, we have identified a new metabolic form which may be present in normal animals.

After several experiments had given evidence that the administration of warfarin results in the accumulation of an unknown radioactive compound in the liver of rats given radioactive vitamin K, we undertook the study shown in Table 25.1. Male rats weighing 350 g were given 3.5 mg of warfarin; 30 min later they received about 40 μg of radioactive phylloquinone, and 30 min or 6 hr later they were killed and the livers were

TABLE 25.1. *Effect of warfarin in livers of rats given ^{14}C phylloquinone-(phytyl-U)*

Time after vitamin K[a]	Warfarin[b]	Lipid[c] (mg)	^{14}C lipid (dpm $\times$ 10^{-5})	^{14}C residue (dpm $\times$ 10^{-5})
0.5 hr	+	1123	11.2	2.8
0.5 hr	—	713	13.9	1.1
6.0 hr	+	756	3.4	3.3
6.0 hr	—	669	3.4	0.8

[a] Vitamin K (41 μg, 1.5 $\times$ 10^6 dpm) administered intracardially.
[b] 1 mg/100 g body weight, given 30 min before vitamin K.
[c] Lipids extracted from liver of 2 rats per group.

* Unpublished bioassays; lactone provided through the courtesy of Hoffmann-LaRoche, Basel.

removed for analysis. Data from rats not given warfarin are also shown. The amount of lipid extracted from the liver was not unusual except 1 hr after warfarin. At that time, the lipid appears to be high, but this observation has not been confirmed. In several experiments, the radioactivity from the vitamin has been observed to distribute itself in a characteristic way between the lipid fraction and the extracted residue. The total radioactivity in the liver 30 min after vitamin K was about the same in both groups, but there was some evidence of more nonextractable material in the livers of rats given the anticoagulant. After 6 hr, the livers from warfarin-treated rats contained nearly twice as much radioactivity as those from control rats, but only half of that radioactivity was extractable.

After chromatography on silicic acid, the fractions containing vitamin K were combined and were chromatographed on a reversed-phase partition column. Data from these columns are shown in Figure 25.10. Radio-

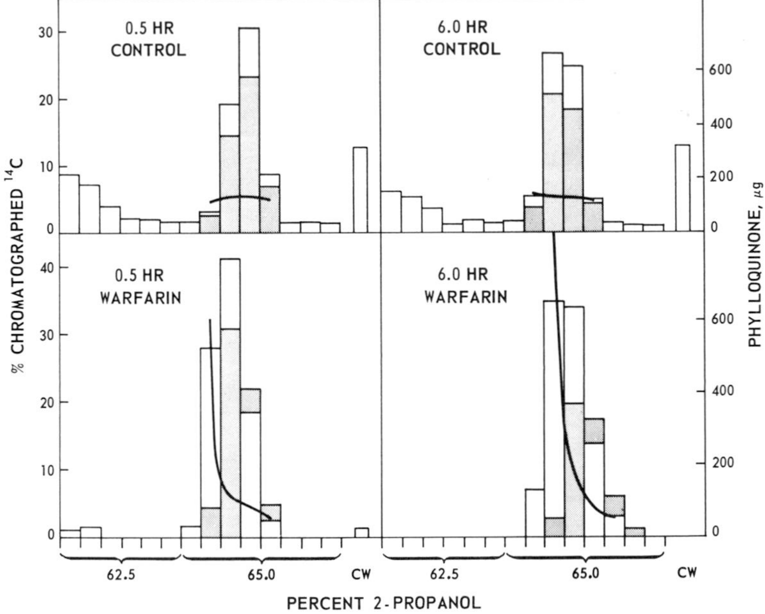

Fig. 25.10. Partition chromatogram (Matschiner and Taggart, 1967) of carrier phylloquinone (shaded bars) and of radioactivity (open bars) from the liver of rats killed 0.5 hr and 6.0 hr after the injection of ^{14}C phylloquinone-(phytyl-U). Warfarin-treated rats were given 1 mg of the anticoagulant per 100 g body weight 0.5 hr before an intracardial injection of the radioactive vitamin. The curved lines show the relative specific activity through the zone of elution of phylloquinone. (Reproduced from *Biochim. Biophys. Acta* 201 [1970] 311 [Fig. 1].)

activity was present in the early fractions and in the column wash if the rats did not receive warfarin, but these fractions contained little if any ^{14}C when lipids from warfarin-treated rats were chromatographed. In the region of elution of phylloquinone, the amount of radioactivity and of vitamin K coincided well if the lipid extracts were from control rats, but did not coincide if the animals received warfarin.

The substance responsible for the radioactivity eluted with the vitamin was purified and was identified as phylloquinone oxide. This compound, probably the 2,3-oxide of phylloquinone, was prepared from phylloquinone by oxidation with H_2O_2, as described by Tishler and associates (1940*b*). The product was purified by chromatography and had the same mobility as the compound isolated from rat liver. The ultraviolet absorption spectra of the natural and the synthetic compounds are shown in Figure 25.11. The mass spectra of these compounds are shown in Figure 25.12. The molecular ion at *m/e* 466 and the unique appearance of a substantial amount of fragment at *m/e* 423 are present in both spectra in Figure 25.12. The formation of fragment *m/e* 423 (which is 43 less than the molecular ion) may result from loss of carbon 2 of the naphthoquinone ring as part of an acylium ion containing the methyl group and the epoxide oxygen. Fragment *m/e* 159 would result from a similar reaction involving carbon 3. The complementary fragments *m/e* 43 and *m/e* 306 also appear. The peak at *m/e* 241 may represent the epoxide of the chroman fragment known to occur from phylloquinone at *m/e* 225 (DiMari et al., 1966). These considerations support the structure already

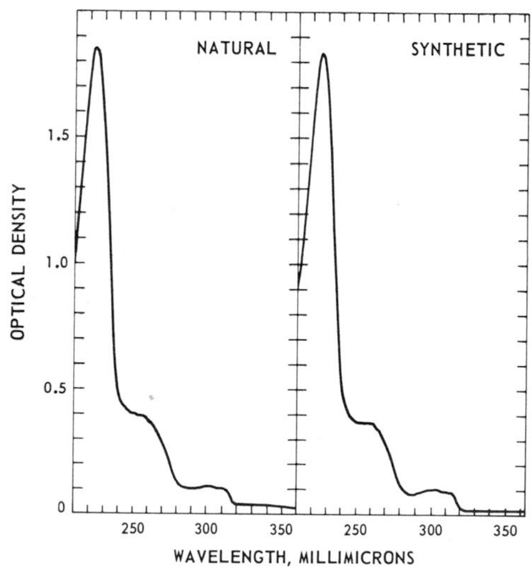

Fig. 25.11. Ultraviolet absorption spectra of synthetic phylloquinone oxide and of the natural oxide isolated from the livers of warfarin-treated rats. (Reproduced from *Biochim. Biophys. Acta* 201 [1970] 312 [Fig. 2].)

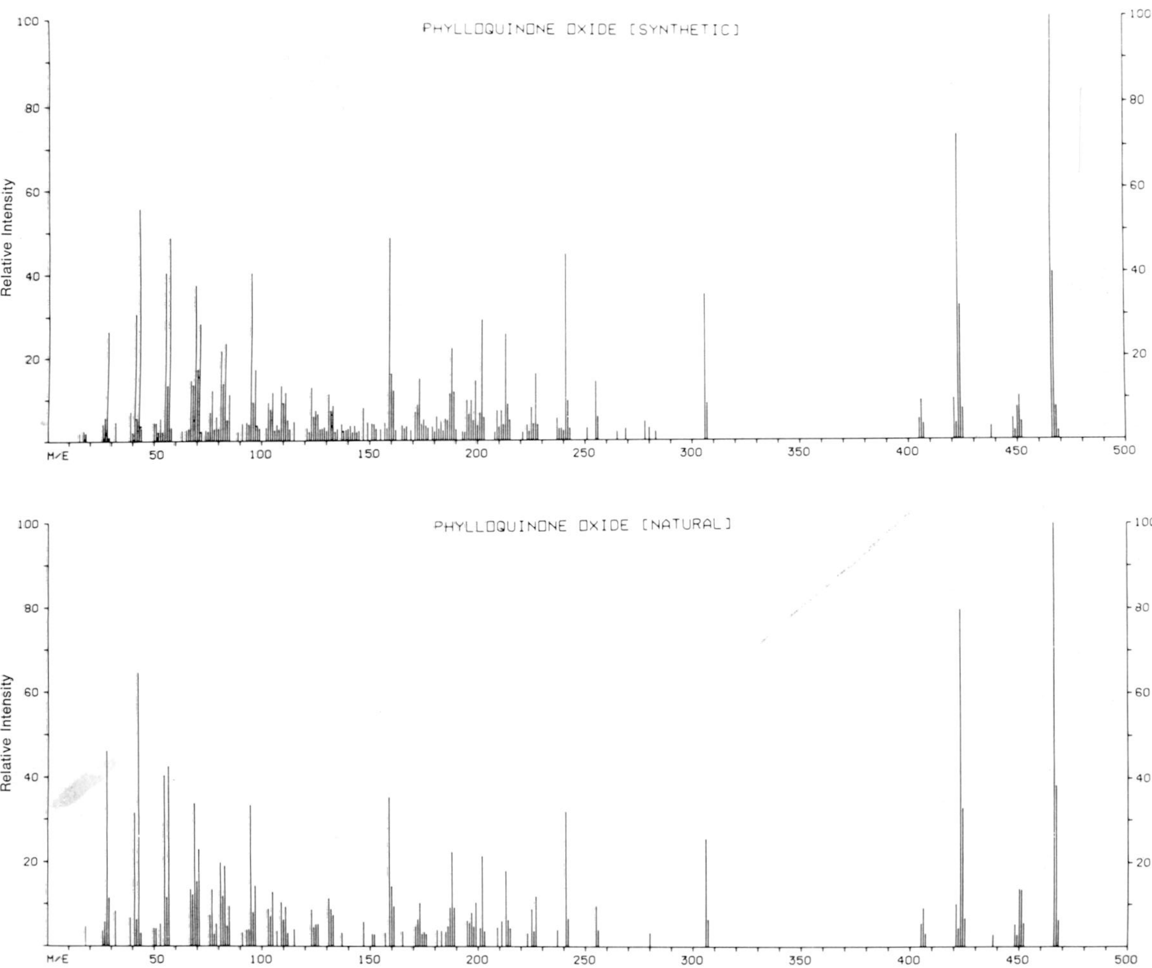
PHYLLOQUINONE OXIDE [SYNTHETIC]
Relative Intensity
M/E
PHYLLOQUINONE OXIDE [NATURAL]
Relative Intensity
M/E

proposed for the oxide of vitamin K (Tishler et al., 1940*b*). The identity of the isolated compound is confirmed by the similarity of these spectra.

The occurrence of phylloquinone oxide in the liver of rats given warfarin is unexplained at present. Before the compound was identified, we imagined the accumulation of a metabolite-inhibitor of the vitamin; but phylloquinone oxide has been reported to be as active as phylloquinone itself (Fieser et al., 1941). If this is a significant observation in relation to the function of vitamin K, the oxide should be present in normal animals. Table 25.2 shows some data obtained from rats fed radioactive

TABLE 25.2. *Partition thin-layer chromatography of phylloquinone fractions from rats fed 6,7-^3H phylloquinone*

	Chromatographed ^3H %		
Band	Liver	Heart	Control
6 (front)	4.1 ± 0.2	3.4 ± 0.4	7.3 ± 0.2
5 (oxide)	3.3 ± 0.1	3.2 ± 0.1	0.9 ± 0.1
4	7.8 ± 1.6	6.9 ± 1.4	9.0 ± 2.3
3 (K)	82.9 ± 2.2	78.5 ± 1.6	76.1 ± 2.2
2	3.1 ± 0.5	2.4 ± 0.5	2.5 ± 0.4
1 (origin)	[a]	[a]	[a]

Note: Silica gel g was impregnated with liquid paraffin and eluted with 92:8 acetone / H_2O.

[a] No ^3H detected.

vitamin K at minimum requirement levels. The tissues were removed, assayed for total radioactivity, and extracted. The extracts were separated by adsorption and by partition chromatography; the phylloquinone fractions were combined and examined for the presence of the oxide by thin-layer chromatography. Small amounts of phylloquinone and the oxide were added as carrier and were visualized in the bands identified in the table. As expected, most of the radioactivity was in the band containing phylloquinone. The control is a sample of the radioactive vitamin which was fed. A comparison with that control would suggest that a small amount of oxide may be present in both liver and heart.

Occurrence of vitamin K outside the liver

Finally, the occurrence of vitamin K and its metabolites is clearly not confined to the liver. The data shown in Table 25.2 concern only liver

Fig. 25.12 (facing page). Mass spectra of synthetic phylloquinone oxide and of the natural oxide isolated from the livers of warfarin-treated rats. Accelerating voltage, 3.5 kv; ion source, 70 ev, 250 C. (Reproduced from *Biochim. Biophys. Acta* 201 [1970] 313 [Fig. 3].)

TABLE 25.3. *Radioactivity in tissues of rats fed 6,7-^{3}H phylloquinone and ^{14}C phylloquinone-(phytyl-U)*

Tissue	Tritium (dpm/mg)	$^{3}H/^{14}C$ ratio
Liver	174	28
Heart	56	45
Kidney	69	48
Muscle	20	47
Blood	19	35
Plasma	30	35
Brain	32	135
Adipose	34	30
Hide	51	33
Lungs	104	59
Spleen	163	61
Testes	58	111
Cartilage	94	53
Sternum	119	120
Skull	67	193
Urine	—	264
Feces	—	56
Diet	*3470*	*66*

and heart, but, whether following a single injection or in rats fed radioactive vitamin K, all tissues become radioactive. Furthermore, the concentrations of radioactivity appear to be specific for several tissues, and, by the use of doubly labeled vitamin – i.e., ^{3}H in the aromatic nucleus and ^{14}C in the side chain – some evidence of metabolite specificity in various tissues has been obtained. In Table 25.3 are data obtained from adult male rats fed a purified diet containing 0.25 μg of phylloquinone per gram, the minimum requirement for maintenance of normal prothrombin levels. The animals had been depleted of vitamin K for ten days and were then fed the radioactive diet for four days. Separate experiments indicate that this period of feeding is sufficient to bring all tissues shown here to a steady isotope concentration. When ^{3}H activity, which is an estimate of the naphthoquinone nucleus, is considered, liver and spleen have approximately the same amount of radioactivity. This radioactivity in the liver, 174 dpm/mg, is equivalent to about 15 ng of vitamin K per gram of tissue, which is among the lowest values we have seen for liver of different species when examined by the chick bioassay. The value for beef liver, for example, is 100 times this amount, or about 1 $\mu g/g$ (Matschiner et al., 1967). In the experiment shown here, surprisingly high concentrations of radioactivity were found in the lung and the cartilage. Of the body tissues, skeletal muscle contained the lowest concentration

TABLE 25.4. *Thin-layer chromatography of menaquinone-4 and phylloquinone fractions from heart tissue of rats fed 6,7-^{3}H phylloquinone and ^{14}C phylloquinone-(phytyl-U)*

	Menaquinone-4			Phylloquinone		
Band [a]	Quinone (μg)	^{3}H (%)[b]	^{3}H/^{14}C ratio	Quinone (μg)	^{3}H (%)[b]	^{3}H/^{14}C ratio
9 (front)	[c]	0.2	[c]	[c]	1.1	31
8 (K)	129	1.7	71	840	85.0	64
7	[c]	0.6	50	[c]	0.3	[c]
6	19	6.8	538	[c]	0.1	[c]
5 (MK–4)	57	42.2	1385	73	0.7	[c]
4	[c]	0.4	39	16	[c]	[c]
3	[c]	1.1	27	[c]	0.2	[c]
2	[c]	1.3	61	[c]	1.0	42
1 (origin)	[c]	16.7	108	[c]	0.8	24

Note: Silica gel g + 1% $AgNO_3$; developing solvent, benzene.

[a] Locations of carrier menaquinone-4 (MK–4) and phylloquinone (K) are shown in bands 5 and 8.

[b] Percent chromatographed ^{3}H.

[c] None detected, or not calculable.

of ^{3}H, but when the amount of that tissue in the whole animal is considered, it comprises one of the largest pools of vitamin K and its metabolites. On the basis of total radioactivity, the three largest pools are hide, muscle, and skeletal structures. Liver contains the fourth largest pool of radioactivity.

This wide distribution of radioactivity confirms and extends earlier experiments, particularly those by Martius (1966), which showed extrahepatic occurrence of vitamin K. The values in Table 25.3, however, are the first estimate of steady-state concentrations of vitamin K and its metabolites in the tissues of a normal animal.

The data in Table 25.3 are preliminary in that we know very little about the structures of the radioactive compounds which may be present, but it seems clear from ^{3}H/^{14}C ratios that the side chain and the nucleus of the vitamin are, at least in part, following separate metabolic paths.* The ^{3}H/^{14}C ratio in urine is higher than expected for the excretion of the lactone, which has about one third of the carbon atoms of the side chain remaining. The high ratios in some tissues may be due to the lactone, but may also reflect the observation made earlier by Billeter and Martius (1960) of exchange of the side chain in the formation of menaquinone-4. That this exchange occurs is confirmed by data in Table 25.4. These data were obtained with fractions of menaquinone-4 and phylloquinone from heart tissue of rats fed both labeled vitamins. The initial

* In pigeons, Billeter and co-workers (1964) recovered the side chain of phylloquinone in the form of an ester of phytanic acid.

separation of the vitamins was achieved on a partition chromatogram. The identification is confirmed here on silica gel containing $AgNO_3$. For phylloquinone, nearly all of the recovered radioactivity was present in the band containing the carrier of phylloquinone, and the $^3H/^{14}C$ ratio was approximately that shown in Table 25.3 for the fed vitamin – 66. For menaquinone-4, most of the recovered ^3H was in the bands with the carrier menaquinone, but the $^3H/^{14}C$ ratio of this material was very high. The value 1385 for the principal fraction is too high to be precise but shows that less than 5% of the ^{14}C originally present in the molecules of phylloquinone could be detected in the metabolite. These data confirm earlier observations by Billeter and Martius on the loss of the side chain and provide a background against which to interpret, at least in part, the ratios shown in Table 25.3.

Summary

These are some of the data which show the steady progress being made toward an understanding of the occurrence of vitamin K in animal tissue. Despite extremely low concentrations of the vitamin, we can progress because of new analytical methods and particularly because highly labeled forms of vitamin K are now available. The vitamin has been isolated and characterized from liver; knowledge of its occurrence in other tissues has been extended and quantitatively estimated by isotopic methods. The question of the active molecular form of vitamin K is not settled, but there is little evidence to suggest that the vitamin is not active in the alkylated form in which we know it. The occurrence of menaquinone-4 as a metabolite in animals (first reported by Martius) has been observed in a number of laboratories, but present evidence does not indicate that that vitamin is specifically required for the synthesis of clotting proteins. The oxide of phylloquinone has been identified in the livers of rats given warfarin and radioactive phylloquinone, but the significance of its occurrence is not clear. Perhaps the most promising experiment is that showing the lag period in rats following the administration of menadione. When the elements of that lag period can be constructed experimentally, we will have substantial information concerning the molecular aspects of the action of vitamin K.

References

Allen, E. V. 1959. My early experience with bishydroxycoumarin (dicumarol). *Circulation 19*:118.

Almquist, H. J., and A. A. Klose. 1939. Synthetic and natural antihemorrhagic compounds. *J. Amer. Chem. Soc. 61*:2558.

Almquist, H. J., and E. L. R. Stokstad. 1935. Dietary haemorrhagic diseases in chicks. *Nature 136*:31.

Billeter, M., W. Bolliger, and C. Martius. 1964. Untersuchungen über die umwandlung von verfütterten K-vitaminen durch austausch der seitenkette und die rolle der darmbacterien dabei. *Biochem. Z. 340*:290.

Billeter, M., and C. Martius. 1960. Über die umwandlung von phyllochinon (vitamin K_1) in vitamin $K_{2(20)}$ im tierkörper. *Biochem. Z. 333*:430.

Binkley, S. B., L. C. Cheney, W. F. Holcomb, R. W. McKee, S. A. Thayer, D. W. MacCorquodale, and E. A. Doisy. 1939. The constitution and synthesis of vitamin K_1. *J. Amer. Chem. Soc. 61*:2558.

Butt, H. R., A. M. Snell, and A. E. Osterberg. 1938. The use of vitamin K and bile in treatment of the hemorrhagic diathesis in cases of jaundice. *Proc. Mayo Clinic 13*:74.

Dam, H. 1929. Cholesterinstoffwechsel in huhnereiern und hühnchen. *Biochem. Z. 215*:475.

Dam, H. 1930. Über die cholesterinsynthese im tierkörper. *Biochem. Z. 220*:158.

Dam, H. 1935*a*. The antihaemorrhagic vitamin of the chick. *Biochem. J. 29*:1273.

Dam, H. 1935*b*. The antihaemorrhagic vitamin of the chick. *Nature 135*:652.

Dam, H., and J. Glavind. 1938*a* Vitamin K in human pathology. *Lancet 243*:720.

Dam, H., and J. Glavind. 1938*b*. The clotting power of human and mammalian blood in relation to vitamin K. *Acta Med. Scand. 96*:108.

Dialameh, G. H., T. S. Najafi, and R. E. Olson. 1968. The relative rates of menaquinone-4 and prothrombin biosynthesis in vitamin K–deficient chicks. *Fed. Proc. 27*:436.

DiMari, S. J., J. H. Supple, and H. Rapoport. 1966. Mass spectra of naphthoquinones. Vitamin $K_{1(20)}$. *J. Amer. Chem. Soc. 88*:1226.

Doisy, E. A., Jr. 1961. Nutritional hypoprothrombinemia and metabolism of vitamin K. *Fed. Proc. 20*:989.

Doisy, E. A., Jr., and J. T. Matschiner. 1965. Nutritional aspects with special reference to hypoprothrombinemia and vitamin K, p. 317. *In* R. A. Morton (ed.), *Biochemistry of Quinones*. Academic Press, London.

Fieser, L. F. 1939. Synthesis of 2-methyl-3-phytyl-1,4-naphthoquinone. *J. Amer. Chem. Soc. 61*:2559.

Fieser, L. F., M. Tishler, and W. L. Sampson. 1941. Vitamin K activity and structure. *J. Biol. Chem. 137*:659.

Gloor, U., J. Würsch, H. Mayer, O. Isler, and O. Wiss. 1966. Stoffwechsel-endprodukte von phyllochinon, menachinon-4, ubichinon-9 und hexahydroplastochinon-4 (phytylplastochinon). *Helv. Chim. Acta 49*:2582.

Griminger, P., and G. Brubacher. 1966. The transfer of vitamin K_1 and menadione from the hen to the egg. *Poultry Sci. 45*:512.

Hamilton, J. W., and R. D. Dallam. 1968. Isolation of vitamin K from animal tissue. *Arch. Biochem. Biophys. 123*:514.

Hjort, P., S. I. Rapaport, and P. A. Owren. 1955. A simple, specific one-stage prothrombin assay using Russell's viper venom in cephalin suspension. *J. Lab. Clin. Med. 46*:89.

Horth, C. E., D. McHale, L. R. Jeffries, S. A. Price, A. T. Diplock, and J. Green. 1966. Vitamin K and oxidative phosphorylation. *Biochem. J. 100*:424.

Isler, O., R. Rüegg, L. H. Chopard-dit-Jean, A. Winterstein, and O. Wiss. 1958. Synthese und isolierung von vitamin K_2 und isoprenologen verbindungen. *Helv. Chim. Acta 41*:786.

Johnson, B. C., M. S. Mameesh, V. C. Metta, and P. B. Rama Rao. 1960. Vitamin K nutrition and irradiation sterilization. *Fed. Proc. 19*:1038.

Langemann, A., and O. Isler. 1965. Chemistry of isoprenoid quinones, p. 89. *In* R. A. Morton (ed.), *Biochemistry of Quinones.* Academic Press, London.

Link, K. P. 1959. The discovery of dicumarol and its sequels. *Circulation 19*:97.

McKee, R. W., S. B. Binkley, D. W. MacCorquodale, S. A. Thayer, and E. A. Doisy. 1939. The isolations of vitamins K_1 and K_2. *J. Amer. Chem. Soc. 61*:1295.

Mameesh, M. S., V. C. Metta, P. B. Rama Rao, and B. C. Johnson. 1962. On the cause of vitamin K deficiency in male rats fed irradiated beef and the production of vitamin K deficiency using an amino acid synthetic diet. *J. Nutr.* 77:165.

Martius, C. 1961*a*. Recent investigations on the chemistry and function of vitamin K, p. 312. *In* G. E. W. Wolstenholme and C. M. O'Connor (eds.), *Quinones and Electron Transport.* Little Brown, Boston.

Martius, C. 1961*b*. The metabolic relationships between the different K vitamins and the synthesis of the ubiquinones. *Amer. J. Clin. Nutr.* 9: (Suppl). p. 97.

Martius, C. 1966. Mode of action of vitamins K in animals. *Vitamins Hormones 24*:441.

Matschiner, J. T., and J. M. Amelotti. 1968. Characterization of vitamin K from bovine liver. *J. Lipid Res. 9*:176.

Matschiner, J. T., and E. A. Doisy, Jr. 1966*a*. Vitamin K content of ground beef. *J. Nutr. 90*:331.

Matschiner J. T., and E. A. Doisy, Jr. 1966*b*. Bioassay of vitamin K in chicks. *J. Nutr. 90*:97.

Matschiner, J. T., and W. V. Taggart. 1967. Separation of vitamin K and associated lipids by reversed-phase partition column chromatography. *Anal. Biochem. 18*:88.

Matschiner, J. T., and W. V. Taggart. 1968. Bioassay of vitamin K by intracardial injection in deficient adult male rats. *J. Nutr. 94*:57.

Matschiner, J. T., W. V. Taggart, and J. M. Amelotti. 1967. The vitamin content of beef liver. Detection of a new form of vitamin K. *Biochemistry 6*:1243.

Mellette, S. J., and L. A. Leone. 1960. Influence of age, sex, strain of rat and fat soluble vitamins on hemorrhagic syndromes in rats fed irradiated beef. *Fed. Proc. 19*:1045.

Metta, V. C., M. S. Mameesh, and B. C. Johnson. 1959. Vitamin K deficiency in rats induced by the feeding of irradiated beef. *J. Nutr. 69*:18.

Meyer, O. O. 1959. Historical data regarding the experiences with coumarin anticoagulants at the University of Wisconsin Medical School. *Circulation 19*:114.

Mitchell, J. S., and D. H. Marrian. 1965. Radiosensitization of cells by a derivative of 2-methyl-1,4-naphthoquinone, p. 503. *In* R. A. Morton (ed.), *Biochemistry of Quinones*. Academic Press, London.

Pyorala, K. 1966. Determinants of the clotting factor response to warfarin in the rat. *Ann. Med. Exp. Biol. Fenn. 43*: Suppl. 3.

Recheigl, M., Jr., and V. E. Price. 1963. The rates and the kinetics of enzyme formation and destruction in the living animal, p. 185. *In* A. A. Albanese (ed.), *Newer Methods of Nutritional Biochemistry*. Academic Press, New York.

Rosenberg, H. R. 1945. *Chemistry and Physiology of the Vitamins*, p. 481. Interscience Publishers, New York.

Schimke, R. T., E. W. Sweeney, and C. M. Berlin. 1964. An analysis of the kinetics of rat liver tryptophan pyrrolase induction: The significance of both enzyme synthesis and degradation. *Biochem. Biophys. Res. Commun. 15*:214.

Segal, H. L., and Y. S. Kim. 1965. Environmental control of enzyme synthesis and degradation. *J. Cell. Comp. Physiol. 66*: Suppl. 1, p. 11.

Taggart, W. V. 1968. The relationship between vitamin K and prothrombin response in vitamin K–deficient rats. *Fed. Proc. 27*:435.

Taggart, W. V., and J. T. Matschiner. 1969. Metabolism of menadione-6, 7-^{3}H in the rat. *Biochemistry 8*:1141.

Tishler, M., L. F. Fieser, and N. L. Wendler. 1940*a*. Nature of the by-product in the synthesis of vitamin K. *J. Amer. Chem. Soc. 62*:1982.

Tishler, M., L. F. Fieser, and N. L. Wendler. 1940*b*. Hydro, oxido and other derivatives of vitamin K_1 and related compounds. *J. Amer. Chem. Soc. 62*:2866.

Waddell, W. W., Jr., D. Guerry, III, W. E. Bray, and O. R. Kelley. 1939. Possible effects of vitamin K on prothrombin and clotting time in newly-born infants. *Proc. Soc. Exp. Biol. Med. 40*:432.

Warner, E. D., K. M. Brinkhous, and H. P. Smith. 1938. Bleeding tendency of obstructive jaundice: Prothrombin deficiency and dietary factors. *Proc. Soc. Exp. Biol. Med. 37*:628.

26

ACTION OF VITAMIN K AT THE CELLULAR LEVEL

Marion I. Barnhart, Sharon M. Noonan, and Gordon F. Anderson

In contrast to the fat-soluble vitamins A and D with their multiple functions and wide biological importance, vitamin K appears to have a more restricted value in promoting prothrombin formation to aid hemostatic mechanisms. This apparent selective influence on only one of the many proteins synthesized by the liver makes vitamin K, its antagonistic drugs, and the prothrombin-synthesis apparatus especially attractive for basic considerations of protein synthesis.

Even though the liver produces and delivers about 80% of the plasma proteins, there is scant information about the intracellular events from loci of protein assembly through packaging and delivery to the circulation. Prothrombin synthesis provides a model system that lends itself to ultrastructural study because of the relative ease of chemical manipulation of the rate and magnitude of synthesis, storage, and release. It might seem that prothrombin, as a trace plasma protein that exists normally at a plasma concentration near 15 mg/100 ml, would be a poor selection for gaining insight into protein synthesis. However, individuals that are essentially depleted of prothrombin because of Coumadin inhibition of synthesis can completely restore their hepatic and blood content within a few hours after receiving vitamin K_1. The magnitude of such synthesis in the prothrombin-deficient dog has approached 80 mg over a few hours of stimulated activity (Barnhart, 1965). With some simple mathematical extrapolations, the rate of prothrombin synthesis can reach 0.5 mg/g hepatocyte per day, which corresponds to the synthesis of at least 21,600

These studies were aided by grants from the National Heart Institute, the National Institutes of Health, the United States Public Health Service, and the Michigan Heart Association.

prothrombin molecules per min per hepatocyte or to the formation of about 10,000,000 peptide bonds per min per hepatocyte.

Thus prothrombin synthesis, with its controlling mechanisms, offers an unique opportunity to explore the cellular synthesis of a protein made for export and hemostatic utilization far from the sites of hepatic origin. Moreover, study of the prothrombin-synthesis model system may also reveal the modes of operation of vitamin K and coumarin drugs. Vitamin K_1 and Coumadin are structurally similar agents (Fig. 26.1) and may interact with the same cellular receptor sites; but this may be too simple a view. Knowledge of the pharmacodynamics of anticoagulant drugs such as warfarin (Coumadin) might be especially valuable because of the extensive use of these drugs, or of those that act in a similar manner, in the medical management of numerous individuals attempting to limit or control thrombus formation and the disability or death resulting from strokes and heart diseases.

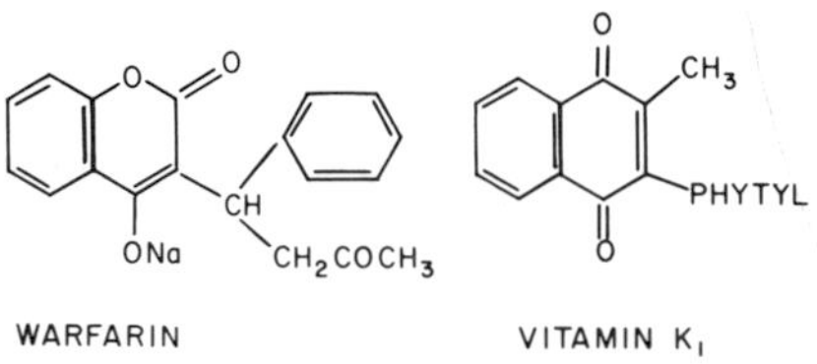

WARFARIN VITAMIN K_1

Fig. 26.1. Similarity of structure of warfarin (Coumadin) and vitamin K_1.

Experimental design

The dynamic state of organ function with accompanying morphologic changes has been established by numerous investigators. The liver may be the most responsive and plastic of all organs by virtue of receiving about 25% of the cardiac output and of having first contact with most materials absorbed from the digestive tract. Not only does the functional state differ from hepatocyte to hepatocyte, but the proportion of hepatocytes to reticuloendothelial cells also varies with age and physiologic state (Daoust, 1958). Intergroup comparison of single samples of subcellular fractions obtained from mixed cell populations may be subject to misinterpretation because of physiologic and morphologic variation within the livers which may be either accentuated or neutralized by pooling of specimens.

To capitalize on these facts and to obtain samples of perhaps greater relevance for interpretation of drug-induced changes, our experimental studies have employed sequential specimens taken from a few, selected, normal individuals. Tissue or cell organization was ordinarily preserved, except in some cell-fractionation work where the subcellular organelles were isolated from a relatively homogeneous hepatocyte fraction previously separated from the other cell types that comprise the liver. Concurrent blood samples were taken serially, so that the concentrations of various blood-clotting substances could be assessed and related to the properties observed in the liver biopsies (morphology by bright-field or electron microscopy, and function evaluated with the aid of specific immunologic or fluorescent antibody tools). This approach seemed likely to provide a dynamic overview of an individual's exact response to the drug manipulation of protein synthesis.

Immunocytofluorescent studies

Previous immunologic work has established that prothrombin is produced exclusively by hepatocytes in cattle (Barnhart, 1960), in dogs (Anderson and Barnhart, 1964*a*), and in humans (Barnhart, 1965). The pattern of prothrombin synthesis, storage, and release is similar for these three species. Although all hepatocytes are capable of prothrombin production, under normal demands, hepatocytes function asynchronously with only 10%–30% active at any one time, and measurement with a specific fluorescent antiprothrombin would indicate that intracellular storage is limited.

Prothrombin is synthesized in the microsomal fraction of hepatocytes and, if present, exists in insufficient quantity to be detected by immunologic aids in microsomes obtained from extremely prothrombin-deficient dogs (Anderson and Barnhart, 1964*b*). Intravenous administration of vitamin K_1 to such dogs restores the prothrombin-synthesizing apparatus of the microsomal fraction, so that prothrombin again becomes measurable at that subcellular locus.

Regulators of prothrombin synthesis

Prothrombin biosynthesis is responsive to at least two controlling mechanisms: (1) the plasma level of prothrombin or its degradation products, and (2) the concentration of vitamin K_1.

The prothrombinemia induced in dogs by plasmapheresis, by experimental microthrombosis initiated by thrombin infusion (Barnhart and Forman, 1963), or by sufficient blood loss is usually followed, unless shock is severe, by restoration to a normal plasma-prothrombin level. Recovery has been the slowest in an admittedly limited experience with plasmapheresis, where one may assume there are few, if any, prothrombin degradation products and where the reduced "native" prothrombin level acts as the stimulus for replenishing the circulation. In contrast, more rapid correction of prothrombin deficiency occurs when prothrombin by-products of blood clotting exist in the blood along with a reduced native prothrombin content.

Four dogs subjected to controlled diffuse intravascular coagulation showed the expected declines in fibrinogen level and platelet numbers and also had their prothrombin levels reduced about 30%. There were prompt additions of prothrombin to the circulation within 2–4 hr. According to immunocytofluorescence with a specific antibody, the hepatocyte population had been stimulated to synthesize and store prothrombin, as both numbers and intensity of fluorescence increased in liver biopsies from 1 hr to 6 hr after the stress. Prothrombin degradation products or derivatives were likely the stimuli for prothrombin synthesis, because sham-operated animals, with presumably few prothrombin degradation products, did not exhibit cytofluorescence typical of a stimulus to prothrombin synthesis.

Prothrombin synthesis can be turned on or up promptly after intravenous administration of vitamin K_1. The increased cytofluorescent response of hepatocytes, which signals their prothrombin content, occurs in the prothrombin deficiency following Coumadin suppression of prothrombin synthesis, in normal dogs, or in humans who provided liver biopsies during corrective surgery for nonhepatic pathology (Barnhart, 1965).

An example follows of the correction of prothrombin deficiency and apparent *de novo* synthesis of prothrombin by hepatocytes after vitamin K_1 treatment (Fig. 26.2). Dog F had a normal control plasma prothrombin of 115 Iowa units (U)/ml plasma as determined by the modified two-stage

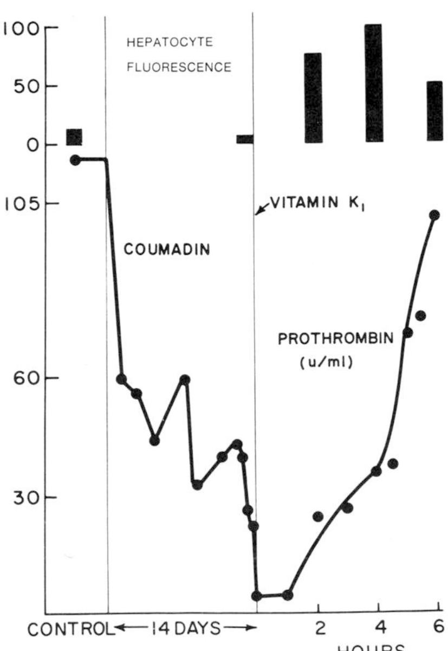

Fig. 26.2. Sequence of events in dog F given Mephyton (K_1) after becoming prothrombin deficient. Hepatocyte fluorescence reflects the prothrombin content of hepatocytes (%) after reacting with a specific fluorescent antiprothrombin.

procedure of Ware and Seegers (1949). When hepatocytes from the control biopsy were treated with rhodamine antidog prothrombin, about 25% of the hepatocytes were found to contain some prothrombin. After recovery from the surgery for control specimens, a series of injections of Coumadin was given over a 14-day period. The priming dose of Coumadin was 1 mg/kg body weight and was followed at intervals by doses of 0.1 mg/kg or 0.2 mg/kg in attempts to reach a stable state whereby the plasma prothrombin would be maintained near 30% of the control level. This objective was not achieved in this particular dog, and he was given vitamin K_1 when his prothrombin measured less than 5 U/ml. The liver biopsy taken immediately before vitamin K_1 (Mephyton, 5 mg/kg) was administered had about 8% of the hepatocytes reactive and a low prothrombin content as judged by immunocytofluorescence. After K_1 treatment, the hepatocytes at 2 hr exhibited increased fluorescent intensity, with about 70% reactive; at 4 hr, essentially 100% of the hepatocytes vividly fluoresced. Very little prothrombin had been released to the circulation during the first 4 hr, although prothrombin synthesis was obviously turned on and turned up by the vitamin K. By 6 hr the hepatocyte fluorescence was diminishing and only about 50% fluoresced—but still brightly. At this time, the plasma prothrombin reached its peak recovery of about 90% of the control level. By 8 hr only 10% of the hepatocytes showed brilliant fluorescence. Thus, the additions to the plasma reflected newly synthesized prothrombin released from the hepatocytes. Although the deficiency existed and there was a demand to replenish the circulation, a lag period of 2–4 hr occurred before the prothrombin that had been visible earlier in hepatocytes was released.

The concentration of vitamin K_1 also serves to regulate prothrombin synthesis, with a certain critical concentration necessary for the occurrence of significant synthesis and storage. This fact has been demonstrated by studies in both dogs (Barnhart, 1965) and humans (Barnhart, 1967).

In cooperation with Dr. Alex Walt (Surgery Department, Wayne State University), a study was made to determine if there was a response to vitamin K_1 in humans as there was in the dog model system. Permission for liver biopsy was obtained from selected subjects with apparently normal livers who were to undergo corrective surgery near the liver. Control liver biopsies were removed surgically, and then vitamin K_1 (Mephyton) was given intravenously. Such patients had the benefit of a plentiful supply of prothrombin to combat any bleeding problems that arose during or after surgery and provided us with an opportunity for a direct cellular study of prothrombin synthesis in man. A second biopsy was taken just before completion of the surgery. Of the 25 patients evaluated, the control biopsies exhibited fluorescence in 20%–35% of their hepatocytes, indicating that they contained prothrombin, when fluorescent antihuman prothrombin was applied to liver-cell imprints. All subjects responded to the administration of vitamin K_1, and there were increases in both the number and the intensity of fluorescent cells, indicating that prothrombin synthesis and storage was stimulated. The second biopsies were taken from 1 hr to 5.75 hr after vitamin K_1. From 60%–86% of the hepatocyte population revealed activation of prothrombin synthesis. A second dose of vitamin K_1 stimulated more hepatocytes. Very little of this newly synthesized and stored prothrombin was released to enrich the plasma during the time observed.

Regulator for prothrombin release

The regulator of the plasma-prothrombin level is a remarkably sensitive, effective homeostatic mechanism that prevents excesses of prothrombin in the circulation. Records from 4 control dogs illustrate this point (Fig. 26.3). These dogs were subjected to sequence analysis of blood and liver to simulate the drug manipulation of the rate of prothrombin synthesis. Dogs A–11 and A–12 were given a mixture of polysorbate 80, which is the vehicle for AquaMephyton. This was preceded by a dose of Benedryl (1 mg/kg) to protect the dog from histamine shock, which can be a troublesome complication in this species where the mast cells are especially sensitive to fatty acid esters (Goth, 1962). The prothrombin level fluctuated

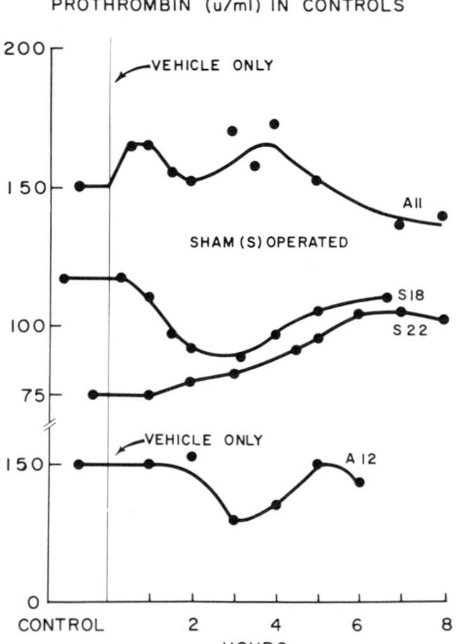

Fig. 26.3. Plasma prothrombin in several control dogs during study for 9–12 hr. Sham-operated dogs did not receive vehicle or other injections.

near ± 10% of the control state in dog A–11. Dog A–12 showed a drop of about 40% in prothrombin, which was restored within 2 hr to the initial control value. Sham operations without any drug administrations were carried on in dogs S–18 and S–22. During the experiment on S–18, there was a 22% drop in circulating prothrombin, which was essentially restored without overshoot of the control value. Dog S–22 had a fairly low control prothrombin level, and during the sham experiment he had a continual, slow rise in plasma prothrombin which leveled off at 25% higher than the control.

These values for prothrombin fluctuation during a sequence study of about 9 hr with concurrent blood and liver sampling are typical of our general laboratory experiences. For example, data from 10 other dogs infused with small amounts of fibrinogen proteolysis products or with doses of thrombin insufficient to produce defibrination in work carried out with other associates showed 8 remained within ± 13% of control prothrombin. Plasma prothrombin in the 2 remaining dogs declined 26% and 17%.

Monitoring of the livers of selected animals (A–11, A–12, S–18, and S–22) with the fluorescent-antibody technique did not reveal that prothrombin synthesis was visibly stimulated. The number of prothrombin-containing cells ranged between 10% and 30% and these cells retained their patchy distribution in the liver. Such findings as these emphasize that storage of prothrombin is limited but is adequate to improve the plasma compartment from 25% to 40%. Furthermore, each dog seems to have his plasma-prothrombin regulator set at a slightly different level but operating as an effective guard against excessive prothrombin.

When the plasma compartment has a normal prothrombin level, vitamin K_1 treatment of either humans or dogs is not followed by a spectacular rise in plasma prothrombin. Even when immunocytology seems to indicate that hepatocytes are full of prothrombin, the addition of prothrombin to the circulation has not exceeded 40% of the control state.

In the human series of sequence liver biopsies and blood samples, the plasma prothrombin retained its control, pre–vitamin K_1 level in 4 subjects and dropped in 3 subjects (9%, 18%, and 28%) over the 2–6 hr of this study. In one subject, a 9% decrease at 3 hr was followed by an increase and an overshoot of 7% by 4.5 hr.

Vitamin K_1 was given to 5 normal dogs, and their blood and liver biopsies were evaluated over 8 hr and were compared to the control state. In each dog, an increased fluorescence in the hepatocytes – indicating a stimulated synthesis and storage of prothrombin in response to the K_1 was apparent at 1 hr. There was no change in the plasma prothrombin in 3 of these dogs and an insignificant increase of 12% in one dog. The other dog improved his plasma prothrombin level by 40%, but a second dose of vitamin K_1 was without effect on the plasma-prothrombin concentration. Apparently unrelated to the actual prothrombin concentration as determined by two-stage analysis, the prothrombin time by one stage was immediately shortened but soon assumed control values in all dogs.

Prothrombin movement within the hepatocyte and its ultimate release to the circulation do not appear to follow a simple concentration gradient. Vitamin K_1 does not appear to be a prothrombin-releasing factor, although vitamin K_1 promotes the immediate release of a procoagulant to alter the prothrombin-time test. The release of prothrombin, per se, must be governed by some substance or mechanism unrelated to vitamin K_1.

On Coumadin

Prothrombin biosynthesis is inhibited by coumarin drugs. With suitable doses and time, a treated dog loses its hepatocyte reactivity to fluorescent antidog prothrombin. Sequence biopsies have been taken up to 28.5 hr after an intravenous dose of Coumadin (4 mg/kg body weight). By 4 hr, the number and the intensity of immunoreactive hepatocytes are reduced. Loss of fluorescence specific for prothrombin is progressive. Depending on the prothrombin stores, the fluorescent response disappears between 6 hr and 12 hr after Coumadin, signifying that the amounts of prothrombin have become too small for visual detection. Clearly, the mechanism of action of Coumadin is not to stabilize membranes so that storage is promoted. Nor is the release of prothrombin prevented, because small additions to plasma prothrombin can be detected which briefly plateau the prothrombin curve that continues to decline.

Coumadin acts in some way to prevent the biosynthesis of prothrombin, as can be shown by the loss of immunochemical reactivity from microsome fractions of dogs treated with Coumadin (Anderson and Barnhart, 1964*b*). The Coumadin block of prothrombin synthesis can be promptly displaced, neutralized, or bypassed by treatment with vitamin K_1. Such restoration of the prothrombin-biosynthesis machinery permits identification of prothrombin by immunoprecipitin reaction. Because the microsome fractions were washed repeatedly, it is likely their prothrombin content reflects prothrombin bound at its site of synthesis.

Prothrombin half-life

Suppression of prothrombin synthesis by Coumadin provides the opportunity to investigate the rate of prothrombin utilization, destruction, or removal from the circulation. Calculation of half-life can be made under appropriate conditions. Hellemans and co-workers (1963) followed prothrombin survival in dogs after blocking with several different coumarin drugs, most given orally. Using a one-stage test to assay prothrombin, they calculated the half-life to be 41 hr.

Our work illustrates that canine prothrombin has a fairly short life in the circulation. In 15 of 20 dogs (75%) given 4–8 mg Coumadin/kg body weight over 2 days, the plasma-prothrombin concentration had decayed to less than 10 U/ml by 1 day after drug administration. The life-span of prothrombin must be less than 72 hr. Data from 5 additional dogs given Coumadin once and followed for 11–30 hr revealed a decrease of 50%–80% of the control plasma prothrombin, so it seems likely that the prothrombin life-span lies between 24 hr and 60 hr.

In another series of 5 dogs, prothrombin survival was followed at 1–2 hr intervals, and sequential liver biopsies were taken following a single intravenous dose of Coumadin (2 or 4 mg/kg). It is unlikely that excessive destruction or utilization of prothrombin were complications in these early hours of inhibition. Essentially complete inhibition of prothrombin synthesis occurred between 6 hr and 12 hr, and the response to fluorescent antiprothrombin indicated that most stored prothrombin was released during that time. Some of these dogs were followed up to 30 hr after Coumadin. In all cases, prothrombin concentration declined, although there were occasional rebounds or brief plateaus in the prothrombin regression curves. Prothrombin half-life was calculated, and it averaged 14.6 hr, with the variation between 12 and 18.2 hr (for dog 40, 14.5 hr; for dog 42, 18.2 hr; for dog 44, 12 hr; for dog A–6, 16.5 hr; for dog A–9, 12 hr).

Pharmacodynamic considerations

At this point, perhaps we should examine the questions of whether or not Coumadin stops prothrombin synthesis completely; or promotes formation of an abnormal prothrombin molecule, as suggested by Carter and co-workers (1961); or prevents the final assembly of the prothrombin complex with its full complement of activities; or favors the production of a prothrombin precursor, or preprothrombin, as suggested by Hemker and co-workers (1963). Although definitive answers cannot yet be supplied by our work, there are three observations that are relevant.

One observation was reported previously (Anderson and Barnhart, 1964*b*) was not placed in context with the posed question of the pharmacodynamics of Coumadin. In our subcellular fraction studies, we noted that the soluble fraction of liver from a dicoumarolized dog gave a weak, but positive, immunoprecipitin reaction when tested in double-diffusion plates. The hepatocytes from this animal had not reacted with the fluorescent antibody to provide a visual difference from autofluorescence by microscopy. Perhaps these differences in response to the two test methods are related to a greater sensitivity of one method. Nonetheless, the positive precipitin reaction indicated the presence of a substance (or substances) that contained antigenic determinant groups that we consider specific for prothrombin, although not necessarily indicative of the biological responsiveness by prothrombin to reagents in the quantitative two-stage assay for prothrombin. These immunologic reactants could reflect translocated material. They were not in the organelle fractions but could have been displaced from microsomes in the fractionation procedure. As this liver was not perfused before fractionation, the immunoprecipitin might represent the prothrombin-poor blood trapped in the liver, which would naturally show up in the soluble fraction. It is also possible that prothrombin synthesis was not completely inhibited in all hepatocytes or that some cells were emerging from this suppression to produce incomplete, abnormal, or even "native" and biologically active prothrombin in minute amounts. Subsequently we applied our quantitative immunoprecipitin assay (Barnhart, 1967) to the blood of several coumadized animals in which we could not detect prothrombin by two-stage assay. The plasmas were unreactive, so it seems unlikely that molecules bearing antigenic determinant groups of prothrombin achieve an appreciable concentration in the circulation of heavily coumadized dogs.

Also pertinent to this discussion is the report by Müller-Berghaus and Seegers (1966) on modification of prothrombin by drugs in rabbits. They compared prothrombin two-stage responsiveness and a quantitation of prethrombin activity in prothrombin-deficient rabbits and following vitamin K_1 corrective treatment. They found an earlier rise in molecules bearing prethrombin activity than in those competent to react in the two-stage. In the coumadized state, about three times as much prethrombin could be measured as prothrombin, although both were low.

The second observation emphasizes the well known finding that vitamin K_1 treatment of prothrombin-deficient animals is promptly followed by some correction of the prothrombin time, which usually precedes detection of increased prothrombin concentration. Of course, the prothrombin-time test is a more accurate measure of procoagulant or accelerator activity than of prothrombin concentration. In our experience with Mephyton to correct prothrombin deficiency after Coumadin, although a prompt change in prothrombin time occurred, correction to control values took 3–5 hr. More recent work with AquaMephyton in Coumadized dogs elicited more striking results, with correction of the prothrombin time to normal by 30 min (Fig. 26.4). However, the prothrombin two-stage assay showed 22 U just before K_1 injection, 22 U at 30 min after, and 28 U at 1 hr. It was

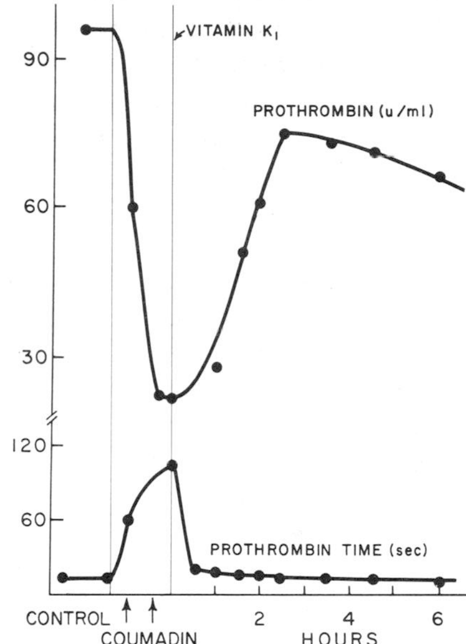

Fig. 26.4. Sequence of events in dog A–2 given AquaMephyton (K_1). Note that prothrombin synthesis and release to circulation occur faster than in dog F (Fig. 26.2).

not until 1.5 hr that the concentration of prothrombin was significantly different (50 U) from that in the Coumadized state. Most investigators have interpreted such results as the emergence or the biosynthesis of one of the procoagulants. Some favor factor VII or autoprothrombin I activity as corrective, while Müller-Berghaus and Seegers (1966) believe correction of prothrombin time after vitamin K_1 treatment is the result of the release of free autoprothrombin III, with its autoprothrombin S or factor X potential. It would be instructive if these procoagulants could be quantitated separately in deficient and in vitamin K_1–stimulated animals.

The third observation is that, after vitamin K_1 administration to a prothrombin-deficient dog, molecules appear in the blood by 1 hr that are reactive in our quantitative immunoprecipitin test that is positive with antigenic groups on the prothrombin complex. It is interesting that the appearance of these molecules precedes the capability of the blood to show significant increases in prothrombin that is biologically active in the two-stage test (Barnhart, 1967). The interpretation is valid that this could be a measure of any one of the subunits (prethrombin or autoprothrombin III) of the prothrombin complex before release of the complete complex that has gained biological activity in the two-stage assay.

The available information continues to encourage the idea that Coumadin turns down (although perhaps not completely off) prothrombin production. None of these observations offer reasonable support for the view that Coumadin favors the production of a prothrombin precursor that builds up in the hepatocyte and simply awaits reconstruction or release. Nor is there support for formation of abnormal prothrombin molecules unless they have antigenic sites as well as biologically reactive sites completely masked on the ribosomal-membrane complexes of the protein-synthesizing apparatus present in the microsome fractions.

The action of vitamin K_1 in correcting the prothrombin defect is as equivocal as the action of Coumadin. None of the findings are incompatible, however, with the concept that vitamin K_1 promotes *de novo* synthesis of one or more molecules valuable in blood clotting. The disparity between correction of the prothrombin-time test and significant increases in prothrombin concentration may imply that two distinctly different molecules are synthesized and released at separate rates. It is not unreasonable to assume, however, that starting up or increasing the activity of the prothrombin-synthesis machinery by administering vitamin K_1 may strip partially completed prothrombin moieties off the assembly line or may transiently favor synthesis of incomplete molecules that have procoagulant power. The apparent dichotomy between the prothrombin one-stage and two-stage tests might then relate simply to the efficiency of the prothrombin-synthesizing machinery. It seems unlikely that the prothrombin one-stage test is so sensitive that minute additions of "native" prothrombin restore clotting times to normal.

Liver ultrastructure

We wondered if careful observation of the fine structure of hepatocytes during drug manipulation of prothrombin synthesis might not contribute to our understanding of the cellular actions of Coumadin and vitamin K_1.

The first studies employed buffered, OsO_4-fixed tissue embedded in Vestapol (Barnhart et al., 1964). We were amazed by the apparent rearrangement of cell organelles after Coumadin and by the even more striking reversal achieved by vitamin K_1 treatment. However, we were concerned that the cell changes might mirror Coumadin toxicity, as we had selected severely deficient dogs (< 5 U), thinking to improve our chances of observing any change.

Most dogs in this series were carefully adjusted in the Coumadin portion of the experiment so that a milder stress applied, and plasma-prothrombin levels thus declined only to 20–30 U/ml (Fig. 26.4). The vitamin K_1 was AquaMephyton, which was given as a single dose (1 mg/kg) or as multiple injections in attempts to further stimulate synthesis and release of prothrombin by prothrombin-deficient dogs. Benedryl was always used as a protective agent preceding the AquaMephyton, as well as in 2 dogs of this series that were vehicle controls and received the polysorbate vehicle without vitamin K_1 included.

Vitamin K_1 in the polysorbate vehicle shortens the lag period noted in our earlier work with Mephyton correction of prothrombin deficiency. Instead of the 4–6 hr required to regain much plasma prothrombin after the Mephyton injection, prothrombin addition was considerable by 1–2 hr after intravenous injection of AquaMephyton into Coumadin-treated dogs.

The present report details our findings when the prothrombin model system was reexamined in 10 dogs, by application of greatly improved electron-microscope technology. Liver specimens were taken from dogs fasted 16–18 hr and were fixed in 0.1 M cacodylate-buffered glutaraldehyde (6.5%), stored in cacodylate-buffered sucrose (0.2 M), and postfixed and stained in veronal acetate buffered OsO_4 (1%), with *p*H maintained in all solutions between 7.2 and 7.4. Following progressive ethanol dehydration, specimens were placed in propylene oxide (absolute) and were ultimately infiltrated with Maraglas. From liver embedded in the polymerized plastic, silver gray sections (200–400Å) were prepared. These were stained with uranyl acetate, washed, and restained with lead citrate. Examination and photography were made on our RCA–EMU IV electron microscope.

GENERAL FEATURES OF A DRUG-MANIPULATED DOG

The pattern of ultrastructural change in the liver resembled that observed in our earlier work but was not so extreme. More cellular constituents were retained and were stained well with the improved technique.

The control biopsy provided normal cell morphology and tissue organization. Hepatocytes were moderately dense, as they contained numerous organelles and substances that were well distributed throughout the cytoplasm (Fig. 26.5). Mitochondria showed typical cristae organization and contained several dense granules. The granular endoplasmic reticulum (gER), the assembly line for protein synthesis, was well organized both around the nucleus and at cell margins and closely associated with mitochondria.

A remarkable alteration of hepatocyte density during the drug modification of prothrombin synthesis could be seen even with ordinary brightfield microscropy on Maraglas thin sections (0.5 μ) stained with toluidine blue (Bennett and Radimska, 1966) and examined at a magnification of 800–1000 (Figs. 26.6–26.8). There was a preponderance of dark or dense hepatocytes in the normal, control biopsies of dogs in this series (Fig. 26.6). On the average, there are 5 dark cells for every light or pale cell. The proportion of dark to light cells changes during the drug manipulation of the rate of prothrombin synthesis. For example, after Coumadin in dog A–2

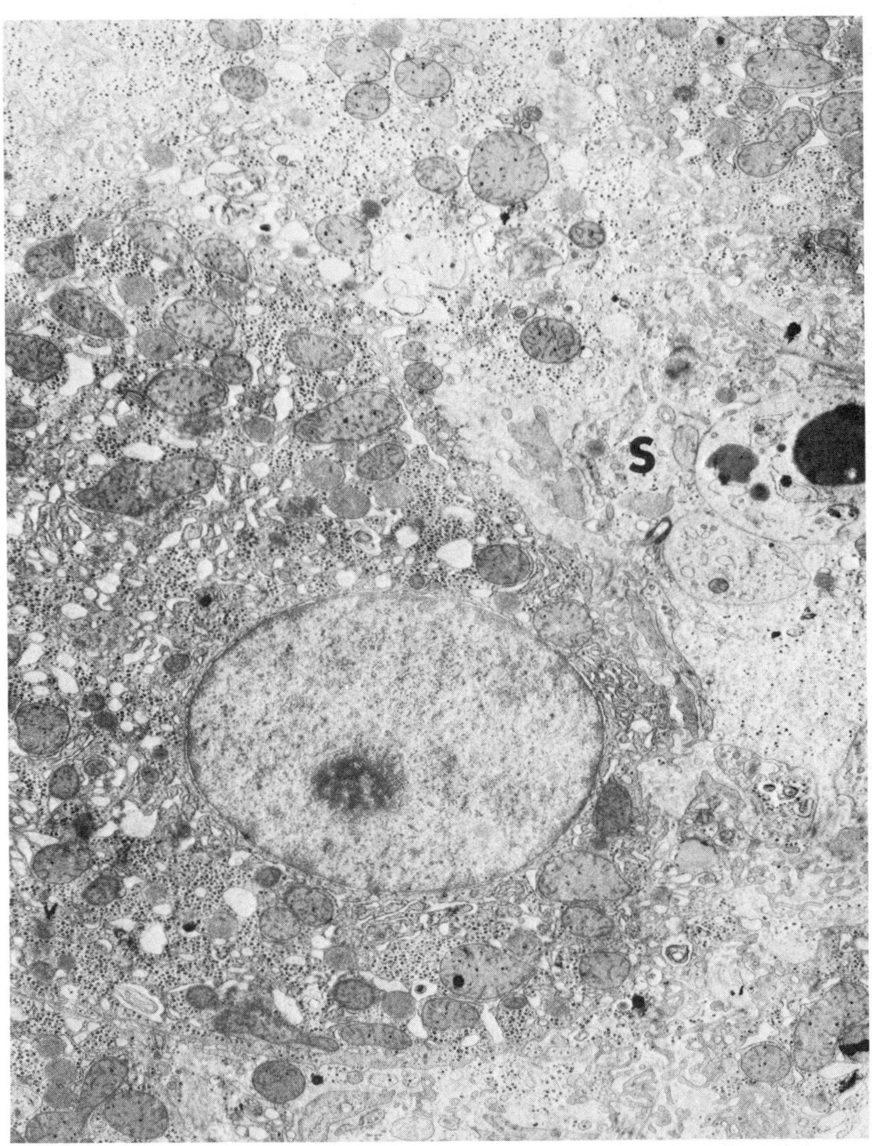

Fig. 26.5. Electron micrograph of control dog liver. Note that the organelles are well distributed in the large hepatocyte containing a nucleus. Numerous mitochondrial granules are present. Sinusoid (S) is designated. × 8000.

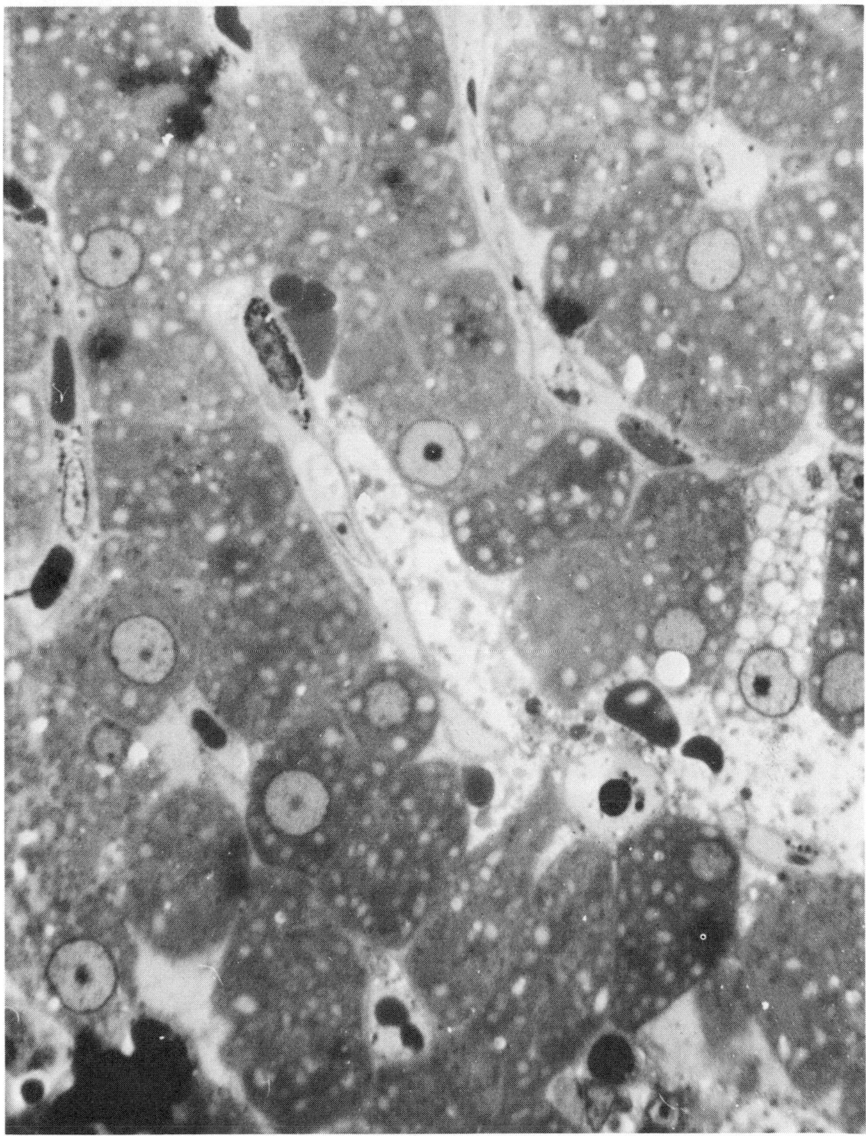

Fig. 26.6. Conventional micrograph of control liver from dog A–2. This glutaraldehyde-fixed, Maraglas tissue was stained with toluidine blue. Note that most hepatocytes are very dense. A pale hepatocyte appears in the upper center. × 800.

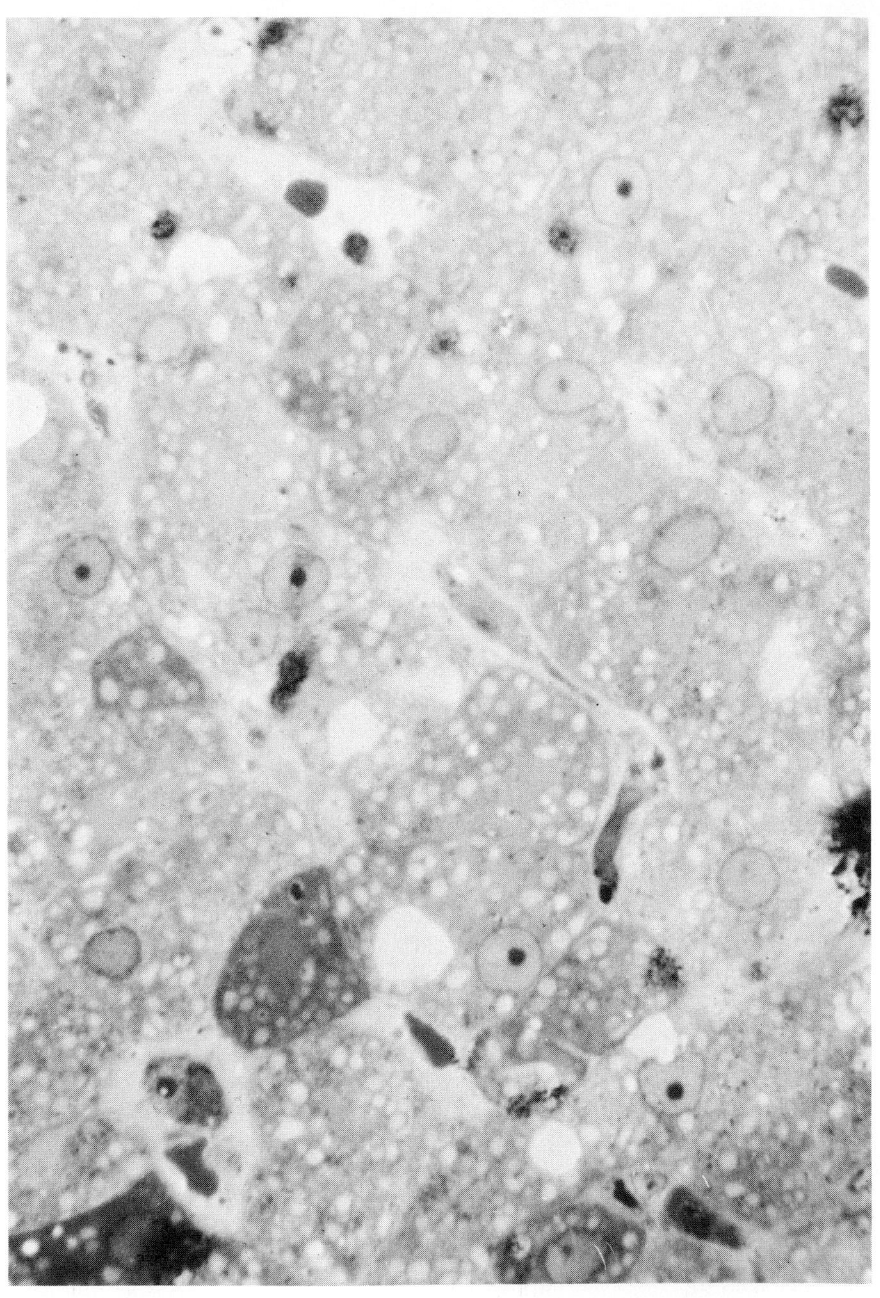

Fig. 26.7. Conventional micrograph of prothrombin-deficient liver of dog A–2, toluidine blue–stained Maraglas tissue. Note that most hepatocytes are pale. × 800.

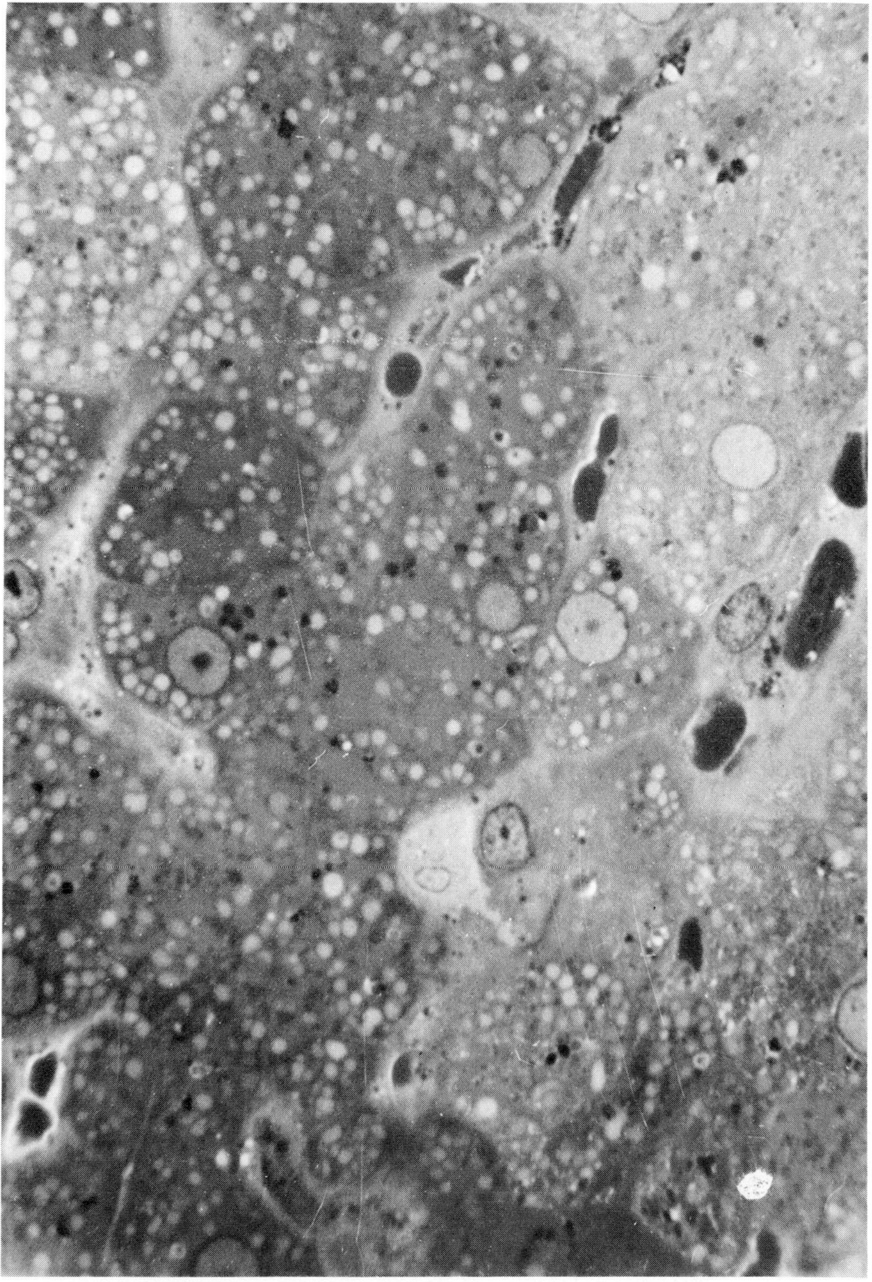

Fig. 26.8. Conventional micrograph of toluidine blue–stained Maraglas liver from dog A–3 taken 5.5 hr after receiving vitamin K_1 to correct his prothrombin-deficient state. Sections of control and Coumadin livers from A–3 were very similar to those seen in Figs. 26.6 and 26.7. Note the reappearance of dark and dense hepatocytes. × 800.

(see Fig. 26.4), there was a preponderance of pale, low-density hepatocytes, and it was rare to find a dark cell (Fig. 26.7). Within 30 min after Aqua-Mephyton was given to dog A–2, more dark cells were seen. By 2.5 hr and later it was rare to find a pale cell (Fig. 26.8).

As noted before and as can be seen in Figure 26.9, after Coumadin there was a marked reorganization of cell organelles resulting in a real or an apparent reduction in cytoplasmic density (cf. Fig. 26.5). Mitochondria exhibited fewer dense granules and also showed a loss of density in the matrix and cristae changes. There was expansion of the endoplasmic reticulum (ER) cisternae. The gER appeared to have some reduction in ribosomal beading, and the matrix of the ER showed increased density in such areas. Associations between gER and mitochondria were not so evident as in controls.

Promptly after vitamin K_1 and continuing for several hours, there were organelle readjustments, with an increased density of the cytoplasm and mitochondria (Fig. 26.10). The gER assumed greater prominence, and ribosomal studding also became more pronounced. The ER cisternae shrank, and deposits could frequently be seen within the cisternae. The number of dense granules increased within mitochondria, and more frequent associations were noted with gER and with lipid drops (Fig. 26.11).

During the drug sequence, there was no readily apparent change in the organization of the nucleus or the nucleolus. Neither microvilli nor bile canaliculi were noticeably different from those of controls. The smooth endoplasmic reticulum (sER) was unremarkable throughout the drug study. Lysosomes of various types were not outstandingly different in number, size, or composition.

ENDOPLASMIC RETICULUM

The sER associated with glycogen formation was apparently unchanged by the concentrations of Coumadin and vitamin K_1 employed. The amount of glycogen remaining in the dogs' livers after a fast of 16–18 hr varies considerably, but, as it is easily identified, it need not confuse interpretation of cytoplasmic density. Also, the evaluations following vitamin K_1 treatment of the prothrombin-deficient dog start from a fasted state, and there is no further opportunity for food intake. Increased density of the matrix of the ER after vitamin K_1 is not due to more glycogen deposition, at least in the typical rosette configuration. The amount and the development of sER varies from dog to dog but, in any one sequence study, was not significantly altered in response to Coumadin or to vitamin K_1.

After Coumadin, there was a marked increase in the number of ER profiles that were expanded (Fig. 26.12). This was especially pronounced along the gER. Furthermore, there was some reduction in the ribosomal

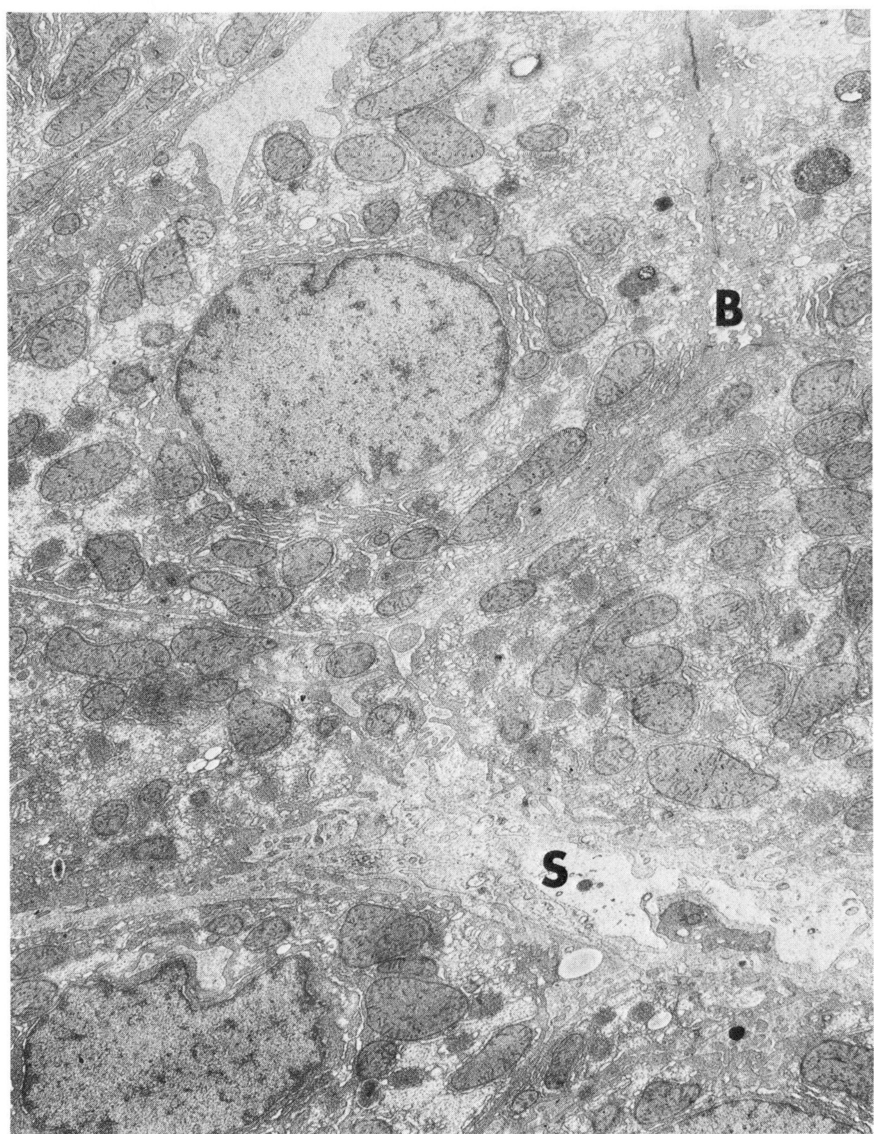

Fig. 26.9. Electron micrograph of prothrombin-deficient liver of dog A–2. Note the paleness of cytoplasms, bizarre mitochondria, and rare dense mitochondrial granules. Sinusoid (S) and bile canaliculus (B) are designated. × 8245.

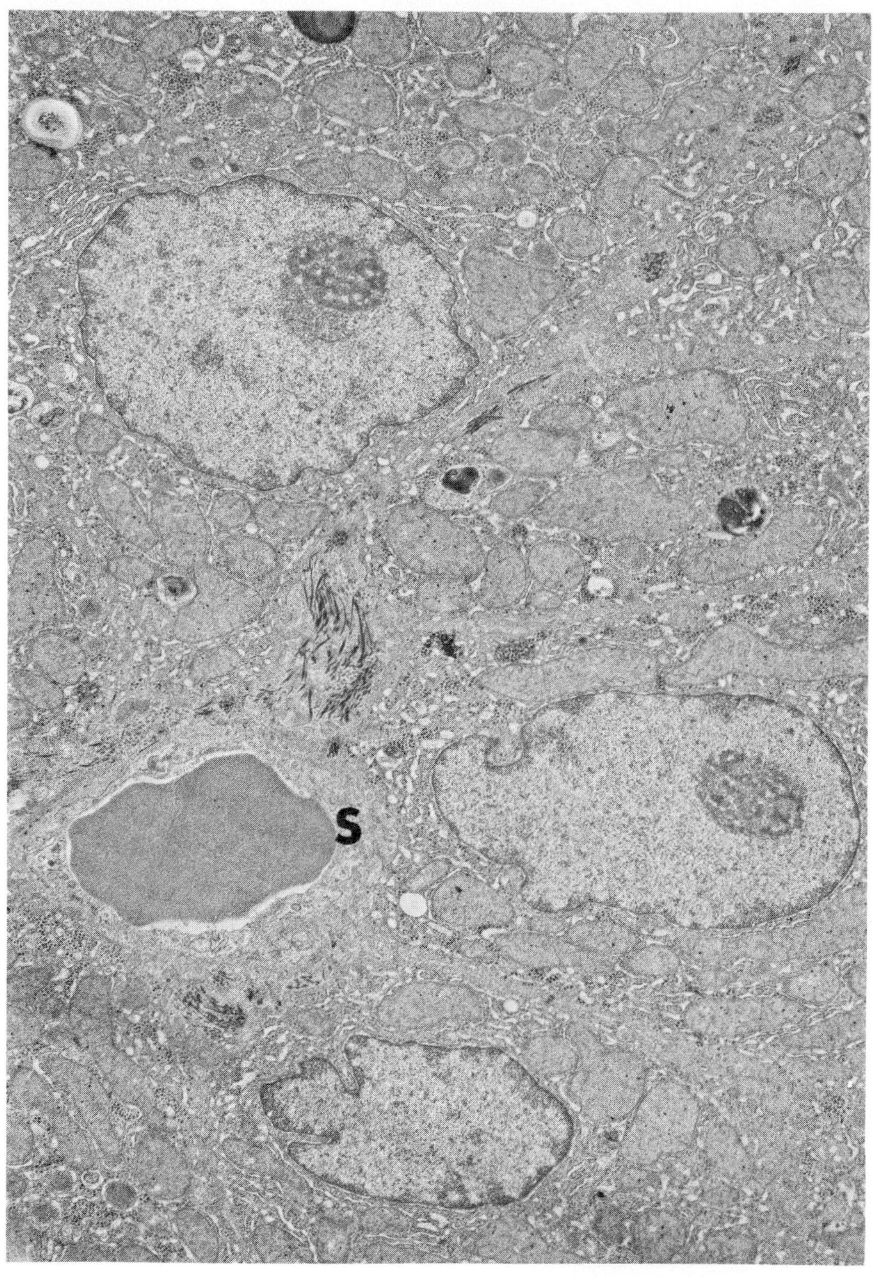

Fig. 26.10. Electron micrograph of liver from dog A–2 taken 2.5 hr after giving Aqua-Mephyton (K_1) to correct prothrombin deficiency. Note the greatly increased cytoplasmic density. Sinusoid (S) is designated. × 8000.

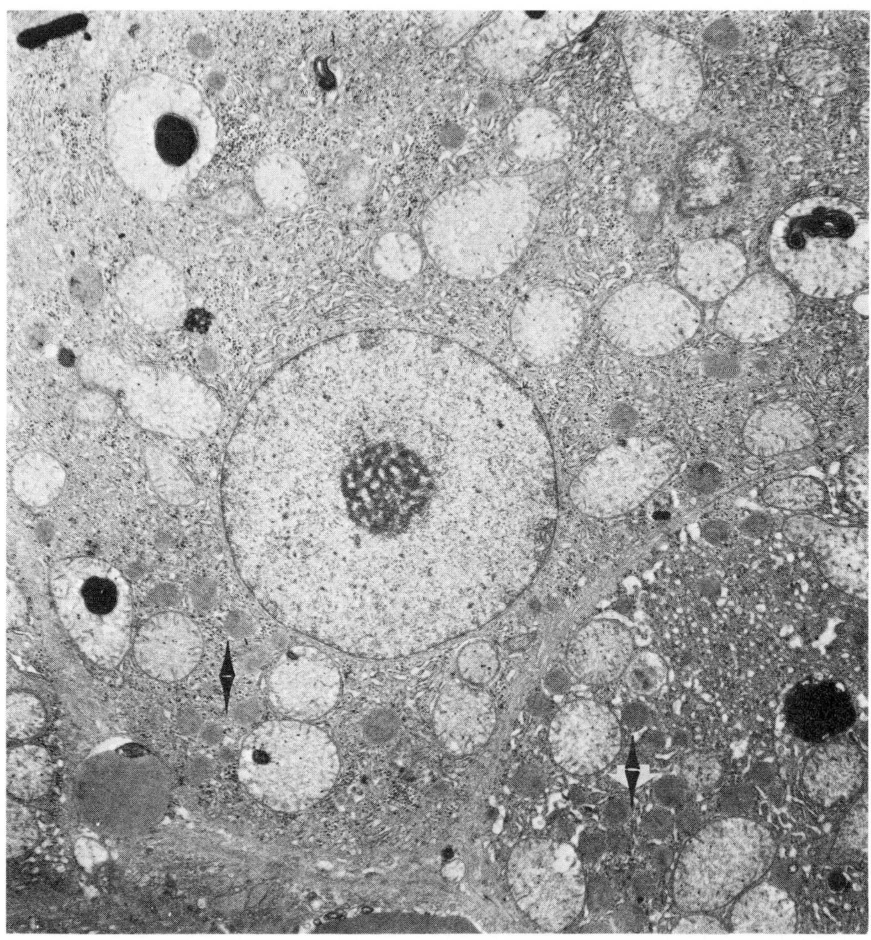

Fig. 26.11. Electron micrograph of liver from dog A–3 taken 5.5 hr after AquaMephyton was given to correct the prothrombin-deficient state. Note the mitochondria-lipid associations, cytoplasmic-density increase, and numerous microbodies at arrows. × 6386.

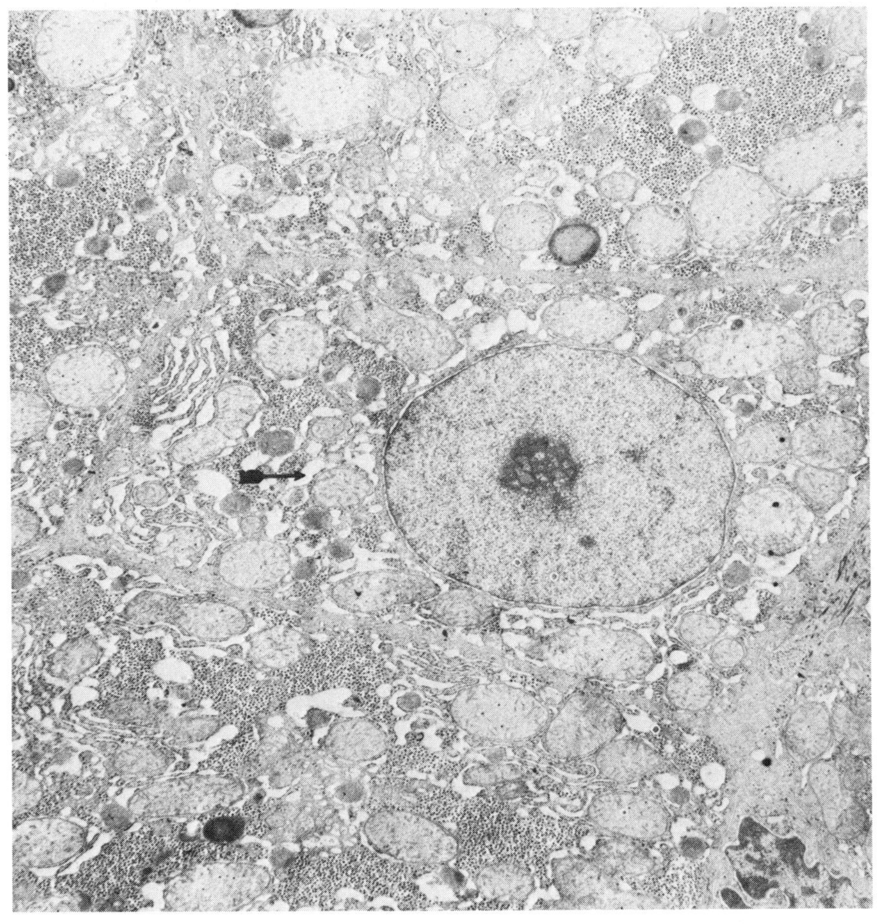

Fig. 26.12. Electron micrograph of liver from dog A–3 during prothrombin-deficient state. Note the expanded cisternae of ER (arrow). × 6017.

arrays along the ER, so that more of the membrane system was sparsely studded with ribosomes. In some areas, the ribosomes appeared to have dissociated from their membranes and were lying free in the ER matrix (Fig. 26.13). These dissociations were not as extensive as those reported by Smuckler and co-workers (1962) after carbon tetrachloride intoxication. Although immunocytofluorescence indicated that prothrombin was not being synthesized and stored in the liver, fibrinogen synthesis and storage was still occurring, and at a stimulated level (Fig. 26.14).

After vitamin K_1 there was shrinkage of the canalicular and cisternal portions of the ER. Ribosomal studding became more prominent by 1 hr. The matrix of the ER became progressively more dense (Fig. 26.15). The gER was prominent throughout the cell, but was especially noticeable near cell margins and nucleus. Loops of gER were frequently seen in association with mitochondria.

MITOCHONDRIA

The intramitochondrial organization was altered in the sequence study and presumably was responding to the drugs, Coumadin, and vitamin K_1. The changes were more evident in some cells than in others. However, the loss in mitochondrial density and changes in cristae organization occurred in a greater proportion of the mitochondria after Coumadin treatment. Mitochondrial shape was more bizarre than that observed in controls, and the impression was that more mitochondria were enlarged. The dimensions and size of the mitochondria was probably not as important, however, as the underlying configurational state which may be illustrated by the cristae-matrix organization — of which density is a reflection. After vitamin K_1, mitochondrial density increased, and cristae profiles were more organized. Thus far it has not been possible to establish a consistent relationship between the numbers of energized and nonenergized mitochondria (Harris et al., 1968; Hackenbrock, 1968), but further examination of enlargements of representative mitochondria may resolve the present difficulty.

The number of mitochondrial transections was reduced after Coumadin treatment. Counts were made from 5×7 or 8×10 prints, with final magnifications of 10,000–20,000. Mitochondria were counted in 4×5 areas of these prints when neither nuclei nor sinusoid area comprised a significant space. Dog A–2 had 58 mitochondria in the control state and 29 mitochondria following Coumadin treatment. Dog A–3 had 30 mitochondria per 4×5 area in the control state and 15 mitochondria following Coumadin treatment. By 5.5–6 hr after vitamin K_1, the mitochondria per 4×5 area had increased in A–2 to 45 and in A–3 to 25.

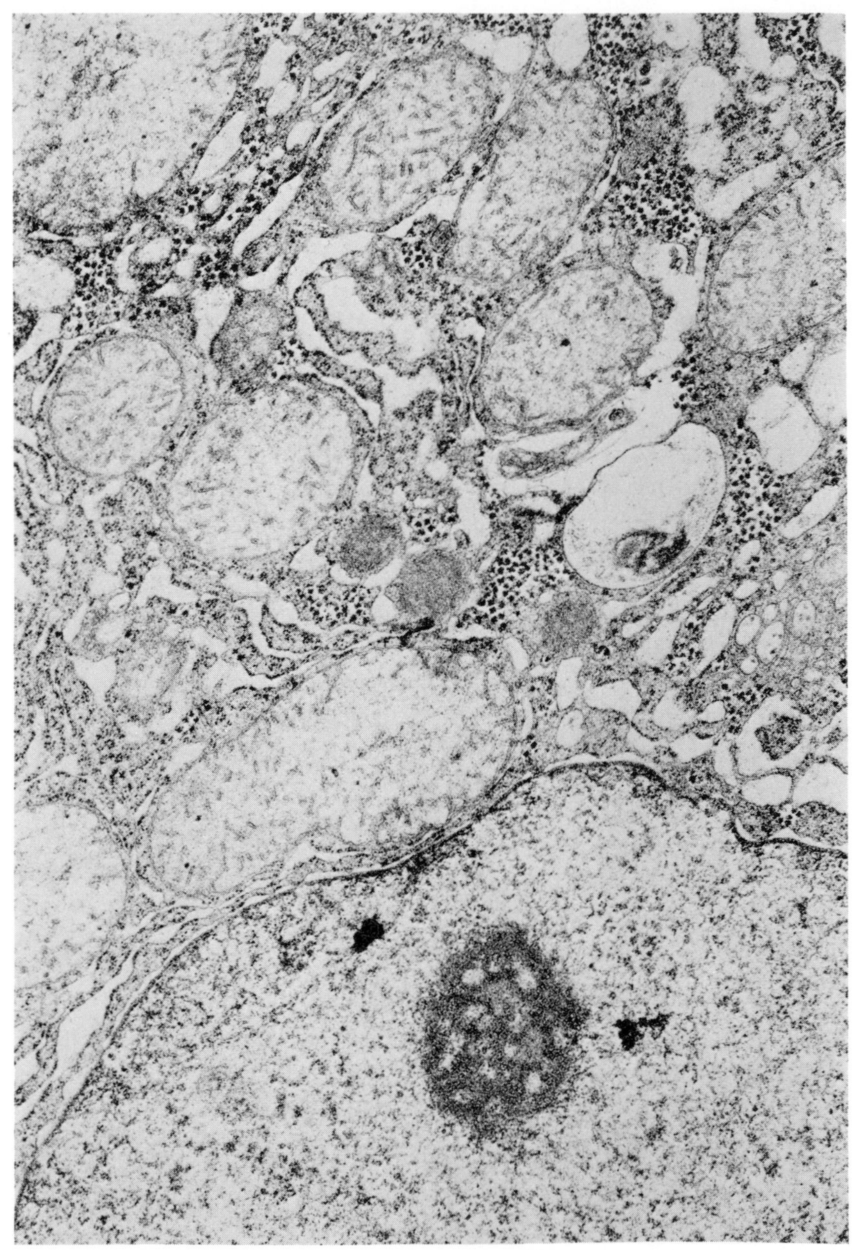

Fig. 26.13. Electron micrograph from another prothrombin-depleted dog. Mitochondria have few dense granules and are of low density. Note the sparsely beaded ER. × 19,733.

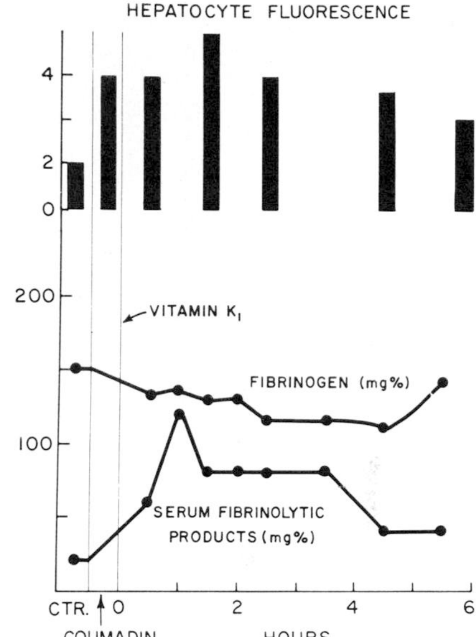

Fig. 26.14. Fibrinogen synthesis and storage in dog A–2, as revealed by treatment with fluorescent antifibrinogen. Probably the elevated level of fibrinolytic products in plasma, rather than the vitamin K_1 was the stimulus.

The most consistent feature was the reduction in number of dense mitochondrial granules after Coumadin and the restoration to control numbers after vitamin K_1. Dog A–2 had 2.3 dense granules per mitochondrion in the control state, 0.5 after Coumadin, and 1 at 1.5 hr after K_1. Dog A–3 had 2.7 dense granules per mitochondrion in the control state; 0.6 after Coumadin; 1.4 at 0.5 hr after K_1; and 2.5 at 5.5 hr after K_1. Vehicle-control dog A–11 had 2.8 dense granules per mitochondrion just before injection of the polysorbate vehicle, and 2.6 after 2 hr and 4 hr. Clearly, the accumulation of calcium and/or the lipid-containing bodies (Pasquali-Ronchetti et al., 1969) is suppressed by the in vivo Coumadin treatment. It has been well documented that calcium uptake into isolated mitochondria is blocked by the uncoupling agents dinitrophenol and dicoumarol. These agents also provoke discharge of calcium ions under suitable conditions (Lehninger, 1965).

There was no indication that either drug fragmented mitochondria or increased budding. Measurements of the space between inner and outer mitochondrial membranes did not reveal significant changes during experimentation in any single animal.

MICROBODIES

Microbodies assume greater prominence in the dogs after Coumadin. As they are especially prominent when glycogen stores are minimal, one wonders if more are present in the normal state and are just obscured by

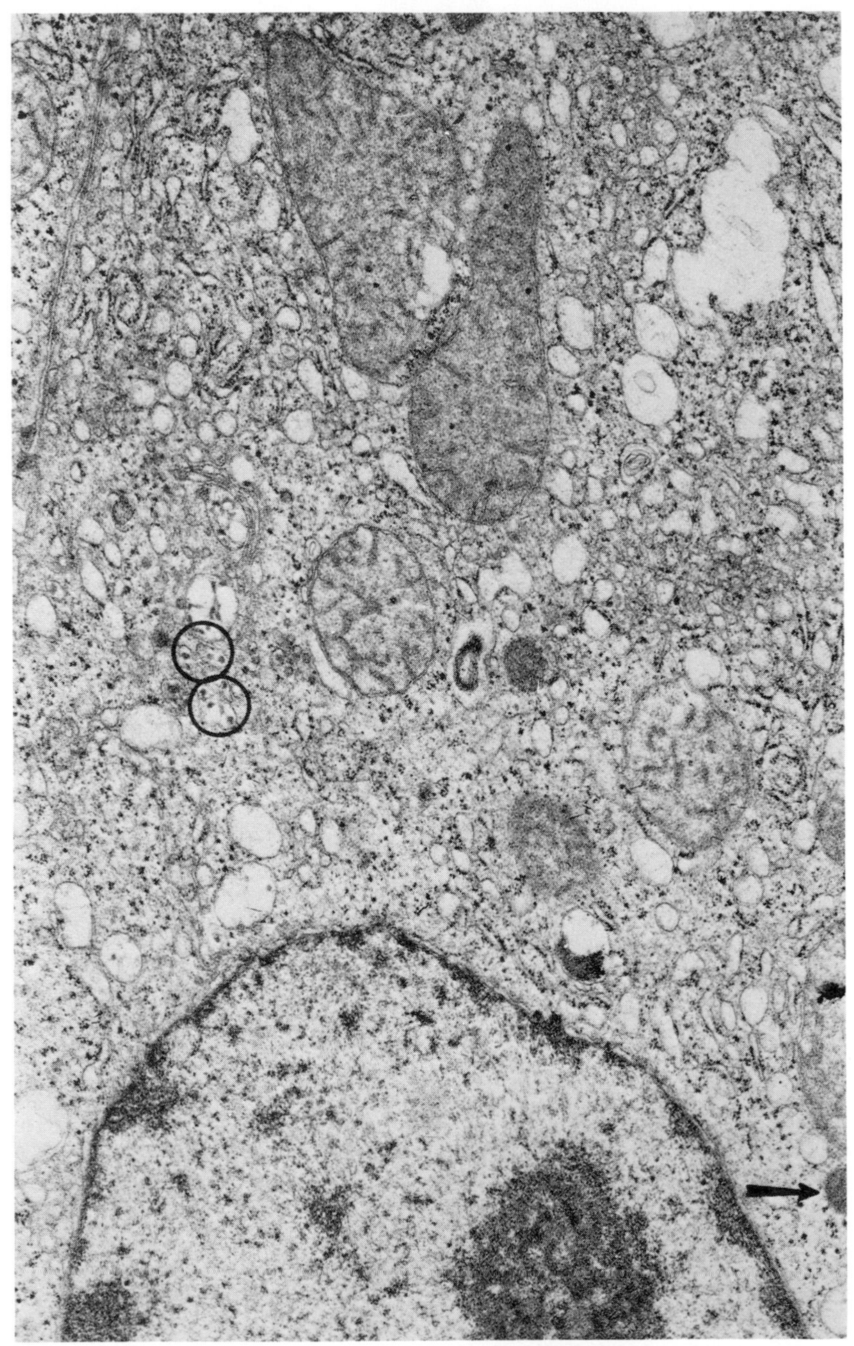

the cytoplasmic density. The increased cytoplasmic density following vitamin K_1 treatment also makes their detection more difficult. Not all of the microbodies have the central crystalloid organization that typifies the peroxisome; however, the plane of section may miss some nucleoids. About half the microbodies counted exhibited the dense core configuration. Many of the microbodies in the drug-treated animals were still associated with the gER, and it was not uncommon to see prominent ribosomal studding encircling the microbody, except at its point of evagination from the matrix of the ER.

The overall number of microbodies within any one sequence study did not change appreciably, although there was considerable variation in the mitochondria-to-microbody proportion. Only one drug-sequence dog has been quantitated thus far and these results, of course, may not reflect the general trend. Dog A–2 had a control of 5.2; after Coumadin the ratio was 3.8, and after vitamin K_1 it was 2.1. In vehicle-control dog A–11 the control just prior to injection of the vehicle was 1.5, at 2 hr it was 2.0, and at 4 hr it was 2.4. Two other control dogs showed mitochondria-to-microbody ratios of 2.4 and 2.0 respectively. One consistent feature—an increased concentration of microbodies near the sinusoidal area and away from the biliary areas—has been noted after vitamin K_1 in 3 of the dogs.

ULTRASTRUCTURE PROJECTION

The sequence study of the drug manipulation of prothrombin synthesis has demonstrated that changes occur in the organization of the fine structure of hepatocytes. These changes illustrate the extreme plasticity of the hepatocyte, reflect the variations in functional state, and indicate how rapidly the control or stimulated state can be regained after vitamin K_1.

The reported impressions and semiquantitative evaluations can be improved by application of Loud's quantitative stereological or morphometric methods (1968). This approach is presently underway in our laboratory on this series of dogs and may add to the understanding of mechanisms of action of Coumadin and vitamin K_1.

However, it has become clear that it is impossible to fit these ultrastructural changes exactly into the functional framework. At the preesnt time, we are unable to bridge the gap between what we see, what is chemically present at that intracellular site, and what is functionally occurring at

Fig. 26.15 (facing page). Electron micrograph of liver from another dog taken 5.5 hr after AquaMephyton was given to correct the prothrombin deficiency (Fig. 26.13). Note the cristae organization in mitochondria. The gER is distributed throughout cell, and ribosomal beading is prominent. Are these accumulations (circles) the newly synthesized prothrombin, is the secretion of prothrombin illustrated at the arrow, or is prothrombin the low-density material in the ER matrix? × 19,380.

that site. After the vitamin K_1 stimulus to prothrombin synthesis, there are obvious cytoplasmic densities, any one or more of which could be accumulations of the newly formed and stored prothrombin. But is the prothrombin for export in the gER matrix, in the ER cisternae, in the microbodies, or elsewhere? Some of the microbodies without cores appear to be moving into the space of Disse, and others seem to be shed into the interstitial fluid compartment. Only in situ work with the discriminative tools of radioisotope labels and/or immunochemical markers applied at the electron-microscopic level is likely to resolve the present dilemma. This approach, too, should yield relevant data for the challenging questions on pharmacodynamics of Coumadin and of vitamin K_1.

Speculations on mechanisms of action

Coumadin and vitamin K_1 are drugs that probably alter cell membranes. Multiple effects on mitochondria and membranes of the ER are suggested by the current work. Because both of these drugs are lipid soluble, they may simply become concentrated in those organelles and structures with the highest lipid content.

Liver, kidney, and heart mitochondria have higher lipid contents than other mitochondria. Anderson (1967) has shown in time studies from 1 hr to 24 hr that ^{3}H Coumadin is concentrated in these three organs, while the liver retains a high order of activity (2–8 times control) for 24 hr. Similar distribution in the organs was earlier shown for ^{14}C Coumadin by Jacques and co-workers (1957). ^{14}C dicoumarol penetrates isolated mitochondria to induce swelling and to uncouple oxidative phosphorylation (Howland, 1968). Wosilait (1968) found that ^{14}C dicoumarol was taken up in vitro by liver slices and that all subcellular fractions bound the dicoumarol.

Our ultrastructure work revealed that mitochondria had fewer dense granules in the matrix, seemed larger, and had shapes that were more bizarre than those in the dogs' control state. These mitochondrial changes could reflect the reduced efficiency of the hepatocyte's power supply. Those mitochondria lacking dense granules may be the ones that have their oxidative phosphorylation blocked by the presence of Coumadin. The power defect following Coumadin is clearly a localized one and does not involve all mitochondria within a single cell. The increased number of microbodies (perhaps peroxisomes) in the Coumadin-treated dog A–2 may illustrate one compensation the hepatocyte makes to a restriction of the mitochondrial power. DeDuve and Baudhuin (1966) suggest one function of the peroxisomes may be to provide an alternate route for oxidation of reduced NAD (nicotinamide amide) and to thus be a support for aerobic metabolism.

Our study also supports the theory that Coumadin and vitamin K_1 act on membranes of the ER. Reversible changes, which could modify the prothrombin assembly line, occurred in attachment of ribosomes and in degree of dilatation of cisternae. According to Lucy (1964), some of the lipid arrangement in membranes may be in the form of micelles. Specificity of membrane function may relate to organization and to physiochemical properties of the contained micelles. As there are set conditions for micelle size, formation, substitution, maintenance, and dissolution, only certain micelle positions may be suitable for Coumadin and/or vitamin K_1 to occupy. Substitution or incorporation of these drugs into the ER membrane micelles may change the stability or the conformation of the ER membranes and thus alter their function. For example, a Coumadin micelle in a gER membrane could change the environment so that mRNA for prothrombin, although present, could not align itself along the membrane to provide instructions for translation of the prothrombin message. However, mRNA for fibrinogen may have affinity for the site, whether or not a Coumadin micelle is present. Immunochemical testing with specific antifibrinogen indicated that fibrinogen clearly was on the protein assembly line (microsome fraction) of prothrombin-depleted and Coumadin-inhibited dogs (Barnhart and Anderson, 1962). Furthermore, in Coumadin-treated dogs, fibrinogen synthesis and storage is actually stimulated, although not much fibrinogen is released to the circulation (Fib. 26.14).

Vitamin K_1 in the vehicle polysorbate is probably already in micelle configuration. In this form it certainly gets to the sensitive or blocked areas to reverse or to bypass the inhibitory effects of Coumadin. The stimulating influence of AquaMephyton is brief, but a second dose promotes further formation and release of prothrombin (Fig. 26.16). Polysorbate alone does not function as a prothrombin-releasing agent when given to normal dogs, because their control plasma-prothrombin levels were not significantly enriched (Fig. 26.3). Vitamin K_1 does not function as a general protein-releasing agent, because stored fibrinogen is not released (Fig. 26.14), nor do normal dogs treated with vitamin K_1 release excess cellular prothrombin.

Vitamin K_1 probably stimulates prothrombin synthesis by improving both the power supply and the prothrombin assembly line. Reappearance and increasing numbers of mitochondrial dense granules signal that such mitochondria are again capable of oxidative phosphorylation. The ER membranes again show prominent arrays of ribosomes frequently in close association with mitochondria. It may be that vitamin K_1 competes with

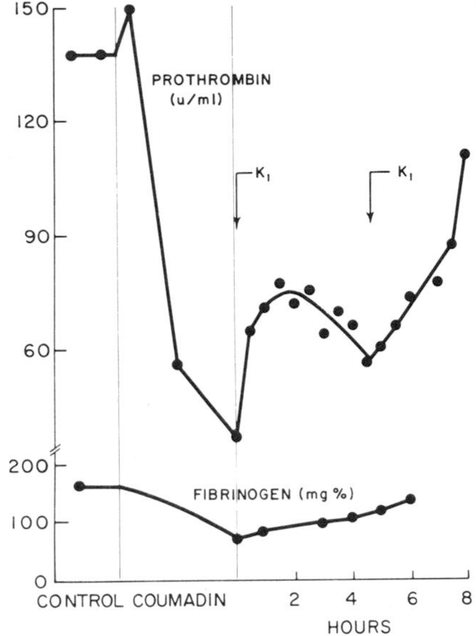

Fig. 26.16. Sequence study of prothrombin-deficient dog A–7 given two doses of AquaMephyton to try to maintain the stimulus to prothrombin synthesis. Note the short lag period after each dose of vitamin K_1. Newly formed prothrombin was promptly released by second injection.

Coumadin for receptor sites and displaces it, or vitamin K_1 may act elsewhere to turn up the power to stabilize gER membranes so that the prothrombin assembly line can run efficiently.

It will be necessary to examine the intracellular distribution of isotopically labeled Coumadin and vitamin K_1 by means of autoradiographs at the electron-microscope level before the cellular mechanisms of action can be precisely stated.

References

Anderson, G. F. 1967. The distribution of warfarin (Coumadin) in the rat. *Thromb. Diath. Haemorrh. 18*:754.

Anderson, G. F., and M. I. Barnhart. 1964*a*. Prothrombin synthesis in the dog. *Amer. J. Physiol. 206*:929.

Anderson, G. F., and M. I. Barnhart. 1964*b*. Intracellular localization of prothrombin. *Proc. Soc. Exp. Biol. Med. 116*:1.

Barnhart, M. I. 1960. Cellular site for prothrombin synthesis. *Amer. J. Physiol. 199*:360.

Barnhart, M. I. 1965. Prothrombin synthesis: An example of hepatic function. *J. Histochem. Cytochem. 13*:740.

Barnhart, M. I. 1967. Immunochemistry. *In* W. H. Seegers (ed.), *Blood Clotting Enzymology*. Academic Press, New York.

Barnhart, M. I., and G. F. Anderson. 1962. Intracellular localization of fibrinogen. *Proc. Soc. Exp. Biol. Med. 110*:734.

Barnhart, M. I., G. F. Anderson, and M. H. Bernstein. 1964. Liver ultrastructure after Coumadin and vitamin K_1. *Fed. Proc. 23*:520. (Abstr.)

Barnhart, M. I., and W. B. Forman. 1963. The cellular localization of fibrinogen as revealed by the fluorescent antibody technique. *Vox Sang. 8*:461.

Bennett, D., and O. Radimska. 1966. Flotation-fluid staining: Toluidine blue applied to Maraglas sections. *Stain Technol. 41*:349.

Carter, J. R., C. V. Nordschow, E. D. Warner, and A. T. Lund. 1961. The in vivo synthesis of defective prothrombin molecules. *Thromb. Diath. Haemorrh. 5*:598.

Daoust, R. 1958. The cell population of liver tissue and the cytological reference base. *In* R. W. Brauer (ed.), *Liver Function.* Amer. Inst. of Biol. Sci., Washington.

DeDuve, C., and P. Baudhuin. 1966. Peroxisomes. *Physiol. Rev. 46*:323.

Goth, A. 1967. Effect of drugs on mast cells, p. 47. *In* S. Garattini and P. A. Shore (eds.), *Advanced Pharmacology,* Vol. 5 Academic Press, New York.

Hackenbrock, C. R. 1968. Ultrastructural bases for metabolically linked mechanical activity in mitochondria. II. Electron transport-linked ultrastructural transformations in mitochondria. *J. Cell Biol. 37*:345.

Harris, R. A., J. T. Penniston, J. Asai, and D. E. Green. 1968. The conformational basis of energy conservation in membrane systems. H. Correlation between conformational change and functional state. *Proc. Nat. Acad. Sci. U.S.A. 59*:830.

Hellemans, J., M. Vorlat, and M. Verstraete. 1963. Survival time of prothrombin and factors VII, IX and X after completely synthesis blocking doses of coumarin derivatives. *Brit. J. Haematol. 9*:506.

Hemker, H. C., J. J. Veltkamp, A. Hensen, and E. A. Loeliger. 1963. Nature of prothrombin biosynthesis: Preprothrombinaemia in vitamin K–deficiency. *Nature 200*:589.

Howland, J. L. 1968. Uptake of Dicoumarol by rat liver mitochondria. *Biochem. J. 106*:317.

Jacques, L. B., E. L. Froese, R. O'Toole, and J. W. T. Spinks. 1957. Relationship between duration of hypoprothrombinemia with Dicoumarol and the level of the drug in the liver. *Arch. Int. Pharmacodyn. 111*:478.

Lehninger, A. L. 1964. *The Mitochondrion: Molecular Basis of Structure and Function.* Benjamin, New York.

Loud, A. V. 1968. A quantitative stereological description of the ultrastructure of normal rat liver parenchymal cells. *J. Cell Biol. 37*:27.

Lucy, J. A. 1964. Globular lipid micelles and cell membranes. *J. Theor. Biol.* 7:360.

Müller-Berghaus, G., and W. H. Seegers. 1966. Some effects of purified autoprothrombin C in blood clotting. *Thromb. Diath. Haemorrh. 16*:707.

Pasquali-Ronchetti, I., J. W. Greenwalt, and E. Carafoli. 1969. The nature of the dense matrix qranules of normal mitochondria. *J. Cell Biol. 40*:565.

Smuckler, E. A., O. A. Iseri, and E. P. Benditt. 1962. An intracellular defect in protein synthesis induced by carbon tetrachloride. *J. Exp. Med. 116*:55.

Ware, A. G., and W. H. Seegers. 1949. Two-stage procedure for the quantitative determination of prothrombin concentration. *Amer. J. Clin. Pathol. 19*:471.

Wosilait, W. D. 1968. The accumulation and distribution of Dicoumarol in rat liver slices. *Biochem. Pharmacol. 17*:429.

27

VITAMIN K ANALOGS AND MECHANISMS OF ACTION OF VITAMIN K

J. Lowenthal

In the course of an investigation aimed at specifying the structural requirements for vitamin K–like activity, we have found a new class of vitamin K antagonists. (Lowenthal et al., 1960; Lowenthal and MacFarlane, 1965; Lowenthal and MacFarlane, 1963.) The new antagonists are structural analogs of compounds with vitamin K activity in which a methyl group has been replaced by a chlorine or a bromine atom. The most active of these compounds is the 2-chloro analog of vitamin K_1 (Fig. 27.1). A single dose of this compound given intravenously to normal

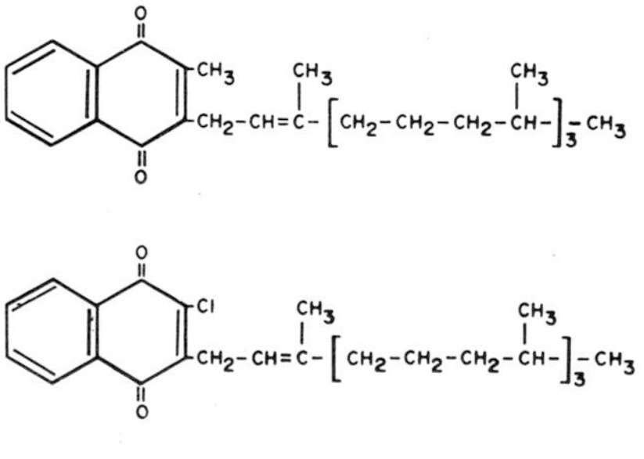

Fig. 27.1. Structure of vitamin K_1 (2-methyl-3-phytyl-1,4-naphthoquinone), above, and its 2-chloro analog (2-chloro-3-phytyl-1,4-naphthoquinone), below.

animals lowers the plasma levels of the vitamin K–dependent clotting factors (prothrombin (or factor II), factors VII, IX, and X), whereas the plasma level of factor V, which does not depend on vitamin K, remains unchanged (Fig. 27.2A). The anticoagulant effect is not only specific, but is also reversible, because the administration of vitamin K_1 promptly returns to plasma levels of the clotting factors to normal (Fig. 27.2B).

This antagonist has been a useful experimental tool for tracing an outline of the mechanism of action of vitamin K. For these experiments, vitamin K–deficient or coumarin anticoagulant–pretreated rats, whose plasma level of factor VII was less than 5% of normal, were used. At zero time, a blood sample was taken by tail-vein puncture, and the substance or sub-

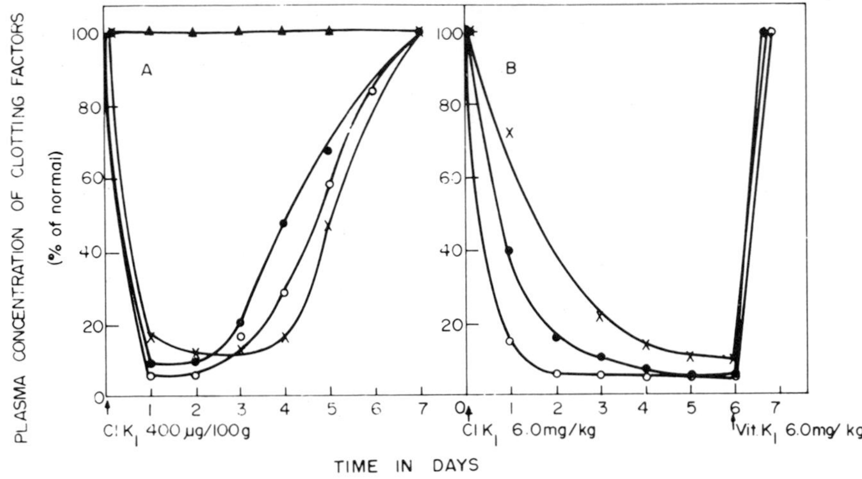

Fig. 27.2. A: Decrease of plasma clotting-factors after a single intravenous dose of the chloro analog of vitamin K_1 to a normal rat. B: Reversal by vitamin K_1 of the anti-coagulant effect in a rabbit pretreated with the chloro analog. O, factor VII; ●, factor X; X, prothrombin; ▲, factor V. (After Lowenthal and MacFarlane, 1965, Fig. 5.)

stances to be tested were injected intravenously. Further blood samples were then taken from the same animal at 30 min, 60 min, 90 min, and 150 min after the injection, and the plasma levels of factor VII were determined by the method of Koller and co-workers (1951). Additional experimental details can be found in the 1967 publication by Lowenthal and MacFarlane.

When the optimal dose of vitamin K_1 in vitamin K–deficient rats (0.5 μg/100 g) and increasing doses of the chloro analog were given together intravenously, the response, as measured by the increase of the plasma level of factor VII, was partially or completely inhibited (Fig. 27.3). While 10 μg/100 g of the chloro analog had no effect on the response, 15 μg/100 g and 20 μg/100 g produced partial, and 80 μg/100 g complete, inhibition. Essentially the same result was obtained with coumarin anticoagulant–pretreated rats, with one notable exception (Fig. 27.3). A 100 μg/100 g dose of vitamin K_1 was required to produce a response in coumarin anticoagulant–pretreated animals that was approximately the same as the response produced by 0.5 μg/100 g in vitamin K–deficient animals, yet the doses of the chloro analog necessary for partial or complete inhibition were nearly the same as in vitamin K–deficient animals, 25–100 μg/100 g compared to 15–80 μg/100 g.

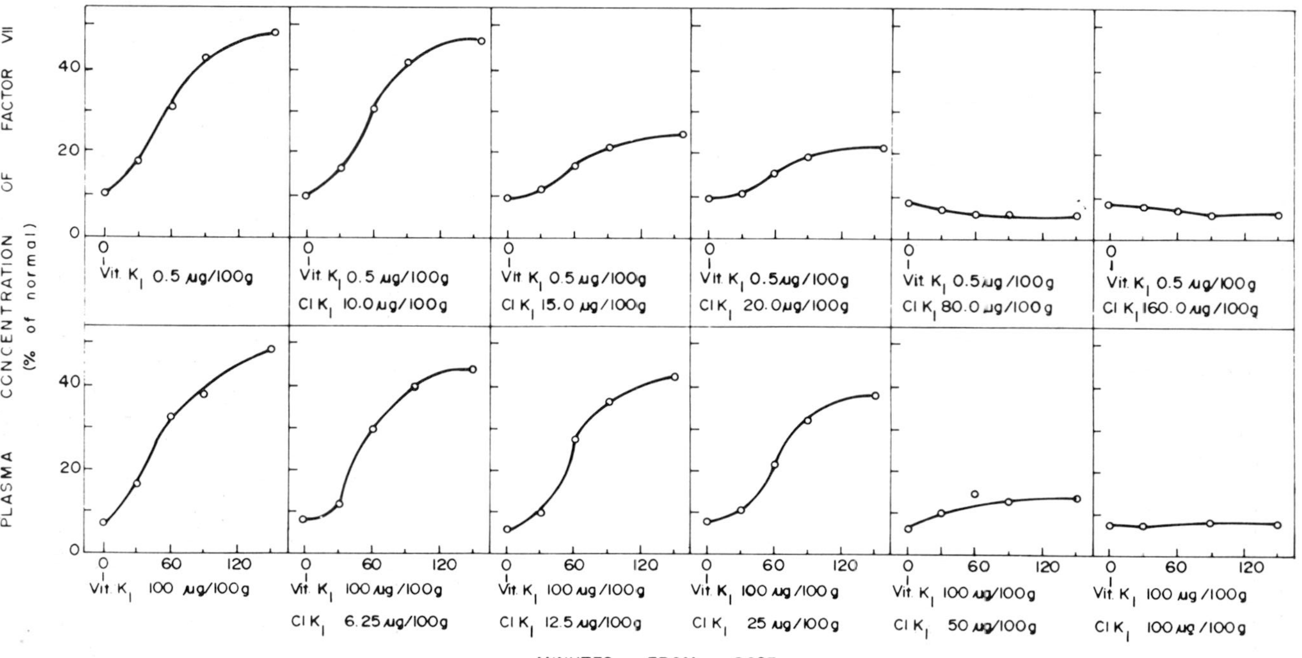

Fig. 27.3. Increase of the plasma level of factor VII by vitamin K_1 inhibited by simultaneous administration of increasing doses of its chloro analog in vitamin K–deficient rats (upper curves) and in coumarin anticoagulant–pretreated rats (lower curves). (After Lowenthal and MacFarlane, 1967, Figs. 1, 2.)

Is this antagonism of the competitive or the noncompetitive type? It is possible to distinguish between the two types of antagonism by testing the effect of increasing doses of constant ratios of the agonist, vitamin K_1, and the antagonist, the chloro analog. The test is based on the assumption that, if the agonist and the antagonist compete for the same receptor sites, the number of sites occupied by the agonist and the antagonist, and therefore the degree of inhibition, will depend on the concentration of the agonist in relation to that of the antagonist at the receptor sites. On the other hand, if the antagonism is of the noncompetitive type, the agonist and the antagonist combine with different sites, and therefore the degree of inhibition produced by the antagonist will be independent of the concentration of the agonist. From these considerations it follows that if the doses are increased by the same factor, so that their ratio remains constant, the degree of inhibition should remain constant if the antagonism is of the competitive type, but should increase if the antagonism is of the noncompetitive type. The validity of this explanation rests on the additional assumption that the relative concentration at the receptor site re-

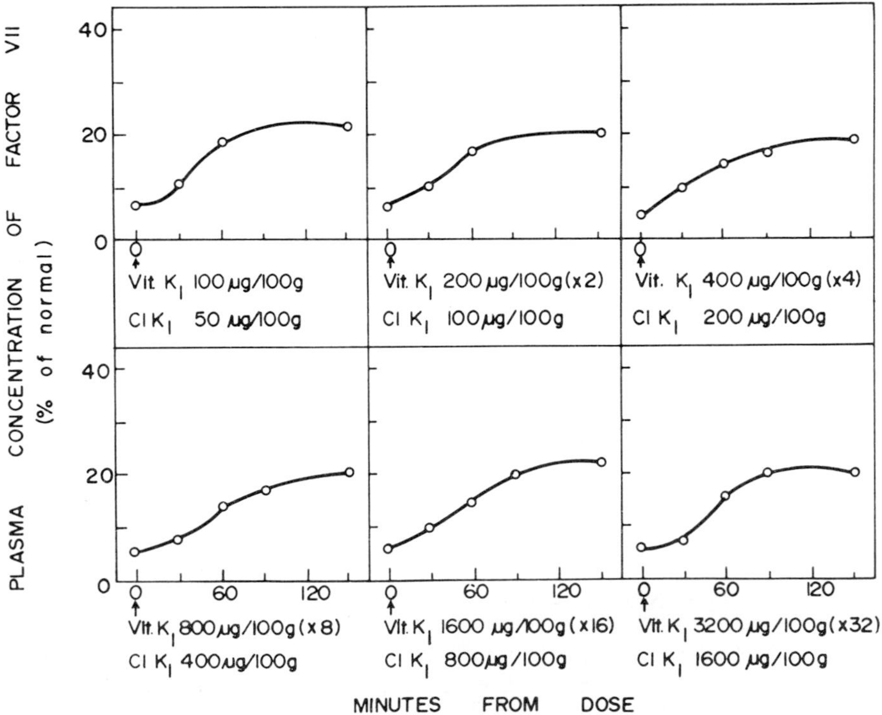

Fig. 27.4. Effect of increasing doses of a constant ratio (2:1) of vitamin K_1 and its chloro analog on the increase of the plasma level of factor VII in coumarin anticoagulant–pretreated rats. (After Lowenthal and MacFarlane, 1967, Fig. 4.)

mains unchanged when the doses are increased but their ratio is kept constant.

When such a test was done in coumarin anticoagulant–pretreated rats for a ratio of vitamin K_1 to the chloro analog of 2 to 1 and a 2-, 4-, 8-, 16-, and 32-fold increase of the doses, it was found that the degree of inhibition does remain constant (Fig. 27.4). When the same test was carried out in vitamin K–deficient rats for ratios of vitamin K_1 to the chloro analog of 1:20 and 1:30 and 8-, 32-, and 64-fold increases of the doses, however, the inhibition did not remain constant, but increased (Fig. 27.5).

It thus appears that the inhibition is of the competitive type in coumarin anticoagulant–pretreated animals but of the noncompetitive type in vitamin K–deficient animals. What is the explanation for this difference? One possible explanation, outlined by the model shown in Figure 27.6, is based on the assumption that, in either vitamin K–deficient or coumarin anticoagulant–pretreated animals, vitamin K acts by combin-

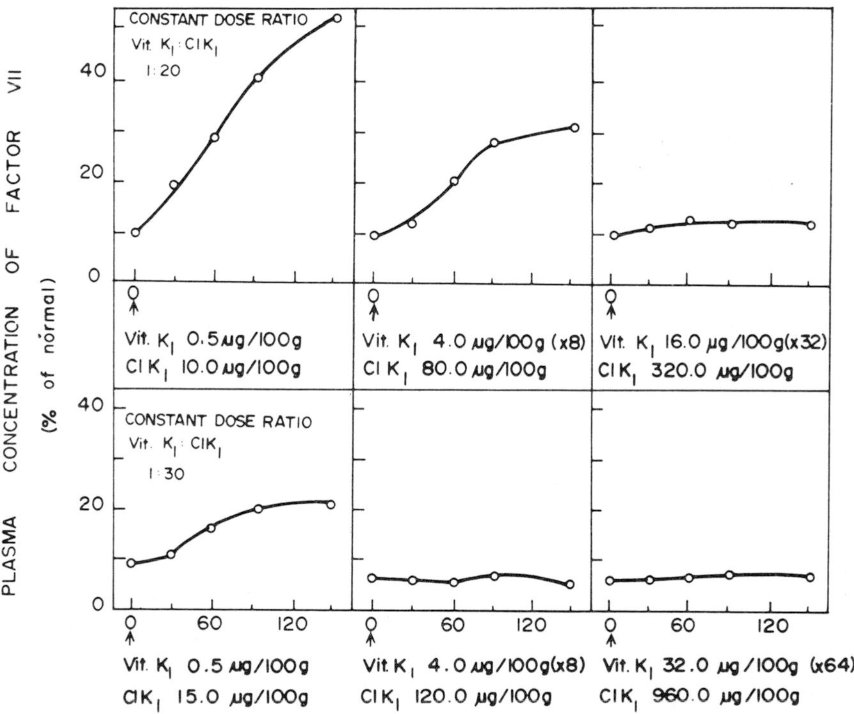

Fig. 27.5. Effect of increasing doses of constant ratios (1:20 and 1:30) of vitamin K_1 and its chloro analog on the increase of the plasma level of factor VII in vitamin K–deficient rats. (After Lowenthal and MacFarlane, 1967, Fig. 3.)

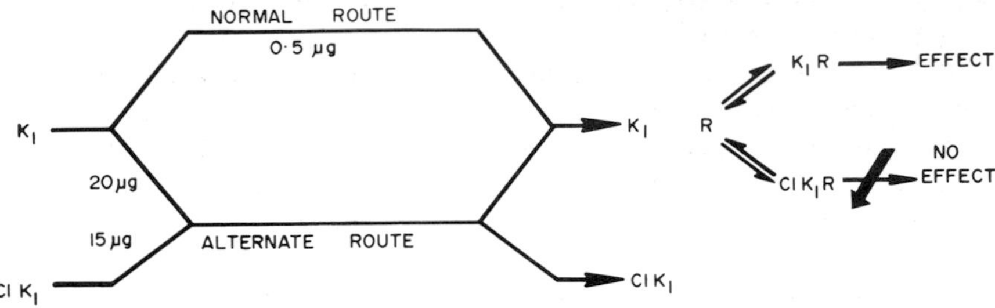

Fig. 27.6. Outline of the model showing the interrelations involved in the mechanism of action of vitamin K_1 and its inhibition by coumarin anticoagulants and the chloro analog of vitamin K_1.

ing reversibly with a complementary receptor site or active center. Normally, that is at physiological concentrations, this site is reached by a route which is of limited capacity, so that it is saturated by an optimal dose of vitamin K_1 in vitamin K–deficient animals, 0.5 μg/100 g. This route can be inhibited irreversibly by coumarin anticoagulants. After irreversible inhibition of this route, however, vitamin K_1, at higher concentrations, can still reach the receptor site by an alternate route, which is not inhibited by coumarin anticoagulants.

The threshold dose of vitamin K_1 for the alternate route is approximately 20 μg/100 g, since this is the lowest dose that will produce a response in coumarin anticoagulant–pretreated animals (Lowenthal and MacFarlane, 1964). Unlike vitamin K_1, the chloro analog cannot make use of the normal route but can reach the receptor site only by the alternate route. Its threshold dose is approximately 15 μg/100 g, since this is the lowest dose of the chloro analog that will produce an inhibitory effect in either vitamin K–deficient or coumarin anticoagulant–pretreated animals. At the receptor site, the chloro analog competes for, and combines reversibly with, the same receptor sites as vitamin K_1, but their combination fails to produce an effect.

Because vitamin K reaches the receptor site by the normal route in vitamin K–deficient animals but by the alternate route in coumarin anticoagulant–pretreated animals, the equipotent doses of vitamin K_1 in vitamin K–deficient animals and in coumarin anticoagulant–pretreated animals are different (0.5 μg/100 g and 100 μg/100 g respectively). In contrast, the chloro analog depends on the alternate route in both vitamin K–deficient and coumarin anticoagulant–pretreated animals. This, therefore, explains why the doses of the chloro analog required for partial or complete inhibition are the same in vitamin K–deficient animals and in coumarin anticoagulant–pretreated animals, although there is a 200-fold difference between the equipotent doses of vitamin K_1.

In coumarin anticoagulant–pretreated animals the normal route is inhibited, and therefore both vitamin K_1 and the chloro analog reach the receptor site by the same path, the alternate route (Fig. 27.6). When increasing doses of a ratio of vitamin K_1 to the chloro analog that produces partial inhibition are tested, the degree of inhibition does not change, because the relative concentration at the receptor site remains constant. This explains why the antagonism is found to be of the competitive type in coumarin anticoagulant–pretreated animals (Fig. 27.4).

A different set of conditions exists in vitamin K–deficient animals (Fig. 27.6). Here, depending on the dose, vitamin K_1 can reach the receptor site by both the normal and the alternate route, whereas the chloro analog can reach the receptor site by only the alternate route. For a ratio which produces partial inhibition — 1:20 (0.5 μg of vitamin K_1 and 10 μg of the chloro analog) or 1:30 (0.5 μg of vitamin K_1 and 15 μg of the chloro analog) — when the doses are increased by a factor of less than 40, the concentration of vitamin K_1 at the receptor site will not increase, because the normal route is already saturated by the initial dose of vitamin K_1 (0.5 μg/100 g), but the threshold dose of vitamin K_1 for the alternate route (20 μg/100 g) has not yet been reached, whereas the concentration of the chloro analog at the receptor site will increase. Therefore, the degree of inhibition will increase. When the doses are increased further — by a factor greater than 40 — vitamin K_1 will begin to reach the receptor site by the alternate route because its threshold dose (20 μg/100 g) has now been attained. Because of the limited capacity of the normal route, however, as the doses are increased, the relative concentration of vitamin K_1 and chloro analog at the receptor site will depend more and more on the relative concentration reaching the receptor site by the alternate route. Since, for ratios of 1:20 and 1:30, the relative concentration is sufficient for complete inhibition, the inhibition will remain complete.

This explains why, in vitamin K–deficient animals, the inhibition appears to be of the noncompetitive type for a ratio of vitamin K_1 to the chloro analog of 1:20 and 1:30. However, from the model, the prediction can be made that, if in vitamin K–deficient animals a ratio of vitamin K_1 to chloro analog were tested for which the relative concentration reaching the receptor site by the alternate route is only sufficient for partial inhibition, the degree of inhibition should remain constant when the doses are increased. This prediction has been tested for a ratio of vitamin K_1 to the chloro analog of 2:1 (Fig. 27.7). With 0.5 μg/100 g of vitamin K_1 and 0.25 μg/100 g of the chloro analog, there was no inhibition.

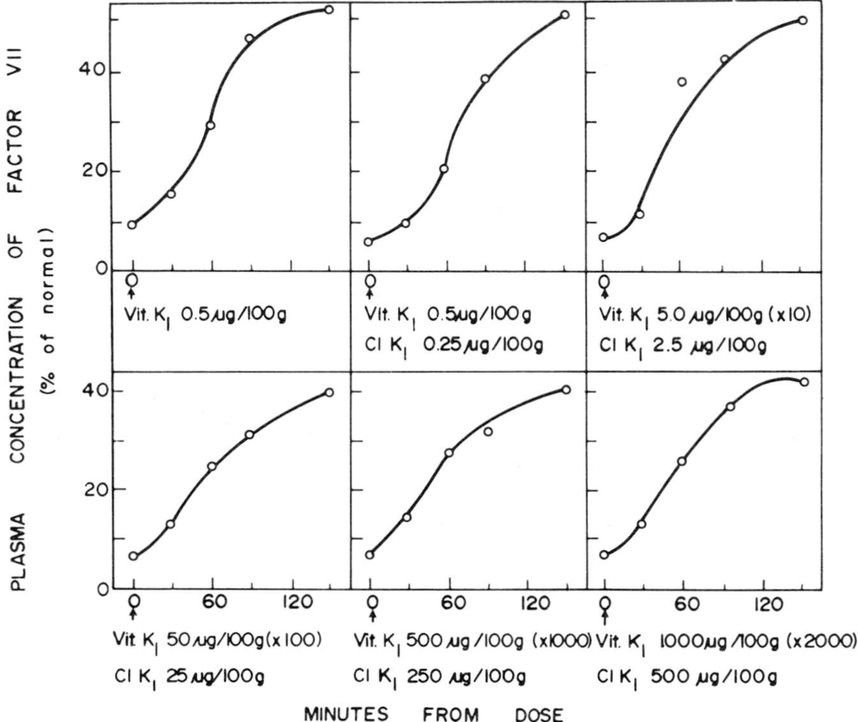

Fig. 27.7. Effect of increasing doses of a constant ratio (2:1) of vitamin K_1 and its chloro analog on the increase of the plasma level of factor VII in vitamin K–deficient rats. (After Lowenthal and MacFarlane, 1967, Fig. 5.)

When doses were increased by a factor of 10 there was still no inhibition, because the threshold dose of the chloro analog (15 μg) for the alternate route had not yet been reached. Inhibition was observed only after a 100-fold increase of the doses, because the threshold dose has now been reached. When the doses were increased 1000- and 2000-fold, however, the degree of inhibition remained constant, because the ratio of vitamin K_1 to the chloro analog (2:1) was only sufficient for partial inhibition.

The model (Fig. 27.6) therefore explains why in vitamin K–deficient animals the antagonism appears to be of the noncompetitive type for some ratios but the competitive type for other ratios.

The validity of the foregoing explanation depends on the assumption that coumarin anticoagulants act as irreversible inhibitors of the normal route but have no effect on the alternate route. If this assumption is correct, simultaneous administration of a coumarin anticoagulant should inhibit the response to vitamin K in vitamin K–deficient animals but should have no effect on the response in coumarin anticoagulant–pretreated animals.

In coumarin anticoagulant pretreated rats, when the largest dose of warfarin (20 mg/100 g) that can be given intravenously without killing the animals was given simultaneously with 20 μg and 40 μg per 100 g of vitamin K_1, the response has been found to be the same as that of vitamin K_1 alone (Fig. 27.8). In contrast, when increasing doses of warfarin and 0.5 μg/100 g of vitamin K_1 were injected simultaneously into vitamin K–deficient rats, the response was found to be partially or completely inhibited (Fig. 27.9).

Moreover, according to the proposed model (Fig. 27.6), if the ratio of vitamin K_1 to warfarin is kept constant, but the doses are increased, the inhibition should begin to disappear once the threshold dose of vitamin K_1 (20 μg) for the alternate route – which is not inhibited by coumarin anticoagulants – is reached, regardless of the simultaneous increase of the dose of warfarin. This prediction has been tested for ratios of 1:20 (0.5 μg of vitamin K_1 to 10 μg of warfarin) and of 1:10 (0.5 μg of vitamin K_1 to 5 μg of warfarin). For both ratios, the inhibition disappeared completely after a 100-fold increase of the doses, because, at a dose of 50 μg/100 g, sufficient vitamin K_1 reaches the receptor site by the alternate route to produce a nearly optimal response (Fig. 27.10).

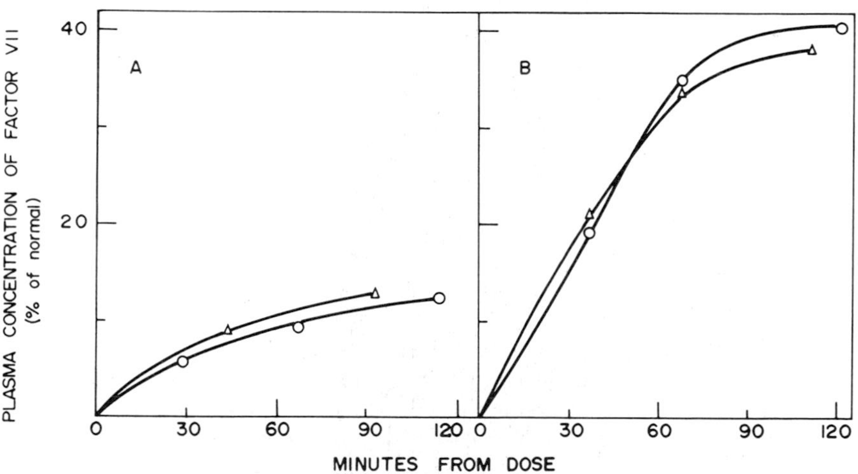

Fig. 27.8. Effect of simultaneous administration of warfarin on the increase of the plasma level of factor VII by vitamin K_1 in coumarin anticoagulant–pretreated rats. A: O, 20 μg vitamin K_1, △, 20 μg vitamin K_1 + 20 mg warfarin. B: O, 40 μg vitamin K_1; △, 40 μg vitamin K_1 + 20 mg warfarin. (After Lowenthal and MacFarlane, 1964, Fig. 5.)

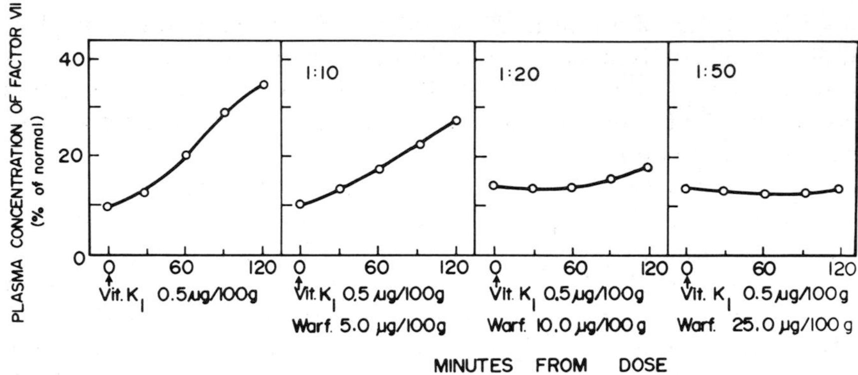

Fig. 27.9. Effect of simultaneous administration of increasing doses of warfarin on the increase of the plasma level of factor VII by vitamin K_1 in vitamin K–deficient rats. (After Lowenthal and MacFarlane, 1964, Fig. 3.)

Furthermore, if coumarin anticoagulants inhibit the normal route by which vitamin K reaches the receptor site but have no effect on its subsequent interaction with the receptor site, their ability to inhibit the response to vitamin K_1 in vitamin K–deficient animals should disappear as soon as vitamin K has reached the receptor site. In vitamin K–deficient

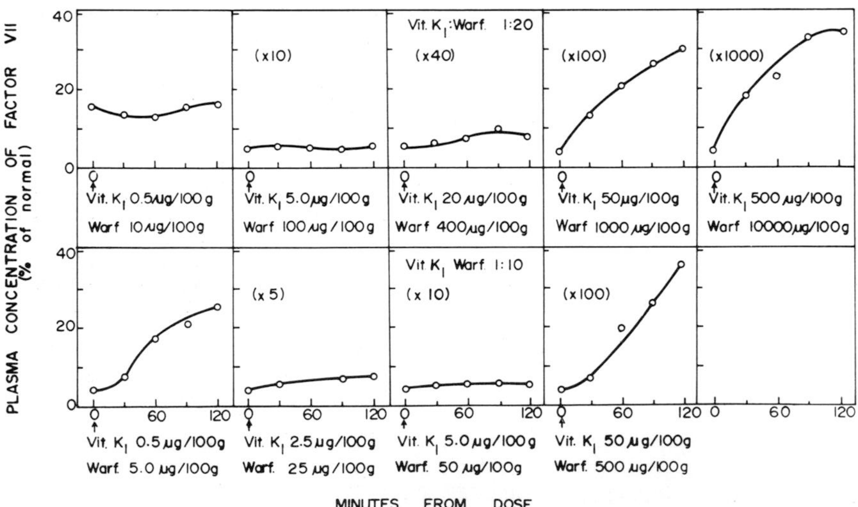

Fig. 27.10. Effect of increasing doses of constant ratios (1:20 and 1:10) of vitamin K_1 and warfarin on the increase of the plasma level of factor VII in vitamin K–deficient rats. (After Lowenthal and MacFarlane, 1964, Fig. 4.)

rats, when a dose of warfarin (20 μg/100 g) sufficient to produce complete inhibition when given simultaneously with vitamin K_1 (0.5 μg/100 g) is instead given 10 min after the administration of vitamin K_1, there was only partial inhibition, and, when given 20 min after vitamin K_1, there was no inhibition (Fig. 27.11).

It has recently been found that, in the presence of vitamin K_1, liver slices from vitamin K–deficient or coumarin anticoagulant–pretreated rats will release vitamin K–dependent plasma clotting-factor VII (Lowenthal and Simmons, 1967). The amount of clotting factor released depends on the concentration of vitamin K_1, and there is an approximately 10-fold to 100-fold difference between equipotent concentrations for slices from vitamin K–deficient animals and from warfarin-pretreated animals (Fig. 27.12).

This finding has made it possible to study the antagonism between vitamin K and coumarin anticoagulants in an in vitro system (Lowenthal and Birnbaum, 1969). Liver slices from vitamin K–deficient rats and from warfarin-pretreated rats were incubated in the presence of ^{14}C L-leucine, and after 4 hr both the concentration of factor VII in the medium and the rate of protein synthesis (as measured by incorporation of ^{14}C L-leucine into the protein of the combined medium and slices) were determined (Fig. 27.13). In the absence of vitamin K_1, little factor VII was found to be released. Addition of vitamin K_1 (10^{-6} M to slices from vitamin K–

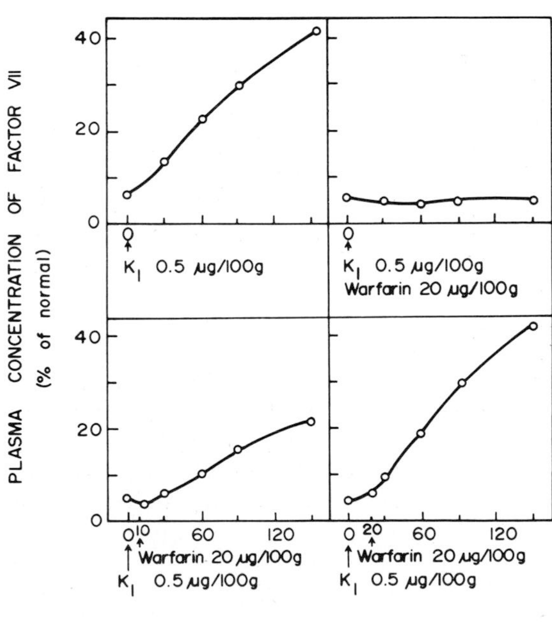

Fig. 27.11. Effect of the time of administration of warfarin on its ability to inhibit the increase of the plasma level of factor VII by vitamin K_1 in vitamin K–deficient rats.

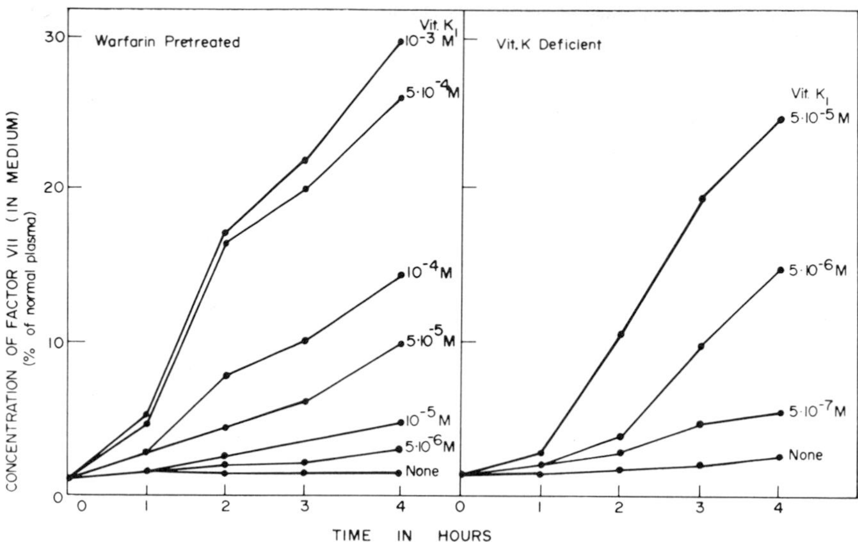

Fig. 27.12. Effect of vitamin K_1 on the release of factor VII by liver slices from warfarin-pretreated rats and from vitamin K–deficient rats. The system consisted of 1.0 g of slices in 10 ml of bicarbonate buffer, *p*H 7.3. The incubation was carried out in a Dubnoff shaker under an atmosphere of 95% oxygen and 5% carbon dioxide at 37 C for 4 hr. The concentration of factor VII in the medium is expressed as the percentage of factor VII, its concentration in normal rat plasma taken as 100%. (After Lowenthal and Birnbaum, 1969, Fig. 1.)

deficient animals or 4×10^{-4} M to slices from warfarin-pretreated animals) produced a significant increase in the release of factor VII. Increasing concentrations of warfarin (10^{-9} M to 10^{-6} M for slices from vitamin K–deficient animals or 10^{-5} M to 10^{-3} M for slices from warfarin-pretreated animals) either partially or completely inhibited the response to vitamin K_1. Although the response in slices from vitamin K–deficient animals was inhibited without inhibition of protein synthesis, the concentration of warfarin required to inhibit the response in slices from warfarin-pretreated animals also inhibited protein synthesis. In slices from vitamin K–deficient animals, when the ratio (1:1) of vitamin K_1 (10^{-6} M) to warfarin (10^{-6} M) was kept constant but the concentrations were increased 10-, 100-, and 1000-fold (Fig. 27.14), the inhibition disappeared because (as in intact animals), at higher concentrations, vitamin K can reach the receptor site by the alternate route, which is not inhibited by coumarin anticoagulants.

Thus, in vitamin K–deficient animals and in slices from such animals, warfarin inhibits the response to vitamin K_1, and this inhibition can be reversed by increasing concentrations of a constant ratio of vitamin K_1 to warfarin.

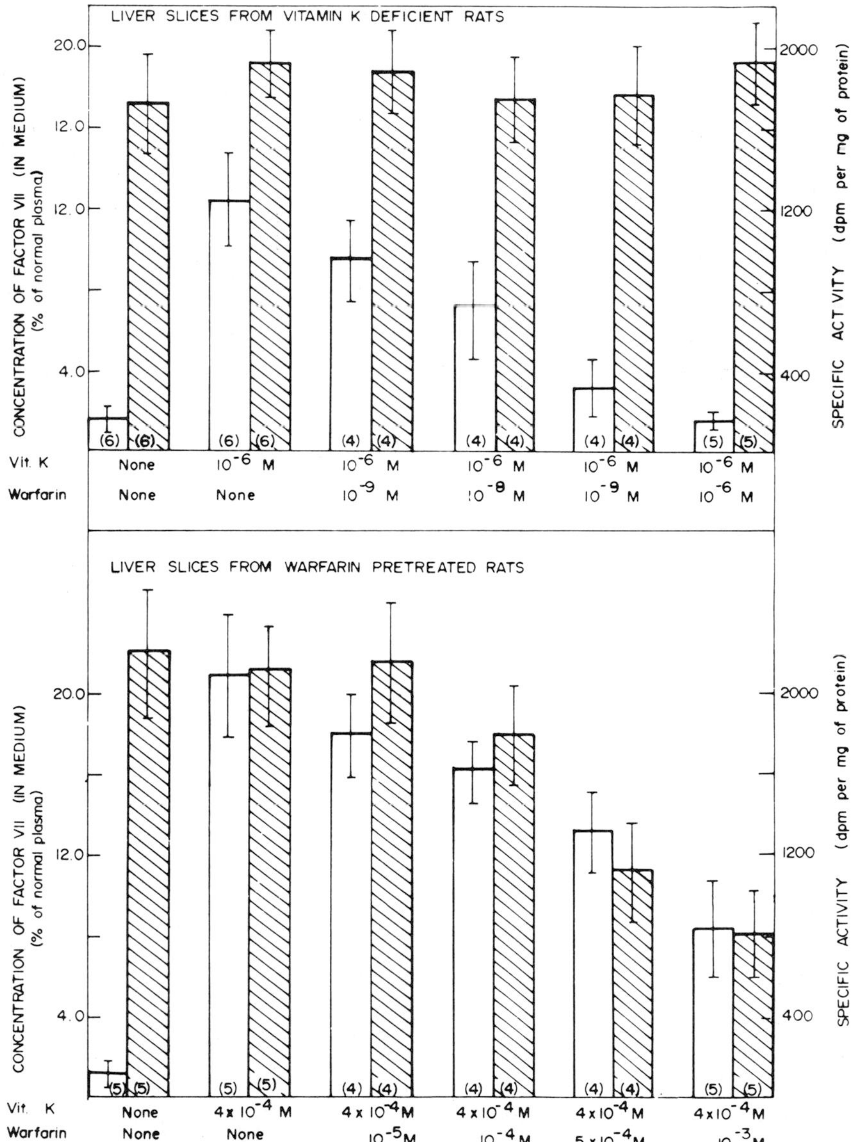

Fig. 27.13. Inhibition by warfarin of the release of factor VII by vitamin K_1 from liver slices of vitamin K–deficient rats and of coumarin anticoagulant–pretreated rats. White columns, concentration of factor VII; striped columns, incorporation of ^{14}C L-leucine into protein. Vertical bars represent standard error of the mean; $^{x}P < 0.05$ and $^{xx}P < 0.10$ compared to the response to vitamin K_1 alone. Numbers in parentheses are the number of animals used. (After Lowenthal and Birnbaum, 1969, Fig. 2.)

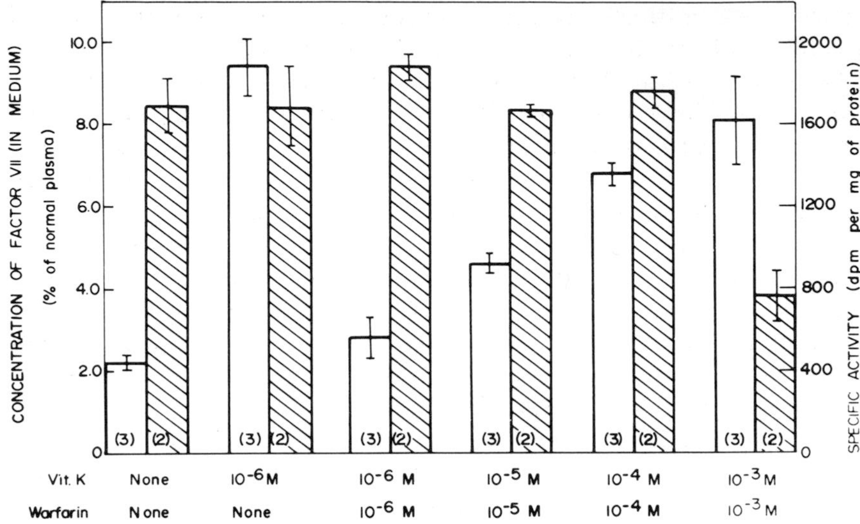

Fig. 27.14. Reversal of the vitamin K antagonism of warfarin by increasing concentrations of a constant dose ratio (1:1) of vitamin K_1 to warfarin in liver slices from vitamin K–deficient rats. In this experiment the incubation period was 3 hr. (See Fig. 27.13 for explanations.)

In contrast, warfarin has no effect on the response to vitamin K in coumarin anticoagulant–pretreated animals, but inhibits the response to vitamin K in slices from such animals.

This difference can be explained by the observation that the concentrations of warfarin (10^{-5} M to 10^{-3} M) required to inhibit the release of factor VII in slices from coumarin anticoagulant–pretreated animals also inhibit protein synthesis, whereas the inhibition of such release in slices from vitamin K–deficient animals is produced by concentrations of warfarin (10^{-9} M to 10^{-6} M) that do not inhibit protein synthesis. The inhibition of the release of factor VII caused by high concentrations of warfarin in slices from coumarin anticoagulant–pretreated animals must therefore be produced by a different and less-specific mechanism than that by which warfarin produces its pharmacological effect in intact animals or in slices from vitamin K–deficient animals. Such concentrations of warfarin, for example, have been reported to inhibit the respiration of liver slices from normal rats (Wosilait, 1961). Doses of warfarin that would produce such high concentrations cannot be administered to intact animals, because such doses cause acute toxic effects.

Therefore, at present, the only in vitro system in which the pharmacological action of coumarin anticoagulants, inhibition of formation or release of vitamin K–dependent clotting factors, can be clearly demonstrated is one in which vitamin K and coumarin anticoagulant are added simultaneously to slices from vitamin K–deficient animals.

While therapeutic doses of warfarin are effective in normal animals, concentrations of warfarin (10^{-9} M to 10^{-6} M) that correspond to such doses have no effect on slices from normal animals, because of the vitamin K already present at the receptor site. This explains, for example, the finding of Pool and Borchgrevink (1964), who reported that slices from anticoagulant–pretreated animals show normal protein synthesis but fail to release vitamin K–dependent clotting factors, while concentrations of warfarin that inhibit clotting-factor release in slices from normal animals also inhibit protein synthesis. From the present results, reinterpretation of the significance of the effects of coumarin anticoagulants on other in vitro systems seems to be indicated.

The proposed model, therefore, not only explains the initial experimental observations, on the basis of which it was introduced, but is also of some predictive value. Other models, based on different assumptions, either do not explain all the experimental observations in a manner free of contradictions or do so only after introducing additional assumptions for which there is, at the moment, no direct evidence. The proposed model, therefore, appears to offer the simplest explanation for the experimental findings available at this time.

It must be pointed out, however, that the evidence is of an indirect nature, and it remains to be established whether the interrelations on which the model is based are of more than formal significance. This applies particularly to the possible functional roles of the "normal" and "alternate" routes. While a specific, saturable transport mechanism for the former and nonspecific diffusion for the latter seem to be likely functional roles, the actual functions of these routes may be of a more complex nature. This appears to be indicated by the observation that the chloro analog acts as a competitive antagonist at the receptor site, yet lacks the structural requirements for interaction at the "normal" route.

Biochemical studies usually start from experiments in intact animals and progress via isolated organs or tissues to cell-free, purified systems. While the final stage of this sequence has not yet been reached in the study of the mechanism of action of vitamin K, the results of the present investigation, by clarifying certain aspects of the problem, may be of some help in the design and the interpretation of experiments directed towards this goal.

References

Koller, F., A. Loeliger, and F. Duckert. 1951. Experiments on a new clotting factor (factor VII). *Acta Haematol. 6*:1.

Lowenthal, J., and H. Birnbaum. 1969. Vitamin K and coumarin anticoagulants: Dependence of anticoagulant effect on inhibition of vitamin K transport. *Science 164*:181.

Lowenthal, J., and J. A. MacFarlane. 1963. The relation between structure and activity of compounds with vitamin K–like activity, p. 333. *In* K. J. Brunings (ed.), *Proceedings of the First International Pharmacological Meeting, Stockholm,* Vol. VII. Pergamon Press, New York.

Lowenthal, J., and J. A. MacFarlane. 1964. The nature of the antagonism between vitamin K and indirect anticoagulants. *J. Pharmacol. Exp. Ther. 143*:273.

Lowenthal, J., and J. A. MacFarlane. 1965. Vitamin K–like and antivitamin K activity of sustituted para-benzoquinones. *J. Pharmacol. Exp. Ther. 147*:130.

Lowenthal, J., and J. A. MacFarlane. 1967. Use of a competitive vitamin K antagonist, 2-chloro-3-phytyl-1,4-naphthoquinone, for the study of the mechanism of action of vitamin K and coumarin anticoagulants. *J. Pharmacol. Exp. Ther. 157*:672.

Lowenthal, J., J. A. MacFarlane, and K. M. McDonald. 1960. The inhibition of the antidotal activity of vitamin K_1 against coumarin anticoagulant drugs by its chloro analogue. *Experientia 16*:428.

Lowenthal, J., and E. Simmons. 1967. Failure of Actinomycin D to inhibit appearance of clotting activity by vitamin K in vitro. *Experientia 23*:421.

Pool, J. G., and C. F. Borchgrevink. 1964. Comparison of rat liver response to coumarin administered in vivo versus in vitro. *Amer. J. Physiol. 206*:229.

Wosilait, W. D. 1961. The effect of anticoagulants on the respiration of rat liver slices. *J. Pharmacol. Exp. Ther. 132*:212.

28

MECHANISM OF ACTION OF VITAMIN K

J. W. Suttie

The existence of a dietary antihemorrhagic factor was first demonstrated by Dam about thirty-five years ago, and that factor was given the name vitamin K. The determination of the structures of phylloquinone and one of the menaquinones within the next few years established that the active compounds were 2-methyl-1,4-naphtoquinones substituted in the 3 position by isoprenoid chains.*

In the years following the discovery of the vitamin, considerable progress was made in identifying active forms of the vitamin and in establishing dietary requirements. The coumarin anticoagulants were discovered by Campbell and Link (1941), and their usefulness as vitamin K antagonists was established. During the period from 1940 until the early 1960's, however, there was little progress made in elucidating the mechanism of action of vitamin K in higher animals. An historical survey of progress in vitamin K research has recently been made by Dam (1966).

It can easily be demonstrated that vitamin K is required to maintain normal plasma levels of the protein prothrombin (factor II) and of three other clotting factors: VII, IX, and X.† Whether the vitamin controls the production of these four separate factors, presumably all proteins, or whether they are all derived from a parent molecule – or if indeed there are four separate factors – is still a subject of disagreement (Seegers et al., 1968). In fact, there is not yet consensus on the basic nature of the coagulation process. Quick (1966) has reviewed three generalized schemes that have been proposed.

* For the currently acceptable nomenclature of the quinones with isoprenoid side chains, see IUPAC–IUB, Commission on Biochemical Nomenclature (1966).

† For a complete list of synonyms for the various clotting factors referred to, see Tocantins and Kazal (1964).

These studies were supported in part by Grant AM–09305 from the National Institutes of Health, United States Public Health Service. Dr. M. Hermodson, Miss M. Thierry, and Mrs. K. Nelson have contributed to some of the unpublished data reported in this paper.

This lack of agreement on the basic nature of the proteins regulated by the vitamin has certainly hampered investigation in the area, but, more important historically, progress in the field had to wait for the better understanding of the biochemical nature of protein biosynthesis which has developed over the past decade. At the present time, the control of prothrombin production by vitamin K is not only of interest as an unsolved problem in the biochemistry of the fat-soluble vitamins, but represents one of the few mammalian systems in which the rate of production of a well-characterized protein can be controlled by the administration of a known chemical compound.

Possible control sites

Anderson and Barnhart (1964) have conclusively demonstrated that the production of prothrombin, and its subsequent release to the plasma, occurs in the hepatic parenchymal cells, but the mechanism by which this synthesis is regulated by vitamin K has not been clarified.

Based on the analogy to the coenzyme function of the water-soluble vitamins, unsuccessful attempts have been made to identify the vitamin as part of the prothrombin molecule (Seegers, 1962). An early postulation of the mechanism of action of the vitamin was that put forth by Martius, who has recently reviewed his contributions (Martius, 1967). He postulated that the vitamin had a function in electron transport in mammalian tissue, as it does in bacterial systems, such that a deficiency results in a defect in oxidative phosphorylation. He then suggested that the rapid turnover of prothrombin would make it particularly sensitive to a decreased energy supply in the cell. Although Martius presented some evidence to support his views on the function of the vitamin in oxidative phosphorylation (Martius and Nitz-Litzow, 1954), there are similar studies which disagree (Paolucci et al., 1963), and Wosilait (1966) has shown that vitamin K–deficient chicks have normal hepatic levels of ATP.

If it is assumed that the vitamin does, in fact, regulate the production of a single protein (or of only a few), current knowledge of the mechanism and the control of mammalian protein biosynthesis leaves open a large number of possible control points. Some, but certainly not all, of these are listed in Table 28.1. Because of the rapid accumulation of data in this field in the past few years, it is not surprising that there is considerable disagreement as to the possible involvement of some of these areas.

Hill and co-workers (1968) have measured prothrombin, or at least some type of clotting activity, in liver-microsomal preparations and have found that this activity is decreased in liver preparations from vitamin K–deficient or from anticoagulant-treated animals. Other studies (Ander-

TABLE 28.1. *Sites where vitamin K could exert an effect on prothrombin biosynthesis*

1. DNA transcription
2. RNA translation:
Polysome formation — chain
Initiation — chain elongation
3. Chain completion:
Nacent peptide release — tertiary
Structure formation — movement to cisternal space
4. Carbohydrate attachment
5. Subunit aggregation
6. Secretion from the cell
7. Rate of prothrombin degradation

son and Barnhart, 1964; Barnhart, 1965) indicate that, in the warfarin-treated dog, the hepatic cells are essentially void of material which will react with a fluorescent antibody prepared against canine prothrombin, indicating that the intact immunoactive protein does not pile up in the presence of the anticoagulant. These data make it unlikely that the completed, functional protein is present in the cells of deficient animals, and they would appear to rule out control of secretion from the cell as the primary site of action of the vitamin.

Bell and Matschiner (1969) have analyzed the prothrombin decay curves obtained when rats are treated with warfarin, cycloheximide, or 2-chloro-3-phytyl-1,4-nathoquinone and have determined that the biological half-life of prothrombin is about 6 hr. This value was decreased somewhat in deficient animals but was unrelated to the degree of severity of the deficiency and was unchanged in warfarin-treated animals. These data would indicate that the effect of the vitamin must be on the rate of synthesis of prothrombin rather than on its degradation rate.

The possibility that the control point might involve attachment of the carbohydrate portion of the molecule, or might involve subunit aggregation, has been alluded to by various workers, but little evidence is available to draw any conclusions at this time. The majority of the recently published work has dealt with efforts to establish a function of the vitamin in nucleic acid or protein biosynthesis. More specifically, three general questions have been asked. First, does the vitamin act by inducing the formation of the specific mRNA molecule for prothrombin synthesis? Second, is the formation of prothrombin in response to the vitamin a completely *de novo* process, or is some precursor involved? Third, if the synthesis is *de novo,* at what point does the vitamin control the process? This chapter will concern itself with these problems, will discuss a new system that might be useful in arriving at some of the answers we are lacking, and will make brief mention of studies designed to determine if proteins other than the clotting factors are influenced by the vitamin K status of the animal.

Involvement of the vitamin in DNA transcription

Based on the ability of actinomycin D to block a vitamin K_3–induced prothrombin response in deficient chicks, Olson (1964, 1965) postulated that the vitamin was functioning as a metabolic inducer at the level of DNA transcription. These observations could not be confirmed by other workers (Suttie, 1967; Johnson et al., 1966) using somewhat different systems. It now appears that the time of administration of the antibiotic, the prothrombin assay used, and the form and mode of administration of the vitamin were all factors involved in the original observations, and Olson has more recently supported an effect of the vitamin at the translational level (Olson et al., 1968).

Further evidence that DNA transcription is not needed for the response came with the demonstration (Suttie, 1967) that an isolated perfused liver from a deficient rat will respond to vitamin K administration by producing and releasing factor VII to the perfusate. This response was not abolished by actinomycin D. Similarly, Lowenthal and Simmons (1967) have shown that actinomycin D is ineffective in blocking a vitamin K–dependent factor VII formation in rat-liver slices prepared from warfarin-treated animals.

Requirement of protein synthesis for clotting-factor formation

Although it can be concluded with some certainty that DNA transcription is not needed to produce a clotting-factor response to the vitamin administration, the requirement for *de novo* protein synthesis to initiate the clotting-factor response is not so clear. The confusing problem has been to determine if there is some unfinished precursor protein in the deficient state that can be converted to prothrombin without the initiation of protein synthesis. Results of numerous experiments testing the effects of the inhibitors of protein biosynthesis, puromycin and cycloheximide, on the vitamin-induced prothrombin response have suggested this possibility, but have been difficult to interpret and compare because of widely differing experimental procedures.

Babior (1966) has indicated that, in a rat-liver-slice system, factor VII production was uninhibited by levels of puromycin that decreased by 98% the total amino acid incorporation into protein in the slices. Prydz (1965), however, found that puromycin was effective in blocking the continual production of factor VII activity in suspensions of hepatic cells obtained from normal rats, although Ranhotra and Johnson (1969) have claimed that puromycin or cycloheximide have little effect in a similar system. In a perfused-liver system, puromycin has been reported to be both effective (Suttie, 1967) and ineffective (J. P. Olson et al., 1966) in blocking a vitamin K response.

The response of intact, hypoprothrombinemic animals to vitamin K in the presence of agents which block protein biosynthesis has also varied. Hill and co-workers (1968) have concluded that a level of cycloheximide which is sufficient to block prothrombin production in normal animals has no effect on the response of the vitamin K–deficient animal to the vitamin. In the same study, puromycin was found to be much more effective than cycloheximide in blocking the vitamin K–induced prothrombin response. Because prothrombin was measured by the one-stage assay in these studies, there is some doubt as to how much actual prothrombin was formed. Bell and Matschiner (1969), using a modified one-stage assay, have also noted that cycloheximide is ineffective in blocking the rapid increase in prothrombin seen when deficient rats are given vitamin K.

Because of our concern that even the modified one-stage prothrombin assay might not be a true measure of prothrombin in the few hours fol-

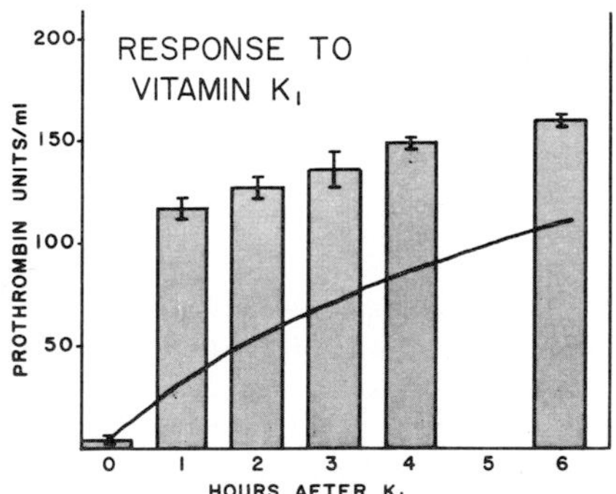

Fig. 28.1. Response of hypoprothrombinemic deficient rats to vitamin K_1. Response was measured in male rats, 150 g, fed a vitamin K–deficient diet in coprophagy-preventing cages for 6–8 days. All rats were given 1 mg of vitamin K_1 intramuscularly at zero time. Values are expressed as Iowa units and were determined in a two-stage assay on blood drawn from the jugular vein or obtained by cardiac puncture. Data from 81 animals are included, and the vertical lines at the top of the shaded bars represent the standard error for 5–26 animals per group. The solid line represents the theoretical curve for the repletion of prothrombin, assuming a biological half-life of 6 hr and a steady-state prothrombin level of 206 units/ml.

lowing the cure of a severe hypoprothrombinemia, we have reinvestigated this response using the classical two-stage assay for prothrombin. The data in Figure 28.1 confirm those of Hill and co-workers (1968) and indicate that the response of prothrombin is extremely rapid. Approximately 50% of the normal circulating level of prothrombin is restored in the first hour following a large intramuscular dose of vitamin K_1 to vitamin K–deficient rats. This rapid response in the first hour is in contrast to the linear response noted in deficient chicks (Olson et al., 1968) and raises the question of whether there might be a species difference or whether other factors are responsible for the differences seen. These data might also suggest that the initial rate of synthesis is much greater than the steady-state rate or that there may be some conversion of an existing precursor. The data in Figure 28.2 indicate that an injected dose of cycloheximide which drastically interferes with the incorporation of radioac-

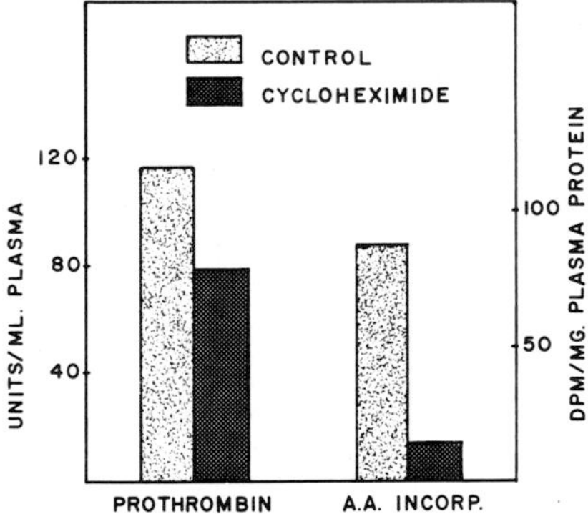

Fig. 28.2. Effect of cycloheximide treatment on the vitamin K–dependent synthesis of prothrombin in deficient rats. Prothrombin response was measured in 150 g, male, vitamin K–deficient rats (avg prothrombin = 13 units/ml) given an intraperitoneal injection of 0.5 mg cycloheximide/100 g body weight at zero time and 1 mg K_1 intramuscularly at 30 min. Blood for a two-stage assay was drawn from the jugular vein at 30 min and by cardiac puncture at 90 min. There were 7 rats per group, and the data are expressed as the increase in prothrombin over the 1-hr period. The effect of this level of cycloheximide on the incorporation of radioactive amino acids into the total plasma proteins was determined in a second group of rats given an intraperitoneal injection of 0.5 mg cycloheximide/100 g body weight or saline at zero time and of 2 μCi ^{14}C amino acid mix at 30 min. Blood was drawn for the radioactivity determination at 90 min. (From Suttie, 1969, Fig. 3.)

tive amino acids into total plasma proteins decreases this initial response in prothrombin formation by only about 30%. Although cycloheximide is rather ineffective in blocking the first-hour response, the preliminary data in Figure 28.3 indicate that the small increase in prothrombin which is seen between 1 hr and 2 hr after vitamin K administration is completely blocked by this antibiotic. Puromycin administration was found (Fig. 28.4) to be more effective than cycloheximide in blocking the initial prothrombin response, but not nearly as effective as it was in blocking total plasma-protein synthesis (see Fig. 28.2). These data, although certainly not conclusive, do indicate that the initial appearance of prothrombin may represent something other than *de novo* synthesis, and they suggest some type of activation of an inactive precursor.

Dulock and Kolmen (1968) have demonstrated a rapid increase in prothrombin activity when vitamin K was given to warfarin-treated dogs whose prothrombin levels had been further depleted by cross circulation with serum. This increase was not seen without prior warfarin treatment and was interpreted as evidence for a precursor in the liver of the warfarin-treated dogs. If such a precursor does exist, it is too large a pool to exist as incompleted nascent peptides on polyribosomes but would have to be present as part of some pool of partially completed or inactivated prothrombin. What relationships these data bear, if any, to the observations of Hemker and co-workers (1963, 1968) is unclear. They have postulated a compound present in the hypoprothrombinemic blood of vitamin K–

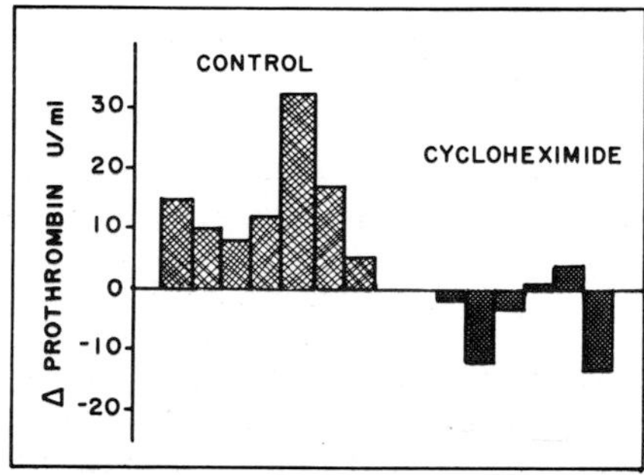

Fig. 28.3. Effect of cycloheximide treatment on prothrombin production 1–2 hr after vitamin K administration. Vitamin K–deficient, male rats, 150 g, were given 1 mg vitamin K_1 intramuscularly at zero time and 0.5 mg cycloheximide/100 g body weight intraperitoneally at 30 min. Blood for a two-stage assay was drawn from the jugular vein at 60 min and by cardiac puncture at 120 min. Data are expressed as the change in prothrombin concentration between the two periods. Each bar represents a single rat.

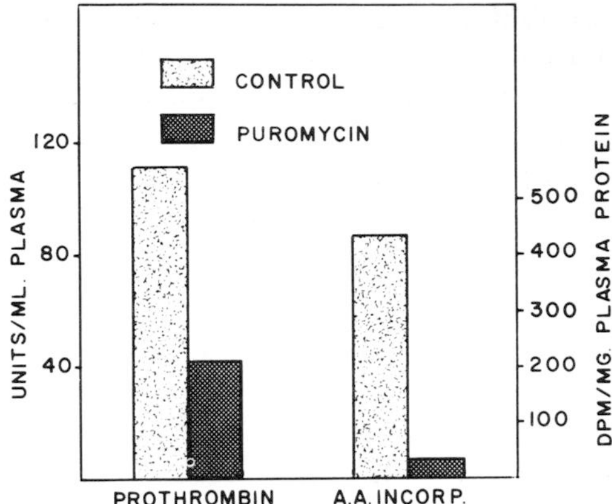

Fig. 28.4. Effect of puromycin treatment on the vitamin K–dependent synthesis of prothrombin in deficient rats. Prothrombin response was measured in male, 150 g, vitamin K–deficient rats (avg prothrombin = 9 units/ml) given an intraperitoneal injection of 10 mg puromycin/100 g body weight at zero time and at 60 min; 1 mg vitamin K_1 intramuscularly at 30 min; and 4 μCi ^{14}C amino acid mix (intraperitoneally) at 30 min. Blood for a two-stage assay was drawn from the jugular vein at 30 min and by cardiac puncture at 90 min. There were 6 rats per group, and the data are expressed as the increase in prothrombin over the 1 hr period. The effect of this level of puromycin on protein synthesis was determined by measuring the incorporation of radioactive amino acids into the total plasma proteins of the 90-min sample.

deficient or warfarin-treated, but not cirrhotic, patients which is a competitive inhibitor of the clotting reaction. The factor, which they have called "Protein Induced by Vitamin K Absence or Antagonists (PIVKA)," is heat labile, has a high molecular weight, and is, as are the vitamin K–dependent clotting factors, absorbed by Ba_2SO_4 or $Al(OH)_3$. It has been suggested (Hemker and Muller, 1968) that in the deficient state the finalization of prothrombin is inhibited, and PIVKA, which they believe to be an analog of factor X, builds up in the liver and reaches the plasma. Losito (1965) has failed to find evidence for this factor in deficient chicks, but we do see some evidence for the factor Hemker and co-workers have described in deficient and in warfarin-treated rats. Seegers and co-workers (1968) have also postulated that different units of the prothrombin molecule are synthesized independently in the liver and may appear in the blood without being combined.

In contrast to these data, which suggest that there may be a precursor of prothrombin present in the hypoprothrombinemic state, both Olson's group (Li et al., 1969) and our own laboratory (Suttie, 1969) have presented data on the kinetics of incorporation of radioactive amino acids into newly synthesized prothrombin which are consistent with de novo synthesis. It would appear that this problem will have to be resolved in a system less complex than the intact animal. It should be emphasized, however, that postulations on the action of the vitamin based on various in vitro or even cell-free systems must continually be viewed in the light of what is known about the response to vitamin K in intact animals.

Vitamin K–warfarin antagonism

Research on vitamin K has been greatly aided by the use of various coumarin-based anticoagulants to produce a hypoprothrombinemic state. Although an alternate hypothesis has been suggested (Lowenthal and MacFarlane, 1967; Lowenthal and Birnbaum, 1969), it has usually been assumed that the coumarin anticoagulants compete directly with vitamin K for a receptor protein, or proteins, at the site where vitamin K is exerting its biological activity. Recent experiments in our laboratory have raised the possibility that at least one such receptor protein can be identified.

Pool and co-workers (1968) have studied the warfarin-resistant strain of rats described by Greaves and Ayres (1967) and have shown that this resistance is heritable as an autosomal dominant gene and that the rates of uptake and excretion of warfarin in the resistant rat are unaltered. O'Reilly and co-workers (1964) studied a similar condition in a human patient and postulated that it could be the result of an altered receptor protein which had an increased affinity for vitamin K and, subsequently, a resistance to the effects of warfarin. The data in Table 28.2 indicate, however, that the warfarin-resistant rat has an increased, not

TABLE 28.2. *Response of depleted male rats to vitamin K_1*

	Prothrombin (units/ml)		
Vitamin K_1 (μg/day)	Normal Holtzman	Heterozygous resistant	Homozygous resistant
0.5	84 ± 15	25 ± 8	—
1.0	159 ± 11	59 ± 13	—
3.0	245 ± 3	198 ± 6	—
6.0	—	209 ± 9	43[a]
10.0	—	—	65 ± 9
20.0	—	—	163 ± 7
30.0	—	—	206 ± 2

Notes: Male rats, 150 g, were fed a low–vitamin K diet in coprophagy-preventing cages for 72 hr, then were given 4 daily subcutaneous doses of phylloquinone. Blood for a two-stage assay was drawn 24 hr after the final dose.
Values are given as mean ± SE for 4–6 rats per group.
[a] One rat.

a decreased, requirement for the vitamin. We have therefore postulated (Hermodson et al., 1969) that the mutation is one which lowers the affinity of some protein binding site for vitamin K slightly but lowers the warfarin binding affinity of this protein greatly.

An alternate hypothesis to explain the increased vitamin K requirement would be that the warfarin-resistant rats are metabolizing the vitamin more rapidly or in a different manner and it is not available to the active site. It has been shown that the whole-body distribution of radioactive menadiol diphosphate seen in normal rats (Thierry and Suttie, 1969) does not differ from the distribution found in the resistant rats, and the data in Table 28.3 indicate that the same is true for the distribution of radioactive

TABLE 28.3. *Localization of vitamin K_1 in normal and in warfarin-resistant rats*

Tissue	Percentage of injected dose	
	Resistant	Normal
Plasma	3.2 ± 0.9	3.0 ± 0.2
Liver	43.6 ± 2.3	50.6 ± 1.9
Lung	1.5 ± 0.6	1.1 ± 0.2
Heart	0.2 ± 0.0	0.2 ± 0.0
Gastrointestinal tract	24.7 ± 1.1	18.9 ± 0.5
Muscle	6.4 ± 0.7	7.2 ± 0.6

Notes: Male rats were killed 3 hr after an intravenous injection of 5 μg of 2-Me-^{14}C vitamin K_1, and distribution of radioactivity in various tissues was determined.

Values are given as mean ± SE for 5 rats per group.

phylloquinone. It is also clear (Fig. 28.5) that the rate of disappearance of an injected dose of radioactive phylloquinone does not differ appreciably in the two types of rats over a 24-hr period. These data would appear to rule out any gross changes in vitamin metabolism as the reason for the altered requirement.

Although the warfarin-resistant rats retain slightly less of an injected dose of vitamin K in the liver, preliminary experiments (Table 28.4) have failed to demonstrate any change in the binding of vitamin K to liver subcellular fractions prepared from rats injected with radioactive vitamin K_1. When normal and warfarin-resistant rats were injected with radioactive warfarin, however, the data on subcellular distribution (Table 28.4) suggested that the receptor might well be a ribosomal protein or at least a protein associated with deoxycholate-prepared ribosomes. Although other cellular organelles were unaffected, the ribosomes isolated from normal rats demonstrated an increased capacity to bind warfarin. Although the amount of warfarin bound to the ribosomes is small, this two- to

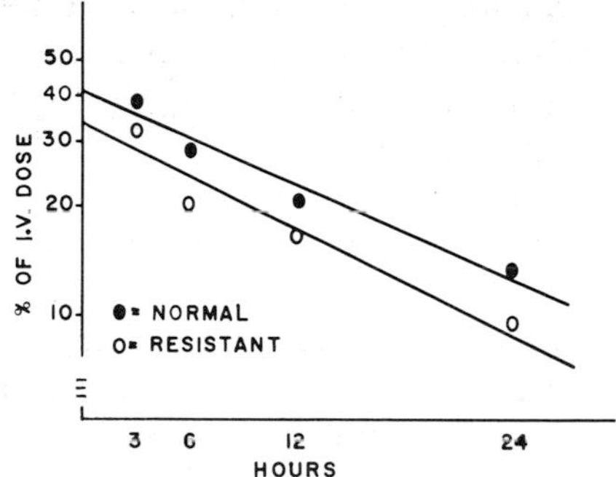

Fig. 28.5. Retention of radioactive vitamin K_1 in rat liver. Male, 350 g, normal or warfarin-resistant rats were given an intravenous injection of 10 μg of 2-Me-^{14}C vitamin K_1 and were killed at various times. The data are the average percentages of the administered dose of radioactivity found in the liver of the three rats killed at each time.

three-fold increase has been consistently seen. The significance of this observation is enhanced by the demonstration that a four-fold increase in warfarin binding to ribosomes from normal rats can be demonstrated when normal and warfarin-resistant rat-liver microsomes are incubated in vitro with radioactive warfarin (Table 28.5). It has also been shown

TABLE 28.4. *Distribution of activity from radioactive phylloquinone or warfarin in the liver of normal or warfarin-resistant rats*

Fraction	Vitamin K_1 (picomoles/mg protein)		Warfarin (picomoles/mg protein)	
	Normal	Resistant	Normal	Resistant
Homogenate	3.6 ± 0.1	3.0 ± 0.3	102 ± 5	111 ± 5
Nuclei	1.9 ± 0.2	1.3 ± 0.1	10 ± 1	6 ± 1
Mitochondria	11.5 ± 2.3	12.9 ± 1.9	33 ± 3	29 ± 7
Microsomes	5.2 ± 0.2	4.9 ± 0.6	108 ± 4	100 ± 10
Ribosomes	2.4 ± 0.4	2.7 ± 0.4	30 ± 1	12 ± 1

Notes: Male rats, 200 g, warfarin-resistant or control, were given an intravenous injection of 5 μg of 2-Me-^{14}C vitamin K_1 and were killed after 3 hr. Subcellular fractions were prepared by standard methods, and radioactivity was converted to molar equivalents of phylloquinone. Similarly, male rats, 350 g, were given an intraperitoneal injection of 1 mg of 4-^{14}C warfarin and were killed at 3 hr; the radioactivity in various fractions was determined and was expressed as molar equivalents of warfarin. The fraction of the radioactivity present as unchanged phylloquinone or warfarin was not determined.

Values are given as mean ± SE for 5–7 rats per group.

TABLE 28.5. *Warfarin binding to rat-liver ribosomes*

Type of rat	Protein (dpm/mg)
Normal Holtzman ($n = 10$)	1866 ± 119
Homozygous resistant ($n = 7$)	436 ± 51

Notes: Microsomes prepared from normal or warfarin-resistant rats were incubated with 10μM 4-^{14}C warfarin for 12 hr at 5 C. Ribosomes were prepared by deoxycholate treatment and were analyzed for protein and bound radioactivity.

Values are given as mean ± SE.

that ribosomes from liver are the only ones affected and that ribosomes prepared from kidney, heart, or spleen show low and presumably nonspecific binding whether they are isolated from normal or from warfarin-resistant rats. Although far from conclusive, these data raise the exciting possibility that we may be dealing with a protein involved in the mutation leading to the development of warfarin resistance. Isolation of the proteins responsible for this binding, and the establishment of their role in the protein-synthesizing function of the ribosome, might give us an important insight into the mechanism of action of the vitamin.

Other effects of the deficiency

The possibility has been raised, originally by Martius in his postulation of an effect of vitamin K deficiency on oxidative phosphorylation, that there might be some generalized metabolic defect in the deficiency (Martius, 1967). Because of the short half-life of the protein, it was thought that the defect might be seen only in a lowering of the concentration of prothrombin. It has been reported both in intact animals (Hill et al., 1968) and in isolated perfused livers (Suttie, 1967) that the rate of total liver protein synthesis is unaffected by a vitamin K deficiency, and Paolucci and co-workers (1964) have shown that a specific protein, tryptophane pyrrolase, may be induced in vitamin K–deficient animals. Although it appears that protein synthesis in general is normal, we have been investigating the possibility that other specific plasma proteins may be influenced by the deficiency. The preliminary data presented in Figure 28.6 suggests that this may be the case. It seems clear from these data that there are differences in the relative rates of synthesis of different plasma proteins in control and in vitamin K–deficient rats. At the present time we have no indication of what plasma proteins are involved. Whether these apparent changes in rates of synthesis of plasma proteins are direct effects of the deficiency state or some secondary response to it has not yet been established, but they are interesting responses that must be further clarified to gain a clear understanding of the deficiency. Similarly, the changes

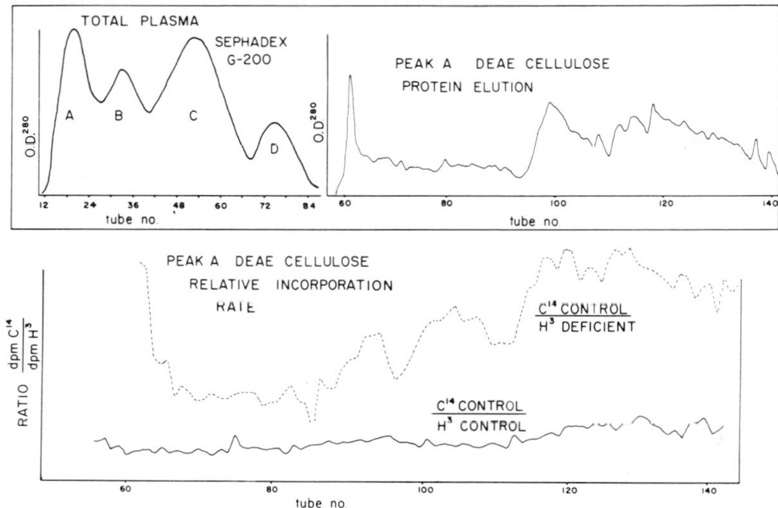

Fig. 28.6. Effect of vitamin K deficiency on the relative rate of synthesis of plasma proteins. Male, 150 g, control or vitamin K–deficient rats were stomach-tubed with 50 μCi of ^{14}C leucine or with 100 μCi of ^{3}H leucine in three equal doses at 0 min, 45 min, and 90 min, and blood was drawn at 135 min. The plasma from three ^{3}H and three ^{14}C rats was pooled and was chromatographed on Sephadex G–200. Each of the major peaks, in this case peak A, was chromatographed on DEAE cellulose, and the ratio of ^{14}C and ^{3}H activity in each fraction was determined. A constant ratio would indicate that the relative rate of synthesis of various plasma proteins was similar in the two groups of animals whose plasma was mixed. This is seen to be the case when plasma from two controls was mixed (solid line). The changing ratio seen (dashed line) when plasma from control and from deficient rats was mixed would indicate that the rate of synthesis of various proteins in the deficient rat was different from the control rate.

induced in pancreatic enzyme levels by vitamin K deficiency or by warfarin reported by Bogdanov and Lider (1967, 1968); the liver microstructural changes seen by Barnhart and co-workers (1964); and the alterations in liver RNA metabolism seen by Olson and co-workers (1968) must be investigated to fully understand the function of the vitamin.

Conclusions

It has been about thirty-five years since it was established that vitamin K is essential in the maintenance of normal levels of the plasma clotting factors, and for about the last ten years it has been possible to approach the mechanism of its action with a sound background knowledge of the biochemical nature of protein biosynthesis. Despite considerable effort, the mechanism of action of the vitamin has not been elucidated. It appears firmly established that the vitamin does not act at the level of DNA transcription. Although much evidence points to an action of the vitamin at the translational level of protein biosynthesis, the acceptance of this explanation still poses some problems. The lack of effect of cycloheximide on the initial burst of prothrombin when the hypoprothrombinemic state is reversed, and the magnitude of this initial response itself, suggests that some type of precursor hypothesis cannot yet be completely ruled out. The studies with warfarin-resistant rats offer what appears to be a new approach to the problem. The resistance seems clearly to be due to an alteration in a protein which interacts with both warfarin and vitamin K, and the interaction of radioactive warfarin with crude ribosomes raises the possibility of actually isolating what might be a regulatory protein. There now appear to be a number of lines of evidence which suggest that there may be metabolic disorders other than the well-recognized decrease in the vitamin K–dependent clotting factors in a vitamin K deficiency. If such disturbances could be verified, it would greatly aid in the search for the mechanism of action of the vitamin. Even though it is not possible to conclusively establish a mechanism of action of the vitamin at this time, the work presented in this volume has demonstrated that there are numerous approaches open and that rapid progress should be made in the next few years.

References

Anderson, G. F., and M. I. Barnhart. 1964. Prothrombin synthesis in the dog. *Amer. J. Physiol. 206*:929.

Babior, B. M. 1966. The Role of vitamin K in clotting factor synthesis. I. Evidence for the participation of vitamin K in the conversion of a polypeptide precursor to factor VII. *Biochim. Biophys. Acta 123*:606.

Barnhart, M. I. 1965. Prothrombin synthesis: An example of hepatic function. *J. Histochem. Cytochem. 13*:740.

Barnhart, M. I., G. F. Anderson, and M. H. Bernstein. 1964. Liver ultrastructure after coumadin and vitamin K_1. *Fed. Proc. 23*:520. (Abstr.)

Bell, R. G., and J. T. Matschiner, 1969. Synthesis and destruction of prothrombin in the rat. *Arch. Biochem. Biophys. 135*:152.

Bogdanov, N. G., and V. A. Lider. 1967. The effect of coumarin derivatives on the activity of some external secreted enzymes. *Farmakol. Toksikol. 30*:727.

Bogdanov, N. G., and V. A. Lider. 1968. Role of vitamin K in biosynthesis of some exoenzymes of the digestive organs. *Biul. Eksp. Biol. Med. 65*:60.

Campbell, H. A., and K. P. Link. 1941. Studies on the hemorrhagic sweet clover disease. IV. The isolation and crystallization of the hemorrhagic agent. *J. Biol. Chem. 138*:21.

Dam, H. 1966. Historical survey and introduction. *Vitamins Hormones 24*:295.

Dulock, M. A., and S. N. Kolmen. 1968. Influence of vitamin K on restoration of prothrombin complex proteins and fibrinogen in plasma of depleted dogs. *Thromb. Diath. Haemorrh. 20*:136.

Greaves, J. H., and P. Ayres. 1967. Heritable resistance to warfarin in rats. *Nature 215*:877.

Hemker, H. C., and A. D. Muller. 1968. Kinetic aspects of the interaction of blood-clotting enzymes. VI. Localization of the site of blood-coagulation inhibition by the protein induced by vitamin K absence (PIVKA). *Thromb. Diath. Haemorrh. 20*:78.

Hemker, H. C., J. J. Veltkamp, A. Hensen, and E. A. Loeliger. 1963. Nature of prothrombin biosynthesis. Preprothrombinaemia in vitamin K–deficiency. *Nature 200*:589.

Hemker, H. C., J. J. Veltkamp, and E. A. Loeliger. 1968. Kinetic aspects of the interaction of blood clotting enzymes. III. Demonstration of an inhibitor of prothrombin conversion in vitamin K deficiency. *Thromb. Diath. Haemorrh. 19*:346.

Hermodson, M. A., J. W. Suttie, and K. P. Link. 1969. Warfarin metabolism and vitamin K requirement in the warfarin-resistant rat. *Amer. J. Physiol. 217*:1316.

Hill, R. B., S. Gaetani, A. M. Paolucci, P. B. RamaRao, R. Alden, G. S. Ranhotra, D. V. Shah, V. K. Shah, and B. C. Johnson. 1968. Vitamin K and biosynthesis of protein and prothrombin. *J. Biol. Chem. 243*:3930.

IUPAC–IUB, Commission on Biochemical Nomenclature. 1966. Tentative Rules. *J. Biol. Chem. 241*:2989.

Johnson, B. C., R. B. Hill, R. Alden, and G. S. Ranhotra. 1966. Turnover time of prothrombin and of prothrombin messenger RNA and evidence for a ribosomal site of action of vitamin K in prothrombin synthesis. *Life Sci. 5*:385.

Li, L. F., R. K. Kipfer, and R. E. Olson. 1969. Immunochemical measurement of vitamin K–induced biosynthesis of prothrombin in the isolated perfused rat liver. *Fed. Proc. 28*:385. (Abstr.)

Losito, R. 1965. Investigations into the presence of a competitive inhibitor (pre-prothrombin) in the plasma of chicks. *Acta Chem. Scand. 19*:2229.

Lowenthal, J., and H. Birnbaum. 1969. Vitamin K and coumarin anticoagulants: dependence of anticoagulant effect on inhibition of vitamin K transport. *Science 164*:181.

Lowenthal, J., and J. A. MacFarlane. 1967. Use of a competitive vitamin K antagonist, 2-chloro-3-phytyl-1,4-naphthoquinone, for the study of the mechanism of action of vitamin K and coumarin anticoagulants. *J. Pharmacol. Exp. Ther. 157*:672.

Lowenthal, J., and E. L. Simmons. 1967. Failure of actinomycin D to inhibit appearance of clotting activity by vitamin K *in vitro*. *Experientia 23*:421.

Martius, C. 1967. Chemistry and function of vitamin K, pp. 551–575. *In* W. H. Seegers (ed.), *Blood Clotting Enzymology*. Academic Press, New York.

Martius, C., and D. Nitz-Litzow. 1954. Oxydative phosphorylierung und vitamin K mangel. *Biochim. Biophys. Acta 13*:152.

Olson, J. P., L. L. Miller, and S. B. Troup. 1966. Synthesis of clotting factors by the isolated perfused rat liver. *J. Clin. Invest. 45*:690.

Olson, R. E. 1964. Vitamin K induced prothrombin formation: antagonism by actinomycin D. *Science 145*:926.

Olson, R. E. 1965. The regulatory function of the fat-soluble vitamins. *Can. J. Biochem. Physiol. 43*:1565.

Olson, R. E., G. Philipps, and N. Wang. 1968. The regulatory action of vitamin K. *Advances Enzyme Regulation 6*:213.

O'Reilly, R. A., P. M. Aggeler, M. S. Hoag, L. S. Leong, and M. L. Kropatking. 1964. Hereditary transmission of exceptional resistance to coumarin anticoagulant drugs. The first reported kindred. *New Engl. J. Med. 271*:809.

Paolucci, A. M., S. Gaetani, and B. C. Johnson. 1964. Vitamin K e sintesi proteica I: Sintesi indotta di triptofano pirrolasi in ratti carenti di vitamina K. *Quad. Nutr. 24*:275.

Paolucci, A. M., P. B. R. Rao, and B. C. Johnson. 1963. Vitamin K deficiency and oxidative phosphorylation. *J. Nutr. 81*:17.

Pool, J. G., R. A. O'Reilly, L. J. Schneiderman, and M. Alexander. 1968. Warfarin resistance in the rat. *Amer. J. Physiol. 215*:627.

Prydz, H. 1965. Studies on proconvertin (factor VII). VII. Further studies on the biosynthesis of factor VII in rat cell suspensions. *Scand. J. Clin. Lab. Invest. 17*:143.

Quick, A. J. 1966. Current blood clotting schemes. *Thromb. Diath. Haemorrh. 16*:318.

Ranhotra, G. S., and B. C. Johnson. 1969. On the site of action of vitamin K. *Fed. Proc. 28*:385 (Abstr.)

Seegers, W. H. 1962. *Prothrombin.* Harvard Univ. Press, Cambridge.

Seegers, W. H., L. McCoy, and E. Marciniak. 1968. Blood-clotting enzymology, three basic reactions. *Clin. Chem. 14*:97.

Suttie, J. W. 1967. Control of prothrombin and factor VII biosynthesis by vitamin K. *Arch. Biochem. Biophys. 118*:166.

Suttie, J. W. 1969. The control of clotting factor biosynthesis by vitamin K. *Fed. Proc. 28*:1696.

Thierry, M. J., and J. W. Suttie. 1969. Distribution and metabolism of menadiol diphosphate in the rat. *J. Nutr. 97*:512.

Tocantins, L. M., and L. A. Kazal (eds.). 1964. *Blood Coagulation, Hemorrhage and Thrombosis: Methods of Study,* p. 519. Grune and Stratton, New York.

Wosilait, W. D. 1966. Effect of vitamin K deficiency on the adenosine nucleotide content of chicken liver. *Biochem. Pharmacol. 15*:204.

29

STUDIES OF THE IN VITRO BIOSYNTHESIS OF VITAMIN K–DEPENDENT CLOTTING PROTEINS

Robert E. Olson

Introduction

The function of the fat-soluble vitamins at the molecular level is still an unsolved problem in biology. Dr. Steenbock was very much aware of the need for a unifying hypothesis for lipid vitamin action. In 1955 he wrote: "In the past, it has been assumed that vitamin D is primarily influential in the absorption and deposition of bone salts but it is suggested by our results . . . that more consideration should be given to the possibility that vitamin D exerts a widespread effect upon organic tissue metabolism of which increased growth is one manifestation" (Steenbock and Herting, 1955). I believe that he would be pleased to see the current developments in this field in which he pioneered.

My own interest in the field of fat-soluble vitamins originated with studies of the role of vitamin E in the prevention of acute hepatic necrosis in the rat. This disorder, independently described in three laboratories (Daft et al, 1942; György and Goldblatt, 1942; Schwarz, 1944), was responsive to cystine supplementation, was partially prevented by some antioxidants (e.g., DPPD) but not by others of equal potency, and was totally prevented by both α-tocopherol and inorganic selenium. Our view of the disorder was that it represented an alteration of sulfur–amino acid metabolism which was corrected at different points by one or more of the pro-

These studies were supported in part by Grant AM–09992 from the National Institute of Arthritis and Metabolic Diseases, U.S. Public Health Service, Bethesda, Maryland.

I am greatly indebted to my colleagues who have carried out the experiments discussed in this report and have been a continuing source of inspiration to me. They are Dr. G. H. Dialameh, Dr. Roger K. Kipfer, Dr. Lan-Fun Li, Dr. G. R Philipps, Mrs. Elizabeth Berry, Mrs. Jeanette Block, Mrs. Katherine Compagno, Mrs. Marilyn Johnston, Miss Lourdes Maglasang, Mr. K. Park, Mr. Dan Walz, and Mrs. Kay Wilbur.

tective agents (Olson and Dinning, 1954). I was at Oxford University on sabbatical leave from the University of Pittsburgh when the paper of Jacob and Monod (1961) appeared, proposing a new hypothesis to account for the induction of β-galactosidase in *E. coli.* This hypothesis, now a dogma in biology, postulates interactions of inducer molecules with a repressor protein, which in turn interacts with the DNA-operon at an operator site and permits the expression or the nonexpression of genetic information. It was soon hailed as a model to account for changes in enzyme level in mammalian systems, particularly those changes occurring under the influence of steroid hormones.*

It suddenly occurred to me that the theory might also account for the changes in concentration of proteins and enzymes observed in association with diseases caused by deficiencies of α-tocopherol and the other fat-soluble vitamins. Such a hypothesis could explain the interaction of a variety of compounds with a regulatory protein. Thus the replaceability of α-tocopherol by selenium and selected antioxidants (if their molecular size and shape permitted association with such a hypothetical repressor protein) could be explained. Further arguments in favor of the hypothesis were completely a priori: (1) The coenzyme theory had failed to explain the action of the lipid vitamins; (2) The action of the fat-soluble vitamins in highly differentiated animals are expressed by biological activities which in many ways are closer to the action of the steroid hormones than to that of the B-complex vitamins; (3) The fat-soluble vitamins are structurally related to the steroid hormones in the sense that all of them, to a greater or lesser extent, are products of isoprene polymerization; and (4) Since nutrient requirements are accidents of evolutionary deletion of biosynthetic enzyme systems, there is no a priori reason for believing that all trace nutrients should function in a predictable manner.

When I returned from Oxford to Pittsburgh in late 1962 and began to design and carry out some preliminary studies of this hypothesis in the vitamin E–deficient rat, some of the experimental difficulties became evident. The most obvious difficulty in testing the hypotheses in vitamin E deficiency was the fact that there was no presumed gene product for which the vitamin could be considered a regulator. In fact, in vitamin E deficiency, many of the enzymes associated with dystrophic and necrotic states are increased, rather than decreased, in the deficient state. These enzymes include an array of lysosomal enzymes and others, such as xanthine oxidase and creatine phosphokinase (Olson, 1967).

* Sir Hans Krebs, who was studying the effects of glucocorticoids on gluconeogenesis, was the first (to my knowledge) to suggest that the Jacob-Monod theory might apply to enzyme induction in mammals; he did so in a lecture at Oxford University on January 29, 1962.

What about the other fat-soluble vitamins? A quick survey indicated that the vitamin K–prothrombin system appeared to be ideal for study of this hypothesis. In this case, a fat-soluble vitamin was indubitably related to the synthesis or the release of several proteins concerned with coagulation. In addition to prothrombin (factor II), three other vitamin K–dependent proteins were known (factors VII, IX, and X). Furthermore, disorders of coagulation were known in which there was genetic deletion of one or more of these factors and resultant insensitivity to vitamin K therapy.

Shortly after the discovery of vitamin K, it was shown by Dam and his co-workers (1936) that the principal effect of vitamin K deficiency in the chick is a reduction in the content of plasma prothrombin. These workers suggested that vitamin K might be a part of the prothrombin molecule, but this postulate has not been confirmed in many laboratories which have sought evidence for it. Subsequently, Martius and Nitz-Litzow (1954) proposed that the defective prothrombin formation in vitamin K–deficient chicks could be explained on the basis of a primary disorder of energy conservation, i.e., the failure to synthesize ATP at an appropriate rate. This analysis was based upon the presumption that vitamin K is involved in electron transport and in the coupling reactions between electron transport and phosphate uptake in avian and in mammalian mitochondria. Martius and Nitz-Litzow argued that coagulation factors would be especially sensitive to ATP lack because they possess biological half-lives of short duration. This imaginative hypothesis has not, however, been confirmed in many studies in which (1) the presence of vitamin K in the mammalian electron-transport system has been sought (Colpa-Boonstra and Slater, 1958); (2) P/O-ratios have been measured in mitochondria from vitamin K–deficient and from dicoumarol-treated rats and chicks (Beyer and Kennison, 1959; Paolucci et al., 1963); and (3) the distribution of adenine nucleotides in the liver of vitamin K–deficient chicks was measured (Wosilait, 1966). All tests of Martius and Nitz-Litzow's hypothesis have given negative results. Therefore, in 1963, we undertook experiments in vitamin K–deficient chicks and rats to implicate the action of vitamin K in the regulation of specific *de novo* protein syntheses.

Hypotheses for the action of vitamin K at the molecular level

The great advances in our understanding of the molecular biology of protein synthesis over the past two decades, summarized in the Cold Spring Harbor Symposium of Quantitative Biology (Crick, 1966), provided a basis for studying the role of vitamin K in the various stages in the transfer of biochemical information from the genome of the liver cell to the ribosome, thence to the cytoplasm, and finally across the cell membrane to the plasma. Figure 29.1 presents a number of possibilities for the action of vitamin K in regulating the synthesis and the secretion of prothrombin and related clotting proenzymes. The steps which are involved and which could be subject to regulation include (1) the transcription of DNA to a messenger RNA (mRNA), (2) the assimilation of this mRNA by the polysome, (3) the translation of this message into a polypeptide sequence by the polysome, (4) the release of the nascent peptide into the medium and its conjugation with its glycid (carbohydrate) moiety, and (5) the secretion of the newly synthesized prothrombin into the circulation. Since pro-

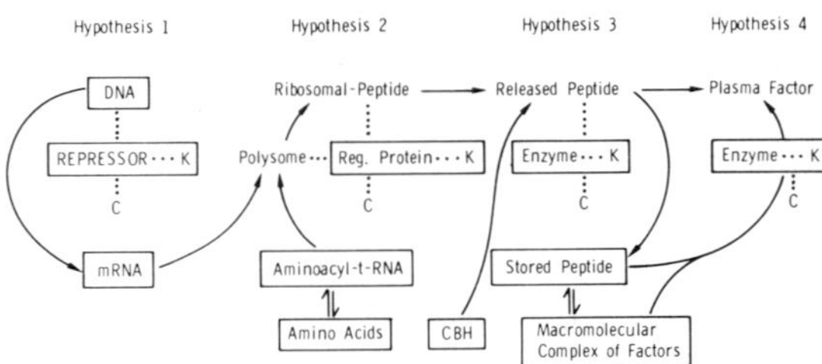

Fig. 29.1. Hypotheses for the mode of action of vitamin K in regulating the biosynthesis and/or the release of vitamin K–dependent clotting factors to plasma. K = vitamin K; C = coumarin anticoagulant drug; CBH = carbohydrate.

thrombin and the other vitamin K–dependent factors are manufactured by the liver for export, it was evident in 1963, as it is now, that there are basically four major steps in the above biosynthetic and secretory sequence which could be regulated by vitamin K. These have become the basis of four, essentially mutually exclusive, hypotheses which have been, and still are, under intensive scrutiny.

The first hypothesis provides that vitamin K and the coumarin drugs react allosterically with a repressor protein to alter the activity of the DNA operator for synthesis of the respective mRNA's for prothrombin and the related vitamin K–dependent coagulation proteins. This mode of action is typical of genetic regulation (Jacob and Monod, 1961) and was the hypothesis first proposed by us (Olson, 1964) for the action of vitamin K in which the response of vitamin K–deficient chicks to that vitamin was altered by actinomycin D. It is now clear that these experiments were misinterpreted by us, since it has been shown subsequently by us and by others that the response of vitamin K–deficient chicks to vitamin K in the presence of actinomycin D is a function of the time which elapses between the administration of the antibiotic and the administration of the vitamin (Johnson et al., 1966; Hill et al., 1968; Prydz, 1965; Olson et al., 1968*b*; Suttie, 1967). In fact, in contrast to the mRNA for hemoglobin, which has a relatively long life (ca. 2 days), the mRNA for prothrombin in the chick is relatively short-lived, having a half-life on the order of 4 hr. In our original experiments, we were blocking synthesis of all mRNA's, including the messenger for prothrombin, and hence were observing reduced responses to vitamin K administration after 4 hr because of the reduced availability of template. Those data did not assist in pinpointing the site of action of vitamin K except to eliminate hypothesis 1 as a likely possibility.

Hypothesis 2 provides for the interaction of a regulatory protein which binds vitamin K and coumarin drugs with some element of the ribosomal-mRNA-tRNA-binding factors complex to facilitate either initiation or termination of specific peptide synthesis. Central to this hypothesis is the view that vitamin K directly regulates specific protein synthesis at the ribosomal level rather than regulating some ancillary event which, in turn, triggers vitamin K–dependent protein synthesis. The fact that puromycin inhibits prothrombin and factor VII synthesis in intact chicks (Olson, 1966), in rats (Johnson et al., 1966), and in the isolated perfused liver (Suttie, 1967; Olson et al., 1968*a*) strongly supports the view that new protein synthesis is involved in the action of vitamin K. If initiation of peptide synthesis is regulated, the regulatory protein in the proper conformation must recognize the prothrombin messenger attached to the 40 *S* ribosome particle. If termination is regulated, the regulatory protein in the proper conformation must recognize a complementary peptide sequence, must combine with it, and must block further synthetic activity (or release of peptide) by the ribosome. The latter idea was first suggested by Vogel (1957) and was elaborated by Cline and Bock (1966). This general type of regulation is also consistent with the studies by Barnhart and Anderson (1962) in which they showed, with the aid of immunofluorescent antibody to prothrombin, that Dicumarol-treated animals show no evidence of prothrombin in parenchymal cells and that prothrombin appeared promptly in these cells (in association with the endoplasmic reticulum) after administration of vitamin K_1.

It seems quite clear from many lines of study in intact animals, in the isolated perfused rat liver, and in microsomes (Hill, et al., 1963, 1968; Berry et al., 1966; Olson et al., 1969*b*) that there is no change in general protein synthesis in vitamin K deficiency or in coumarin-induced anticoagulant states in vivo. The action of vitamin K in the regulation of protein synthesis is thus confined to the control of the vitamin K–dependent proteins.

Hypothesis 3 provides for the interaction of vitamin K (or its coenzyme derivative) and an enzyme that is involved in the conversion of the nascent peptide into its final folded (and complete) structure. Action at this point might include the step in which the glycid moiety is added to the peptide chain. This action of vitamin K, which does not occur until *after* the peptide has been converted into its final structure on the ribosome, has been proposed by B. C. Johnson and his co-workers (Hill et al., 1968) as best explaining the action of vitamin K. This conclusion was based in part upon the failure of cycloheximide to prevent the action of vitamin K in vivo, which may have another explanation (Olson et al., 1969*a*).

Hypothesis 4 provides for an action of vitamin K concerned not with protein synthesis, but rather with the release of preformed clotting proenzyme or a complex thereof from the liver. The link between the release of peptide from hepatic stores and the subsequent activation of protein synthesis has not been defined. The hypothesis has been supported by Babior (1966), by Leon Miller and his associates (Olson et al., 1966) and by Lowenthal and Birnbaum (1969). For poorly understood reasons, these investigators found little, if any, effect of inhibitors of protein synthesis upon output of factors from their in vitro preparations. A related hypothesis by Hemker and co-workers (1963) postulates that in vitamin K deficiency there is an accumulation of preprothrombin in liver and plasma which disappears on the administration of vitamin K.

In all four hypotheses shown in Figure 29.1, the antagonism between vitamin K and the coumarin drugs is accounted for by postulating an allosteric interaction of the two effectors with a single protein or enzyme (Olson et al., 1966). Most investigators (Babson et al., 1956; Woolley, 1947; Lowenthal and MacFarlane, 1964) agree that the antagonism between vitamin K and the 4-hydroxy-coumarins is not a classical competitive one, although Quick and Collentine (1950), and more recently Hermodson and co-workers (1969), have postulated a competitive antagonism between the two agents. Lowenthal and MacFarlane (1964) prefer a dual transport system to account for the anomalous competition between warfarin and vitamin K. In any event, much of the evidence bearing on these alternative hypotheses obtained from whole animals, and even from in vitro systems, is controversial and conflicting.

It appeared to us that the problem could not be advanced by further studies in whole animals, and thus we undertook the study of the biosynthesis of prothrombin and related vitamin K–dependent clotting proteins in isolated systems in vitro. In this chapter I wish to report experiments carried out in two such systems. The first is the isolated perfused rat liver, which, as first demonstrated by Mattii and co-workers (1964), is an excellent system for the study of the elaboration of clotting factors under the influence of vitamin K. The second is a cell-free system of light microsomes from rat liver which is capable of vigorous general protein synthesis and in which the specific syntheses of plasma prothrombin and plasma albumin have been demonstrated by immunochemical means.

Studies of vitamin K–dependent protein biosynthesis in the isolated perfused rat liver

Livers from normal rats and from vitamin K–deficient rats were isolated and perfused by the basic technique of Miller and co-workers (1951). The medium was Krebs-Ringer bicarbonate containing 20% washed red cells, 3% bovine-serum albumin, all the L-amino acids in a concentration totaling 80 mg percent, and glucose at 300 mg/100 ml (Olson et al., 1966). Heparin (10 U.S.P. units/ml) was added to effect in vitro anticoagulation, and it was removed at the termination of the experiment by titration with protamine. Terramycin (10 mg/100 ml was added to prevent bacterial growth. In given experiments, puromycin, cycloheximide, warfarin, and vitamin K_1 (as AquaMephyton) were added to the perfusion medium at given times. The *p*H of the system was kept constant by automatic infusion of 0.15 M $NaHCO_3$ by a radiometer *p*H meter set at 7.4. Prothrombin was assayed at intervals by the method of Hjort and co-workers (1955), which is a simple one-stage prothrombin assay that depends upon the action of Russell's viper venom (RVV). Stuart's factor X was determined by the method of Denson (1961), factor VII was determined by the method of Owren and Aas (1951), and factor IX was determined by the method of Stapp (1965). In some experiments, the prothrombin was also detected immunochemically by a specific antibody. Antisera against pure rat prothrombin were prepared in rabbits according to the method of Li and Olson (1967) and Li and co-workers (1970*b*). The rat prothrombin assayed 3600 Iowa units per milligram of protein and gave a single band on polyacrylamide-gel electrophoresis. The antibody formed in the rabbit gave a single line by double diffusion on an Ouchterlony plate and a single line by immunoelectrophoresis. The antibody also formed a good precipitin. The radioactivity of biosynthesized prothrombin was measured by precipitating the prothrombin from the perfusate with its specific antibody for 4 days at 4 C. The final precipitates were collected by centrifugation, washed with physiologic saline, and counted in Bray's solution in a Packard scintillation spectrometer.

The study of metabolites during the perfusion described above revealed that the glucose concentration remained relatively constant at 300 ± 50 mg/100 ml during the 6-hr period. Total amino acid nitrogen increased slightly from 8 mg/100 ml to 10 mg/100 ml. When individual amino acids were studied by ion-exchange chromatography, it was observed that certain amino acids increased in concentration during the course of the perfusion and that certain others decreased. The amino acids that increased were glutamic acid, isoleucine, leucine, and valine. Amino acids remaining relatively constant were serine and threonine. Amino acids declining in concentration during the 6-hr period were alanine, glycine, aspartic acid, phenylalanine, and proline. Of particular interest is the fact that the leucine concentration increased about five-fold during the 6-hr incubation (Li et al., 1970*a*).

When radioactive leucine was introduced at the beginning of the experiment, the concentration of radioactivity in the protein-free fractions declined exponentially with time, whereas the radioactivity of the total protein increased linearly with time (Fig. 29.2). The rising free-leucine concentration indicates that the specific activity of the leucine was decreasing more rapidly than the total radioactivity during the 6-hr period. Lactate also rose from 2 μM/ml to 7 μM/ml during the period of perfusion and accounted for 50% of the free acid produced during the 6-hr

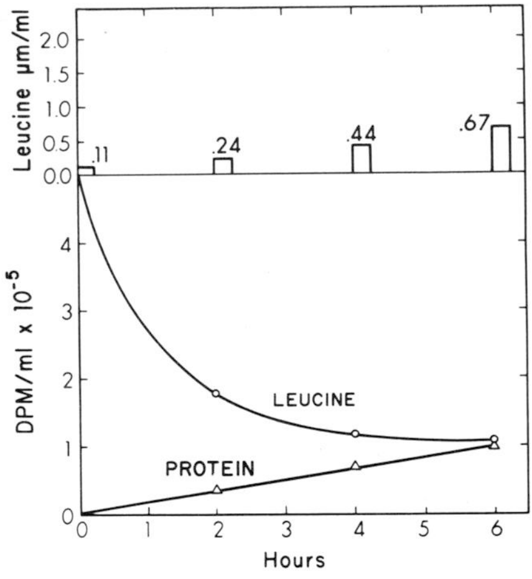

Fig. 29.2. Metabolism of $1\text{-}^{14}C$ L-leucine in the isolated, perfused rat liver. The top panel shows the changes in concentration of free leucine at various times.

period. The presence or the absence of vitamin K_1 did not affect the disappearance of leucine radioactivity from the plasma, the total protein synthesis, or the appearance of lactate.

To determine the response of vitamin K–dependent clotting proenzymes to the addition of vitamin K to the perfusate of the isolated rat liver, we have carried out experiments with three rat-liver preparations: (*1*) livers from normal rats, without warfarin in the perfusate; (*2*) livers from normal rats, with warfarin added to the perfusate; and (*3*) livers from vitamin K–deficient rats, without warfarin in the perfusate. In the experiments with the third preparation, we have discovered an enormous variability in various strains of rats to induction of vitamin K deficiency. Even rats of the same strain inbred in separate colonies may show variable retention of endogenous vitamin K and variable sensitivity to vitamin K added in vitro. Certain Sprague-Dawley rats appear to be best suited for these studies.

Figure 29.3 presents the results of a sample perfusion of a normal rat liver without warfarin. Note that the yield of prothrombin is relatively low (i.e., 3% of normal values), in agreement with Kazmeier and coworkers (1968). If vitamin K is added after 2 hr in amounts of 1 mg to yield a concentration in the perfusate of 5 μg/ml, the output of prothrombin is increased, but not dramatically, to a level of about 5%. Higher doses (50 μg/ml) of vitamin K had no additional effect in the normal liver. The "zero time" value (taken 10 min after the liver is in the circuit) of 2% of the normal plasma value of prothrombin is characteristic of normal rats not pretreated with warfarin or subjected to depletion of vitamin K. This initial prothrombin apparently represents preformed prothrombin which leaks out of the liver within minutes of the initiation of perfusion.

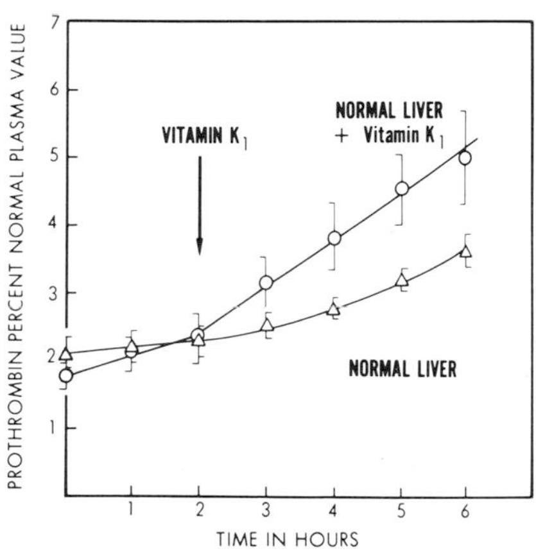

Fig. 29.3. Effect of vitamin K_1 (5 μg/ml) upon prothrombin production over a 6-hr period in an isolated, perfused, normal rat liver. The lower curve shows the production without the addition of vitamin K_1. Values for prothrombin production, measured as the percentage of the normal plasma value, are given as mean ± SE.

Figure 29.4 shows that normal rats treated in vitro with warfarin at concentrations of 10 μg/ml show no release of prothrombin. When vitamin K_1 is given, there is a very brisk increase in prothrombin concentration to values higher than those observed in the normal rat liver. It would appear that the potential rate of production of prothrombin is enhanced by treatment with warfarin. The presence of puromycin at concentrations of 200 μg/ml abolished the response to vitamin K under these conditions (Olson et al., 1969*b*).

At higher concentrations of warfarin, larger amounts of vitamin K are required. Figure 29.5 illustrates the effect of adding various doses (from 1 mg to 15 mg, i.e., 5–75 μg/ml) of vitamin K_1. When the concentration of warfarin in the medium was 10 μg/ml, there was a steep slope to the vitamin K–response curve over the range 0–5 μg/ml. On the other hand, with a warfarin concentration of 30 μg/ml, higher doses of vitamin K_1 are required to reach a maximum response: 5 μg/ml of vitamin K_1 had a negligible effect, but 50 μg/ml was highly effective. The dose-response

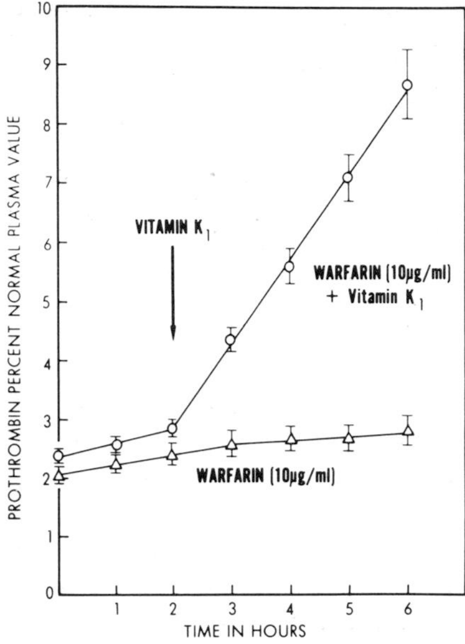

Fig. 29.4. Effect of vitamin K_1 (5 $\mu g/ml$) upon prothrombin production over a 6-hr period in an isolated, perfused, normal rat liver that had been incubated with 10 $\mu g/ml$ of warfarin. The lower curve shows the effect of warfarin alone. Values for prothrombin production, measured as the percentage of the normal plasma value, are given as mean ± SE.

curve is clearly sigmoid, thus pointing to an allosteric interaction of the coumarin drug and vitamin K_1 with a single regulatory protein in the system.

Much lower doses of vitamin K are required in vitro to stimulate maximum factor synthesis in the isolated liver from a vitamin K–deficient animal. Figure 29.6 presents the results of a study of an isolated liver ob-

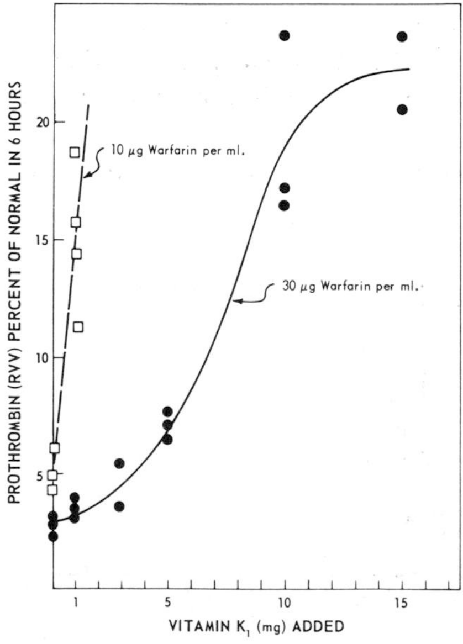

Fig. 29.5. Effect of vitamin K_1 dosage on prothrombin production over a 6-hr period in isolated rat liver to which 10 $\mu g/ml$ and 30 $\mu g/ml$ of warfarin had been added initially.

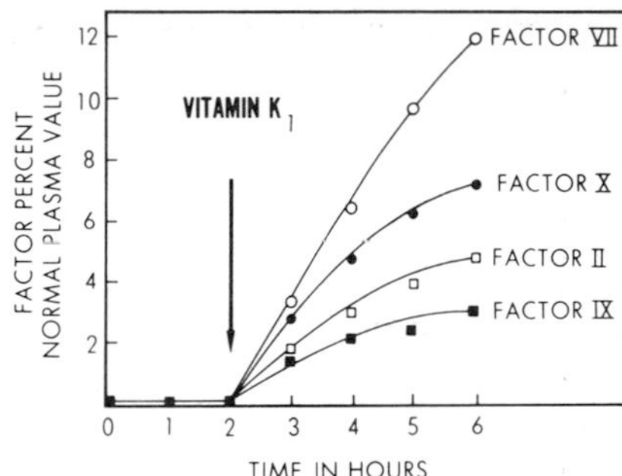

Fig. 29.6. Effect of vitamin K_1 (0.5 μg/ml) upon the elaboration of the vitamin K–dependent coagulation factors by isolated, perfused liver derived from a vitamin K–deficient rat.

tained from a vitamin K–deficient rat in which all of the vitamin K–dependent clotting factors are reduced to less than 10% of normal plasma values. Under these conditions, there was no "blank value" of clotting factors detectable in the perfusate before the addition of the vitamin. Upon the addition of vitamin K_1 in a dose exceeding 0.5 μg/ml, all the vitamin K–dependent factors appeared promptly after the addition of the vitamins. Factor VII was produced in the largest relative amount, reaching 12% of normal plasma values in the rat. Factor X (7%) was next best synthesized, followed by factor II (5%) and factor IX (3%).

The threshold for the appearance of the four factors in this system also varied. The doses of vitamin K required to give half maximum responses for the various vitamin K–dependent factors were as follows: factor VII, 0.001 μg/ml; factor II, 0.002 μg/ml; factor X, 0.005 μg/ml; factor IX, 0.1 μg/ml. Saturation kinetics were observed in most instances, independent of the elaboration of other factors. In the case of factor X, however, inhibition of response by high doses of vitamin K was noted. At 0.005 μg/ml of vitamin K, factor X synthesis reached 10% of normal plasma values in 4 hr, whereas at 50 μg/ml, it was reduced to a maximum of 4% in the same period.

Figure 29.7 represents the dose-response curve for prothrombin in the

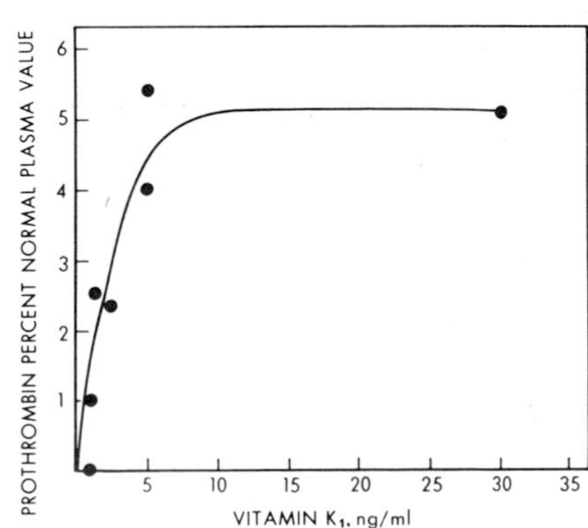

Fig. 29.7. Prothrombin output (in 4 hr) as a function of vitamin K_1 concentration in isolated, perfused liver from a vitamin K–deficient rat.

isolated vitamin K–deficient rat liver. It can be seen that the concentration required to reach half maximum activity is approximately 2 ng/ml, and the curve has a classical shape representing Michaelis-Mentlen kinetics, even though it represents interaction between whole cells and factors in the perfusion medium.

Of great interest was the discovery in our laboratory (Olson et al., 1969*a*) that cycloheximide blockade of general protein synthesis in the isolated perfused liver can be overcome for the vitamin K–dependent proteins by large doses of vitamin K_1. A series of experiments showing the degree of inhibition of prothrombin synthesis at two concentrations of cycloheximide in the presence of various concentrations of vitamin K are presented in Figure 29.8. The kinetic data are presented in a semilogarithmic fashion, the prothrombin production in 4 hr being plotted against the logarithm of the vitamin K_1 dose. The response in the presence of no inhibitor shows typical sigmoid kinetics that are characteristic of an enzyme-

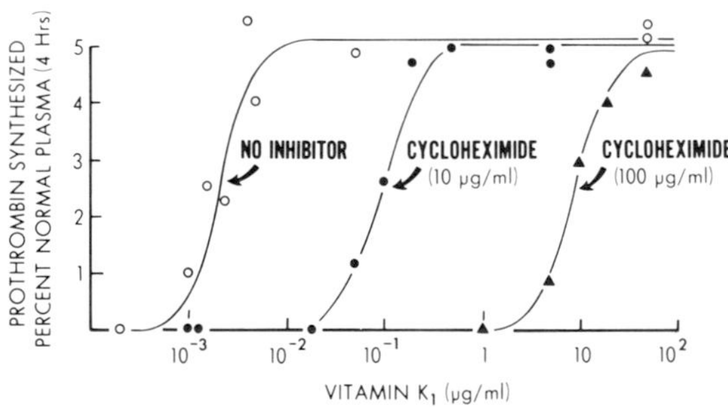

Fig. 29.8. Effect of two concentrations of cycloheximide on the dose-response relationship between vitamin K_1 and prothrombin in isolated, perfused liver from a vitamin K–deficient rat.

substrate interaction. When cycloheximide was added to the perfusate at 10 μg/ml, the dose of vitamin K_1 required to overcome the inhibition had to be increased about two orders of magnitude. When the cycloheximide was further increased to 100 μg/ml, the concentration of vitamin K required to reach half maximum response was increased another two orders of magnitude. Nonetheless, V_{max} was ultimately reached in the presence of inhibitor, signaling a competitive inhibition. Double reciprocal plots of these data, confirm the competitive nature of the antagonism between vitamin K and cycloheximide (Fig. 29.9). Since calculation of the K_1 value for the two inhibitor concentrations gave different values, however, it is believed that the antagonism is of the partially competitive, or pseudocompetitive, type rather than of the type representing competition of two ligands for a single site on a protein. This interpretation, in fact, is consistent with the model presented in Figure 29.14.

1-^{14}C L-leucine was added to isolated, perfused livers from vitamin K–deficient rats in the presence and in the absence of 100 μg/ml of cyclo-

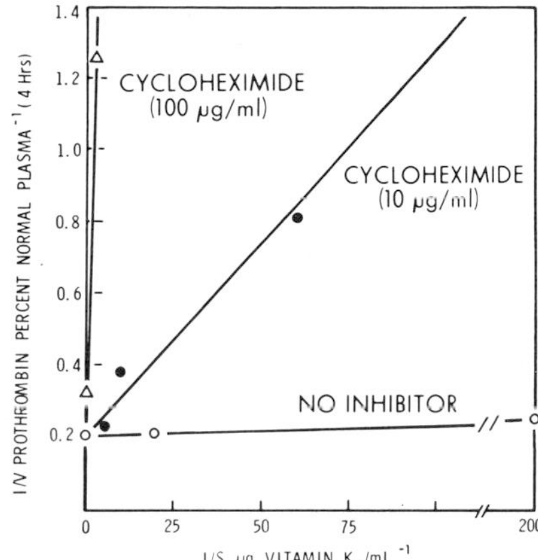

Fig. 29.9. Double reciprocal plots of velocity as a function of vitamin K_1 concentration in the presence and in the absence of cycloheximide, observed in isolated, perfused liver from vitamin K–deficient rats.

heximide. In the presence of the antibiotic general protein synthesis was markedly inhibited to the extent of 97% (Table 29.1). The effect was visible in the liver as well as in the perfusate. In the presence of small doses of vitamin K_1, the distribution of radioactivity was unaffected. In the presence of vitamin K_1 in amounts large enough to reverse the block of vitamin K–dependent factor synthesis, the radioactivity of both liver and plasma proteins was significantly increased after 6 hr. It is likely that this increase in radioactivity represents the manufacture and release of the vitamin K–dependent clotting proteins.

The contrast in the action of puromycin and of cycloheximide in the isolated liver from vitamin K–deficient rats is shown in Figure 29.10. The cycloheximide blockade is removed when the concentration of vitamin K_1 in the perfusate reaches 50 μg/ml, whereas the blockade imposed

TABLE 29.1. *Effect of vitamin K and cycloheximide on protein synthesis in the isolated perfused liver from vitamin K–deficient rats*

Experiment	Vitamin K_1 (μg/ml)	Cycloheximide (μg/ml)	Plasma protein[a] (dpm/ml)[b]	Liver protein (dpm/ml)[b]
1	[c]	0	25,200 ± 1610	1770 ± 204
2	[c]	100	508 ± 89	70 ± 9
3	50	100	801 ± 65	228 ± 18

Note: 10 μCi of 1-^{14}C L-leucine was added to the perfusate at zero time. Cycloheximide was added at zero time; vitamin K_1 was added at 2 hr.

[a] Each milliliter of perfusion fluid contained about 35 mg of protein, of which 30 mg was bovine-serum albumin.

[b] Measured at 6 hr. Values are given as mean ± SE.

[c] Vitamin K_1 was added at 5μg/ml or was not added. Protein synthesis was not affected at this dose.

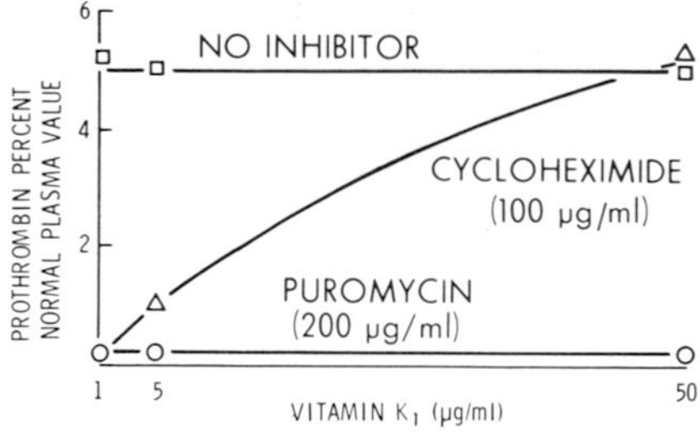

Fig. 29.10. Effect of puromycin and of cycloheximide on the synthesis of prothrombin by isolated, perfused liver from vitamin K–deficient rats.

by puromycin is irreversible. Since puromycin blocks protein synthesis by chain termination and cycloheximide blocks protein synthesis by stopping chain initiation and elongation, the reversibility of cycloheximide action by vitamin K points to a mechanism of regulation involving chain initiation.

If vitamin K controls prothrombin biosynthesis at the translational level, it seemed important to demonstrate that the product of vitamin K action was newly synthesized from amino acids available to the liver polysome. As already pointed out, when 1-^{14}C L-leucine was added to the perfusate at zero time, the rat liver takes up the isotopic amino acid rapidly and engages in general protein synthesis, including the elaboration of plasma proteins at a rate not affected by the presence or absence of vitamin K. In order to study the incorporation of radioactive leucine into prothrombin in the presence or absence of vitamin K, samples were taken at the end of 6-hr experiments in which 50 μCi of radioactive leucine had been added during the period of perfusion. Excess radioactive amino acids were removed from the protein fraction by Sephadex G–25 chromatography, and the protein fraction was treated with antibody to rat prothrombin at 4 C for 4 days.

The results of three such experiments are shown in Table 29.2. Each experiment consisted of a pair of perfusions, one to which vitamin K was added and one to which no vitamin K was added. The first two experiments were with normal animals in which the livers were warfarinized in vitro with 10 μg/ml. The third experiment was with livers from vitamin K–deficient animals. In all cases, the radioactivity found in the antibody precipitate per milliliter of perfusate correlated roughly with the amount of prothrombin determined by clotting assay. The data from experiment 1 have been plotted as a function of time in Figure 29.11, in which the specific activity of free 1-^{14}C L-leucine in the perfusate and of prothrombin-bound leucine are plotted on the same scale. The increase in total prothrombin is also shown. Specific activity of free leucine in this experiment declined from 3×10^6 dpm/μmole to 1.5×10^5 dpm/μmole at the end of 6 hr. This marked change is due to both a decline in total

TABLE 29.2. *Immunochemical measurement of prothrombin biosynthesized by rat liver perfused with radioactive amino acids*

Vitamin K_1	Prothrombin activity (% of normal)	Perfusate prothrombin (dpm/ml)
Warfarinized liver (Exp. 1)[a]		
25 μg/ml	14.0	4237
0 μg/ml	2.0	828
Warfarinized liver (Exp. 2)[a]		
25 μg/ml	8.2	1020
0 μg/ml	2.0	168
Vitamin K–deficient liver		
1 μg/ml	5.5	1800
0 μg/ml	0.1	120

Note: 50 μCi of 1-^{14}C L-leucine was used. Blanks obtained by the use of indifferent precipitins were subtracted from the total dpm.

[a] Liver from normal animals, with 10 μg/ml of warfarin added to the perfusate.

radioactivity and a rise in leucine content during the perfusion. The amount of prothrombin-bound leucine can be calculated from the content of prothrombin and the known amino acid composition of the molecule. When the prothrombin-bound leucine is related to the differences between the treated and the untreated perfusate, it can be seen that the prothrombin-bound leucine has a specific activity, as shown, of about 1.7×10^6 dpm/μmole, suggesting that the pool of radioactive leucine from which this prothrombin was derived was more radioactive than the perfusate at the time of incorporation into prothrombin. The correspondence between the radioactivity of prothrombin and the total concentration of the prothrombin suggests very strongly that vitamin K influences the *de novo* biosynthesis of the coagulation protein in the isolated perfused rat liver. Experiment 3 was conducted on a liver from a vitamin K–defi-

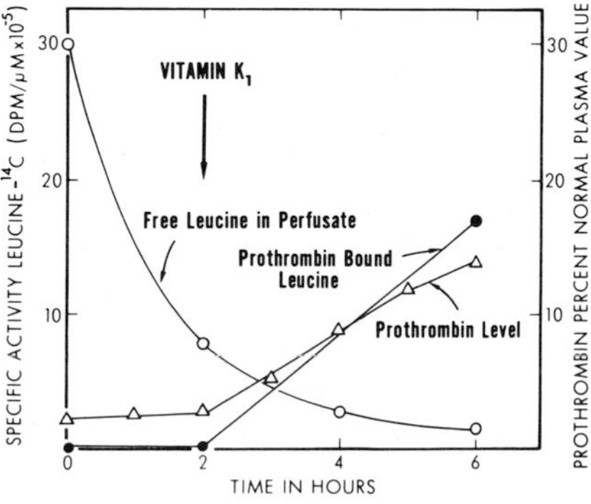

Fig. 29.11. Specific activity of free and of prothrombin-bound 1-^{14}C L-leucine and total prothrombin production during 6 hr of perfusion of an isolated rat liver. Warfarin was present at 10 μg/ml. The dose of vitamin K was 5 mg.

cient animal, and similar results were obtained with a somewhat lower dose of the vitamin.

These studies demonstrate (1) that vitamin K_1 stimulates the appearance of prothrombin in the perfusate of the isolated rat liver when added in vitro, (2) that the prothrombin appears to be derived from free amino acids which are present in the liver at the time of the addition of vitamin K_1, and (3) that this process is inhibited irreversibly by puromycin and reversibly by cycloheximide. These observations constitute good evidence that the action of vitamin K is to stimulate *de novo* biosynthesis of prothrombin before its release from the liver.

Prothrombin biosynthesis in a cell-free system

Attempts to demonstrate the biosynthesis of prothrombin and of related vitamin K–dependent clotting factors in cell-free systems have been equivocal and, in some instances, irreproducible. Lasch and Roka (1953) reported that rat-liver mitochondria, in the presence of serum, would synthesize factor VII and convert it to prothrombin. Pool and Robinson (1959) could not confirm this observation and observed that intact liver cells were required for factor VII synthesis. Goswami and Munro (1962), employing the Allington reagent (1958) for the detection of prothrombin, observed that heavy microsomes isolated from rat liver contained appreciable amounts of assayable prothrombin, which increased upon incubation in Krebs-Ringer bicarbonate medium for 3 hr. These results were confirmed by Hill and co-workers (1968), using the same clotting assay. They also observed that assayable prothrombin appeared to be markedly decreased in microsomes from vitamin K–deficient or from coumarin-drug-treated rats.

In our attempts to confirm and extend the observations of Goswami and Munro (1962), some of the limitations of the Allington reagent for the detection of prothrombin became evident (Johnston et al., 1968). Originally modified from the method of Owren and Aas (1951) for use in the clinic, the Allington reagent uses as a component an incompletely adsorbed bovine plasma containing residual prothrombin. We found 15 rat units (1 ml of rat plasma contains 100 rat units) of prothrombin per milliliter of reagent. This reagent shortens the clotting times in the clinic but also poses some problems for investigators studying tissue extracts. When adsorbed serum fortified with fibrinogen was substituted for the Allington reagent, no prothrombin could be detected in microsomes from normal liver. Likewise, the two-stage method of Ware and Seegers (1949) gave no detectable prothrombin in microsomes from normal rat liver. The questions then arose, What factor caused the apparent increase in prothrombin with incubation? and Why did vitamin K–deficient rats seem to have less of this mystical factor? It occurred to us that lysosomal enzymes, known to be present in the heavy-microsome fraction, might be instrumental in activating the prothrombin present in the reagent, since it had been demonstrated by Purcell and Barnhart (1963) that cathepsin C will convert prothrombin to thrombin. It was then demonstrated that levels of cathepsin C in various microsomal fractions isolated from liver derived from normal and from vitamin K–deficient rats paralleled the apparent clotting activity (Johnston et al., 1968). The technique of Wettstein and co-workers (1963) was used to make comparisons also of the ability of various microsomal fractions to carry out general protein synthesis (Table 29.3). As has already been noted in the heavy-microsomal fraction the Allington method gave apparent prothrombin values which increased with incubation for 3 hr. The two-stage method of Ware and Seegers (1949) gave no assayable prothrombin in either fraction at either time. In the high-sodium medium, in which the incubation for "prothrombin synthesis" were carried out, neither microsomal fraction synthesized any significant amount of protein. In a more conventional high-potassium medium, protein synthesis in the light-microsome fraction was considerably superior to that in the heavy-microsome fraction.

In view of these results, a fresh approach to the problem seemed to be indicated. It was decided to develop an active system for general protein synthesis in rat-liver microsomes and then to apply immunochemical techniques to identify specific products of protein biosynthesis. Campbell and co-workers (1960) were able to demonstrate the specific biosynthesis of

TABLE 29.3. *Measurement of rates of protein synthesis and prothrombin content of heavy and light microsomes from rat liver*

	Prothrombin (clotting-assay)				Protein Synthesis[a]	
	Before incubation		After incubation		High sodium	High potassium
Microsomes	One stage[b]	Two-stage[c]	One stage[b]	Two-stage[c]	(dpm/mg)	(dpm/mg)
Heavy[d]	3.5	0	9.0	0	34	450
Light[e]	1.5	0	3.6	0	44	1460

[a] Protein synthesis was measured according to Wettstein et al. (1963), with 3 mg of ribosomal protein and 0.3 μCi/ml of 1-^{14}C L-leucine.

[b] Method used was that of Allington (1958), whose reagent contained 15 units prothrombin/ml.

[c] As described by Ware and Seegers (1949).

[d] Obtained by centrifugation of homogenates of rat liver in 0.25 M sucrose at 18,000 $\times$ *g* for 1 hr.

[e] Obtained by spinning the supernatant from the preparation of heavy microsomes at 105,000 $\times$ *g* for 60 min.

rat-serum albumin by immunochemical techniques applied to sonicated rat-liver microsomes which had engaged in protein synthesis. By following the guidelines set down by these authors, we have been able to identify both prothrombin and serum albumin in sonicated extracts of light microsomes after incubation of these microsomes with radioactive 1-^{14}C L-leucine.

Rat livers from normal, from warfarinized, and from vitamin K–deficient rats were perfused *in situ* at 5 C, first with heparinized Krebs-Ringer bicarbonate buffer in order to remove all preformed plasma proteins from the organ, and then with an extracting solution (0.25 M sucrose in 0.05 M tris (hydroxymethyl) amino methane, *p*H 7.8, 0.04 M potassium chloride and 0.005 M magnesium acetate) in order to remove the heparin and the high-sodium medium. The liver was then excised and was homogenized with 2.5 volumes of extracting solution in a Potter-Elvehjem homogenizer. Heavy particles and unbroken cells were removed by centrifuging the solution at 27,000 × *g* for 20 min. The pellet was discarded, and the supernatant was spun at 105,000 × *g* for 1 hr. The pellet from this step, which consisted of light microsomes, was washed with buffer and used or stored at −70 C. The supernatant was a source of transfer factors and of tRNA for studies of protein synthesis. The requirements of this system for total protein synthesis are shown in Table 29.4 The need for an energy-generating system and microsomes is clearly shown.

In order to identify specific proteins synthesized by this system, the protein-synthesizing mixture was sonicated at the end of the 20-min period of incubation and centrifuged at 105,000 × *g* for 4 hr. Then ovalbumin and rabbit antiovalbumin were added to the supernatant to cause a nonspecific precipitin reaction. This reaction removed nonspecific radioactive materials which are adsorbed on such precipitates. Then carrier rat pro-

TABLE 29.4. *Requirements of the rat-liver microsomal system for protein synthesis*

Experimental system	Protein synthesized	
	dpm/mg	Percentage
Full system [a]	34,500	100
Full system less ATP, CP, and CPK	3,700	11
Microsomes	300	1

[a] The full system consists of 10 ml of 0.03 M Tris (*p*H 7.8), 0.005 M magnesium acetate, 0.08 M KCl, 0.001 M ATP, 0.02 M CP, 0.0004 M GTP, 0.0025 M GSH, 3 μg/ml CPK, complete amino acid mixture, 100 IU/ml penicillin G, 1 mg/ml supernatant enzymes, 3 mg ribosomal protein/ml, 10 nmole/ml L-leucine U-^{14}C (specific activity, 311 mCi/mmole; total activity, 30 μCi/10 ml).

The reaction mixture was incubated 20 min at 37 C in a Dubnoff shaker.

TABLE 29.5. *Biosynthesis of albumin and of prothrombin by microsomes from normal rats*

Measurement	Protein-synthesized[a] dpm/mg	Percentage
Blank	582 ± 40	100 ± 7
Albumin	2,620 ± 37	450 ± 31
Prothrombin	888 ± 47	153 ± 8
Total protein	29,900 ± 4,200	—

[a] Values are given as the mean ± SE. The means are for 12–16 determinations in 4 experiments.

thrombin (40 μg) and carrier rat-serum albumin (60 μg) were added, and multiple precipitations were carried out with nonspecific ovalbumin-antiovalbumin, with specific prothrombin-antiprothrombin, and with specific rat-serum albumin-antialbumin. The radioactivity found in the nonspecific precipitin at this stage served as the blank for the specific precipitins. The results of four experiments with normal rat liver are shown in Table 29.5. Triplicate precipitations were carried out for both albumin and prothrombin in each experiment. In normal rats it was demonstrated that both prothrombin and albumin were synthesized, albumin incorporating 3 times more radioactivity than prothrombin.

In order to further demonstrate that prothrombin was a genuine product of microsomal biosynthesis, the supernatant from one incubation medium after sonication was adsorbed onto barium citrate with carrier, eluted with dilute ammonium sulfate, fractionally precipitated with additional ammonium sulfate, desalted on Sephadex G–25, and subjected to acrylamide-gel electrophoresis. The gel was cut into 1 mm slices and counted. As shown in Figure 29.12, all of the radioactivity migrated with the single prothrombin spot on the gel.

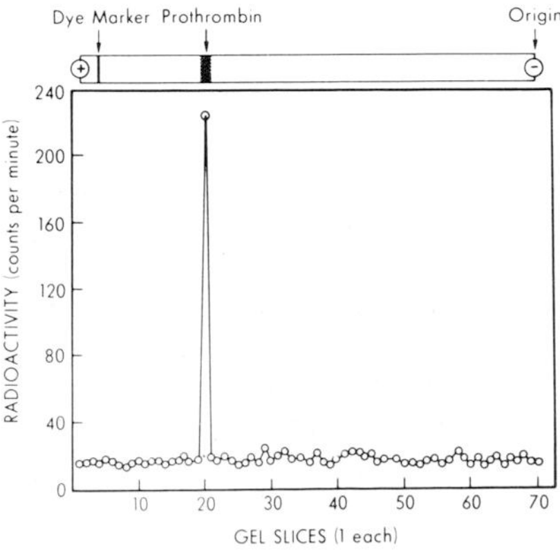

Fig. 29.12. Acrylamide-gel electrophoresis of biosynthesized prothrombin. The top panel shows the position of prothrombin on the gel after electrophoresis. The bottom panel presents the radioactivity of sequential 1-mm sections of the gel.

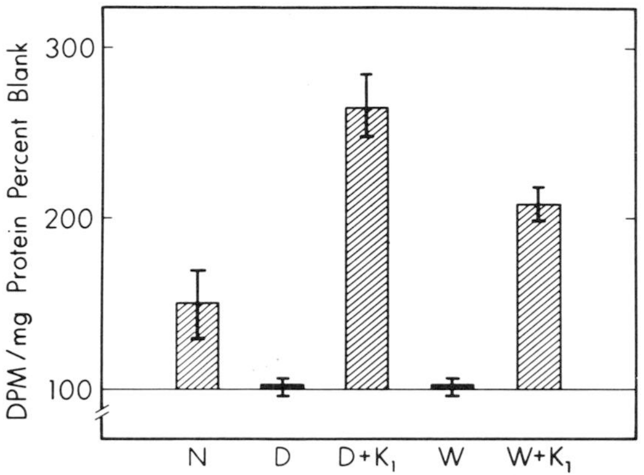

Fig. 29.13. Biosynthesis of prothrombin by light microsomes from various rats. N = normal; D = vitamin K deficient; D + K_1 = vitamin K deficient treated with vitamin K_1; W = warfarin treated; W + K_1 = warfarinized and treated with vitamin K_1.

The capacity of light microsomes from vitamin K–deficient rats, from vitamin K–deficient rats treated with vitamin K_1 (300 μg), from warfarinized rats (2 mg/day for 2 days), and from warfarinized rats treated with vitamin K_1 (300 μg) to synthesize prothrombin was next compared with that of normal rats (Fig. 29.13). Both the vitamin K–deficient and the warfarinized rats demonstrated a negligible synthesis of prothrombin, although their total protein synthesis and their synthesis of albumin were within normal limits. Vitamin K–deficient rats given vitamin K_1 and warfarinized rats given vitamin K_1 showed much better incorporation of ^{14}C leucine into prothrombin than did the normal rats. This more exuberant biosynthesis of prothrombin in deficient animals given vitamin K_1 is consistent with observations of the isolated perfused rat liver and suggests that more polysomes are involved in the biosynthesis of prothrombin under these conditions than under normal steady-state conditions. It is possible that this result in the deficient state is caused by the accumulation of mRNA for prothrombin, which is assimilated into polysomes when vitamin K is added. It has been demonstrated that liver RNA, including the messenger fraction, turns over more rapidly in vitamin K–deficient chicks than in normal ones (Olson et al., 1968*b*).

Summary and conclusions

Of these hypotheses for the action of vitamin K presented earlier, experiments reported from our laboratory definitely favor hypothesis 2, i.e., that vitamin K acts to regulate the biosynthesis of prothrombin and other vitamin K–dependent clotting proteins at the ribosomal level. Our experiments have demonstrated (*1*) that vitamin K_1 stimulates the prompt appearance of prothrombin in the perfusate of the isolated rat liver when added in vitro; (*2*) that the prothrombin that appears is derived from free amino acids which were present in the liver at the time of the addition of the vitamin K_1; (*3*) that this process is inhibited irreversibly by puromycin and reversibly by cycloheximide, but is not inhibited by actinomycin D; and (*4*) that the ability of a cell-free system to synthesize prothrombin is dependent upon the vitamin K–coumarin status of the animal from which the microsomes were isolated. A model for this regulatory process is presented in Fig. 29.14.

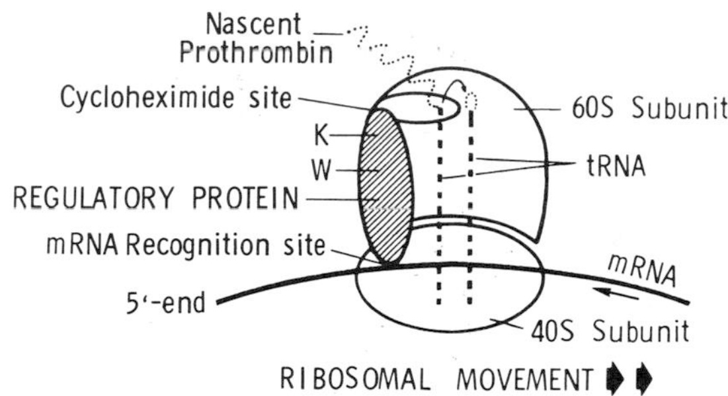

Fig. 29.14. Hypothetical model of a ribosome which is synthesizing prothrombin. The action of vitamin K and warfarin in regulating prothrombin biosynthesis is pictured as the result of an interaction of these ligands (K and W) with a regulatory protein.

This model provides for a regulatory protein that binds vitamin K and 4-hydroxy-coumarin drugs at separate sites, associates with the 60 *S* particle of the ribosome, and has a recognition site for the prothrombin mRNA (probably attached to the 40 *S* subunit of the ribosome). Although the existence of a regulatory (binding) protein for vitamin K and the coumarin drugs is hypothetical at the present time, support for its existence is based upon the following evidence: (1) Thus far, only proteins have been found to mediate the effects of small molecules upon the macromolecular events of protein synthesis. This generalization applies to (a) repressor proteins that affect transcription, (b) proteins that bind tRNA's to the ribosome, (c) proteins that bind GTP to the ribosome and provide for translocation in protein synthesis, and (d) initiation factors that bind f-Met-tRNA to the ribosome. (2) Binding proteins have been identified for 17β-estradiol (Jensen et al., 1968) and for aldosterone (Fanestil and Edelman, 1966). (3) The kinetic relationship between the coumarin drugs and vitamin K, as measured in intact chicks and in isolated perfused liver, appears to be an allosteric one. (4) There exist coumarin-drug-resistant rats (Greaves and Ayres, 1967; Pool et al., 1968) and humans (O'Reilly et al., 1964) that are not insensitive to vitamin K and demonstrated no altered drug metabolism. These data, in our opinion, warrant a search for the regulatory protein along the lines followed by Gilbert and Müller-Hill (1966, 1967), who revealed the existence of the *lac* repressor protein by studies of the binding of radioactive isopropyl-1-thio-β-D-galactoside (IPTG) to the repressor protein. They subsequently showed that the repressor, labeled isotopically, would also bind specifically to the *lac* operon captured in 35S *dlac* phage DNA. Taggart and Matschiner (1969) have observed that the physiologic concentration of vitamin K_1 in normal rat liver is 10 picomoles/g, or 10^{-8} M. If one assumes that the regulatory protein is saturated at this concentration, the association constant with vitamin K_1 must be on the order of 10^{-9}. The half-activity (i.e, the amount necessary to depress coagulation factors to 50%) of warfarin in the rat is about 3 mg/liter of plasma, or on the order of 10^{-5} M. Experiments are in progress to identify this regulatory (binding) protein for vitamin K and the coumarin drugs by carrying out double-labeling experiments that employ ^{14}C warfarin and ^{3}H phylloquinone.

The most important argument bearing on this model is the antagonism between cycloheximide and vitamin K (Olson et al., 1969*a*). It has been demonstrated by others (Siegel and Sisler, 1965; Rao and Grollman, 1967) that cycloheximide binds to the 60S particle in the mammalian ribosome and arrests the peptide synthetase required to elongate the peptide chain. This tends to freeze polysomes undergoing protein synthesis in a fixed state of aggregation (Wettstein et al., 1964) and to prevent completion of polypeptide chains. Felicetti and co-workers (1966) observed that cycloheximide is a reversible inhibitor of the peptide synthetase in reticulocytes and could be washed out with restoration of protein synthesis. Munro and co-workers (1968) noted that cycloheximide inhibited both chain initiation and chain elongation in ribosomes prepared from rat liver and that the block in elongation could be reversed by the addition of high concentrations of glutathione. Munro and co-workers concluded that the site of action of cycloheximide was transferase II (translocase) (Skogerson and Moldave, 1967), which is a sulfhydryl enzyme. It is likely, furthermore, that sensitivity to cycloheximide is a function of the protein structure of the ribosome, since a wide range in sensitivity is associated with genetic variation in yeasts (Cooper et al., 1967. Sensitivity to streptomycin is clearly a function of the protein structure of the 30S particle of bacterial ribosomes (Leboy et al., 1964; Ozaki et al., 1969).

In the model presented in Figure 29.14, the cycloheximide-binding protein is shown lying across the peptide-synthetase site and overlapping the vitamin K–regulatory protein. The antagonism noted in the isolated perfused liver between cycloheximide and vitamin K_1 is of the partially competitive type in which the inhibitor influences the association between ligand and protein. This could only happen if there was some crossover between the binding proteins for cycloheximide and for vitamin K. Since the reversal of cycloheximide inhibition by vitamin K applies only to vitamin K–dependent proteins, it follows that the vitamin K–regulatory protein affects only a small percentage of the total ribosomes.

Finally, it appears from all the evidence available that vitamin K (and the coumarin drugs) are most likely to influence the initiation of peptide synthesis of their dependent proteins. The vitamin K–regulatory protein may thus be regarded as an initiation factor in the mammal. Both the reversible inhibition by cycloheximide and the findings in the cell-free system favor this view. It follows, also from these considerations, that the regulatory protein must have a mRNA recognition site in order to permit the combination of the mRNA–40 *S* subunit–tRNA complex with suitably programmed 60 *S* subunits. In many respects, therefore, the postulated regulatory protein for prothrombin synthesis (and others specific for the other vitamin K–dependent proteins) share properties with the group of repressor proteins that act to regulate protein synthesis at the transcriptional level. The repressor proteins also have allosteric sites for effector molecules and a recognition site for nucleic acid (DNA operator).

There is still much to learn about the mode of action of vitamin K and the coumarin drugs in affecting the synthesis of the vitamin K–dependent clotting proenzymes. It is believed, however, that the model presented may serve as a useful working hypothesis for continuing investigation of the problem.

References

Allington, M. J. 1958. Owren's method for the control of anticoagulant therapy. *J. Clin. Pathol. 11*:62.

Babior, B. M. 1966. The role of vitamin K in clotting factor synthesis. I. Evidence for the participation of vitamin K in the conversion of a polypeptide precursor to factor VII. *Biochim. Biophys. Acta 123*:606.

Babson, A. L., S. Malament, G. H. Mangun, and G. E. Phillips. 1956. The effect of simultaneous administration of vitamin K_1 and dicumarol on the prothrombin in rat plasma. *Clin. Chem. 2*:243.

Barnhart, M. I., and G. F. Anderson. 1962. Cellular study of drug alteration of prothrombin synthesis. *Biochem. Pharmacol. 9*:23.

Berry, D., E. Berry, and R. E. Olson. 1966. Site of antagonism between vitamin K and dicumarol. *Fed. Proc. 25*:542. (Abstr.)

Beyer, R. E., and R. D. Kennison. 1959. Relationship between prothrombin time and oxidative phosphorylation in chick liver mitochondria. *Arch. Biochem. Biophys. 84*:63.

Campbell, P. N., O. Greengard, and B. A. Kernot. 1960. Studies on the synthesis of serum albumin by the isolated microsome fraction from rat liver. *Biochem. J. 74*:107.

Cline, A. L., and R. M. Bock. 1966. Translational control of gene expression. *Quant. Biol. 31*:321.

Colpa-Boonstra, J. P., and E. C. Slater. 1958. The possible role of vitamin K in the respiratory chain. *Biochim. Biophys. Acta 27*:122.

Cooper, D., D. V. Banthorpe, and D. Wilkie. 1967. Modified ribosomes conferring resistance to cycloheximide in mutants of *Saccharomyces cerevisiae. J. Mol. Biol. 26*:347.

Crick, F. H. C. 1966. The genetic code — Yesterday, today, and tomorrow. Cold Spring Harbor Symposium. *Quant. Biol. 31*:3.

Daft, F. S., W. H. Sebrell, and R. D. Lillie. 1942. Prevention by cystine or methionine of hemorrhage and necrosis of the liver. *Proc. Soc. Exp. Biol. Med. 50*:1.

Dam, H., F. Schønheyder, and E. Tage-Hansen. 1936. Studies on the mode of action of vitamin K. *Biochem. J. 30*:1075.

Denson, K. W. 1961. The specific assay of Prower-Stuart factor and factor VII. *Acta Haematol. 25*:105.

Fanestil, D. D. and I. S. Edelman. 1966. Characteristics of the renal nuclear receptors for aldosterone. *Proc. Nat. Acad. Sci. U.S.A. 56*:872.

Felicetti, L., B. Colombo, and C. Baglioni. 1966. Inhibition of protein synthesis in reticulocytes by antibiotics. II. The site of action of cycloheximide, streptovitacin A and pactamycin. *Biochim. Biophys. Acta 119*:120.

Gilbert, W., and B. Müller-Hill. 1966. Isolation of the *lac* repressor. *Proc. Nat. Acad. Sci. U.S.A. 56*:1891.

Gilbert, W., and B. Müller-Hill. 1967. The *lac* operator is DNA. *Proc. Nat. Acad. Sci. U.S.A. 58*:2415.

Goswami, P., and H. N. Munro. 1962. The role of ribonucleic acid in the formation of prothrombin activity by rat-liver microsomes. *Biochim. Biophys. Acta 55*:410.

Greaves, J. H., and P. Ayres. 1967. Heritable resistance to warfarin in rats. *Nature 215*:877.

György, P., and H. Goldblatt. 1942. Observations on the conditions of dietary hepatic injury (necrosis, cirrhosis) in rats. *J. Exp. Med. 75*:355.

Hemker, H. C., J. J. Veltkamp, A. Hensen, and E. A. Loeliger. 1963. Nature of prothrombin biosynthesis: Preprothrombinaemia in vitamin K–deficiency. *Nature 200*:589.

Hermodson, M. A., J. W. Suttie, and K. P. Link. 1969. Warfarin resistance in the rat. *Fed. Proc. 28*:386.

Hill, R. B., S. Gaetani, and B. C. Johnson. 1963. Vitamin K and liver microsomal prothrombin. *Fed. Proc. 22*:620.

Hill, R. B., S. Gaetani, A. M. Paolucci, P. B. Rama Rao, R. Alden, G. S. Ranhotra, D. V. Shah, V. K. Shah, and B. C. Johnson. 1968. Vitamin K and biosynthesis of protein and prothrombin. *J. Biol. Chem. 243*:3930.

Hjort, P., S. I. Rapaport, and P. A. Owren. 1955. A simple, specific one-stage prothrombin assay using Russell's viper venom in cephalin suspension. *J. Lab. Clin. Med. 46*:89.

Jacob, F., and J. Monod. 1961. Genetic regulatory mechanisms in the synthesis of proteins. *J. Mol. Biol. 3*:318.

Jensen, E. V., T. Suzuki, T. Kawashima, W. E. Stumpf, P. W. Jungblut, and E. R. DeSombre. 1968. A two-step mechanism for the interaction of estradiol with rat uterus. *Proc. Nat. Acad. Sci. U.S.A. 59*:632.

Johnson, B. C., R. B. Hill, R. Alden, and G. S. Ranhotra. 1966. Turnover time of prothrombin and of prothrombin messenger RNA and evidence for a ribosomal site of action of vitamin K in prothrombin synthesis. *Life Sci. 5*:385.

Johnston, M. F. M., R. K. Kipfer, and R. E. Olson. 1968. Effect of lysosomal enzymes on apparent prothrombin synthesis by microsomes from normal and vitamin K deficient rats. *Fed. Proc. 27*:436.

Kazmeier, F. J., J. A. Spittell, Jr., E. J. W. Bowie, J. H. Thompson, Jr., and C. A. Owen, Jr. 1968. Release of vitamin K–dependent coagulation factors by isolated perfused rat liver. *Amer. J. Physiol. 214*:919.

Lasch, H. G., and L. Roka. 1953. Mechanism of formation of the coagulation factors, prothrombin and factor VII. *Hoppe-Seyler's Z. Physiol. Chem. 294*:30.

Leboy, P. S., E. C. Cox, and J. G. Flaks. 1964. The chromosomal site specifying a ribosomal protein in *Escherichia coli*. *Proc. Nat. Acad. Sci. U.S.A. 52*:1367.

Li, L. -F., J. Block, R. K. Kipfer, and R. E. Olson. 1970. [Li et al., 1970*a*.] Amino acid metabolism and the biosynthesis of prothrombin in the perfused rat liver. *Proc. Soc. Exp. Biol. Med. 133*:168.

Li, L. -F., R. K. Kipfer, and R. E. Olson. 1970. [Li et al., 1970*b*] Immunochemical measurement of vitamin K induced biosynthesis of prothrombin in the isolated perfused rat liver. *Arch. Biochem. Biophys. 137*:494.

Li, L. -F., and R. E. Olson. 1967. Purification and properties of rat prothrombin. *J. Biol. Chem. 242*:5611.

Lowenthal, J., and H. Birnbaum. 1969. Mechanism of action of vitamin K in plasma clotting factor synthesis: Evidence from "in vitro" experiments that the action is not at the level of polypeptide formation. *Fed. Proc. 28*:385. (Abstr.)

Lowenthal, J., and J. A. MacFarlane. 1964. The nature of the antagonism between vitamin K and indirect anticoagulants. *J. Pharmacol. Exp. Ther. 143*:273.

Martius, C., and D. Nitz-Litzow. 1954. Oxydative phosphorylierung und vitamin K Mangel. *Biochim. Biophys. Acta 13*:152.

Mattii, R., J. L. Ambrus, J. E. Sokal, and I. Mink. 1964. Production of members of the blood coagulation and fibrinolysin systems by the isolated perfused liver. *Proc. Soc. Exp. Biol. Med. 116*:69.

Miller, L. L., C. G. Bly, M. L. Watson, and W. F. Bale. 1951. The dominant role of the liver in plasma protein synthesis: A direct study of the isolated perfused rat liver with the aid of lysine-ε-^{14}C. *J. Exp. Med. 94*:431.

Munro, H. N., B. S. Baliga, and A. W. Pronczuk. 1968. *In vitro* inhibition of peptide synthesis and GTP hydrolysis by cycloheximide and reversal of inhibition by glutathione. *Nature 219*:944.

Olson, J. P., L. L. Miller, and S. B. Troup. 1966. Synthesis of clotting factors by the isolated perfused rat liver. *J. Clin. Invest. 45*:690.

Olson, R. E. 1964. Vitamin K induced prothrombin formation: Antagonism by actinomycin D. *Science 145*:926.

Olson, R. E. 1966. Studies on the mode of action of vitamin K. *Advances Enzyme Regulation 4*:181.

Olson, R. E. 1967. Are we looking at the right enzyme systems? *Amer. J. Clin. Nutr. 20*:604.

Olson, R. E., and J. S. Dinning. 1954. Enzyme abnormalities associated with dietary necrotic liver degeneration in rats. *Ann. N.Y. Acad. Sci. 57*:889.

Olson, R. E., R. K. Kipfer, and L. -F. Li. 1969*a*. Evidence for a ribosomal site of action for vitamin K. *Clin. Res. 2*:465.

Olson, R. E., R. K. Kipfer, and L. -F. Li. 1969*b*. Vitamin K–induced biosynthesis of prothrombin in the isolated, perfused rat liver. *Advances Enzyme Regulation 7*:83.

Olson, R. E., L. -F. Li, G. Philipps, and R. K. Kipfer. 1968. [Olson et al., 1968*a*.] The mode of action of vitamin K in stimulating prothrombin synthesis. *Thromb. Diath. Haemorrh. 19*:611.

Olson, R. E., G. Philipps, and N. -T. Wang. 1968 [Olson et al., 1968*b*.] The regulatory action of vitamin K. *Advances Enzyme Regulation 6*:213.

O'Reilly, R. A., P. M. Aggeler, M. S. Hoag, L. S. Leong, and M. Kropatkin. 1964. Hereditary transmission of exceptional resistance to coumarin anticoagulant drugs: the first reported kindred. *New Engl. J. Med. 271*:809.

Owren, P. A., and K. Aas. 1951. The control of dicumarol therapy and quantitative determination of prothrombin and proconvertin. *Scand. J. Clin. Lab. Invest. 3*:201.

Ozaki, M., S. Mizushima, and M. Nomura. 1969. Identification of the ribosomal protein controlled by the streptomycin resistant locus in *E. coli*. *Fed. Proc. 28*:725.

Paolucci, A. M., P. B. R. Rao, and B. C. Johnson. 1963. Vitamin K deficiency and oxidative phosphorylation. *J. Nutr. 81*:17.

Pool, J. G., R. A. O'Reilly, L. J. Schneiderman, and M. Alexander. 1968. Warfarin resistance in the rat. *Amer. J. Physiol. 215*:627.

Pool, J. G., and J. Robinson. 1969. *In vitro* synthesis of coagulation factors by rat liver slices. *Amer. J. Physiol. 196*:423.

Prydz, H. 1965. Studies on proconvertin (factor VII). VII. Further studies on the biosynthesis of factor VII in rat cell suspensions. *Scand. J. Clin. Lab. Invest. 17*:143.

Purcell, G. M., and M. I. Barnhart. 1963. Prothrombin activation with cathepsin C. *Biochim. Biophys. Acta 78*:800.

Quick, A. J., and G. Collentine. 1950. The role of vitamin K in the formation of prothrombin. *J. Lab. Clin. Med. 36*:976.

Rao, S. S., and A. P. Grollman. 1967. Cycloheximide resistance in yeast: a property of the 60S ribosomal subunit. *Biochem. Biophys. Res. Commun. 29*:696.

Schwarz, K. 1944. A fatal dietary-induced liver damage and the occurrence of liver-protecting substances. *Physiol. Chem. 281*:101.

Siegel, M. R., and H. D. Sisler. 1965. Site of action of cycloheximide in cells of

Saccharomyces pastorianus. III. Further studies on the mechanism of action and the mechanism of resistance in *Saccharomyces species*. *Biochim. Biophys. Acta 103*:558.

Skogerson, L., and K. Moldave. 1967. The binding of aminoacyl transferase II to ribosomes. *Biochem. Biophys. Res. Commun. 27*:568.

Stapp, W. F. 1965. The assay of factor IX: With a note on the use of a bentonite suspension in the preparation of an artificial substrate system for factor IX assay. *Scand. J. Clin. Lab. Invest. 17*: Suppl. 84, 109.

Steenbock, H., and D. C. Herting. 1955. Vitamin D and growth. *J. Nutr. 57*:449.

Suttie, J. W. 1967. Control of prothrombin and factor VII biosynthesis by vitamin K. *Arch. Biochem. Biophys. 118*:166.

Taggart, W. V., and J. T. Matschiner. 1969. Metabolism of menadione-6,7-^{3}H in the rat. *Biochemistry 8*:1141.

Vogel, H. J. 1957. Repression and induction as control mechanisms of enzyme biogenesis: The adaptive formation of acctylornithinasc, p. 276. W. D. McElroy and B. Glass (eds.), *A Symposium on the Chemical Basis of Heredity*. Johns Hopkins Press, Baltimore.

Ware, A. G., and W. H. Seegers. 1949. Two-stage procedure for the quantitative determination of prothrombin concentration. *Amer. J. Clin. Pathol. 19*:471.

Wettstein, F. O., H. Noll, and S. Penman. 1964. Effect of cycloheximide on ribosomal aggregates engaged in protein synthesis *in vitro*. *Biochim. Biophys. Acta 87*:525.

Wettstein, F. O., T. Staehelin, and H. Noll. 1963. Ribosomal aggregate engaged in protein synthesis: Characterization of the ergosome. *Nature 197*:430.

Woolley, D. W. 1947. Recent advances in the study of biological competition between structurally related compounds. *Physiol. Rev. 27*:308.

Wosilait, W. D. 1966. Effect of vitamin K deficiency on the adenosine nucleotide content of chicken liver. *Biochem. Pharmacol. 15*:204.

30

STUDIES ON THE SITE OF ACTION OF VITAMIN K IN THE SYNTHESIS OF CLOTTING PROTEINS IN THE MAMMALIAN SYSTEM

B. Connor Johnson

Our work on vitamin K started in 1958, when we observed that many of our male rats fed irradiated-beef diets were dying of hemorrhage (Metta et al., 1969; Mameesh et al., 1962). We soon found that this was caused by the low vitamin K content of meat and that the disease could be cured or prevented by vitamin K. From this first observation of a dietary vitamin K deficiency in the rat, we proceeded to develop a vitamin K–free diet (Mameesh and Johnson, 1959; Johnson et al., 1960) and, in order to consistently produce a vitamin K deficiency in the rat, developed a tubular cage to prevent coprophagy (Metta et al., 1961). Using this diet and this cage, we routinely have been able to produce vitamin K deficiency in male rats in from 6 to 10 days and have determined that the vitamin K requirement of the noncoprophagic male rat is about 0.1 μg of vitamin K_1 per gram of diet (Mameesh and Johnson, 1960). It was early observed that male rats were particularly susceptible to the deficiency and that female rats on the same diet could be maintained even through a reproductive cycle without any significant incidence of vitamin K defi-

The work reported here was carried out partly in the Division of Nutritional Biochemistry, University of Illinois, Urbana, Illinois, and partly at Oklahoma. The work has been carried out by M. S. Mameesh, P. B. Rama Rao, V. C. Metta, A. M. Paolucci, S. Gaetani, R. B. Hill, G. S. Ranhotra, and H. V. Johnson, postdoctoral fellows; by F. Paul, V. K. Shah, D. V. Shah, G. Forsyth, and G. Valkovich, graduate students; and by R. Alden, L. Nash, E. Everett, and C. Boyd, technicians.

This work has been supported in part by National Institutes of Health grants AM–06005 and AM–10282 and by Department of Defense contract DA–49–193 MD–2830 with the Office of the Surgeon General. The opinions expressed herein are those of the author and not necessarily those of the Department of Defense.

ciency. Having found that we could routinely produce vitamin K–deficient rats, we set about to study the deficiency and have directed our research toward gaining an understanding of the molecular-level function of vitamin K.

The role of vitamin K has been of interest for many years. In the animal, the only observed effects of vitamin K deficiency are a decrease in the clotting proteins: prothrombin (factor II), factor VII (proconvertin), factor IX (Christmas factor), and factor X (Stuart factor). One of the first mechanisms proposed for the effect of vitamin K on these clotting proteins was that of Martius and Nitz-Litzow (1954). Their work with vitamin K–deficient chickens indicates that vitamin K functions in oxidative phosphorylation, and they postulated that the role of vitamin K in prothrombin synthesis is a manifestation of this indirect role of vitamin K in all protein synthesis. The inhibition was postulated to be caused by a lack of ATP for amino acid activation as a result of the block in oxidative phosphorylation, and the specific effect on the four vitamin K–dependent clotting proteins was suggested to be caused only by their more rapid turnover. However, we were unable to demonstrate any effect of vitamin K deficiency in the rat on either oxidative phosphorylation (Table 30.1) (Paolucci et al., 1963) or general protein synthesis as indicated by amino acid incorporation into protein of various tissues of the rat and by the induced synthesis of the enzyme tryptophan oxygenase (Paolucci et al., 1964). Since vitamin K does not appear to be a part of the prothrombin molecule (Ray et al., 1962) it must be functioning in a regulatory role in prothrombin formation.

Thus, while vitamin K does not function in general protein synthesis, it might function at a control site for the formation of the four specific vitamin K–dependent proteins. Such control sites could be: (1) at the genetic level of specific DNA transcription, (2) in the regulation of translation of specific message for these four proteins, (3) at some site after the formation of the peptide precursor, or (4) in the transport of the active protein out of the cell. Site 4 can be eliminated on the basis of studies which used the fluorescent antibody technique and in which a very rapid

TABLE 30.1. *Oxidative phosphorylation by rat liver mitochondria*

	Glutamate as substrate		β-hydroxybutyrate as substrate	
Treatment	Prothrombin time (sec)	P/O [a]	Prothrombin time (sec)	P/O [a]
Control	15	2.46 ± 0.22	15	2.68 ± 0.26
Vitamin K–deficient diet	40–200	2.30 ± 0.37	32–> 360	2.38 ± 0.42
Dicoumarol-treated [b]	190–> 360	2.27 ± 0.44	—	—

[a] Values are given as mean ± SD for 10–13 rats per group.
[b] 0.25% in vitamin K-free diet.

appearance of prothrombin in liver cells of dicoumarol-treated dogs was observed after administration of vitamin D (Barnhart and Anderson, 1962; Anderson and Barnhart, 1964).

Vitamin K and transcription regulation

ACTINOMYCIN D EXPERIMENTS

Olson (1964, 1965*a*, 1965*b*) and Berry and co-workers (1966) have proposed that vitamin K functions at the genetic level in the specific transcription of the part of the DNA molecule involved as template for the biosynthesis of the vitamin K–dependent proteins. On the basis of actinomycin D experiments, we reported in 1965 that vitamin K does not appear to be involved in RNA formation (Johnson et al., 1965).

The normal picture of the response of vitamin K–deficient rats to the administration of vitamin K_1 is shown in Figure 30.1. As measured by the single-stage prothrombin assay, the deficient rat responds very rapidly (within 1 hr) to vitamin K, in contrast to the considerably slower response of warfarin-treated rats. This delayed response to vitamin K in the pres-

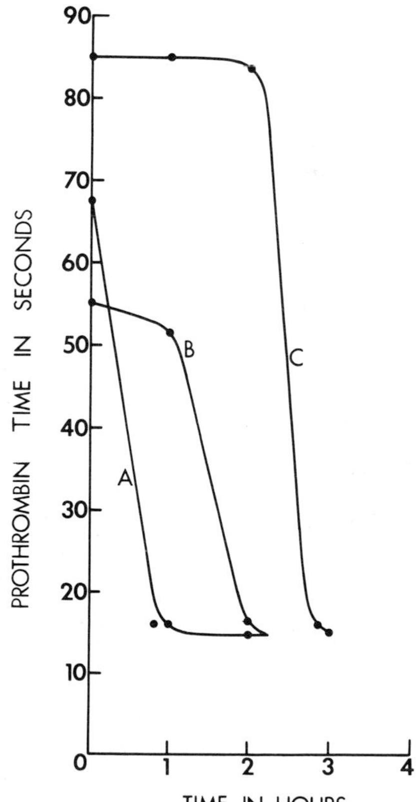

Fig. 30.1. Prothrombin activity in 5 vitamin K–deficient rats given 100 μg of vitamin K_1 at zero time (*A*), compared with that of warfarinized rats (*B* and *C*). Curve *B* shows the response of 4 normal rats that were treated with 0.2 mg of sodium warfarin 24 hr before zero time and given 20 μg of vitamin K_1 at zero time. Curve *C* shows the response of 8 normal rats that were treated with 2.5 mg of sodium warfarin 24 hr before zero time and given 1 mg of vitamin K_1 at zero time.

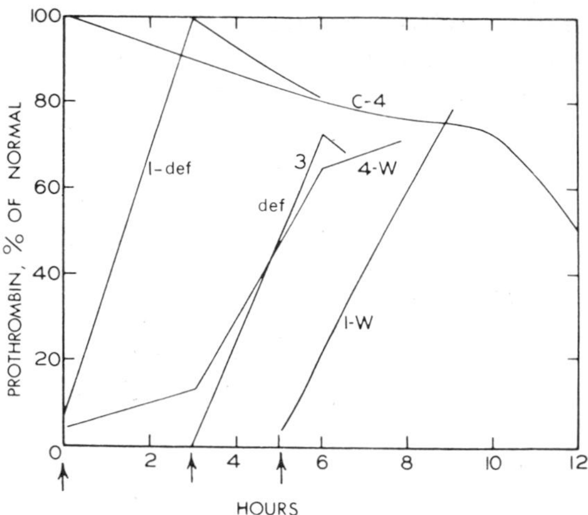

Fig. 30.2. Prothrombin activity of vitamin K–deficient rats treated with actinomycin D (*def*), compared with that of control (*C*) and warfarin-treated (*W*) rats. Rats were given 500 μg of actinomycin D per 100 g of body weight at zero time, then given 40 μg of vitamin K_1 at zero time, at 3 hr, and at 5 hr (arrows). Warfarin-treated rats had received 1 mg of warfarin per 100 g of body weight 24 hr before zero time. The numbers represent the number of rats for each curve. (Hill et al., 1968. Reproduced by permission of the American Society of Biological Chemists.)

ence of warfarin is presumably due to the necessity of displacing warfarin by vitamin K at the binding site on the vitamin K–regulator protein.

Figure 30.2 shows that vitamin K–deficient and warfarin-treated rats respond to vitamin K_1 in the presence of levels of actinomycin D high enough to completely block prothrombin biosynthesis in control animals (Johnson et al., 1966; Hill et al., 1968). This nondependence of the formation of prothrombin or of factor VII on RNA synthesis has been confirmed by Suttie (1967), by Lowenthal and Simmons (1967), and by Olson and co-workers (1968).

From data on the time course of the blocking of prothrombin synthesis by actinomycin D, the lifetime of mRNA for prothrombin synthesis can be estimated (Johnson et al., 1966). At the highest level of actinomycin D used, prothrombin levels remained relatively stable for about 6 hr, after which there was a very rapid decline. This indicates an approximate 6-hr lifetime for prothrombin message.

ETHIONINE EXPERIMENTS

Experiments carried out with ethionine also indicated a response to vitamin K, independent of the blocking of RNA synthesis (Hill et al., 1968).

Vitamin K and translation regulation

CYCLOHEXIMIDE EXPERIMENTS

Since it appeared that the site of action of vitamin K was not related to DNA transcription, our efforts were next directed to the study of a possible role of vitamin K at the level of translation of specific mRNA, that is, at some step in *de novo* peptide-bond formation. To do this, protein-synthesis blocking agents were again used, but, in this case, agents were used which block at the level of peptide-bond formation.

Fortunately, I believe, the first of these protein-synthesis (peptide-bond formation) blocking agents we used was cycloheximide. It was found that, at doses of 50–750 μg per 100 g of body weight, cycloheximide blocked further prothrombin synthesis, and prothrombin dropped rapidly to a very low level. The rate of decrease indicated that the turnover time for active prothrombin in the blood was 6–7 hr. When cycloheximide was given to vitamin K–deficient rats, the subsequent response to vitamin K administration depended very much on the level of cycloheximide which had been given.

When 750 μg of cycloheximide per 100 g of body weight was given nutritionally vitamin K–deficient rats, only a very small response to vitamin K_1 was seen (Fig. 30.3). In the same way, when this level or lower levels of cycloheximide were used with warfarin-treated rats, only a small, transitory response to vitamin K_1 was obtained.

However, as can be seen from the graphs in Figure 30.4, when 50 μg of cycloheximide per 100 g of body weight was used, then essentially complete responses were obtained after vitamin K_1 was administered to either nutritionally vitamin K–deficient rats or warfarin-treated rats. In all cases, these responses were obtained well within the 6-hr period during which a total block of prothrombin synthesis occurs in normal animals. While the 750 μg level was lethal, the 250 μg and 50 μg levels were not.

These data led us to ask the question, Is cycloheximide a vitamin K antagonist at the levels used? In order to answer this question, some five or six years ago we treated normal animals with 50 μg cycloheximide per 100 g of body weight, observed the rapid decline in 6 hr in plasma prothrombin, and attempted unsuccessfully to reverse this by administration of high levels (1 mg) of vitamin K.

Also, while the highly active vitamin K antagonist, warfarin, required 24 hr to produce a marked hypoprothrombinemia, cycloheximide did this (by blocking protein synthesis) in 6 hr. If higher levels of warfarin were used, the animals died sooner (in 2–4 hr at 50 mg per 100 g of body weight), without showing any hypoprothrombinemia. (Death was possibly caused by uncoupling of oxidative phosphorylation or by interference with electron transport.) These data indicate that the site of action of cycloheximide was not the vitamin K function site.

The rapid cures obtained in the presence of 50 μg of cycloheximide indicated that the site of action of vitamin K is beyond that of cycloheximide. The very poor response to vitamin K in the presence of high levels

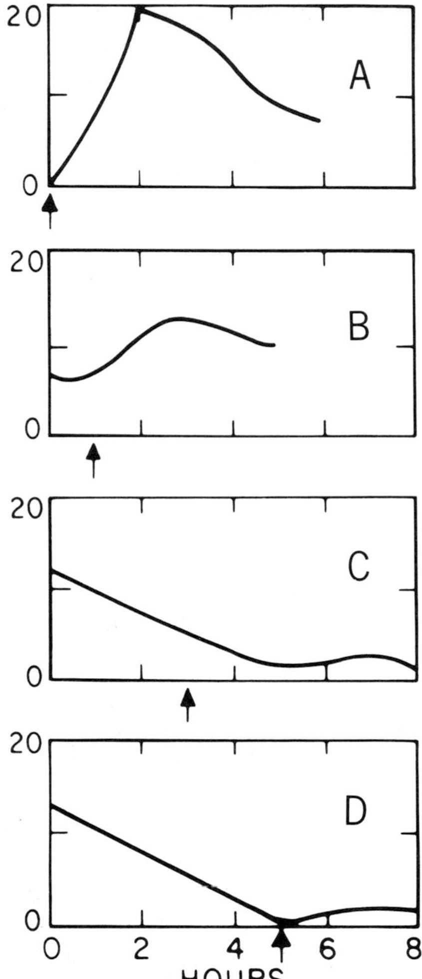

Fig. 30.3. Prothrombin activity, expressed as percent of normal, of vitamin K–deficient rats given cycloheximide and treated with vitamin K_1. The rats were given 750 μg of cycloheximide per 100 g of body weight at zero time. Vitamin K_1 was given as follows: 40 μg at zero time to 5 rats (*A*); 40 μg at 1 hr to 6 rats (*B*); 40 μg at 3 hr to 2 rats (*C*); and 500 μg at 5 hr to 4 rats (*D*). (Johnson et al., 1966. Reproduced by permission of Pergamon Press.)

of cycloheximide is, however, difficult to understand, but it must be related to the mechanism of action of cycloheximide. Godschaux and co-workers (1967) have shown very different ribosomal effects of high and low concentrations of cycloheximide, and Baliga and co-workers (1968*a*) have observed that much smaller doses of cycloheximide are needed to inhibit polysome aggregation than to prevent chain elongation. Cycloheximide has been variously reported not to inhibit polyribosome formation, but to prevent conversion of polysomes to single ribosomes (Wettstein et al., 1964; Baliga et al., 1968*b*) and to inhibit polysome aggregation.

Munro and co-workers (1968) have recently indicated that the action of cycloheximide is to block transferase II (translocase) and thus the translo-

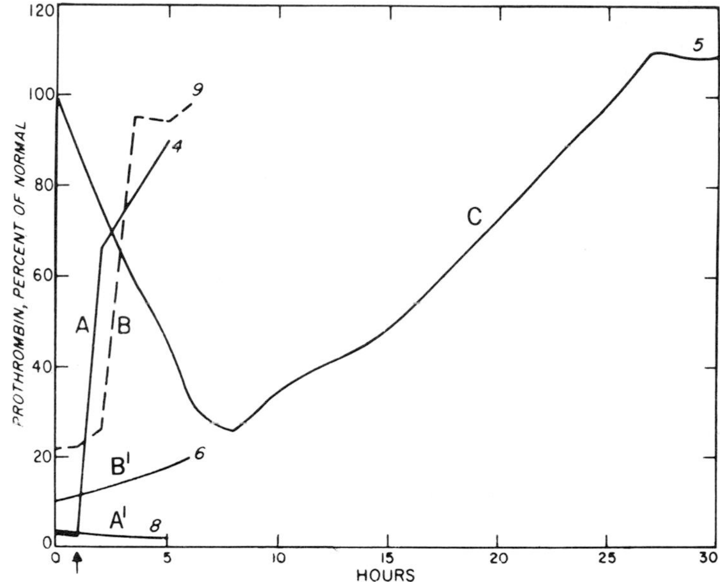

Fig. 30.4. Prothrombin activity in rats given 50 μg of cycloheximide per 100 g of body weight at zero time, showing effect of treatment with 40 μg of vitamin K_1 at 1 hr. Curves show the results for vitamin K–deficient rats (*A′*) and vitamin K–deficient rats given vitamin K (*A*); for warfarin-treated rats (*B′*) for warfarin-treated rats given vitamin K (*B*); and for normal rats without vitamin K treatment (*C*). The numbers represent the number of rats in each group. (Johnson et al., 1966. Reproduced by permission of Pergamon Press.)

cation of charged tRNA from site A to site P on the ribosome; this action therefore blocks peptide-chain elongation. Cycloheximide inhibits incorporation of amino acids into nascent peptide chains that were initiated in intact cells and remain attached to ribosomes during their isolation (Lin et al., 1966). If the nascent peptide still attached to the ribosome cannot be released at high levels of cycloheximide, this might offer an explanation of the difference in response to vitamin K at different levels of cycloheximide.

As one considers the results of vitamin K treatment of the animals given the higher levels of cycloheximide, one other fact appears evident. From Figure 30.3B it can be seen that when vitamin K was administered simultaneously with the high level of 750 μg of cycloheximide per 100 g of body weight to vitamin K–deficient rats, there was an immediate response to vitamin K. However, this response was not maintained, and prothrombin levels decreased. Similar data were seen when prothrombin levels were reduced by warfarin treatment. These data seem to indicate that there is a prothrombin precursor which is converted to active prothrombin in a vitamin K–dependent step and that, once the amount of this precursor present in the liver cells is consumed, no further prothrombin synthesis can take place because of the block in protein synthesis. Such a suggestion cannot be deduced from the experiments involving low levels of cycloheximide, because the responses in these experiments during the first hour after vitamin K therapy were essentially complete. Suttie (1969) reported that, in experiments with vitamin K–deficient rats, cycloheximide did not block an early response to vitamin K, but that there was no further response after 1 hr. Similar results were also reported by Lowenthal and Birnbaum (1969).

PUROMYCIN EXPERIMENTS

Another protein-synthesis blocking agent used was puromycin. Puromycin blocks protein synthesis by terminating peptide synthesis, becoming itself incorporated into the growing peptide chain (Allen and Zamecnik, 1962; Allen and Schweet, 1962; Smith et al., 1965). Puromycin is thus inactivated, and large amounts must be used to completely block protein synthesis. This action of puromycin is accompanied by a rapid breakdown of liver polysomes to a new steady-state level characterized by a shift to smaller aggregates (Villa-Trevino et al., 1964). Thus, after treatment with the high levels of puromycin which must be used, one might expect responses to vitamin K similar to those found in the presence of high levels of cycloheximide. The puromycin data shown in Figure 30.5 indicate that,

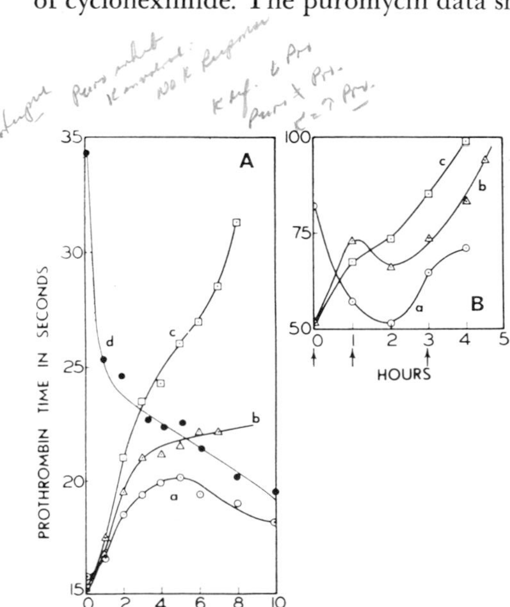

Fig. 30.5. Prothrombin activity in rats given puromycin at zero time, showing response of vitamin K–deficient rats to vitamin K_1.

A: Prothrombin activity in vitamin K–deficient rats given 20 mg of puromycin per 100 g of body weight and 40 μg of vitamin K_1 at zero time (*d*), compared with that of normal rats given 20 mg (*a*), 30 mg (*b*), or 40 mg (*c*) of puromycin per 100 g of body weight at zero time.

B: Prothrombin activity in vitamin K–deficient rats given 40 mg of puromycin per 100 g of body weight at zero time and 40 μg of vitamin K_1 per 100 g of body weight at zero time (*a*), at 1 hr (*b*), or at 3 hr (*c*). (Hill et al., 1968. Reproduced by permission of the American Society of Biological Chemists.)

in fact, this is true. While responses to vitamin K are seen in the presence of blocking levels of puromycin, they are incomplete. Together, the data on high levels of cycloheximide and the puromycin data indicate the necessity for normal polysome aggregation before vitamin K function can take place.

Very conflicting data have resulted from work with puromycin in different laboratories. Using liver-perfusion methods, J. P. Olson and co-workers (1966) found no effect of puromycin in blocking of prothrombin biosynthesis. In contrast, Suttie (1967) and R. E. Olson and co-workers (1968), in liver-perfusion experiments, found that puromycin completely blocked the vitamin K action of stimulating factor VII formation. Using isolated liver cells, Prydz (1965) found that puromycin blocked factor VII biosynthesis, while Babior (1966) and Lowenthal and Birnbaum (1969) found that in vitro addition of puromycin did not inhibit formation of factor VII activity in liver slices.

In vitro isolated-liver-cell experiments

In an attempt to understand this confusion, we have carried out experiments with liver cells isolated from vitamin K–deficient and from normal rats. Liver-cell suspensions were prepared by the method of Jacob and Bhargava (1962). The cells were counted in a hemacytometer and were examined for their structural integrity. Respiratory activity of the cells was measured, and oxygen uptake was found to continue in both normal and vitamin K–deficient rat-liver cells for 90 min (Ranhotra and Johnson, 1969). In these experiments, factor VII activity rather than prothrombin activity was measured. Three to four million cells suspended in 1 ml of Tris KCl buffer (containing 1.25 mM $CaCl_2$) were incubated at 37 C in a Dubnoff shaker under an atmosphere of 95% oxygen and 5% carbon dioxide. At intervals during incubation, 0.1 ml of cell suspension was removed, diluted with 0.9 ml of cold dilution fluid, and centrifuged; and the supernatant was immediately assayed for factor VII activity by the method of Pechet (1964), using charcoal-filtered bovine plasma (Adamis et al., 1956) and commercial Simplastin.

For normal and vitamin K–deficient rats, factor VII activity in the liver-cell suspensions increased continuously for 90 min, that is, during the time that cell respiration was normal. For vitamin K–deficient rats, the amount of factor VII synthesis depended on vitamin K_1 administration. When vitamin K_1 was administered before the rats were killed, factor VII activity in the liver-cell suspensions was higher than in liver-cell suspensions derived from normal rats; when no vitamin K_1 was given or when vitamin K_1 was added in vitro, there was essentially no factor VII synthesis.

TABLE 30.2. *In vitro effect of cycloheximide and puromycin on the production of factor VII activity*

Treatment	Factor VII (units per 10^6 cells)			
	30 min	60 min	90 min	120 min
Vitamin K–deficient rats[a] ($n = 4$)				
Control	1.8 ± 0.1	3.7 ± 0.4	4.2 ± 0.4	3.7 ± 0.4
Cycloheximide[b]	1.8 ± 0.1	3.7 ± 0.4	4.3 ± 0.7	4.4 ± 0.6
Puromycin[c]	2.2 ± 0.2	4.3 ± 0.6	4.7 ± 0.7	4.8 ± 0.6
Normal rats ($n = 4$)				
Control	2.2 ± 0.2	3.7 ± 0.2	5.2 ± 0.5	3.9 ± 0.2
Cycloheximide[b]	1.2 ± 0.3	4.3 ± 0.3	5.0 ± 0.0	4.2 ± 0.2
Puromycin[c]	1.8 ± 0.4	3.8 ± 0.3	4.2 ± 0.1	4.3 ± 0.2

Notes: Liver-cell suspensions from normal and vitamin K–deficient rats were prepared as described in the text. The incubation mixture contained 3–4 × 10^6 cells in 1 ml of Tris-KCl buffer. Factor VII activity was assayed by the method of Pechet (1964). Values are given as mean ± SE.

[a] Vitamin K_1 was administered intracardially to the deficient rats 25 min before they were killed.

[b] 1 mg of cycloheximide was added to 1 ml of incubation mixture.

[c] 5 mg of puromycin was added to 1 ml of incubation mixture.

IN VITRO ADMINISTRATION OF CYCLOHEXIMIDE OR PUROMYCIN

Further experiments (Ranhotra and Johnson, 1969) indicated that the in vitro addition of cycloheximide or puromycin to isolated liver cells from vitamin K–deficient rats treated in vivo with vitamin K or from normal rats did not affect factor VII synthesis (Table 30.2). This lack of in vitro effect of puromycin confirms the results in liver slices (Babior, 1966; Lowenthal and Birnbaum, 1969).

IN VIVO ADMINISTRATION OF PUROMYCIN

The in vivo effects of puromycin were markedly different from its in vitro effects. When puromycin and vitamin K were simultaneously administered in vivo, the later synthesis of factor VII by the subsequently isolated liver-cell suspension was blocked (Table 30.3). The failure of puromycin and now also of cycloheximide to inhibit the in vitro continuing synthesis of factor VII in liver slices has been interpreted to indicate that the vitamin K–dependent step in factor VII formation does not occur during *de novo* protein synthesis. It appears that this conclusion may be open to question. In contrast to the results reported by Pool and Brown (1962), Lowenthal and Simmons (1967) were able to initiate factor VII synthesis in liver slices in vitro. However, we were not able to obtain stimulation of factor VII activity by vitamin K_1 in liver-cell suspensions in vitro, and thus it was

TABLE 30.3. *In vivo effect of puromycin on the production of factor VII activity by vitamin K–deficient rats*

Treatment	Factor VII (units per 10^6 cells)			
	30 min	60 min	90 min	120 min
Control ($n = 4$)	1.8 ± 0.1	3.7 ± 0.4	4.2 ± 0.4	3.7 ± 0.4
Puromycin[a] ($n = 3$)	0.7 ± 0.4	1.2 ± 0.3	1.1 ± 0.4	1.1 ± 0.3

Notes: Liver-cell suspensions from vitamin K–deficient rats given vitamin K in vivo were prepared as described in the text. The incubation mixture contained $3–4 \times 10^6$ cells in 1 ml of Tris-KCl buffer. Factor VII activity was assayed by the method of Pechet (1964).

Values are given as mean ± SE.

[a] 30 mg of puromycin per 100 g of body weight was administered in vivo simultaneously with vitamin K_1.

not possible for us to test the effect of these protein-synthesis blocking agents on initiation of factor VII formation in vitro. Since puromycin given in vivo simultaneously with vitamin K does block the initiation and any subsequent formation of factor VII activity, this must indicate that there is some step in the formation of factor VII activity after vitamin K is administered which is in some way dependent on the synthesis of protein, even though continued vitamin K–stimulated formation of factor VII in isolated liver cells or in liver slices is independent of protein synthesis.

SIGNIFICANCE OF THE PUROMYCIN-LIVER CELL RESULTS

It is possible that this requirement for protein synthesis for the formation of factor VII activity after vitamin K is administered may involve a requirement for synthesis of a "vitamin K enzyme" which is unstable in the absence of vitamin K. This vitamin K enzyme may then function in the formation of active factor VII from a precursor (as suggested above), independently of peptide-bond synthesis. In the case of vitamin A in the eye, Dowling and Wald (1960) found opsin to be unstable and to disappear in the absence of retinal.

Another possibility is that vitamin K is in some way involved in chain completion, termination, or release from the ribosome. This final step would be blocked, if it involves any peptide-bond formation, when puromycin is administered to the intact animal but could already have been carried out in the case of the animal given only the vitamin. The continued release of active factor VII into the medium during the subsequent incubation of the cells would then not be affected by puromycin, the puromycin-blocked step having already been accomplished. This would also be a possible explanation of results of liver-perfusion studies by Suttie (1967) and by R. E. Olson and co-workers (1968), who found a complete block by puromycin of factor VII formation when both vitamin K and puromycin were included in the liver-perfusion medium.

Antithrombin and the Ware and Seegers two-stage prothrombin assay as applied to vitamin K–deficient plasma

Our early work on the effect of protein-synthesis blocking agents on prothrombin biosynthesis in the intact animal was carried out with the Allington (1958) modification of the Quick single-stage prothrombin assay (Quick et al., 1935) – although we were well aware, and frequently reminded of the fact, that it is less specific than the two-stage assay of Ware and Seegers (1949). However, since four of the clotting proteins are vitamin K dependent, specificity seems less important than response to vitamin K. When we decided to try and investigate the in vitro biosynthesis of prothrombin and factor VII by cell-free systems in rat-liver microsomes (Hill et al., 1963), however, we required a more sensitive and more specific assay and so substituted the standard two-stage assay for the single-stage assay method used earlier.

RECOVERY OF ADDED PROTHROMBIN

The application of this two-stage assay to microsomes, to microsomal supernatant, and to plasma has led to a number of interesting findings. Various supernatant preparations from the livers of normal and of vitamin K–deficient rats were assayed for prothrombin by the two-stage procedure. It was found that the microsomal supernatant from livers of vitamin K–normal animals did contain small amounts of prothrombin – about $\frac{1}{10}$ the amount in blood. In contrast to the results of Goswami and Munro (1962), liver microsomes from both normal and vitamin K–deficient rats contained no measurable prothrombin activity. Attempts were made to increase the sensitivity of the assay by adding known amounts of prothrombin in order to bring the amount present within the range of the assay. Data for the recovery of one level of added prothrombin (of the two levels used) are given in Table 30.4. It can be seen that not only did these additions fail to increase the sensitivity, but the added prothrombin could not be recovered – apparently because the microsomes of the normal liver and, to a greater extent, the microsomes of the vitamin K–deficient liver, contained an inhibitor which interfered with the two-stage prothrombin assay (Johnson and Johnson, 1968). Hemker and co-workers (1963) and Loeliger and Hemker (1968) have reported the presence of a prothrombin inhibitor which interfered with recovery assays of added prothrombin in the plasma of dicoumarol-treated patients. They stated that this inhibitor was a prothrombin precursor which is an antagonist of pro-

TABLE 30.4. *Inhibition of prothrombin activity in microsomes of normal and vitamin K–deficient rats*

Levels of microsomal protein in suspension (mg)	Prothrombin recovered (%)	
	Normal rats	Vitamin K–deficient rats
1.55	0	4
0.775	42	0
0.390	75	44
0.195	88	66

Note: 0.250 Iowa units of prothrombin was added per assay.

thrombin and that this "pre-prothrombin" piles up in the liver of the vitamin K–deficient individual to such an extent that it spills over into the blood, where it acts as an inhibitor of prothrombin activity. We therefore next examined vitamin K–deficient rat plasma which contained no discernible prothrombin activity by the two-stage method to determine the extent of recovery of prothrombin. The data from a representative experiment are given in Table 30.5. Prothrombin added to the plasma was not recovered, and the blood of vitamin K–deficient rats apparently contains an inhibitor of the two-stage prothrombin assay. This inhibition was not found when prothrombin was added to normal plasma. However, because of the high content of active prothrombin in normal plasma, high dilutions must be used in recovery experiments. We used 6.2×10^{-4} ml and 3.1×10^{-4} ml plasma volumes for each assay, and thus recovery of 0.25 units, of 0.125 units, and even of 0.06 units was essentially complete re-

TABLE 30.5. *Recovery of prothrombin added to the plasma of vitamin K–deficient rats*

Plasma added (10^{-4} ml)	Prothrombin recovered (Iowa units)	
	0.500 units [a]	0.250 units [a]
250	0.0	0.0
125	0.065	0.031
62.5	0.171	0.094
31.2	0.265	0.184
15.6	0.410	0.212
7.8	0.420	0.240
3.9	0.470	0.260

Note: The two-stage prothrombin assay did not detect prothrombin in the plasma of vitamin K–deficient rats. A purified preparation of bovine prothrombin, 0.500 Iowa units or 0.250 Iowa units, and plasma, in the amounts indicated, were added to the standard two-stage assay for prothrombin.

[a] Iowa units added per assay.

covery. If deficient plasma is diluted to the same extent, no inhibition of the recovery of added prothrombin by the two-stage assay occurs (Table 30.5).

ANTIPROTHROMBIN VS. ANTITHROMBIN INHIBITOR

Because of Hemker's claim (Loeliger and Hemker, 1968) of a pre-prothrombin-inhibitor present in vitamin K–deficient plasma, it was important to pursue this further. Antithrombin is a known protein which occurs naturally in the blood (Monkhouse, 1967) but which does not interfere with the prothrombin assay at the high dilutions normally run. Antithrombin is not adsorbed on barium sulfate, whereas prothrombin is. Hemker and co-workers (1963) have claimed that their pre-prothrombin prothrombin-inhibitor was adsorbable on barium sulfate; however, we have never been able to obtain significant adsorption of this inhibition on barium sulfate. In order to determine whether the inhibition of recovery of added prothrombin was due to inhibition of prothrombin (first stage) or of thrombin (second stage), we carried out thrombin-recovery experiments on vitamin K–deficient plasma. The results show clearly that prothrombin-free plasma can inhibit thrombin activity and hence that the inhibition seen is caused by antithrombin.

PRESENCE OF THE INHIBITOR IN NORMAL PLASMA AS WELL AS IN DEFICIENT PLASMA

Normal plasma was therefore freed of prothrombin by barium sulfate adsorption, and prothrombin-recovery determinations were made at the same low dilutions used with the vitamin K–deficient plasma. Figures 30.6 and 30.7 give the comparative recoveries of prothrombin added to vitamin K–deficient plasma (Fig. 30.6) and to normal plasma treated with

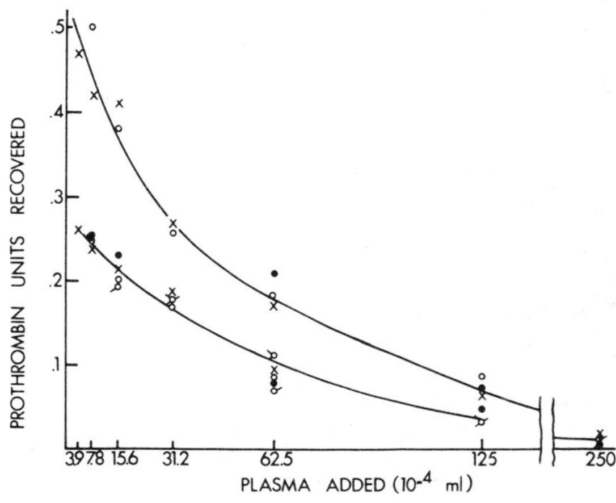

Fig. 30.6. Recovery of prothrombin added to the plasma of vitamin K–deficient rats. Two levels of bovine prothrombin, 0.5 units (upper curve) and 0.25 units (lower curve), were added to different dilutions of plasma. The vitamin K–deficient rat plasma alone contained no assayable prothrombin.

$BaSO_4$ to remove the prothrombin (Fig. 30.7). It appears that both plasmas contain the same amount of inhibitor of the two-stage prothrombin assay. No evidence was found of a pre-prothrombin prothrombin-inhibitor in vitamin K–deficient plasma. We were able to separate antithrombin from prothrombin by using Sephadex columns, and, from a Sephadex G–200 column, we determined that the molecular weight of antithrombin is over 200,000, in confirmation of previous reports (Monkhouse, 1967).

ELIMINATION OF ANTITHROMBIN INTERFERENCE

A method that would not be subject to antithrombin interference was then developed for the actual determination of prothrombin in vitamin K–deficient plasma. Previous investigations (Monkhouse, 1967) had indicated that ether extraction will destroy antithrombin activity; however, even five ether extractions did not completely remove antithrombin activity from the plasma. For this reason, we used barium sulfate adsorption. The vitamin K–dependent proteins were adsorbed on barium sulfate and were eluted with sodium citrate, and the eluate was assayed for prothrombin activity. This procedure proved usable in determining protein content and prothrombin activity in plasma from normal and vitamin K–deficient rats (Table 30.6). Using this procedure and the two-stage assay, we were also able to show the presence of low levels of prothrombin ac-

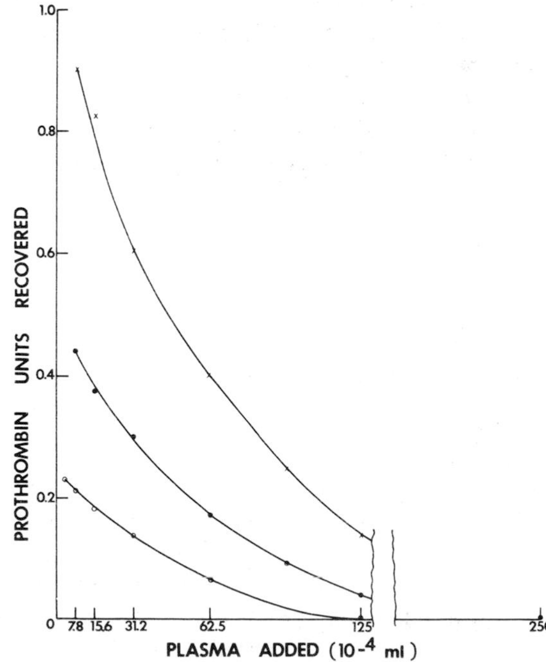

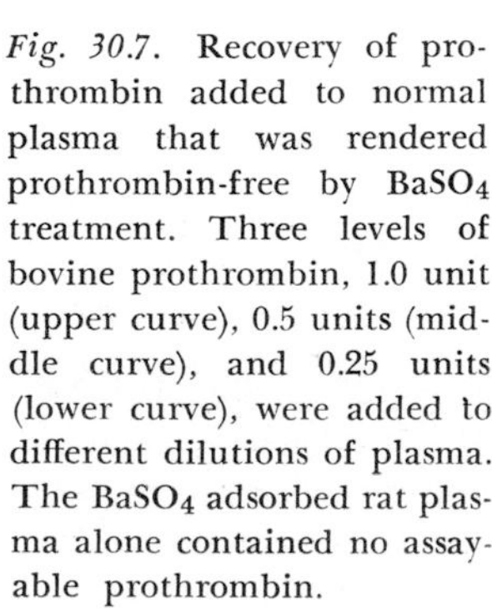
Fig. 30.7. Recovery of prothrombin added to normal plasma that was rendered prothrombin-free by $BaSO_4$ treatment. Three levels of bovine prothrombin, 1.0 unit (upper curve), 0.5 units (middle curve), and 0.25 units (lower curve), were added to different dilutions of plasma. The $BaSO_4$ adsorbed rat plasma alone contained no assayable prothrombin.

TABLE 30.6. *Protein content and prothrombin activity of eluates from $BaSO_4$ adsorbates of normal and vitamin K–deficient plasma*

Characteristic	Normal plasma	Vitamin K–deficient plasma
OD at 280 mμ[a]	0.155	0.135
Protein content (mg protein per 10 ml plasma)[b]	2.9	2.0
Prothrombin activity (sec)	14.4 (1:200)[c]	24:7 (1:10)
	19.4 (1:400)	35.0 (1:20)
	28.4 (1:800)	50.9 (1:40)
Prothrombin units per 10 ml plasma[b]	2298	44.7

Note: 10 ml of normal plasma and 10 ml of vitamin K–deficient plasma were collected from 2–4 rats in each group. 1.25 g $BaSO_4$ was added to each 10 ml of plasma, and the mixture was stirred 60 min in the cold room. The $BaSO_4$ adsorbate was washed twice with 0.5 plasma volume of cold 0.1 M potassium oxalate in 0.15 M NaCl and once with 0.5 plasma volume of cold 0.15 M NaCl. The $BaSO_4$ adsorbate was stirred twice with 1 ml of 0.17 M sodium citrate to elute the prothrombin.

[a] The eluate was diluted with 0.9% NaCl in the ratio 1:10.

[b] Based on 2 ml of eluate representing 10 ml of plasma.

[c] Ratios in parentheses give the ratio of the eluate to the diluent used for prothrombin determination.

tivity in plasma from warfarin-treated rats and, in some cases, from vitamin K–deficient rats.

Purification of prothrombin

PURIFICATION AND DISC-GEL ELECTROPHORESIS

In order to have a primary standard in adequate quantity for various types of experimentation, we prepared bovine prothrombin first by the method of Moore and co-workers (1965) and later by the modification of Malhotra and Carter (1968). Disc-gel electrophoresis of these preparations of prothrombin shows only very small amounts of other, contaminating proteins (Fig. 30.8). Starting with a commercial preparation, Ingwall and Scheraga (1969) have recently obtained bovine-prothrombin preparations free of traces of other proteins. Our prothrombin preparations assayed approximately 3000 Iowa units per milligram of protein.

NUMBER OF DISULFIDE BONDS

No free sulfhydryl groups are detectable by dithionitrobenzoate (DTNB) assay in this native prothrombin. An estimate of the number of disulfide bonds present was made by incubating prothrombin in 8 M urea with 10^{-3} M 2-mercaptoethanol at *p*H 8.5. After acidification and removal of urea and mercaptoethanol by Sephadex G–25 gel filtration, the reduced

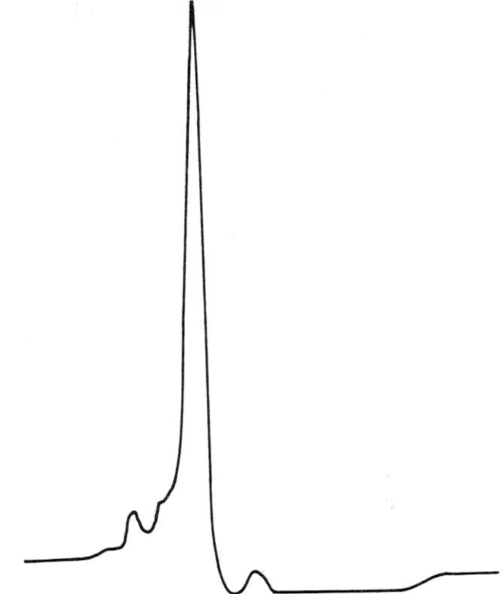

Fig. 30.8. Densitometer scan of an amido black-stained polyacrylamide electrophoresis gel of purified bovine prothrombin.

material was assayed with DTNB for free –SH groups. The results indicated 10 disulfide bonds per prothrombin molecule, based on a molecular weight of 68,000 for prothrombin (Forsyth, 1967). Ingwall and Scheraga (1969) report 20, half cystines, per molecule, based on a molecular weight of 74,000.

REDUCED PROTHROMBIN AND ITS SUBUNIT STRUCTURE

The structure of the reduced prothrombin molecule was investigated for possible prothrombin subunits, since the thrombin molecule is thought to have a molecular weight of only about 10,000. The sedimentation characteristics of prothrombin in 8 M urea, 10^{-3} M 2-mercaptoethanol, and sufficient 5% aqueous methylamine to bring the *p*H to 8.5, were studied in the analytical ultracentrifuge (Forsyth, 1967) and gave molecular-weight data for the reduced prothrombin which did not indicate any subunit structure. This value has just been elegantly confirmed by Ingwall and Scheraga (1969).

A liver microsomal supernatant enzyme which will partially reactivate reduced prothrombin has been demonstrated (Forsyth, 1967; Forsyth and Johnson, 1967).

Incorporation of labeled amino acids

Let us now return to the line of investigation which has established that vitamin K function is not blocked by the in vitro addition of cycloheximide or of puromycin to a liver-cell system, nor is it blocked by in vivo low levels of cycloheximide given to intact rats (these levels, however, would completely block synthesis of prothrombin in normal rats). On the other hand, an in vitro liver-cell system cannot make factor VII if the vitamin K–deficient animal is given puromycin in vivo along with the vitamin K. Also, high levels of cycloheximide in vivo almost completely blocked vitamin K function in prothrombin formation. All these findings together indicate that the site of action of vitamin K either is very late in translation or immediately follows translation in which a precursor is activated in a vitamin K–dependent step.

INCORPORATION OF AMINO ACID INTO BARIUM SULFATE ADSORBATE

In order to really test the suggestion that the site of action of vitamin K might in fact be beyond peptide-bond formation and *de novo* synthesis of the protein molecule, we carried out experiments on the incorporation of labeled amino acid. For these experiments, a tritium-labeled amino acid mixture was given to normal rats, to vitamin K–deficient rats, and to vitamin K–deficient rats treated with vitamin K_1. The amino acids were administered 1 hr before the blood withdrawal, and the vitamin K–treated rats received the vitamin at the same time. The prothrombin and other vitamin K–dependent clotting proteins of the plasma were adsorbed on barium sulfate, and the protein was eluted from the barium sulfate by sodium citrate and was counted in the scintillation counter,. The results of these experiments are given in Table 30.7. Prothrombin time returned from a very low level to normal during the 1 hr after the vitamin K treatment, and yet, during that same hour, the incorporation of amino acid into the $BaSO_4$-adsorbed, vitamin K–dependent proteins was not increased by the administration of vitamin K to the deficient animals.

INCORPORATION OF AMINO ACID INTO PROTHROMBIN

However, since barium sulfate adsorbs proteins other than prothrombin and the vitamin K–dependent proteins (Voss, 1967*a*), we further purified the proteins adsorbed in a second experiment. In this experiment, a tritium-labeled L-amino acid mixture was given to normal rats, to vitamin K–deficient rats, and to vitamin K–deficient rats treated with vitamin K_1. Again, vitamin K_1 and the labeled amino acids were given 1 hr before blood withdrawal. The time used in these experiments was 1 hr because, from the earlier cycloheximide data, it appeared that new protein synthesis is required after 1 hr, a possible precursor having been consumed. The vitamin K–dependent clotting proteins were adsorbed on barium sulfate and were eluted from the barium sulfate with sodium citrate. The individual eluates were then fractionated by analytical polyacrylamide-gel eletrophoresis and were stained with amido black, and the prothrombin band was counted. In order to identify the prothrombin band, pure bovine prothrombin was added as a carrier to some eluates. As can be

TABLE 30.7. *Incorporation of labeled amino acids by plasma proteins adsorbed on* $BaSO_4$

Plasma prothrombin (% of normal)[a]	dpm/mg protein in $BaSO_4$ eluate
NORMAL RATS (N = 4)	
100 ± 4	260
	64
	64
	237
DEFICIENT RATS + VITAMIN K_1[b] (N = 4)	
100 ± 5	120
	191
	154
	31
DEFICIENT RATS (N = 4)	
5 ± 5	120
	69
	26
	75

Notes: All rats were administered, intraperitoneally, 5 μCi of labeled amino acids per 100 g body weight. The amino acids used were L Amino Acids-^{3}H(G) mixture (28.9 mCi/mg) from New England Nuclear (Boston, Mass.). Blood was withdrawn 1 hr later by heart puncture.

Plasma proteins were adsorbed on $BaSO_4$, and the protein was eluted from the $BaSO_4$ by sodium citrate and was counted in the scintillation counter.

Values are given as mean ± SE.

[a] Measured at time of blood withdrawal by the method of Quick et al. (1935).

[b] 1 mg of vitamin K_1 was given with the labeled amino acids, 1 hr before blood withdrawal.

seen from Figure 30.9, the same "prothrombin" band appeared in all plasmas, whether from vitamin K–deficient rats, from vitamin K–normal rats, or from vitamin K–deficient rats treated with vitamin K_1.

This finding of the same apparent amount of prothrombin protein in vitamin K–normal and –deficient plasmas was a great surprise, since assays of vitamin K–deficient plasma have been interpreted as indicating the absence of prothrombin; however, these assays have been for prothrombin activity. Figure 30.9 indicates that a "prothrombin" protein was present at essentially the same level in all cases. Elution of the prothrombin band from the gels yielded prothrombin activity in the plasma from the vitamin K–treated rats, but not in that from the deficient rats. More recent work (Johnson et al., 1970) has proven that this apparent prothrombin band is separable into two bands and that the amount of true prothrombin does in fact depend on the vitamin K status.

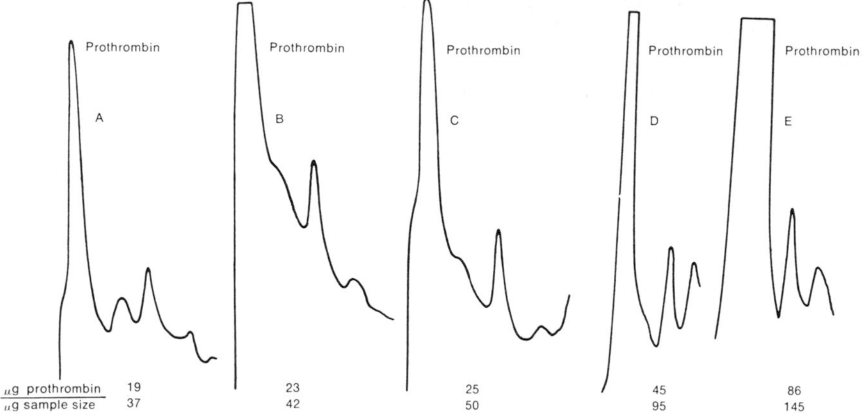

Fig. 30.9. Densitometer scans of polyacrylamide electrophoresis gels of the proteins from various rat plasmas. The proteins were adsorbed on $BaSO_4$ and were eluted from the $BaSO_4$ with sodium citrate; the eluates were then electrophoresed and stained with amido black. Scans are shown for: (*A*) normal rat; (*B* and *D*) vitamin K–deficient rat treated with vitamin K_1; (*C*) vitamin K–deficient rat not treated with vitamin K_1; and (*E*) vitamin K–deficient rat treated with vitamin K_1, with bovine prothrombin added to the eluate as a carrier. (Johnson et al., 1966. Reproduced by permission of Pergamon Press.)

The extent to which radioactive amino acid was incorporated into the prothrombin band again indicates no increase in the incorporation of amino acid into prothrombin in 1 hr under the influence of vitamin K_1 (Table 30.8). The results indicate that prothrombin synthesis is taking place continuously in the vitamin K–deficient animals as well as in the vitamin K–normal animals and that, in 1 hr, there appears to be no increase of *de novo* synthesis of prothrombin as a result of vitamin K_1 administration to vitamin K–deficient animals. Table 30.9 shows that, in an experiment in which ^{14}C–uniformly labeled L-amino acids were given, incorporation of amino acids into the proteins adsorbed on $BaSO_4$ and into the other plasma proteins both occurred in the 1-hr period (Table 30.9). It appears that prothrombin and related vitamin K–dependent proteins turn over somewhat faster than do the other plasma proteins.

Column chromatography of $BaSO_4$-adsorbable proteins

From the data indicating that the vitamin K–dependent clotting proteins are synthesized *de novo* in the absence of vitamin K and are converted to enzymatically active proteins in a vitamin K–dependent step, we were led to continue the column chromatography we had carried out

TABLE 30.8. *Amount and radioactivity of prothrombin in $BaSO_4$ eluate*

Plasma volume [a] (ml)	Total protein [b] (μg/10 μliter $BaSO_4$ eluate)	Prothrombin protein [c] (μg/10 μliter $BaSO_4$ eluate)	dpm/mg prothrombin
	NORMAL RATS (N = 4)		
4.0	37	19	630
3.5	25	12	500
4.0	25	11	1363
5.0	35	15	200
	DEFICIENT RATS + VITAMIN K_1 (N — 4)		
5.0	42	23	783
5.0	80	35	171
4.5	45	21	429
6.0	95	45	131
	DEFICIENT RATS (N = 4)		
5.0	50	25	360
4.0	95	40	150
3.0	35	17	529
4.5	45	22	273

[a] 0.01 plasma volume of sodium citrate was used to elute proteins adsorbed on $BaSO_4$.
[b] Determined by method of Lowry.
[c] Determined by scanning stained gels.

TABLE 30.9. *Incorporation of labeled amino acids by plasma proteins*

dpm/mg protein in $BaSO_4$ eluate	dpm/mg protein in $BaSO_4$-treated plasma
NORMAL RATS + VITAMIN K_1[a] (N = 2)	
420	258
337	172
NORMAL RATS (N = 2)	
314	200
302	220
DEFICIENT RAT + VITAMIN K_1[a] (N= 1)	
416	283

Notes: All rats were administered, intraperitoneally, 5 μCi of labeled amino acids per 100 g of body weight, 1 hr before blood withdrawal. The amino acids used were L Amino Acids-^{14}C(U) mixture (14.3 mCi/mg) from New England Nuclear (Boston, Mass.). The plasma was treated as described in the note to Table 30.7.

[a] 1 mg of vitamin K_1 was given with the labeled amino acids, 1 hr before blood withdrawal.

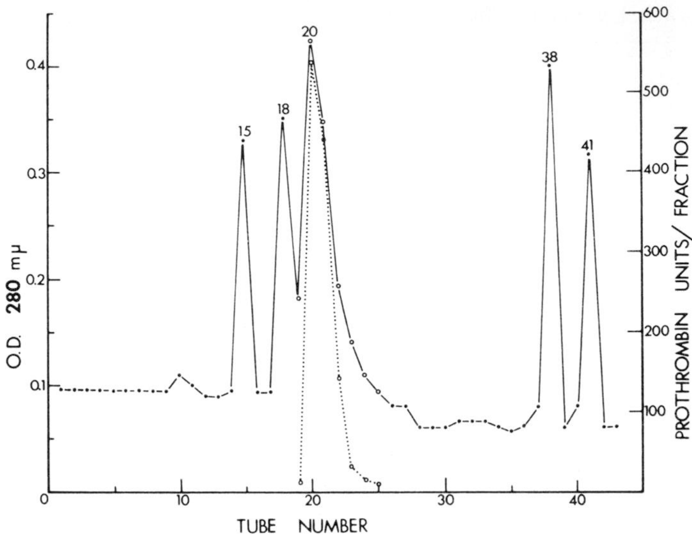

Fig. 30.10. DEAE-cellulose chromatography of the $BaSO_4$-adsorbable proteins from 10 ml of normal rat plasma. Shown are the optical density at 280 mμ (solid lines) and the prothrombin activity in units per 2.5 ml of fraction (dotted lines). The proteins were adsorbed on $BaSO_4$ and eluted with 0.17 M sodium citrate; the eluates were dialyzed and chromatographed in a 0.01 M imidazole buffer (*p*H 8) with a 0.15–0.25 M NaCl gradient.

to separate antithrombin from prothrombin. Chromatographic separation of the vitamin K–dependent clotting proteins which are adsorbed on $BaSO_4$ was carried out for both vitamin K–deficient and vitamin K–normal animals. DEAE-cellulose columns (Voss, 1967*b*) with NaCl gradient elution were run. Scans for optical density at 280 mμ and for prothrombin activity of the effluent fractions from the DEAE-cellulose columns were made of the $BaSO_4$ eluates of plasma from normal and from vitamin K–deficient rats (Figs. 30.10, 30.11). It appears from these very preliminary chromatograms that similar protein bands are present in the eluates from both deficient and normal plasma. When the prothrombin band from the normal animals was assayed for prothrombin, high activity was found on the order of 3000 Iowa units/mg, while the same band from the vitamin K–deficient rats showed very low prothrombin specific activity (see Table 30.6).

Relationship to previous antibody data

A number of years ago, Anderson and Barnhart (1964) demonstrated clearly that administration of vitamin K initiates formation of prothrom-

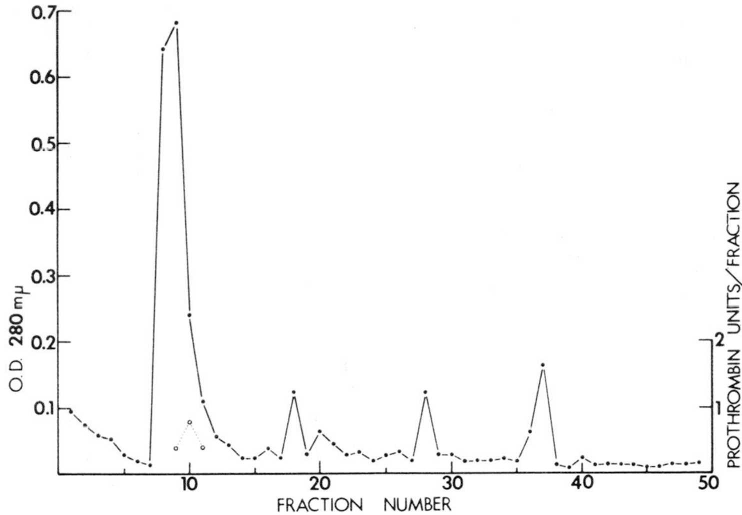

Fig. 30.11. DEAE-cellulose chromatography of the $BaSO_4$-adsorbable proteins from 10 ml of vitamin K–deficient rat plasma. Shown are the optical density at 280 mμ (solid lines) and the prothrombin activity in units per 2.5 ml of fraction (dotted lines). The proteins were adsorbed on $BaSO_4$ and eluted with 0.17 M sodium citrate; the eluates were dialyzed and chromatographed in a 0.01 M imidazole buffer (*p*H 8) with a 0.15–0.25 M NaCl gradient.

bin in the parenchymal cells of the liver; this prothrombin cross-reacts with prothrombin antibody. A possible explanation is that the vitamin K–dependent step changes the protein molecule so that antigenic activity is changed and so that antibody prepared against active prothrombin does not cross-react with inactive prothrombin. Li and co-workers (1969) have reported that *de novo* synthesis depends on vitamin K; in their antibody experiments, the prothrombin antigen was precipitated by rabbit antibody prepared against active rat prothrombin. This experiment was of 6-hr duration, and during this period of time a considerable amount of radioactivity was incorporated into prothrombin. Using cycloheximide, however, we demonstrated earlier that the total turnover time for prothrombin appears to be on the order of 6 hr, so one would expect labeling in such an experiment. We also had indications that a possible precursor was consumed in 1 hr after vitamin K was administered, so any further active prothrombin synthesis would be dependent on protein synthesis in the vitamin K–treated, deficient rat. Furthermore, if the antibody did not precipitate non-vitamin K–dependent inactive prothrombin, little incorporation of radioactivity would be found in such controls. Josso and co-workers (1968) have reported different molecular states of prothrombin and suggest that a lack of vitamin K leads to synthesis of an inactive prothrombin.

The site of action of vitamin K, as suggested by studies on amino acid incorporation and on prothrombin separation

Our data indicate that vitamin K functions at the site beyond the majority of peptide-bond formation. It appears that a nonfunctional form of prothrombin is released into the plasma of the vitamin K–deficient animal. This action suggests that the liver contains an inactive precursor which is converted to active prothrombin in a vitamin K–dependent step. Hemker and co-workers (1963) have suggested that a pre-prothrombin prothrombin-inhibitor occurs in the plasma of the vitamin K–deficient rat and is converted into prothrombin in a vitamin K–dependent step. However, recently they have proposed that this postulated inhibitor (now termed PIVKA) is an analog of factor X rather than a pre-prothrombin (Hemker et al., 1968; Hemker and Muller, 1968). Dulock and Kolmen (1968) have suggested that vitamin K functions in completeing the formation of prothrombin from a pre-prothrombin precursor present in the liver; however, this suggestion is based only on the rapidity of cures of dogs that had been given warfarin and had had 50% of their blood exchanged for an erythrocyte serum infusate.

We have previously suggested (Johnson et al., 1966) that vitamin K, as a quinone, functions in a specific pattern of —S—S— bond formation. Twenty-five years ago, Lyons (1945) proposed a close relationship between vitamin K and prothrombin and —SH to —S—S— conversion. The fact that prothrombin contains 10 —S—S— bonds suggests many possibilities of control at the level of the folded structure.

Summary

In summary, we believe we have demonstrated that the site of function of vitamin K is in the activation of an inactive prothrombin precursor in the liver cell. It is possible that this precursor may still be incomplete and attached to the ribosome. There are several possible sites of action of vitamin K at this level of specific protein synthesis.

1. It is possible that the vitamin K–dependent step involved chain termination — perhaps the addition of final amino acids before release of the polypeptide from the ribosome. This would be consistent with the data from high levels of cycloheximide and from puromycin administered in vivo.

2. It is possible that the vitamin K–dependent step involves the release of the nascent peptide chain from the ribosome. Hawtrey and Biedron

(1966) have reported that release is a complex process, and it appears (Godschaux et al., 1967) that high levels of cycloheximide block this peptide-chain release.

3. The addition of the carbohydrate portion (Kowarzyk et al., 1965) of the prothrombin molecule requires intact ribosomes (Molnar and Sy, 1967), and vitamin K dependency at this step need not involve the incorporation of amino acid.

4. While the folding of newly formed polypeptide chains to meet their most stable state thermodynamically appears to occur spontaneously, it is possible that prothrombin must be folded into a less stable state to be functional and that this requires the vitamin K regulation.

5. It is possible that vitamin K as a quinone functions in active polymer formation.

6. Possibly vitamin K as a quinone functions in cleavage of a precursor protein.

It appears certain that the function of vitamin K does not involve regulation of total *de novo* synthesis of the prothrombin molecule. It appears probable that the picture is similar with regard to the three other vitamin K–dependent proteins. As we stated some five years ago, it appears to us that vitamin K is acting in some way as an electron-transport agent (Hill et al., 1966) in the production of the proper conformation for function of this series of proteins. The question of whether these four proteins — prothrombin, factor VII, factor IX, and factor X — have a common protein precursor (perhaps factor VII–proconvertin) that is activated in a vitamin K–dependent step and is then converted to these four proteins in hydrolytic steps or whether they are four closely related proteins made independently and activated independently by the vitamin K–dependent step must await much more thorough knowledge of these four proteins.

It appears to us that further work on the site of action of vitamin K will also depend on further work on the structure of the active and the inactive vitamin K–dependent protein molecules and on the structure of the functional form of vitamin K and of the protein to which it binds and with which it functions.

References

Adamis, D., H. S. Sise, and D. M. Kimball. 1956. Proconvertin test. Its application to the study of anticoagulant processes. *J. Lab. Clin. Med.* *47*:320.

Allen, D. W., and P. C. Zamecnik. 1962. The effect of puromycin on rabbit reticulocyte ribosomes. *Biochim. Biophys. Acta* *55*:865.

Allen, E. H., and R. S. Schweet. 1962. Synthesis of hemoglobin in a cell-free system. *J. Biol. Chem.* *237*:760.

Allington, M. J. 1958. Owren's method for the control of anticoagulant therapy. *J. Clin. Pathol. 11*:62.

Anderson, G. F., and M. I. Barnhart. 1964. Prothrombin synthesis in the dog. *Amer. J. Physiol. 206*:929.

Babior, B. M. 1966. The role of vitamin K in clotting factor synthesis. I. Evidence for the participation of vitamin K in the conversion of a polypeptide precursor to factor VII. *Biochim. Biophys. Acta 123*:606.

Baliga, B. S., A. W. Pronczuk, and H. N. Munro. 1968*a*. Site of action of cycloheximide on protein synthesis by liver polysomes. *Fed. Proc. 27*:776. (Abstr. 3089.)

Baliga, B. S., A. W. Pronczuk, and H. N. Munro. 1968*b*. Regulation of polysome aggregation in a cell-free system through amino acid supply. *J. Mol. Biol. 34*:199.

Barnhart, M. I., and G. F. Anderson. 1962. Cellular study of drug alteration of prothrombin synthesis. *Biochem. Pharmacol. 9*:23.

Berry, D., E. Berry, and R. E. Olson. 1966. Site of antagonism between vitamin K and dicumarol. *Fed. Proc. 25*:542. (Abstr. 1993.)

Dowling, J. E. and G. Wald. 1960. The biological function of vitamin A acid. *Proc. Nat. Acad. Sci. U.S.A. 46*:587.

Dulock, M. A., and S. N. Kolmen. 1968. Influence of vitamin K on restoration of prothrombin complex proteins and fibrinogen in plasma of depleted dogs. *Thromb. Diath. Haemorrh. 20*:136.

Forsyth, G. W. 1967. Vitamin K and prothrombin. Ph.D. thesis. University of Oklahoma.

Forsyth, G., and B. Connor Johnson. 1967. Studies on a new enzyme which reactivates prothrombin. *Indian J. Biochem. 4*: Suppl. 2, p. 22.

Godschaux, W., S. Adamson, and E. Herbert. 1967. Effects of cycloheximide on polyribosome function in reticulocytes. *J. Mol. Biol. 27*:57.

Goswami, P., and H. N. Munro. 1962. The role of ribonucleic acid in the formation of prothrombin activity by rat liver microsomes. *Biochim. Biophys. Acta 55*:410.

Hawtrey, A. O., and S. I. Biedron. 1966. Release of peptide chains from rat-liver polysomes by the *N,N*-dimethyl-*p*-methoxy-L-phenylalanyl analogue of puromycin. *Nature 211*:187.

Hemker, H. C., and A. D. Muller. 1968. Kinetic aspects of the interaction of blood-clotting enzymes. VI. Localization of the site of blood-coagulation inhibition by the protein induced by vitamin K absence (PIVKA). *Thromb. Diath. Haemorrh. 20*:78.

Hemker, H. C., J. J. Veltkamp, A. Hansen, and E. A. Loeliger. 1963. Nature of prothrombin biosynthesis. Preprothrombinaemia in vitamin K–deficiency. *Nature 200*:589.

Hemker, H. C., J. J. Veltkamp, and E. A. Loeliger. 1968. Kinetic aspects of the interaction of blood-clotting enzymes. III. Demonstration of an inhibitor of prothrombin conversion in vitamin K deficiency. *Thromb. Diath. Haemorrh. 19*:346.

Hill, R. B., S. Gaetani, and B. C. Johnson. 1963. Vitamin K and liver microsomal prothrombin. *Fed. Proc. 22*:620.

Hill, R. B., S. Gaetani, A. M. Paolucci, P. B. Rama Rao, R. Alden, G. S. Ranhotra, D. V. Shah, V. K. Shah, and B. Connor Johnson. 1968. Vitamin K and biosynthesis of protein and prothrombin. *J. Biol. Chem. 243*:3930.

Hill, R. B., F. Paul, and B. C. Johnson. 1966. Oxygen consumption and NADPH oxidation in microsomes from vitamin K–deficient, Warfarin- and dicumarol-treated rats. *Proc. Soc. Exp. Biol. Med. 121*:1287.

Ingwall, J. S. and H. A. Scheraga. 1969. Purification and properties of bovine prothrombin. *Biochemistry 8*:1860.

Jacob, S. T., and P. M. Bhargava. 1962. A new method for the preparation of liver cell suspensions. *Exp. Cell. Res. 27*:453.

Johnson, B. C., R. H. Hill, R. Alden, and G. S. Ranhotra. 1966. Turnover time of prothrombin and of prothrombin messenger RNA and evidence for a ribosomal site of action of vitamin K in prothrombin synthesis. *Life Sci. 5*:385.

Johnson, B. C., R. B. Hill, G. S. Ranhotra, and R. Alden. 1965. Control of prothrombin synthesis by vitamin K. *Fed. Proc. 24*:453. (Abstr. 1801.)

Johnson, B. C., M. S. Mameesh, V. C. Metta, and P. B. Rama Rao. 1960. Vitamin K nutrition and irradiation sterilization. *Fed. Proc. 19*:1038.

Johnson, H. V., K. Boyd, G. Valkovich, A. C. Cox, and B. C. Johnson. 1970. *Fed. Proc.* 29. (Abstr. 1887.)

Johnson, H., and B. C. Johnson. 1968. Prothrombin inhibitor in vitamin K deficient rat liver microsomes. *Fed. Proc. 27*:678. (Abstr. 2600.)

Josso, F., J. M. Lavergne, M. Gonault, O. Prou-Wartelle, and J. P. Soulier. 1968. Différents états moléculaires du facteur II (prothrombine). Leur étude à l'aide de la staphylocoagulase et d'anticorps anti-facteur II. I. Le facteur II chez sujets traités par les antagonistes de la vitamine K. *Thromb. Diath. Haemorrh. 20*:88.

Kowarzyk, H., W. Mejbaum-Katzenellenbogen, B. Czerwinska-Kossobudzka, H. Jakobi, J. Skrzypczyk, and L. Czerchawski. 1965. The sialic acid of prothrombin. *Bull. Acad. Pol. Sci.* [*Biol.*] *13*: No. 6, p. 317.

Li, Lan-Fun, R. K. Kipfer, and R. E. Olson. 1969. Immunochemical measurement of vitamin K–induced biosynthesis of prothrombin in the isolated perfused rat liver. *Fed. Proc. 28*:385. (Abstr. 716.)

Lin, S.-Y., R. D. Mosteller, and B. Hardesty. 1966. The mechanism of sodium fluoroide and cycloheximide inhibition of hemoglobin biosynthesis in the cell-free reticulocyte system. *J. Mol. Biol. 21*:51.

Loeliger, E. A., and H. C. Hemker. 1968. The principles of the mode of action of coumarin congeners, p. 13. *In* G. V. R. Born (ed)., *Drugs in Relation to Blood Coagulation, Haemostasis and Thrombosis.* (Third International Pharmacological Meeting, Sao Paulo, July, 1966). Vol. 6. Pergamon Press, New York.

Lowenthal, J., and H. Birnbaum. 1969. Mechanism of action of vitamin K in plasma clotting factor synthesis. Evidence from "in vitro" experiments that the action is not at the level of polypeptide formation. *Fed. Proc. 28*:385. (Abstr. 718.)

Lowenthal, J., and E. L. Simmons. 1967. Failure of actinomycin D to inhibit appearance of clotting activity by vitamin K *in vitro. Experientia 23*:421.

Lyons, R. J. 1945. Thiol–vitamin K mechanism in the clotting of fibrinogen. *Nature 155*:633.

Malhotra, O. P., and J. R. Carter. 1968. Modified method for the preparation of purified bovine prothrombin of high specific activity. *Thromb. Diath. Haemorrh. 19*: Suppl., p. 178.

Mameesh, M. S., and B. C. Johnson. 1959. Production of dietary vitamin K deficiency in the rat. *Proc. Soc. Exp. Biol. Med. 101*:467.

Mameesh, M. S., and B. C. Johnson. 1960. Dietary vitamin K requirement of the rat. *Proc. Soc. Exp. Biol. Med. 103*:378.

Mameesh, M. S., V. C. Metta, P. B. Rama Rao, and B. C. Johnson. 1962. On the cause of vitamin K deficiency in male rats fed irradiated beef and the production of vitamin K deficiency using an amino acid synthetic diet. *J. Nutr. 77*:165.

Martius, C., and D. Nitz-Litzow. 1954. Oxydative phosphorylieurung und vitamin K Mangel. *Biochim. Biophys. Acta* 13:152.

Metta, V. C., M. S. Mameesh, and B. C. Johnson. 1959. Vitamin K deficiency in rats induced by the feeding of irradiated beef. *J. Nutr. 69*:18.

Metta, V. C., L. Nash, and B. C. Johnson. 1961. A tubular coprophagy-preventing cage for the rat. *J. Nutr. 74*:473.

Molnar, J., and D. Sy. 1967. Attachment of glucosamine to protein at the ribosomal site of rat liver. *Biochemistry 6*:1941.

Monkhouse, S. C. 1967. *In* W. H. Seegers (ed.), *Blood Clotting Enzymology*, Ch. 7, p. 323. Academic Press, New York and London.

Moore, H. C., S. E. Lux, O. P. Malhotra, S. Bakerman, and J. R. Carter. 1965. Isolation and purification of bovine and canine prothrombin. *Biochim. Biophys. Acta 111*:174.

Munro, H. N., B. S. Baliga, and A. W. Pronczuk. 1968. "In vitro" inhibition of peptide synthesis and GTP hydrolysis by cycloheximide and reversal of inhibition by glutathione. *Nature 219*:944.

Olson, J. P., L. L. Miller, and S. B. Troup. 1966. Synthesis of clotting factors by the isolated perfused rat liver. *J. Clin. Invest. 45*:690.

Olson, R. E. 1964. Vitamin K induced prothrombin formation. Antagonism by actinomycin D. *Science 145*:926.

Olson, R. E. 1965*a*. The regulatory function of the fat-soluble vitamins. *Can. J. Biochem. Physiol. 43*:1565.

Olson, R. E. 1965*b*. Effect of inhibitors of protein synthesis upon vitamin K induced prothrombin formation. *Fed. Proc.* 24:623. (Abstr. 2728.)

Olson, R. E., G. Phillips, and N. Wang. 1968. The regulatory action of vitamin K. *Advances Enzyme Regulation 6*:213.

Paolucci, A. M., Gaetani, and B. C. Johnson. 1964. Vitamin K_1 sintesi proteica. I. Sintesi indotta di triptofano pirrolasi in ratti carenti di vitamina K. *Quad. Nutr. 24*:275.

Paolucci, A. M., P. B. Rama Rao, and B. C. Johnson. 1963. Vitamin K deficiency and oxidative phosphorylation. *J. Nutr. 81*:17.

Pechet, L. 1964. *In* L. M. Tocantis and L. A. Kazal (eds.), *Blood Coagulation, Hemorrhage and Thrombosis,* p. 213. Grune and Stratton, New York.

Pool, J. P., and M. B. Brown. 1962. Effects of vitamin K_1 and warfarin on factor VII synthesis by rat liver slices, p. 401. *Proceedings of the 8th Congress of the European Society of Haematology* (Vienna, 1961), Pt. II. Karger, Basel and New York.

Prydz, H. 1965. Studies on proconvertin (factor VII). VII. Further studies on the biosynthesis of factor VII in rat cell suspensions. *Scand. J. Clin. Lab. Invest. 17*:143.

Quick, A. J., M. Stanley-Brown, and F. W. Bancroft. 1935. A study of the coagulation defect in hemophilia and in jaundice. *Amer. J. Med. Sci. 190*:501.

Ranhotra, G. S., and B. Connor Johnson. 1969. Vitamin K and the synthesis of factors VII–X by isolated rat liver cells. *Proc. Soc. Exp. Biol. Med. 132*: No. 2, p. 509.

Ray, G., N. N. Chakravarty, and S. C. Roy. 1962. Prothrombin. The position of vitamin K as a component of prothrombin. *Ann. Biochem. Exp. Med. 22*:319.

Smith, J. D., R. R. Traut, G. M. Blackburn, and R. E. Monro. 1965. Action of puromycin in polyadenylic acid. Directed polylysine synthesis. *J. Mol. Biol. 13*:617.

Suttie, J. W. 1969. Control of clotting factor biosynthesis by vitamin K. *Fed. Proc. 28*:1696.

Suttie, J. W. 1967. Control of prothrombin and factor VII biosynthesis by vitamin K. *Arch. Biochem. Biophys. 118*:166.

Villa-Trevino, S., E. Farber, T. S. Staehelin, F. O. Wettstein, and H. Noll. 1964. Breakdown and reassembly of rat liver ergosomes after administration of ethionine or puromycin. *J. Biol. Chem. 239*:3826.

Voss, D. 1967*a*. Untersuchungen am Prothrombin-Komplex I. Das Verhalten von Prothrombin, Faktor II, IX und X an Bariumsulfat. *Hoppe-Seyler's Z. Physiol. Chem. 348*:1163.

Voss, D. 1967*b*. Untersuchungen am Prothrombin-Komplex II. Das Verhalten von Prothrombin, Faktor VII, IX und X bei der Säulenchromatographie an Anionen-Austanschern. *Hoppe-Seyler's Z. Physiol. Chem. 348*:1172.

Ware, A. G., and W. H. Seegers. 1949. Two-stage procedure for the quantitative determination of prothrombin concentration. *Amer. J. Clin. Pathol. 19*:471.

Wettstein, F. O., H. Noll, and S. Penman. 1964. Effect of cycloheximide on ribosomal aggregates engaged in protein synthesis *in vitro. Biochim. Biophys. Acta 87*:525.

INDEX